CEREBRAL CORTEX

Volume 8B
Comparative Structure
and Evolution of
Cerebral Cortex, Part II

CEREBRAL CORTEX
Edited by Edward G. Jones and Alan Peters

Advisory Committee

J. C. Eccles, *Contra, Switzerland*
H. H. Jasper, *Montreal, Canada*
V. B. Mountcastle, *Baltimore, Maryland*
W. J. H. Nauta, *Cambridge, Massachusetts*
S. L. Palay, *Boston, Massachusetts*
F. Plum, *New York, New York*
R. D. Terry, *La Jolla, California*
P. Ulinski, *Chicago, Illinois*

CEREBRAL CORTEX

Volume 8B
Comparative Structure
and Evolution of
Cerebral Cortex, Part II

Edited by

EDWARD G. JONES
California College of Medicine
University of California, Irvine
Irvine, California

and

ALAN PETERS
Boston University School of Medicine
Boston, Massachusetts

Plenum Press · New York and London

Library of Congress Cataloging in Publication Data

(Revised for vol. 8a—8b)
Cerebral cortex.

Vol. 2, 5–   edited by Edward G. Jones and Alan Peters.
Includes bibliographies and indexes.
Contents: v. 1. Cellular components of the cerebral cortex—v. 2. Functional properties of cortial cells—[etc.]—v. 8. Comparative structure and evolution of cerebral cortex, Parts I and II.
1. Cerebral cortex. I. Peters, Alan, 1929–   II. Jones, Edward G., 1939–   . [DNLM: 1. Cerebral Cortex—anatomy and histology. 2. Cerebral Cortex—physiology.
QP383.C45   1984   612′.825   84-1982

ISBN 0-306-43635-3

© 1990 Plenum Press, New York
A Division of Plenum Publishing Corporation
233 Spring Street, New York, N.Y. 10013

Contributors

Mary Carlson　　　Department of Neurobiology, Harvard Medical School, Boston, Massachusetts 02115

Christine Gall　　　Department of Anatomy and Neurobiology, University of California–Irvine, Irvine, California 92717

Ilya I. Glezer　　　Neuroscience Program, The City College of New York Medical School, New York, New York 10031; and Osborn Laboratories of Marine Sciences, New York Aquarium, Brooklyn, New York 11224

Lewis B. Haberly　　　Department of Anatomy, University of Wisconsin Medical Sciences Center, Madison, Wisconsin 53706

Myron S. Jacobs　　　New York University Dental Center, New York University, New York, 10010; and Osborn Laboratories of Marine Sciences, New York Aquarium, Brooklyn, New York 11224

John Irwin Johnson　　　Anatomy Department and Neuroscience Program, Michigan State University, East Lansing, Michigan 48824

Peter J. Morgane　　　Laboratory of Neurobiology, Worcester Foundation for Experimental Biology, Shrewsbury, Massachusetts 01545

Mark Rowe　　　School of Physiology and Pharmacology, University of New South Wales, Sydney, Australia 2033

Wally Welker　　　Department of Neurophysiology, University of Wisconsin, Madison, Wisconsin 53706

Preface

The cerebral cortex, especially that part customarily designated "neocortex," is one of the hallmarks of mammalian evolution and reaches its greatest size, relatively speaking, and its widest structural diversity in the human brain. The evolution of this structure, as remarkable for the huge numbers of neurons that it contains as for the range of behaviors that it controls, has been of abiding interest to many generations of neuroscientists. Yet few theories of cortical evolution have been proposed and none has stood the test of time. In particular, no theory has been successful in bridging the evolutionary gap that appears to exist between the pallium of nonmammalian vertebrates and the neocortex of mammals. Undoubtedly this stems in large part from the rapid divergence of nonmammalian and mammalian forms and the lack of contemporary species whose telencephalic wall can be seen as having transitional characteristics. The monotreme cortex, for example, is unquestionably mammalian in organization and that of no living reptile comes close to resembling it. Yet anatomists such as Ramón y Cajal, on examining the finer details of cortical structure, were struck by the similarities in neuronal form, particularly of the pyramidal cells, and their predisposition to laminar alignment shared by representatives of all vertebrate classes. In later years, other anatomists, in studying the connectivity of the pallium in nonmammals, have been able to identify putative homologues of the mammalian hippocampal formation and possibly of other cortical territories as well. These observations lend credence to the belief in a fundamental commonality from which has emerged in the course of evolution the radical differences in structure of the telencephalic wall exhibited by fish, amphibians, birds, and mammals.

The present pair of volumes cannot be regarded as a complete study in the evolution of the cerebral cortex. However, they do set out in some detail the range of telencephalic and especially cortical structure and connectivity exhibited by the five major classes of vertebrates, and contain many insights into the special characteristics of each. Volume 8A deals largely with nonmammalian vertebrates. It starts with three chapters by Wilhelmus J. A. J. Smeets and by R.

Nieuwenhuys and J. Meek on the brains of fish, in which telencephalic evolution seems to have emphasized the development of a large central nucleus at the expense of a pallium. It then includes chapters by Timothy J. Neary and Philip S. Ulinski on the telencephalic wall of amphibia and reptiles, in which a rudimentary and, in some regions, relatively advanced cortical structure is seen. This part concludes with an essay by Philip S. Ulinski and Daniel Margoliash on birds, in which the functions of a cortex per se seem to have been largely subsumed by the enormous expansion of that unique structure, the hyperstriatum. The latter part of Volume 8A serves as an introduction to the detailed studies of mammals presented in Volume 8B. It includes our analysis of the fossil record of neocortical evolution by Harry J. Jerison, and essays by John Allman and Edward G. Jones on the fundamental elements of cortical structure and cortical development upon which the evolutionary process must exert its effects. Volume 8B deals solely with the cerebral cortex of mammals and includes chapters on comparative structure of particular regions, such as the olfactory cortex (by Lewis B. Haberly) and the hippocampal formation (by Christine Gall), and considerations by Peter J. Morgane, Ilya I. Glezer, and Myron S. Jacobs, and Mark Rowe, of cortical structure in orders as diverse as marsupials and dolphins. The evolutionary development of some particular functional areas of the neocortex is pursued by Mary Carlson and John Irwin Johnson in their chapters. A study by Wally Welker on the determinants of sulci and gyri in living forms nicely complements that by Harry J. Jerison in Volume 8A.

The editors are again grateful for the efforts and forbearance displayed by the contributors to this wide-ranging pair of volumes, and feel confident that the high quality of their chapters will be as widely recognized.

Edward G. Jones
Alan Peters

Irvine and Boston

Contents

Volume 8B

III. Mammals

Chapter 10

Why Does Cerebral Cortex Fissure and Fold? A Review of Determinants of Gyri and Sulci

Wally Welker

Chapter 11

Comparative Aspects of Olfactory Cortex

Lewis B. Haberly

Chapter 12

Comparative Anatomy of the Hippocampus: With Special Reference to Differences in the Distributions of Neuroactive Peptides

Christine Gall

Chapter 13

**Comparative and Evolutionary Anatomy of the Visual Cortex
of the Dolphin**

Peter J. Morgane, Ilya I. Glezer, and Myron S. Jacobs

Chapter 14

Organization of the Cerebral Cortex in Monotremes and Marsupials

Mark Rowe

Chapter 15

Comparative Development of Somatic Sensory Cortex

John Irwin Johnson

Chapter 16

The Role of Somatic Sensory Cortex in Tactile Discrimination in Primates

Mary Carlson

III

Mammals

Why Does Cerebral Cortex Fissure and Fold?

A Review of Determinants of Gyri and Sulci

WALLY WELKER

1. Introduction

The most striking, interesting, yet poorly understood gross morphological features of the cerebral hemispheres in mammals are the diverse and complex arrangements of their cortical gyri and sulci (Fig. 1). Among mammals, the spinal cord and brain-stem nuclei are morphologically quite similar, despite variations in size. However, during evolution, the cerebrum and cerebellum have undergone marked variations in size, shape, and convolutional complexity (Fig. 2). External morphological features of mammalian brains have long been utilized to judge not only the degree of phylogenetic development, but also the nature and level of complexity of brain functions. The great variety of living mammals exhibit a corresponding variety of brain shapes, sizes, and patterns of fissuration and convolution of the cerebral neocortex. The view has consistently been expressed that animals with brains having greater amounts of convoluted cerebral neocortex were more intelligent as well as perceptually and behaviorally more complex.

It is recognized early in comparative studies of cerebral cortex that cortical thickness and columnar and laminar architecture differ relatively little in different mammals, whereas the cortical surface area varies over an enormous range

WALLY WELKER • Department of Neurophysiology, University of Wisconsin, Madison, Wisconsin 53706.

3

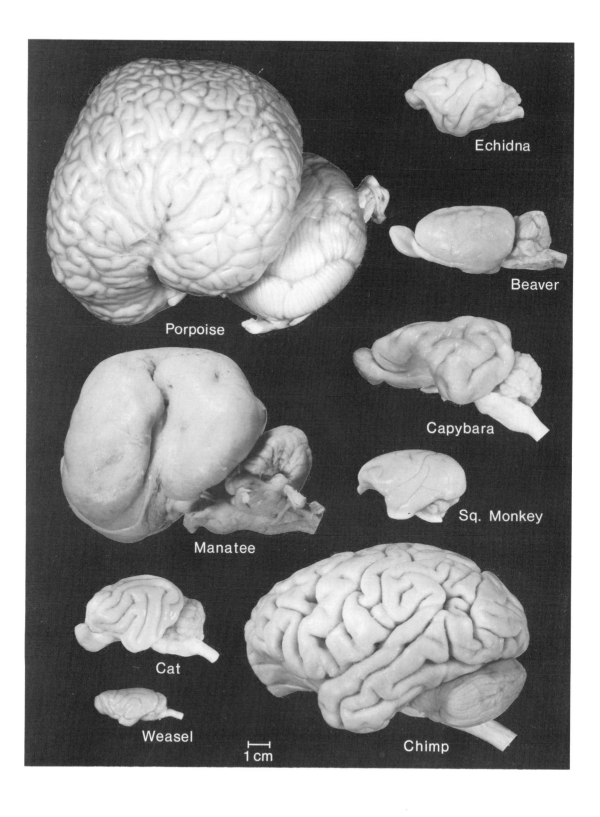

Porpoise

Manatee

Cat

Weasel

1 cm

Echidna

Beaver

Capybara

Sq. Monkey

Chimp

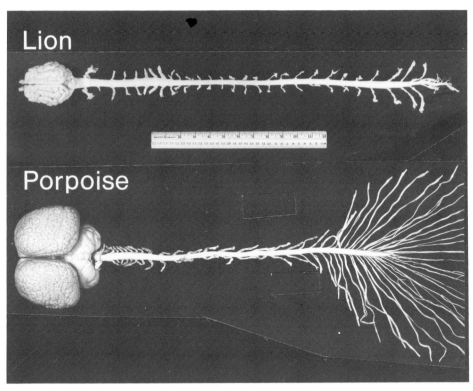

Figure 2. In different mammals of similar body size, the spinal cord is similar in size and morphology, whereas the cerebrum and cerebellum are markedly different with respect to their size and in complexity of cortical convolutions. (Top) African lion (*Panthera leo*, #62-566). (Bottom) Atlantic dolphin or porpoise (*Tursiops truncatus*, #66-127). Both brains to same scale.

(Jerison, 1973; Tables I, VIII, X).* In the larger and more complex brains the gyri and sulci exhibit elaborate, contorted, and irregular three-dimensionally complex convolutional patterns.

    An enduring belief has it that during evolution of functionally more complex mammals, a greater number and diversity of brain functions were achieved by increasing the surface area of cerebral neocortex (Jerison, 1973). This view

---

*In this chapter most statements of fact or conjecture are not followed by in-text citations of relevant references. This was done to produce a more free-flowing text. Interested readers will have to find pertinent references by referring to the tables of references that accompany each section.

Figure 1. Diverse brain conformations and gyral and sulcal patterns in nine different mammals. (Left) A cetacean (porpoise, *Tursiops truncatus*, #62-127), a sirenian (manatee, *Trichechus manatus*, #85-32), and two carnivores (domestic cat, *Felis cattus*, #65-255; least weasel, *Mustela nivalis*, #63-107). (Right) A monotreme (echidna, *Tachyglossus aculeatus*, #62-455), two rodents (North American beaver, *Castor canadensis*, #63-168; capybara, *Hydrochoerus hydrochoerus*, #62-621), and two primates (squirrel monkey, *Saimiri squirius*, #61-672; chimpanzee, *Pan paniscus*, #63-397). Note large, but lissencephalic cerebrum of manatee, small, but gyrencephalic brain of least weasel, the highly fissured monotreme brain, two large rodent brains, one with fissured cerebrum (capybara) and the other unfissured (beaver). The two carnivores exhibit similar patterns of their primary gyri and sulci as do those of the two primates. These specimens are from the Wisconsin Comparative Mammalian Brain Collection.

Table I.   References to Historical Reviews of Gyri and Sulci

Ackerknecht and Vallois (1956)	Edinger (1899)
Anker *et al.* (1987)	Harman (1947)
Ariëns Kappers *et al.* (1936)	Haymaker and Schiller (1982)
Bay (1964)	Hofman (1989)
Bok (1959)	Jefferson (1913, 1915)
Broca (1878b)	Karplus (1905)
Brodmann (1909)	Magoun and Anker (1987)
Clarke and Dewhurst (1972)	Obersteiner (1890)
Clarke and O'Malley (1968)	Riley and Riley (1921)
Clemente and Marshall (1987)	Schiller (1965)
Cole (1911, 1944)	Smith (1907b)
Creutzfeldt (1975)	Temkin (1947)
Cunningham (1890a–c)	Tizard (1959)
Dareste (1852)	Wilder (1895)
Ecker (1873)	Young (1970)
Economo (1927)	

emphasizes the role of mechanical buckling, infolding, and fissuring in providing for the greater expanses of cortex "needed" in both larger and perceptually and behaviorally more complex mammals. Such fissuring, it is maintained, would increase the number of functional modules of cortex without increasing the size of the cerebrum (and head) beyond biologically feasible limits (Jerison, 1973). Fissuration would allow cortex to increase in areal extent in order to keep pace with increases in volume of the rest of the telencephalon. Implicit in this formulation of cortical convolutions is the assumption that modules of cortex in all parts of a convolution are equivalent in their structure, connections, and function, and that fissuration increased cortical potency additively. The view that cortical fissuration is mainly a mechanical process was inferred from normative comparative data and from mathematical evaluations of cortical architecture, cell density, lamination, surface area, and volume in mammals of different body sizes from different taxonomic groups (Tables I, VIII, X).

This notion of fissure formation has received little critical evaluation or experimental test. As a result, how and why cortex becomes convoluted and fissured in the various ways that it does in different mammals are not well understood (Clarke and O'Malley, 1968).

Historically, there was a time when the ventricular system was conceived as the seat of cerebral activity (Clarke and Dewhurst, 1973; Clarke and O'Malley, 1968). The cortical convolutions that covered the deeper structures were not believed to have important psychic or mental function and, in addition, like loops of small intestines seemed to lie in no particular order. However, in the early 1800s attention was drawn to the possibility of localizing specific mental faculties to specific gyri by Gall and his followers (Clarke and O'Malley, 1968). Although the specific beliefs of the phrenologists did not endure, their initial stimulus prompted numerous descriptive studies of cerebral convolutions, both in humans and in a variety of other mammals (Table I). Species-specific gyral patterns were identified (Table VIII), and their ontogenetic development was studied (Table V). In keeping with the growing appreciation of the importance of biological evolution, trends were proposed for the evolution of gyral and fissural patterns, particularly among primates (Table VIII). After the 1860s, this descriptive period waned as interest in microscopic structure and architecture of cerebral cortex increased (Table VI). As a result, experimental interest in localizing specific functions to specific convolutions diminished.

The major interest in cerebral cortex during the last 50 years has been in defining finer and finer details of projections and connections of sensory and motor circuits using an increasing variety of precise mapping methods (Table VII). In the last two decades, neuroscience has entered a time during which wiring diagrams of great hierarchic complexity, precision, and diversity are being disclosed. These microcircuits are highly ordered in their columnar, patchy, striped, and laminar patterns of organization and connectivity (Table VI; Constantine-Paton, 1983; Hubel & Wiesel, 1965; Mountcastle, 1978). Study of correlations between such microstructures and subtle details of function has accelerated.

Understandably, with all this detailed knowledge of cortical circuitry, there has been little interest in the functional morphology of the larger structural entities, the gyri and convolutions themselves. This is evident in the minimal consideration given to these gross features in the previous volumes in this series. One reason for this lack of interest has been that it is commonly assumed that the gyrification and fissuration of cortex is simply a mechanical outcome of increases in extent of cortext and that they have no architectural, connectional, or functional significance.

Historically, an enormous literature has accumulated during the last century on the subject of gyri and sulci (Tables I, V, VI, VIII). Much of this has been purely descriptive, and proposals regarding the determinants of cortical folding and fissuring have been largely speculative. However, as experimental methods evolved, there have been scattered groups of structural, connectional, and functional studies that reveal correlates of gyri and sulci that now provide the basis for the development of testable hypotheses.

It is appropriate and timely, therefore, to summarize a variety of lines of evidence regarding gyri and sulci and their determinants. Accordingly, I will review evidence that *gyrus building* consists of numerous constructional processes during cortical development which differ in gyral crowns, sulcal walls, and fundi, and that cortex in these different parts of convolutions exhibit different architectural, connectional, and functional features. Evidence also indicates that the developmental processes which produce such differences generate multiple microforces which determine the form and pattern of gyri and sulci.

There is already sufficient evidence to suggest the general working hypothesis that crown–wall–fundic complexes, and gyral–sulcal aggregates may be analogous to the nuclei and nuclear complexes in the rest of the brain, with the exception that these cortical complexes are structural–functional entities of greater hierarchic complexity.

2. Definitions and Nomenclature

Gyri and sulci exhibit varied forms, patterns, and arrangements in different mammals (Fig. 1). When cortex is viewed in depth by dissection, or in serial sections, gyri and sulci appear much more complex in three-dimensional perspective than would appear from their external morphology.

Probably because fissures and sulci are perceptually sharp and discrete, as well as simpler to describe and measure, most discussions of the external morphology of cerebral cortex have emphasized *sulcal patterns* rather than *gyral patterns*. This focus on fissures and sulci tends to deflect attention from the gyri themselves, which are the anatomically and functionally significant morphological entities.

Given the enormous number and variety of gyral forms and patterns among mammals with convoluted brains, it is easy to see why it has been difficult to achieve a unified conception regarding these three-dimensionally diverse entities. Because of this inherent morphological complexity, experimental study of buried cortex in convoluted brains has not been easy. As a consequence, many investigators have often chosen to study smaller smooth-surfaced brains.

A prerequisite to useful discussion of the salient features of gyri and sulci is the designation of a descriptive vocabulary. In this section I will review the kinds of terminology and sets of definitions that are generally applied to major features of gyri and sulci. Table II lists many of these terms (together with their identifying criteria) that are commonly found in the literature. The determinants and significance of these varied gyral and sulcal features are discussed in subsequent sections.

2.1. Gyral Nomenclature

The terms *gyri* and *convolutions* refer to the smooth rounded elevations or *folds* of cortical tissue lying between two sulci or fissures. Gyri vary in width, length, height, and shape. The names of gyri usually refer to their geometric form or their topographic relationships to sulci (Figs. 3–8, Table II). The *shapes*

Table II.   Nomenclature: Identifying Criteria for Gyral and Sulcal Terminology[a]

Resemblance to features and forms: angular, angulus, annectant, ansate, arcuate, bridge, calcarine, cingulate, cleft, convexity, convolution, coronal, crown, cruciate, crus, cryptogyrus, cryptosulcus, culmen, cuneate, cuneus, dimple, eminence, fissure, fork, fossa, fundus, furrow, genu, gyrus, hummock, incisure, insula, limb, lingual, lingula, lip, lobe, lobule, lunate, nodulus, notch, operculum, pachygyria, pocket, process, prominence, ramus, sagittal, splenial, spur, torus, ulegyria, uvula, vallecula, wart, wing, wulst

Topographic orientation or direction: anterior, ascending, axial, central, confluent, collateral, diagonal, dorsal, ectopic, inferior, lateral, longitudinal, marginal, medial, middle, orbital, posterior, rectus, rhinal, superior, temporal, terminal, transitional, transverse, triradiate, ventral

Positional prefixes: ectopic, ectosylvian, interparietal, intraparietal, paracentral, paragyral, parahippocampal, parasulcal, perfissura, pericentral, postcruciate, precentral, pseudosylvian, retrosplenial, semilunar, subcallosal, superior, supracallosal, supramarginal

Alphanumeric, size, sequential order, and fractionation: alpha, beta, gamma, . . . , 1, 2, 3, . . . , I–X, microgyria, pachygyria, polygyria, primary, secondary, semilunar, tertiary

Authorship[b]: Sylvian fissure, central sulcus of Rolando, island of Reil

Relation to overlying bone[c]: frontal, occipital, parietal, temporal

Structural–functional neural criteria[d]: interbrachial, labiar, limiting, rhinal

Degree of fissurization and convolution: gyrencephalic, lissencephalic

---

[a]This is a list of terms given to features of gyri or sulci as viewed externally, or in cross section. Terms applied to gyri and sulci are intermingled in alphabetical order under each category of defining criteria. In this table, and throughout the text, English equivalents of the proper Latin and Greek names are used (Hogben, 1971). The use of one or the other language form varies in the literature and there is formal agreement on only a few descriptive terms for human cerebral cortex (see reference to *Nomina Anatomica*).
[b]Some fissures have been named for the person who first described them.
[c]First proposed by Gratiolet (see Clarke and O'Malley, 1968).
[d]See Johnson (1980).

and orientations of most gyri and of gyral formations differ in predictable ways in different species, as well as in different cortical regions in any one species (see Section 6). There are gyri (and sulci) that have transverse, radial, longitudinal, coronal, diagonal, rectilinear, curvilinear, and concentric arrangements. Developmental defects, such as those that result in *porencephaly,* produce spokelike convergent arrangements of gyri and sulci (see Section 3).

Gyri often are arranged in groups or *formations.* Large topographical regions of cortical outgrowth containing several gyral groups are referred to as *lobes* (frontal, parietal, occipital, temporal), whereas smaller groups of gyri within a lobe are called *lobules.* Gyri or gyral formations that grow outward, bend over, and overlie adjacent, slower-developing cortex are called *opercula.* In some locations, groups of gyri "effloresce" or "mushroom" outward from a slender stalk of white matter, expanding in all directions laterally at their summits (Figs. 3, 5, 6, 28, 30). *Buried gyri* lie within sulci and are hidden from external view, either bulging out from sulcal walls or up from the fundus. An *annectant gyrus* is a *transitional* or *bridging gyrus* between two adjacent gyri. Such a gyrus may be buried within a fissure, or be partially or fully exposed at the surface of the brain (Connolly, 1936, 1950). In different mammals, gyri vary in complexity from *simple* to *compound* and occur in many different shapes, sizes, lengths, depths, patterns, orientations, and arrangements (see Section 6).

Brains that are smooth or relatively unconvoluted (and unfissured) are called *lissencephalic* or *semilissencephalic,* whereas highly convoluted brains are referred to as *gyrencephalic.* Many relatively lissencephalic brains exhibit slight *bulges, eminences,* or *hummocks* that regularly appear in species-typical locations. An unusual example of this is seen in the brains of manatees where such cameolike prominences are common over most of the cerebral surface (Fig. 7; Smith, 1902a–c). A further subtle cortical feature is revealed in myeloarchitectonic studies of small lissencephalic brains such as in mice, which led Kreiner (1973) to use the term *cryptogyri* to refer to smooth cortical zones that are fiber-rich, a feature which characterizes gyral crowns in convoluted brains (Fig. 8).

Terms which describe several kinds of anomalies of cortical development in humans and animals include: *agyria* (lacking gyri), *pachygyria* (broad gyri with thick cortex), *ulegyria* (narrow, distorted, and scarred gyri), *microgyria* (abnormally narrow gyri), *micropolygyria* (supernumerary tiny gyri), *polygyria* (an unusually large number of gyral formations), and *schizogyria* (gyri with disrupted continuity). *Ectopic gyri* are those that occur in unusual locations. Cortical *warts* are small innervated cellular protrusions of cortex occasionally seen on the cortical surface. They are usually considered to be focal cortical anomalies (*verrucose dysplasia*). They exhibit, in miniature, some of the features of gyral crowns (Fig. 27; see Section 3.7; Table V).

2.2 Sulcal Nomenclature

The terms *fissure* and *sulcus* are often used interchangeably, although the former is usually used to refer to the deeper, longer, or developmentally earlier, cortical *grooves* or *furrows.* A sulcus may split to form two or more *limbs, forks,* or *wings,* and a *spur, notch,* or *process* may project from its side. A *processus acuminus* is a small sulcal spur which occurs where a major sulcus makes a sharp bend. An *incipient sulcus* refers to a small slightly depressed cortical zone. When such a zone is somewhat deeper, it is called a *dimple* or *fissuret.* Kreiner (1973) referred

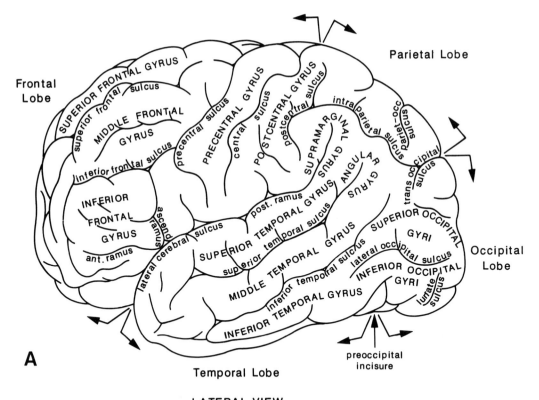

A

Frontal Lobe

Parietal Lobe

Occipital Lobe

Temporal Lobe

LATERAL VIEW

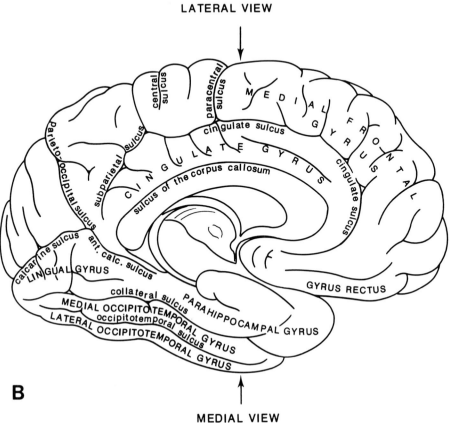

B

MEDIAL VIEW

to the fiber-sparse zones in the smooth cortex of mice as *cryptosulci* (Fig. 8). These zones appear in locations which, in larger rodents (Fig. 63), exhibit clear sulci.

In a variety of cortical locations on any brain, *vascular impressions* in cortex should not be mistaken for an incipient sulcus or dimple. Vascular impressions vary in size with the size of the overlying blood vessel. Such impressions are distinguished in cross section by the fact that, if small, they usually distort only the superficial one or two cortical layers, or if large, the underlying laminar and columnar cyto- and myeloarchitecture do not differ from those in cortex on either side of the vascular impression. Cortex underlying true incipient sulci, on the other hand, exhibits architectural differences from cortex on either side (see Section 4).

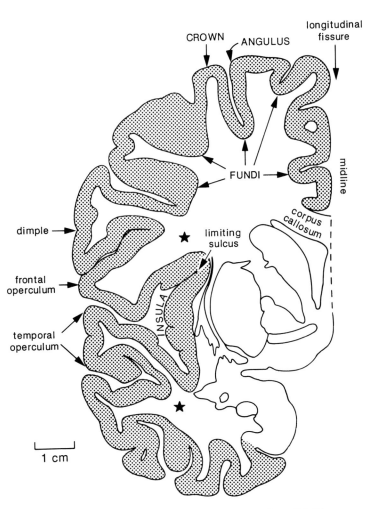

Figure 3. Diagrams of human cerebrum from left lateral (A) and medial (B) aspects, and in transverse section (C). Major gyri and sulci are labeled by conventional terms for primates. Location of major lobes indicated by arrows. (C) Transverse section of human brain taken from rostrocaudal level indicated by arrows in B. (C) The several gyri that compose part of the frontal and temporal opercula mushroom out over the insula from slender stalks of white matter (indicated by stars). (A and B, revised and reproduced with permission from Clemente, 1985, Figs. 11-93 and 11-98. C, modified and reproduced with permission from Roberts *et al.*, 1987, coronal plate 1.5.)

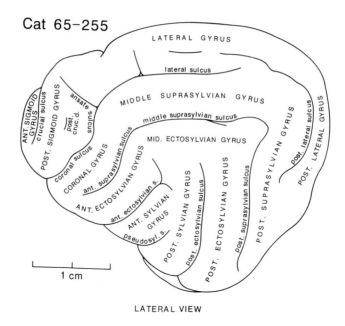

Cat 65-255

LATERAL VIEW

Figure 4. Diagram of cerebrum of domestic cat from left lateral aspect. Gyri and sulci are labeled by terms that are conventional for carnivores (Papez, 1929). ant., anterior; d, dimple; mid., middle; post., posterior; s., sulcus.

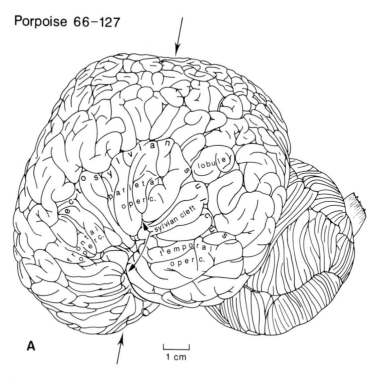

Porpoise 66-127

A

Figure 5. Diagram of highly convoluted brain of porpoise (*Tursiops truncatus*) from left lateral aspect (A) and in cross section (B) at location indicated by arrows in A. (B) Note multigyrated and multi-lobulated mushroom appearance of frontal and temporal opercula overlying the insula from slender stalks of white matter (indicated by stars). Large separation between these two sets of opercula is more appropriately named the Sylvian *cleft* rather than fissure. Other operculated gyral regions mushrooming from slender fiber stalks (indicated by stars) are also seen.

Like gyri, sulci vary in complexity from *simple* to *compound* and occur in many shapes, patterns, orientations, depths, and lengths in different mammals. If the walls of a simple sulcus are spread apart, they are usually deepest at its middle, with its bottom, or *fundus*, gradually coming to the surface of the cerebral mantle at both ends. In compound sulci, one or more sulci that are separate and distinct early in development, may later merge at the surface and thereby appear superficially as a single sulcus or fissure. Some of the deeper sulci may contain *buried sulci* that are hidden from view and which separate gyri within the sulcal walls or at the fundus (Figs. 5, 28). Such compound sulci vary widely in complexity in different animals. Like gyri, several sulci often appear in groups or *formations*.

Superfissures, Opercula, and Cortical Islands (Insulae)

In the larger mammalian brains, a large fissural complex develops where the frontal, parietal, and temporal cortical gyral regions grow outward farther than does the *island* of cortex just lateral to the basal ganglia, and in so doing, they bulge toward each other as *opercula* over this *insula* (Figs. 3, 5). This large fissure,

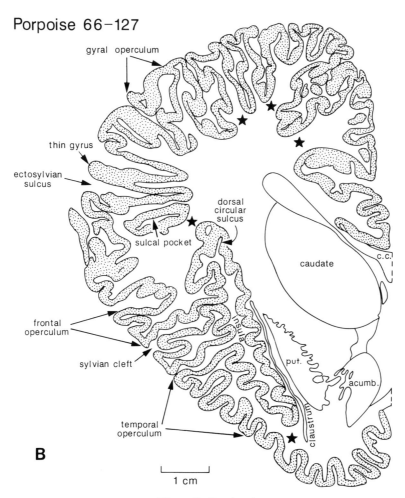

Figure 5. (*Continued*)

cleft, or fossa is called the *Sylvian* or *lateral* fissure. The buried sulci formed at the margins of the insula, between it and the overlying opercula, are called the *limiting* sulci of the insula. The fundi of some sulci within the Sylvian fissure are so thoroughly buried from all directions by operculated cortex that a *sulcal pocket* and *fundic pocket,* surrounded by fibers, can be seen in certain cross sections (Fig. 5). The term *per fissurae* has been used to refer to these very large or deep fissures which are formed by the operculation of large adjacent gyral formations. The result is an extensive fissural complex which is unlike simple sulci, in that it is produced by regional operculation of gyral aggregates rather than by local gyrogenesis (see Section 3). In some animals the Sylvian fissure is small, being no more than a sulcal spur which ascends at its typical location from the rhinal sulcus above claustrocortex. In such cases it is often referred to as the *pseudosylvian* sulcus. In other cases, the three major cortical opercula do not come together and the gap between them appears as a *cleft* or *fossa,* or more specifically, the Sylvian or lateral fossa (see manatee brains in Figs. 1 and 7). In small brains with a smooth cortical surface the lateral sulcus may be absent or appear

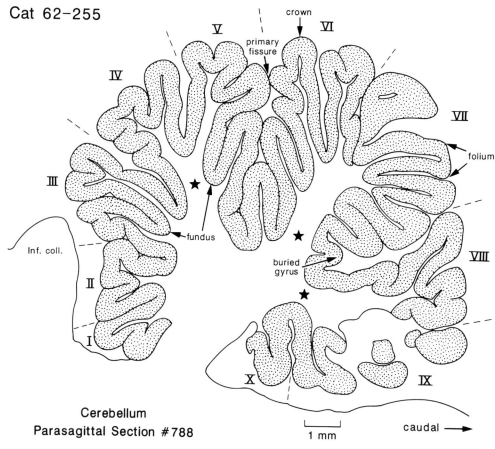

Cat 62–255

Cerebellum
Parasagittal Section #788

1 mm

caudal ⟶

Figure 6. Drawing of parasagittal section of cerebellar vermis of domestic cat showing multifoliated lobules that effloresce, like gyral blooms, from slender fiber stalks (indicated by stars). Vermal lobules (demarcated by dashed lines) are conventionally identified by roman numerals (I–X; Larsell and Jansen, 1970). Gyral crowns are called folia in the cerebellum because when viewed externally they lie adjacent to one another as long sheaves of slender folded ridges lying in parallel arrays. Inf. col., inferior colliculus.

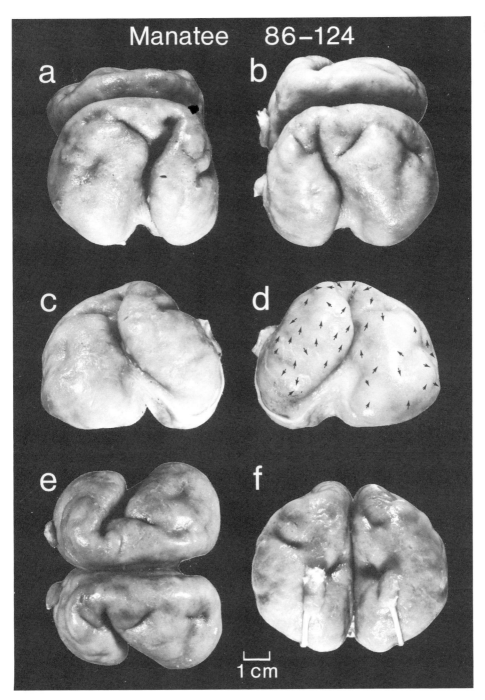

Figure 7. Cerebral hemispheres of Florida manatee (*Trichechus manatus*) from six views: right dorsolateral (a), left dorsolateral (b), right lateral (c), left lateral (d), dorsal (e), and frontal (f). Note large Sylvian (lateral) fossa and cleft in c. The relatively large cerebrum of manatees is remarkably unconvoluted. Yet, there are several shallow sulci clearly visible in frontal, parietal, temporal, and occipital cortex. Even more striking is the common appearance of numerous slight cortical prominences or *hummocks* (indicated by arrows in d).

only as an incipient sulcus or cryptosulcus. Operculated cortex which forms superfissures, as well as buried gyral formations that appear as islands, are common in several locations in large, highly convoluted brains. The submerged island of visual cortex that spreads out at the base of the *calcarine fissure* is a well-known example of such a cortical island in primates.

Another large special fissure is the *sagittal fissure,* which separates the two hemispheres of the brain at the midline. It differs from other cortical sulci and fissures in that its cortex is not continuous across the midline at its base (except in holoprosencephaly, Fig. 24). Rather, cortex either comes to an end at the corpus callosum (in eutherian mammals) or is transitional with the allocortex or hippo-campal formation on the same side in monotremes and marsupials. In all mammals, midline cortex is continuous ipsilaterally with dorsal and inferior cortex at the frontal and occipital poles of the forebrain.

2.3. Cross-Sectional Morphology of Gyri and Sulci

Viewed in transverse, sagittal, or horizontal cross section (Figs. 3, 5, 6), the *crown* of a gyrus refers to its *convexity.* The crown varies in degree of curvature and

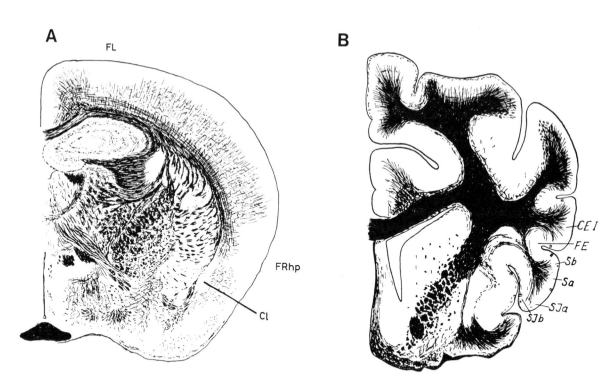

Figure 8. Comparison of myeloarchitecture of cerebral cortex of (A) mouse (Kreiner, 1973, Fig. 1d) and (B) dog (Kreiner, 1964c, Fig. 2A). In the dog (B), fundi of sulci are fiber-sparse, whereas gyral crowns are richly innervated. In the mouse (A), Kreiner called fiber-sparse zones *cryptosulci,* whereas fiber-rich regions in the mouse are referred to as *cryptogyri.* FL, fissura lateralis; FRhp, fissure rhinalis posterior; Cl, claustrum. FE, ectosylvian fissure; other abbreviations refer to Kreiner's designations of cortical architectonic areas. (Modified and reproduced with permission from the publications mentioned above.)

extent of lateral expansion. In some gyri the surface at the middle of a gyrus is flat, except at its margins, where it curves into the adjacent sulci. Each curved margin of a gyrus is usually sharply convex and is referred to as the *lip, angulus,* or *paragyral cortex.* The *wall* of a sulcus is that cortex along either of the two apposing sides of adjacent gyri. The *fundus,* or floor of a sulcus, is the cortex at that point deepest or farthest from the surface. On either side of a fundus the *parafundic* cortex curves concavely upward. A buried gyrus may emerge from the fundus of a sulcus, so that the latter exhibits two *limiting fundi.* The gyri of some gyral formations or lobules seem to effloresce or "mushroom" up and outward from a relatively slender *gyral stem* or *peduncle* (Figs. 3, 5, 6). The fiber mass within a gyrus (containing its afferent and efferent axons) is referred to as the *stalk* or *core* of the gyrus.

2.4. Standardization of Nomenclature

Study of the gyral and sulcal terms listed in Table II and depicted in Figs. 3–8 should provide the reader with an understanding of the descriptive criteria customarily used to name and identify specific gyri and sulci. It should be clear by now that these structures are named mainly on the basis of rather superficial criteria such as shape, size, orientation, grouping, and topographical location. Attempts to standardize nomenclature for gyri and sulci have had limited success. There is a general consensus regarding descriptive terms only for some of the better studied brains such as those of humans (Clemente, 1985; *Nomina Anatomica,* 1983) and a few other primates (Connolly, 1950). A different set of terms is in use for the most frequently studied carnivores (Papez, 1929). For most other mammals, a variety of descriptive naming conventions have been used (Smith, 1902a–c; Table VIII).

There are several reasons for the existence of different nomenclatural schemes: (1) There are species differences in gyral and sulcal location, shape, and pattern; (2) gyral and sulcal homologues (if any) in different animals are usually unknown; (3) different authors, independently, have applied different names to the same gyri and sulci in a particular animal type, and done so using different criteria; (4) tradition, custom, and training also influence the use of specific terms by different investigators; (5) finally, there is usually no consensus regarding the architectural, connectional, or functional significance of gyri and sulci. As a result of such factors, the development of a standard nomenclature based on rational, uniform sets of criteria does not yet seem practicable, or possibly even wise.

A consistent terminology might be developed if gyri in different animals could be identified as *homologues* on the basis of their similarity with respect to several neurobiological criteria, such as might be obtained in studies of developmental, architectural, connectional, physiological, and chemical features of different specific gyri in different mammals. Such data are simply not yet available for most regions of cerebral cortex. Even if the existence of homologous gyri could be determined, it seems unlikely that a new and valid neurobiologically based terminology could quickly or easily displace the descriptive nomenclature with which we all have become familiar.

3. Ontogeny of Convoluted Cortex

How gyri and sulci are formed is best seen during ontogeny. I will briefly review those major events and processes that are either known or hypothesized to underlie the ontogeny of gyri and sulci. The pertinent literature on this topic is extensive and covers a period of over a century (Table V). Discussions of developmental determinants of convoluted cortex have centered around four general subject areas: normal development, the role of nonneural tissues in development, experimental alterations of development, and developmental pathology.

3.1. Normal Macroscopic Developmental Events

Four major types of macroscopic change occur contemporaneously in the development of cortex in convoluted brains: *gyrogenesis, operculation, expansion,* and *lobation* (Figs. 10, 11). These developments transform the small, smooth cortical surface of the embryonic or fetal forebrain into that of the large convoluted and fissured cortical configuration of the adult brain. The primary constructional changes occur in *gyrogenesis,* in which localized regions of cortex differentiate, expand, and grow outward more rapidly than do adjacent zones which lag behind as the walls and fundi of sulci (Figs. 11–13). *Operculation* occurs when actively developing cortical regions grow outward over an adjacent slowly developing or nonexpanding region (Fig. 10). *Expansion* of cortex occurs when the cellular components of the thalamus, basal ganglia, and of the underlying fiber tracts, as well as those of the cerebral cortex grow and differentiate. These developments contribute to the outward expansion of the entire cortical sheet, gyri and fundi alike. In *lobation,* large regions of the telencephalon expand: (1) rostrally against the frontal and sphenoidal plates of the skull, pressing forward toward the face and over the eyes and nasopharynx (*frontal lobe*), (2) dorsally and dorsolaterally against the parietal cranial vault (*parietal lobe*), (3) laterally against the parietal and temporal bony plates as well as ventrally against the basocranial aspects of the temporal bone and along the outside of the deep basal forebrain and midbrain (*temporal lobe*), and (4) dorsocaudally over the midbrain and, in some cases, over the cerebellum toward the occipital bony plate (*occipital lobe*).

Together, gyrus building, operculation, expansion, and lobation increase the volume and surface area of the entire cortical sheet of each hemisphere as well as the number, complexity, and spatial configuration of convolutions in gyrencephalic mammals.

3.2. Initial Formation of the Cortical Mantle: Migration

Cerebral cortex has its origin in the postmitotic cells of the ependyma which migrate radially outwards in contact guidance with a transient population of elongated astroglial cells of the embryonic telencephalon (Fig. 9). The cells within these migrating sheets of neuroblasts are topographically organized in register with their ventricular and subventricular progenitors, and maintain the same

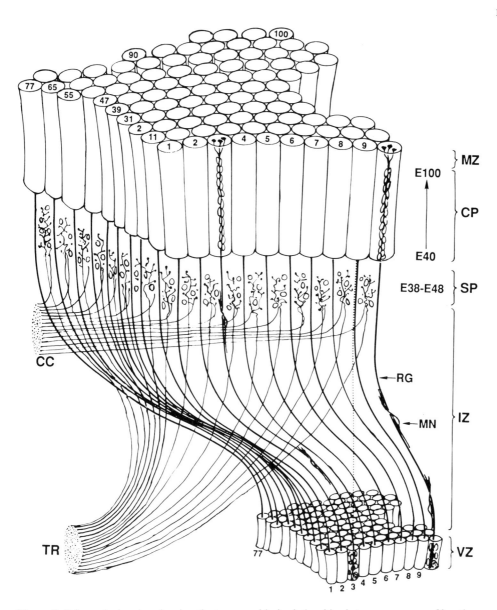

Figure 9. Schematic drawing showing the topographical relationships between an array of locations (numbered) within a small patch of proliferative cells in the ventricular zone (VZ) and its corresponding columnar locations in the cortical plate (CP) between embryonic days E40 and E100 of a macaque monkey. These topographical relationships are maintained during ontogeny as the cortical surface expands, shifts, and convolutes. These relationships are established as embryonic neurons migrate in succession along the same radial guides (RG) and stack up from deep to superficial within each developing cortical column. MN, migrating neuron; IZ, intermediate zone; SP, subplate, within which (at embryonic days E38–E48) are interstitial cells and the waiting afferents of thalamic radiations (TR) and contralateral corticocortical (CC) connections; MZ, marginal zone of cortical plate. (Reproduced with permission from Rakic, 1988, Fig. 2.)

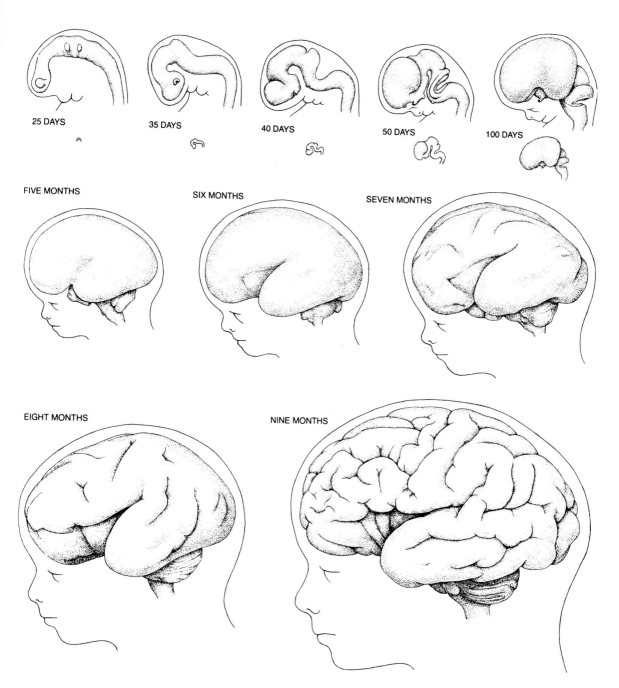

Figure 10. Development of the human brain viewed from the left side showing a succession of embryonic and fetal stages. The top row of drawings of embryonic stages are enlarged to an arbitrary common size to clarify their structural details. This figure nicely illustrates the relatively greater increase of the telencephalon, the smooth oval shape of the cerebrum at 100 days, the beginning of operculation over the insula at 6 months, and the progressive gyrification and lobation from 7–9 months. (Reproduced with permission from Cowan, 1979, p. 59; illustrated by Tom Prentiss.) Similar portrayals can be seen in Retzius (1891), Patten (1968), Noback and Demarest (1975), and Sidman and Rakic (1982).

topographical relationships as they ascend into the cortical plate of the small, round, and smooth early fetal brain (Fig. 9; Rakic, 1985, 1988). This migration occurs from the dorsolateral aspects of the two lateral ventricles and results in two bilaterally symmetrical hemispheres that are separated by the large sagittal interhemispheric fissure. Outward migration of sheets of topographically organized neurons occurs in successive waves. The earliest young neurons to reach the cortical plate are separated into a superficial layer I and a deep layer VII (Marin-Padilla, 1971, 1972, 1978, 1984, 1988; Rickmann *et al.*, 1977) soon after their arrival by later waves of migrations which fill in the bulk of neurons of the early developing cortical plate. In these later migrations, the neurons in each new wave come to rest radially outward just above the cortical neurons already set in place at the deeper layers of the cortical plate by previous migrating waves. In this way, the columnar architecture of the middle layers of cerebral cortex are built up successively from its deep layer VI to its superficial layer II (Table V). When the last born neurons migrate away from the ventricular plate, the surface of the cortex on each side of the brain is still smooth. Neurons and glia are arranged in columns vertical to the cortical surface, are small and densely packed, and lamination has just begun. As the last neurons move out of the subplate into the cortical plate, afferent axons from several sources are already waiting in the subplate (Fig. 9). The smooth rounded external morphology of the cerebrum is similar in all mammals at this early stage (Figs. 10, 11), whether it occurs during late embryonic, fetal, or early neonatal life (depending on the species). At this stage, cerebral cortex exhibits little regional architectural or cellular heterogeneity. From this point onward the brains of different species achieve different sizes, shapes, and patterns of gyri and sulci. Gyrogenesis now begins.

3.3. Gyrogenesis

Several active processes are hypothesized to occur in cerebral cortex during gyrogenesis (Figs. 12–15; Table III): (1) *Neuronal differentiation and dendrogenesis.* Neurons differentiate and increase in size, shape, and degree of elaboration of their dendrites sooner and more extensively in gyral crowns than in fundi. (2) *Neuronal orientation.* In crown cortex, future pyramidal cell bodies elongate vertically, extending their apical dendrites perpendicular to the cortical surface and parallel to, and interspersed with, the bundles of afferent axons. In fundic cortex, such cell bodies and their basal dendrites often extend tangentially, although their apical dendrites ascend perpendicular to the cortical surface at the base of the beginning sulci (Fig. 33). (3) *Afferent arrival, penetration, fasciculation, and arborization.* Thalamocortical axons arrive before gyrogenesis begins (Rakic, 1975b, 1976, 1979, 1988), followed by corticocortical axons from several different sources in the same and opposite hemispheres. These axons penetrate cortex between vertical columns of cell bodies. Then local intracortical axons begin to increase in number, density, diameter, and degree of myelination. The terminal plexuses of the axons from different sources arborize more profusely at certain specific laminar levels, and probably do so at different times. All these axonal proliferative events appear to be more profuse in gyral crowns than in fundi.

RACCOON

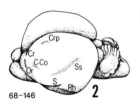

68-146   **2**

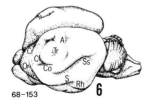

68-153   **6**

68-158   **10**

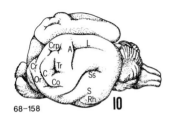

68-163   **14**

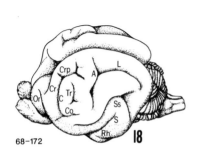

68-172   **18**

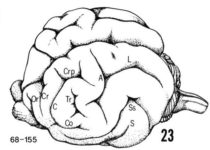

68-155   **23**

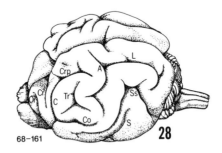

68-161   **28**

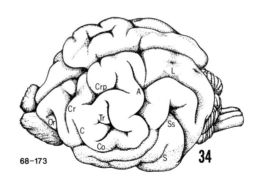

68-173   **34**

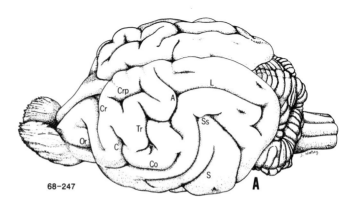

68-247   **A**

DORSOLATERAL SURFACE

|—| 1 CM

Moreover, different myeloarchitectural patterns commonly develop in different gyri (Fig. 36). (4) *Synaptogenesis.* As dendrites and axons arborize and multiply in proximity to one another, they form synapses of various kinds. Dendritic spines, synaptic knobs, and endbulbs differentiate and increase in size and number. These developments appear to be more profuse and voluminous in gyral crowns than in sulcal walls. (5) *Glial proliferation and ensheathment.* Glial cells play prominent roles in neuronal migration, development of myelin sheaths, formation of segregated specialized neuronal assemblies or glomeruli, synaptogenesis, and in maintaining intercellular and extracellular ionic balances (Kandel and Schwartz, 1985). Such events are hypothesized to be more profuse in gyral crowns than in sulcal walls and fundi. (6) *Laminar aggregation and segregation.* As cell bodies, dendrites, afferent axon arbors and synaptic neuropil differentially assemble at different depths, cerebral cortex develops several distinct cellular and neuropil laminae (Armstrong-James and Fox, 1988; Rakic, 1981). In three-dimensional perspective, these layers appear as sheets of cells stacked parallel to the cortical surface. Such laminar differentiation begins earlier and is more pronounced in crown cortex than in sulci and fundi (Smart and McSherry, 1986b). (7) *"Plasticity" changes.* Cortex in crowns, walls, and fundi probably undergoes further shaping as differential cell death, axonal sprouting, retraction and resorption of neurites, dendritic extension, and rearrangement and establishment of local circuit components (synapses, axonal arbors, dendritic spines) occur within different laminae and in different cortical areas at different times (Armstrong-James and Fox, 1988; Rakic and Goldman-Rakic, 1982; Rakic *et al.*, 1986). Such rearrangements are likely influenced by the presence or absence of neurelectric activity afferent to, and within, the local neural networks (Diamond *et al.*, 1966; Merzenich *et al.*, 1988). A testable hypothesis is that these finer sculpting processes occur differentially in the crowns, walls, and fundi, but there is little direct evidence on this point. (8) *Rearrangement of cell adhesion molecules and related membrane structures.* The architectural alterations of gyral crowns, walls, and fundi associated with migration, innervation, axonal and dendritic proliferation and arborization, and synaptogenesis involve structural changes in interneuronal contacts which are regulated by intracellular and intercellular processes (Edelman, 1986; Palade, 1985; Rakic, 1985). The actions of cell adhesion molecules produce intercellular attachments which affect the strength and rigidity of cortical tissue. Changes in conformation of cortex presumably require the active dissolution, rearrangement, and re-formation of such intercellular bonds. Even simple mechanical alterations in cortical architecture that are associated with gyrogenesis such as expansion, compression, stretching, bending, changes in cell size, reorientation, displacement and final positioning of cortical neurons and glia, and alterations in shape of cell columns and laminae very likely involve such processes. (9) Although only a few studies specifically address the issue, it seems likely that the active transformations listed above have *different timetables*, not only in gyral

Figure 11. Ontogeny of cerebral convolutions of raccoon brain. Left dorsolateral views of external morphology of raccoons at postnatal days 2, 6, 10, 14, 18, 23, 28, 34, and adult (A). All animals from different litters. Homologous sulci are labeled: A ansate, C central sulcus, Co coronal, Cr cruciate, Crp postcruciate, L lateral, Or orbital, Rh rhinal, S Sylvian, Ss suprasylvian, and Tr triradiate sulci. Animal numbers (e.g., 68–146) indicate year and animal sequence.

crowns, fundi, and parasulcal cortex, but also in different gyri and gyral formations.

I propose that the nine sets of developmental factors or parameters listed above produce the several known distinctive differences between cortex in gyral crowns, sulcal walls, and fundi (described in Section 4). Elaborating on this proposal, I suggest that as a result of factors 2 and 3 above, the *height of cortical columns* increases in developing gyral crowns more than it does in fundic and parasulcal cortex. Consequently, *cortical thickness* is greater in gyral crowns than in sulcal walls, and is thinnest in fundi.* In gyral crowns, because of the unusually dense cortical penetration by afferents, and the elaboration of dendritic bundles and arbors, *the volume of neuropil* increases and *cortex expands tangentially*

*There are "apparent exceptions" to this rule in certain planes of section where a fundus comes to the surface as its sulcus becomes shallow (Fig. 28). In such cases, the fundus is being cut obliquely rather than at right angles to its axis.

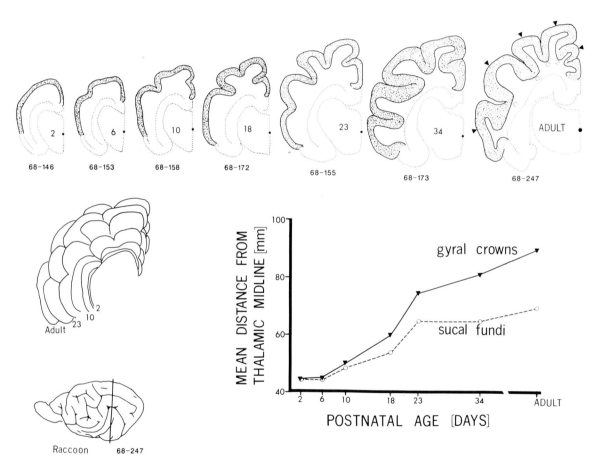

Figure 12. Gyrogenesis of raccoon cortex during ontogeny. Transverse sections taken from the same animals as in Fig. 11. Approximate plane of these sections indicated on drawing of adult brain at lower left. (Left center) Superimposed outlines of cortex of all animals (only four developmental stages identified). The graph at right plots development of the average distance of crowns and fundi of cortex from a midthalamic midline point (black dot). This graph shows that both gyral crowns and sulcal fundi move away from the center of the brain during development.

as cell columns move apart, both transversely across the gyral crown, and longitudinally along the long axis of the gyrus. This tangential spreading of cortex is more pronounced in gyral crowns than in sulcal walls, and is least evident in parafundic and fundic cortex. A corollary of the above is a lesser *perikaryal density* in gyral crown cortex than in cortex of sulcal walls and fundi. Thus, cell bodies

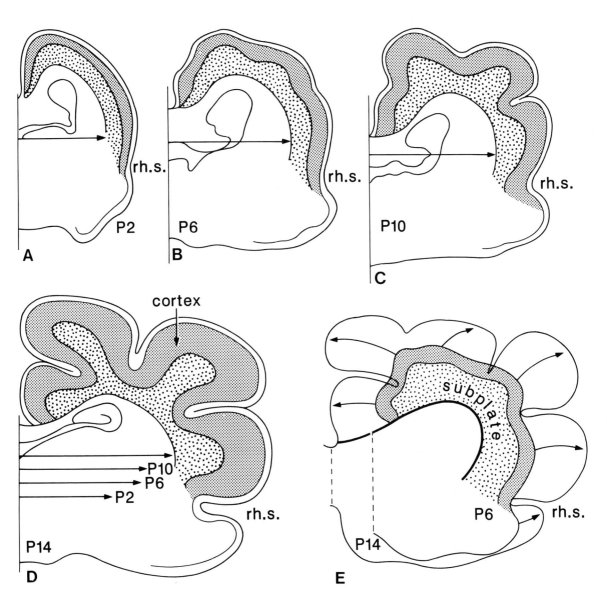

Figure 13. Gyrogenesis of ferret cerebral cortex during ontogeny. (a–d) Drawings of transverse sections of ferret brains at 2, 6, 10, and 14 postnatal days. All sections at level of the interventricular foramen. Subplate indicated by coarse dots. Cortex (except marginal layer) indicated by fine dots. Arrows in d indicate distance of subplate from the midline at the indicated postnatal ages. This figure shows that the core of the hemisphere expands and contributes to the outward movement of the cortical surface. (e) Outline of the 14-day-old section superimposed on the outline of 6-day-old brain (cortex = fine dots, subplate = coarse dots) with the deep surface of the 6-day and 14-day subplates superimposed. This shows that the gyral crowns grow outward (arrows) to a greater extent than do the sulcal fundi. (Modified and reproduced with permission from Smart and McSherry, 1986b, Fig. 17.)

are most densely packed within the fundus. From the perspective of external morphology, *differential development of different gyri and lobules* affects their relative width, height, shape, orientation, and spatial pattern.

In summary, the macroscopic and microscopic data reviewed so far suggest that gyral crowns, sulcal walls, and fundi are constructed differently and according to different developmental timetables.

3.4. Mechanical Forces Generated during Gyrogenesis

Historically, contrasting views, at least superficially so, have been proposed to account for the folding and fissuring of cerebral cortex (Barron, 1950; Goldman-Rakic, 1980, 1981; Hofman, 1989; Jacobson, 1978; Jefferson, 1913, 1915; Smart and McSherry, 1986a,b). In one view, the structural differences between cortex of gyral crowns, sulcal walls, and fundi are seen as secondary to mechanical folding, and therefore functionally insignificant. In the other view, these

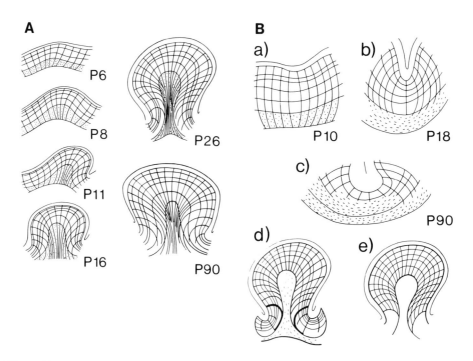

Figure 14. (A) Drawings of coronal sections of coronal gyrus of the ferret at postnatal days 6, 8, 11, 16, 26, and 90, schematically showing developmental changes in radial orientation of fiber bundles and cell columns, as well as tangential orientation of cortical layers (drawn from hematoxylin–eosin-stained sections). Stippling indicates the subplate region. Note that radial columns are progressively bent toward the parasulcal and parafundic regions. (B, a–c) Drawings of three stages in development of suprasylvian sulcus at three postnatal ages (P10, 18, and 90), showing increasing curvature of parasulcal radial lines and decreasing distinctiveness of cellular laminae. (d) Redrawing of section P26 from A, to show (in heavy line, which is omitted in e) the last curved radial column in the sulcus that is equally long as is a column in the gyral crown. (Modified and reproduced with permission from Smart and McSherry, 1986a, Figs. 3 and 5.)

differences are conceived as being structurally, connectionally, and functionally significant. I discuss these opposing views briefly below.

3.4.1. Primary (Active) Determinants (Table III)

The processes discussed in the previous paragraphs necessarily generate numerous miniature mechanical forces which, together, constitute the primary, active, or *intrinsic determinants* of gyrus building (Rakic, 1985). Gyri and sulci are not simply the result of purely passive mechanically induced infolding, buckling, bunching up, and stretching as a result of local structural weaknesses of cortex under stress of transverse forces (Bok, 1929, 1959, 1960; Clark, 1945). Moreover, fundi of sulci do not sink into depth (Figs. 12, 13), nor are they restrained from outward movement by the deep structures of the forebrain (Barron, 1950; Goldman-Rakic and Rakic, 1979).

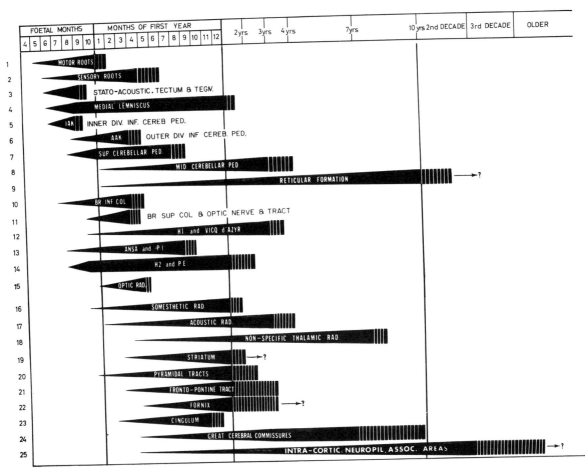

Figure 15. Timetable of development of myelinated fiber bundles in humans. Relative times of onset, rate of increase, and durations of myelination of 25 different major fiber tracts, bundles, or innervated nuclear structures indicated by location, slope, and length of bar graphs with respect to the time axis. Degree of myelination estimated by relative intensity of staining and density of myelinated fibers in human brains from fetal to adult stages of life (age is indicated at top of graph). (Modified and reproduced with permission from Yakovlev and Lecours, 1967, Fig. 1.)

Table III. Gyrogenesis: Differential Development of Gyral Crowns Compared with Sulcal Walls and Fundi[a]

1. *Cytoarchitectural differentiation:* increase in cell size; change in cell shape; elaboration of dendrites and axons; (all these increase cortical thickness)
2. *Neuronal orientation:* elongation of pyramidal cells; extension of dendrites; (these increase cortical thickness)
3. *Afferent innervation:* penetration; fasciculation; terminal arborization; myelination; increase in number and diameter; (all these increase volume of neuropil, decrease cell density, and expand cortex tangentially)
4. *Synaptogenesis and local circuit proliferation* (these also increase neuropil volume, expand cortex tangentially, and decrease cell density)
5. *Glial Proliferation* (also increases neuropil volume, expands cortex tangentially, and decreases cell density)
6. *Lamination:* differential segregation and aggregation of cell bodies, axon terminals, dendritic arbors, and synapses
7. *Plasticity effects:* differential cell death, growth, retraction, resorption, rearrangement of local circuit components and cell adhesion molecules
8. *Differential timetables of 1–7*

[a]Gyrogenesis involves *active intrinsic processes* which produce multiple *miniature mechanical forces.*

3.4.2. Secondary (Passive) Mechanical Effects (Table IV)

Nevertheless, several morphological features of gyri and sulci appear to reflect *passive mechanical effects* that are accessory outcomes of the intrinsic forces generated during gyrogenesis. (1) First of all, the *abuttal of sulcal walls* is probably a passive outcome of the gradual lateral bulging of the actively growing crowns and gyral stalks. (2) The *operculation* of rapidly differentiating cortex out over cortex that is developing more slowly, or that has stopped growing, is also a passive result of localized regional gyrogenesis. (3) To some extent *lobation* of cortex into spaces and regions unapposed by other tissue is probably a passive mechanical outcome of regional gyrogenesis. (4) *Cerebral enlargement and expansion.* Cortex of crowns, walls, and fundi alike are passively pushed away from the center of the brain as deep nuclei and fiber tracts grow and increase in size (Smart and McSherry, 1986a; Figs. 12, 13). (5) In some cases, it seems likely that *late-developing buried gyri* would tend to compress subjacent white matter inward, as well as push overlying gyral walls and crowns outward. In addition, the lateral ventricles may be compressed, bent, or distorted by gyrogenesis in deep-lying cortex. This occurs on the medial surface of the posterior horn of the lateral ventricles where the developing island of visual cortex in the depths of the calcarine fissure compresses the ventricle to form the *calcar avis* in humans (Clemente, 1985). (6) The species-typical *spatial form, pattern, and orientation of specific gyri and sulci* also may be partly due to several passive mechanical effects of brain development. At least three factors may be involved: (a) *differential enlargement of different cortical regions* in different mammals, will passively displace adjacent gyral regions; (b) *different trajectories of migrating axons,* e.g., thalamocortical afferents, may be differently deflected from a direct course to their cortical targets by the contemporaneous development, growth, and displacement of basal ganglia, thalamic nuclei, other fiber tracts, and the ventricles; (c) interspecies differences in timetable of later-arriving *interhemispheric and intercortical fiber tracts and bundles* also may affect the form and arrangement of developing gyri and sulci.

Table IV.   Passive Mechanical Forces[a]

A. Effects of gyrogenesis
   1. Abuttal of sulcal walls
   2. Operculation
   3. Lobation
   4. Cerebral enlargement and expansion
   5. Differential regional enlargement
   6. Compression by late-developing buried gyri
   7. Differential bending of cell columns in crown, angulus, wall, and fundus
   8. Differential curvature of cortical layers in crown, angulus, wall, and fundus
   9. Displacement of trajectories of fiber tracts
B. Variable effects of developing nonneuronal structures: skull plates, meninges, vertricles, cerebrospinal fluid, eyes, ethmoid and nasal bones and cavities, maxilla, mandible, middle ear, oropharyngeal structures
C. Effects of flexure of the neuraxis

[a]These determine form, spatial pattern, and orientation of gyri and sulci.

In addition to such passively induced gross morphological features, there are also finer structural features within the cortex of crowns, walls, and fundi, which, I propose, reflect the influence of passive mechanical forces involved in gyrogenesis. Two such features are the most obvious: (1) *Columnar orientation.* Although cell columns, fiber fascicles, and dendritic bundles are oriented vertically in the middle of gyral crowns, the differential increase in axonal and dendritic neuropil in crown cortex is typically associated with a progressive *bending* of those columns toward the margins of the crown (at the lip or angulus) down into the upper sulcal walls (Fig. 14; Smart and McSherry, 1986b). Within parafundic cortex, the cell columns (as well as their interpolated fiber bundles) curve downward deeper within cortex near the underlying white matter than they do near the cortical surface (Fig. 14). Development of curvilinear cortical columns within the deeper laminae of parafundic cortex suggests either (a) that the more superficial cortex in parafundic regions expands more than does cortex of the deeper laminae, or (b) that the more numerous and thickly myelinated fibers entering cortex of the crown and angulus displace the fiber and cell columns at the deeper laminar levels of parafundic cortex. (2) *Curvature of cortical laminae* at the angulus of gyral crowns and within the fundic and parafundic cortex is probably also a passive mechanical outcome without functional significance.

There are undoubtedly numerous other instances of secondary effects of gyrogenesis including stretching, bending, compression, submersion, and torsion of local regions of cortex, all of which might be secondary or passive outcomes of the spatiotemporally complex mosaic of intrinsic developmental forces being generated during gyrogenesis.

3.5. Role of Nonneural Structures in Cortical Development (Table V)

Skull. It has been argued that the skull imposes mechanical constraints on the expanding cerebrum so as to induce folding of the cortical surface. That the skull is not a major restraining factor is suggested by several facts: (1) The

Table V. Literature on Ontogeny of Cerebral Cortex

Historical
  Bischoff (1870)
  Cunningham (1890a)
  Donaldson (1895)
  Economo and Koskinas (1925)
  Glasser (1916)
  Hochstetter (1924)
  Huxley (1932)
  Huxley *et al.* (1941)
  Jacobson (1978)
  Schmidt (1862)
  Thompson (1942)
  Weiss (1955)

General
  Connolly (1950)
  Di Benedetta *et al.* (1980)
  Dodgson (1962)
  Edelman (1986)
  Edelman and Thiery (1985)
  Edelman *et al.* (1985)
  Farkas-Bargeton and Diebler (1978)
  Gould (1977)
  Hamburger and Oppenheim (1982)
  Meisami and Brazier (1979)
  H. Meyer (1937)
  Minkowski (1967)
  Noback and Moss (1956)
  Palade (1985)
  Passingham (1985)
  Purves (1988)
  Purves and Lichtman (1985)
  Rakic (1979, 1988)
  Rakic and Goldman-Rakic, (1982)
  Rakic *et al.* (1986)
  Thatcher *et al.* (1987)
  Van der Loos (1979)
  Weiss (1970)
  Williams and Herrup (1988)
  Williams *et al.* (1987)
  Willier *et al.* (1955)
  Wolff (1978)
  Yakovlev and Lecours (1967)

Migration and corticogenesis
  Friede (1954)
  Galaburda (1979)
  Goldman and Nauta (1977)
  König and Marty (1981)
  Mangold-Wirz (1966)
  Marin-Padilla (1971, 1972, 1978, 1984, 1988)
  M. Miller (1988)
  Rakic (1974, 1975b, 1976, 1978, 1981, 1985)
  Rakic and Yakovlev (1968)
  Rickmann *et al.* (1977)
  Schaffer (1923)
  Sidman and Rakic (1973)
  Sievers and Raedler (1981)

Gyrogenesis
  Chi *et al.* (1977)
  Harde (1957)
  Kruska (1975)
  Schaffer (1918b)
  Smart and McSherry (1986a,b)
  Zecevic and Rakic (1985)

Experimental studies
  Barron (1950)
  Goldman and Galkin (1978)
  Goldman-Rakic (1980, 1981)
  Goldman-Rakic and Rakic (1979)
  Greenough and Chang (1988)
  Millen and Woollam (1959)
  Moss (1957)
  Moss and Young (1960)

Role of nonneural structures
  Abbie (1947)
  Ariëns Kappers (1932)
  Biegert (1957)
  Bonin (1934)
  Camosso *et al.* (1980)
  de Beer (1937)
  DuBrul (1958)
  DuBrul and Laskin (1961)
  Hofer (1952, 1969)
  Kier (1977)
  Klatt (1949)
  Miller (1923)
  Moss (1957, 1960)
  Neubauer (1925)
  Pickering (1930)
  Starck (1953)
  Washburn (1947)
  Weidenreich (1940)

Neuropathology
  Bielschowsky (1915, 1923)
  Black (1913)
  Blackwood and Corsellis (1976)
  Bruce (1889)
  Jacob (1936a,b, 1940)
  Jellinger and Rett (1976)
  Kalter (1968)
  Larroche (1977)

Table V. (*Continued*)

Brun (1965)	Lierse and Beck (1981)
Buchwald and Brazier (1975)	Loeser and Alvord (1968)
Cameron (1907)	Malamud and Hirano (1974)
Caviness and Williams (1979)	Merritt (1959)
Caviness *et al.* (1988)	Morel and Wildi (1952)
Courville (1971)	Myers *et al.* (1973)
Douglas-Crawford (1906)	Probst (1979)
Dvořák *et al.* (1978)	Ranke (1910)
Evrard *et al.* (1978)	Richman *et al.* (1973, 1974)
Ferrer (1984)	Schaffer (1918a)
Ferrer *et al.* (1987)	Stewart *et al.* (1975)
Fox *et al.* (1965)	Thompson and Green (1985)
Friede (1975)	Vinken *et al.* (1977)
Greenfield and Wolfsohn (1935)	Volpe (1987)
Hanaway *et al.* (1968)	Williams *et al.* (1976)
Haymaker and Adams (1982)	Yakovlev (1959, 1968)
Hefftler (1878)	Yakovlev and Wadsworth (1946a,b)

Physiological data
Armstrong-James and Fox (1988)	Merzenich *et al.* (1988)
Johnston (1988)	Payne *et al.* (1988)
Leavitt *et al.* (1981)	Ray and Craner (1988)

calvarium grows and is shaped in response to forces generated by the growing convolutions and expanding opercula and lobes. (2) Indeed, the expanding crowns of many gyri make impressions on the endocranial surface in many mammals, a fact which makes endocranial casts useful in evaluating the pattern of gyrification of many extinct mammals (see Table VIII; Radinsky, 1976b). (3) Skull sutures do not ossify normally until the brain has ceased growing. (4) If any portions of the cerebrum fail to develop and grow, due either to experimental or pathological causes, the skull tends to conform to the size and shape of the cerebral remnant.

Meninges, ventricles, and cerebrospinal fluid (CSF). Like the cranial vault, the dura also appears to develop in conformation with the subjacent cortical structures. So too do the pia–arachnoid membranes. The ventricles appear to be largely shaped by the development of the cerebral lobes, lobules, and, to a lesser extent, by deep fissures, such as the calcarine. The ventricles are relatively large early in development, but become narrower (possibly being compressed) as cortex and the brain develop (Kier, 1977). CSF maintains a steady pressure not only from within the ventricles but subdurally against the surface of the brain. There is no evidence to indicate that any of these structures or fluids exert significant differential forces that might affect the development of gyri, or of the adult conformation of the convolutions.

Vasculature. No longer is it believed that major blood vessels induce fissuration during development. Without question, blood vessels commonly lie at the fundus of sulci, but the alignment of such vessels with sulci seems to occur secondarily to gyral and sulcal formation during development. Mechanical impressions on cortex by blood vessels are typically minor features, and when seen in fixed material are superficial and do not alter the underlying architecture (see beaver brain in Fig. 63). Capillarization is much more dense in cerebral cortex when compared with underlying white matter, a fact that reflects greater metabolic activity of cortex. Although the capillary net has a different pattern in gyral crowns, sulcal walls, and fundi, it appears similar to that of cell and fiber columns and is probably secondary to the different neuronal architecture in these different zones (Miodoński, 1974).

Structures of the head. The form of the brain and the development of the overall gyral–sulcal patterns are certainly influenced by the contemporaneous development of other nonneural structures within the head such as the eyes, ethmoid and nasal bones and their cavities, maxilla, mandible, middle ear, oropharyngeal structures, and muscles of the skull (DuBrul, 1958; Washburn,

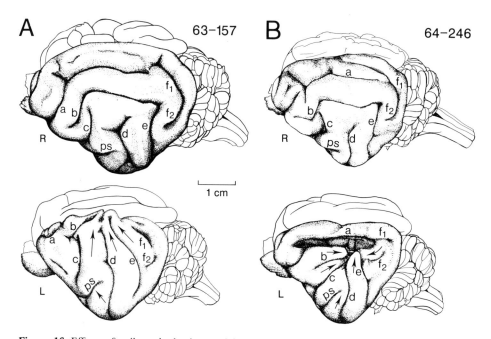

Figure 16. Effects of unilateral selective partial ablation of cerebral cortex in neonatal kittens on the development of gyral and sulcal patterns into adulthood. Ablated hemisphere (left side = L) is compared with the unoperated hemisphere (right side = R, reversed for ease of comparison to appear as the left). Drawings of the two hemispheres for each animal are shown in pairs: Top = right hemisphere, bottom = left hemisphere. (A) Aspiration of marginal (lateral) gyrus. (B) Aspiration of left suprasylvian gyrus. (C) Aspiration of left sigmoid gyrus (pre- and postcruciate gyri). (D) Aspiration of left posterolateral gyrus and portion of posterior suprasylvian gyrus. (E) Aspiration of left middle ectosylvian gyrus (auditory areas I and II). (F) Decortication of left hemisphere. Note the shift (indicated by arrows) of normal cortex that has occurred toward the smaller operated hemisphere in both dorsal (D) and ventral (V) views. This shift was seen also in basal brain structures and was reflected in the basocranium, which was skewed to the side of the aspirated hemisphere. Letters (on normal and operated sides) indicate specific major sulci that typify the brains of cats. Arrows on the operated side in A–E, and unoperated side in (F), indicate direction of movement and reorientation of gyri on the operated side that has occurred during development. Question marks indicate atypical (ectopic) sulci. In all cases the spared cortex moved toward the region of the original defect.

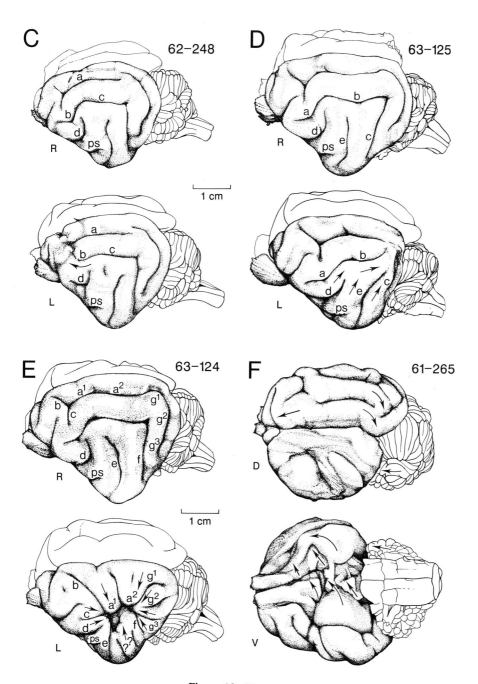

Figure 16. *(Continued)*

1947). The development of these structures probably affects the conformation of basocranial brain structures primarily. The cerebral vault, within which most cortex develops, is relatively free to expand.

Cranial–vertebral flexure. It has been proposed that flexure of the neuraxis associated with development of erect posture has determined the typical gyral–sulcal patterns of many primates (Moss and Young, 1960). Clearly, such flexure primarily affects the relative placement and orientation of the medulla, cerebellum, brain stem and thalamus, and their constituent nuclei. A secondary effect on the cerebrum might be the caudal protrusion of the occipital lobe in such animals. To what extent gyral and sulcal patterns are influenced by cranial–vertebral flexure remains to be determined experimentally in gyrencephalic mammals.

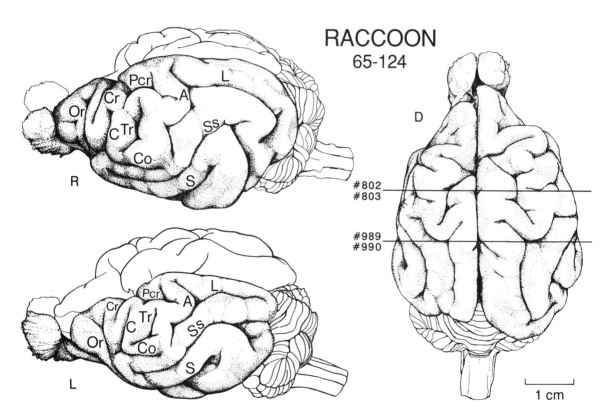

Figure 17. Effects of unilateral (left) subcortical aspiration of internal capsule, basal ganglia, amygdala, most of the hippocampus, and most of the interhemispheric (callosal) fibers and thalamic radiations in a neonatal raccoon on the subsequent development of gyri and sulci of the overlying cortex. Ipsilateral cerebral cortex and subjacent fibers were spared, except for a portion of cortex of the occipital lobe where the aspiration pipette was introduced in the 10-day- old raccoon. The brain was perfused at adulthood. Comparison of the operated left (L) hemisphere with the unoperated right hemisphere (R, reversed to appear as left) reveals smaller hemisphere and gyri on the left, despite normal pattern of gyrification. Numbers (802, 803, 989, 990) on dorsal view (D) indicate planes of sections depicted in Fig. 18. Abbreviations for sulci as in Fig. 11.

3.6. Experimental Alterations of Developing Gyri and Sulci

Determinants of gyral and sulcal form and pattern can be assessed to some extent experimentally by producing selective partial removals or destructions of specific neural structures and connections early in development while cerebral cortex is still relatively smooth. At such times, migration of neurons into the cortical mantle is completed (Goldman-Rakic and Rakic, 1979; Rakic and Goldman-Rakic, 1982) and most major fiber connections are already in place.

In the early 1960s, we performed a variety of aseptic selective partial unilateral aspirations of cerebral cortex, or unilateral aspiration of basal forebrain

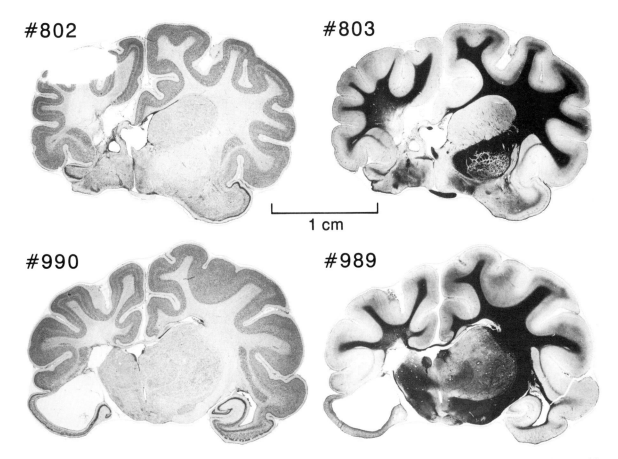

Figure 18. Effects of left unilateral neonatal subcortical aspiration of deep nuclei and fiber tracts in a raccoon (described in Fig. 17) on development of cortical cytoarchitecture and myeloarchitecture in the adult. Two pairs of adjacent coronal sections, stained for cells and myelinated fibers—sections 802 and 803—are from the level of the basal ganglia; 990 and 989 are from the midthalamic level. When compared with cortex of the unoperated (right) hemisphere, gyri on the left are narrower, cortex is thinner (with thinner cellular layers), sulci are shallower, and gyral fiber stalks and intracortical fiber bundles are smaller and not as pronounced. Note that the thalamus is spared on the operated side (sections 990 and 989), but is markedly reduced in size. Only a small fragment of the corpus callosum remains posteriorly.

and fibers of the internal capsule in newborn kittens and in early postnatal raccoons. Our results, most of which are published here for the first time, showed that aspiration of basal ganglia and transection of all thalamocortical connections did not affect the general pattern of cortical folding and fissuring (Chow and Leiman, 1970; Figs. 16–18). However, the orientations and patterns of spared gyri and sulci were predictably altered by selective removal of medial, rostral, caudal, or central portions of cerebral cortex of one hemisphere (Fig. 16). In all these early cortical ablations, the gyri and sulci tended to reorient toward the defect, as is common in porencephaly (Fig. 16; Malamud and Hirano, 1974; Yakovlev and Wadsworth, 1946a,b). When stained sections were examined microscopically, we found that, despite such gyral reorientation, the spared cortex and thalamic sources of spared afferents appeared normal, similar to those of comparable structures on the opposite, unoperated side. However, the widths of gyri and depths of sulci appeared somewhat altered. In these experiments, ectopic sulci were observed in some cases in cortex near the defect (Fig. 16E), but their microscopic features were not examined in detail.

Goldman and Galkin (1978) and Goldman-Rakic (1980) found that aspiration of cerebral cortex in macaque monkey fetuses, before thalamocortical and corticocortical connections have become established, resulted in aberrant sulcal development not only near the region of the lesion, but also at more distant cortical locations, sometimes even on the opposite unoperated hemisphere, with which the aspirated site normally has no connections (Fig. 20). Another relevant experimental discovery was Rakic's (1988) discovery of the development of multiple gyri and sulci in normally smooth occipital cortex on one side following removal of the contralateral eye in a fetal monkey (Fig. 19). From these and other results of studies of generation and migration of cortical neurons, and of thalamocortical and corticocortical connections, these authors conclude that ". . . cerebral fissuration begins at about the same time that thalamocortical afferents

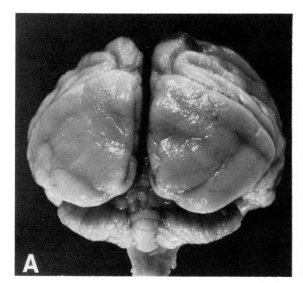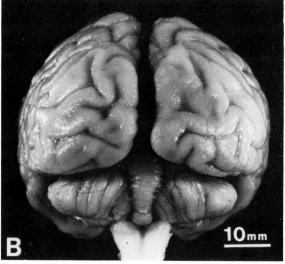

Figure 19. Effect of bilateral enucleation, at embryonic day 60, on the development of gyri and sulci of the occipital lobe. Posterior views of cerebrum in a normal 3-year-old rhesus monkey (A) and a monkey of the same age that was enucleated (B). Note presence of a new pattern of gyri and sulci in the operated animal (B) when compared with the normal, relatively smooth dorsolateral occipital cortex (A). (Reproduced with permission from Rakic, 1988, Fig. 4.)

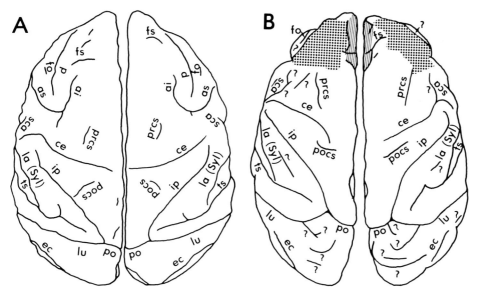

Figure 20. Experimental modification of gyral patterns. Dorsal view of drawing of fissural pattern of normal 2½-year-old rhesus monkey (A) and a monkey at the same age in which frontal cortex was aspirated on embryonic day 106 (B). Note presence of numerous ectopic sulci (indicated by question marks) in the prefrontal, temporal, and occipital lobes in B. (Reproduced with permission from Goldman and Galkin, 1978, Fig. 11.)

invade the cortex and assumes its mature pattern during the major ingrowth of corticocortical connections" (Goldman-Rakic and Rakic, 1979). They believe that interruption of any of these fiber systems before they have innervated their normal cortical targets may produce disrupted, as well as abnormal innervations which may affect gyral and sulcal development in distant regions. The detailed nature of such connectional and architectural disruptions is not known.

Work of this latter kind is needed to ascertain specific developmental correlates of gyrus building and formation. In such studies, gyral and sulcal development would be studied following selective partial interruption of afferent and efferent circuits before, during, and after (1) generation and migration of specific cortical neurons, and (2) arrival of different specific afferent circuits. These and other authors have laid the groundwork for such studies by their autoradiographic studies of normal development of several different laminar cortical architectonic areas (Rakic, 1975b, 1976, 1981, 1988).

3.7. Pathological Gyral and Sulcal Patterns

A wide variety of developmental anomalies of the human brain had already been identified by the early 1900's (Clarke and O'Malley, 1968). Abnormalities of cortical development that produce alterations in form and pattern of gyri and sulci are now well documented (Table V; Figs. 21–26). Many of these came to attention because they were associated with sensory, motor, cognitive, and motivational disorders. Agyria (lissencephaly), pachygyria, microgyria, micropolygyria, ulegyria, schizogyria, hemiatrophy, status verrucosis, heterotopia, and agenesis of the corpus callosum all exhibit features which indicate abnormalities

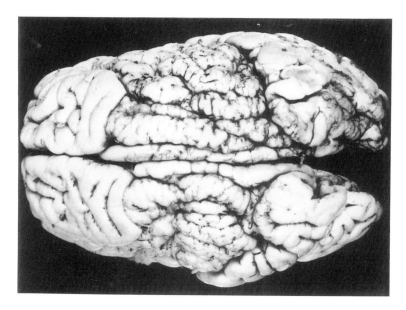

Figure 21. Micropolygyria. Dorsal view of external morphology of cerebral cortex of brain (875 g) of a 2-year-old retarded female infant. This brain exhibits numerous small gyral elevations separated by shallow sulci or dimples, localized in this case to the frontoparietal convolutions. Central sulcus is absent. In cross section, cortex of this specimen was greatly convoluted with a deeply penetrating molecular layer, with a narrowed deep zone of white matter which contained scattered heterotopic cell clusters. This cortex also lacked normal lamination. In other cases, this defect occurs in different locations and degrees of severity. (Reproduced with permission from Malamud and Hirano, 1974, Fig. 205A.)

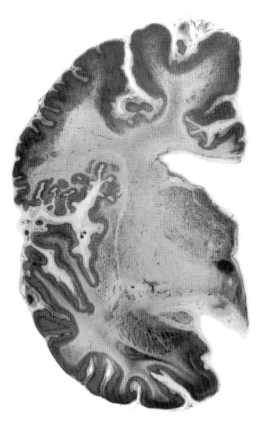

Figure 22. Developmental anomalies of cortical gyri in a 35-day-old human infant with Zellweger syndrome. Coronal section at midsylvian level of left hemisphere showing increased width of gyri dorsally and decreased width of gyri laterally. Convolutions in opercular regions, as well as in insula, were more numerous and much shallower than normal. Defect was bilateral and approximately symmetrical. Dorsally, the cortex became pachygyric (abnormally broad, thick, and fewer in number). Disruptions in migration resulted in incomplete formation of layers II and III as well as heterotopic neurons subjacent to the abnormally convoluted cortex. Brain weight 460 g. Size and general shape of cerebral hemispheres were normal. Cresyl violet stain. (Reproduced with permission from Evrard *et al.*, 1978, Fig. 1A.)

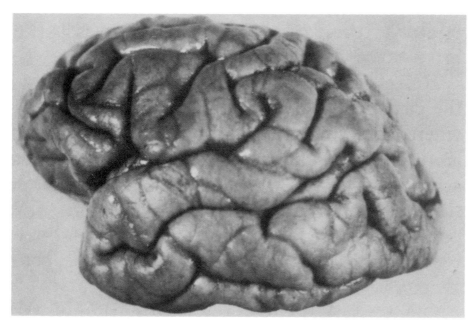

Figure 23. Microcephalic human brain showing simple convolutional pattern with relatively broad gyri. (Reproduced with permission from Blackwood and Corsellis, 1976, Fig. 10.15 and Adams *et al.*, 1984, Fig. 10.38.)

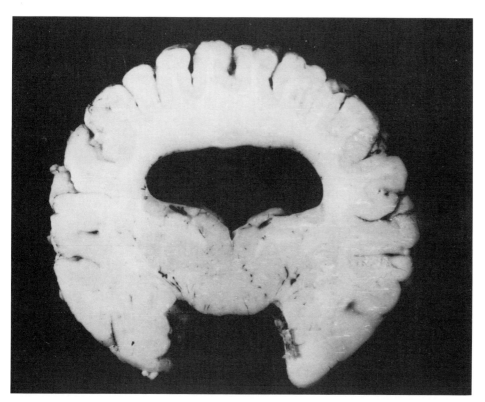

Figure 24. Holoprosencephaly of brain of 8-month retarded human infant female. Fusion of cerebral hemisphere occurs dorsally across the midline, with abnormal gyral and sulcal patterns. (Reproduced with permission from Malamud and Hirano, 1974, Fig. 206b.)

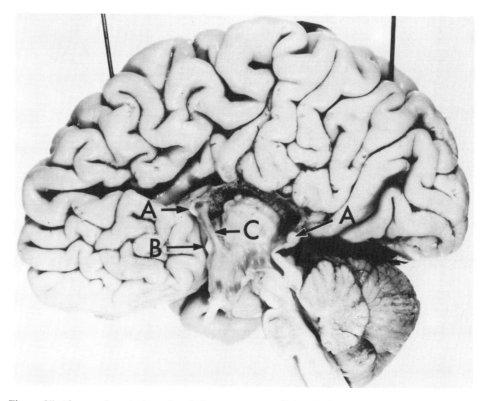

Figure 25. Abnormal cortical gyral–sulcal patterns on medial wall of human brain with agenesis of the corpus callosum. There is no clear-cut demarcation of the cingulate gyrus by a callosomarginal gyrus. Instead, gyri and sulci tend to be oriented vertically toward the callosal site. Rudiments of a genu and splenium of the corpus callosum persist (A). In such cases, Probst's bundle contains fibers otherwise destined to pass through the corpus callosum. This deficit is associated with a defect in development of the upper part of the lamina terminalis. This brain weighed 860 g. The patient was a retarded 10-year-old boy. (Reproduced with permission from Malamud and Hirano, 1974, Fig. 213b.)

in migration, maturation, and connectivity (Bruce, 1889; Cameron, 1907; Douglas-Crawford, 1906; Loeser and Alvord, 1968). Most of these abnormalities are of unknown etiology. In most of these cases, several different levels of the nervous system are usually affected, and all such defects probably involved disruptions in genesis, migration, maturation, and connectivity of neurons (Rakic and Yakovlev, 1968). Malformations of other tissues often accompany such disorders. Many causative factors are known or suspected. These include anoxia, hypoxia, ischemia, carbon dioxide or bilirubin poisoning, alcohol or drug toxicity, metabolic diseases, nutritional deficiencies, viral or bacterial infections, vascular disease, and trauma. Genetic disorders also are known which produce widespread disruptions of the nervous system. Many of these factors may occur perinatally or postnatally and may produce disruptions of cortical architecture which affect the formation of gyri and sulci. Because so little is usually known of the actual determinants, time of occurrence, or developmental course of most of these anomalies, most such tragic cases provide little help in understanding how gyral and sulcal patterns come to be arranged as they are in normal animals or humans.

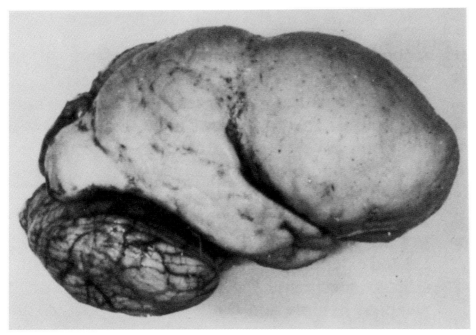

Figure 26. Agyria of human brain (right lateral view) showing absence of gyri and sulci. This case also had an abnormally thick cortex (pachygyria) as well as subcortical heterotopic islands of neurons. (Reproduced with permission from Blackwood and Corsellis, 1976, Fig. 10.29 and Adams *et al.*, 1984, Fig. 10.25.)

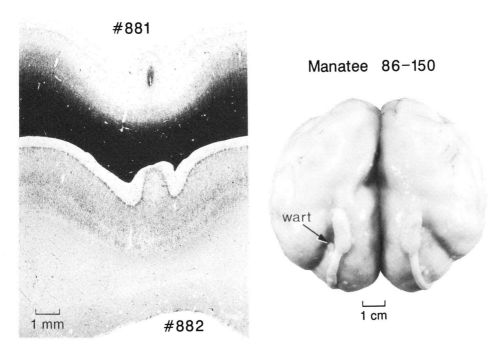

Figure 27. Cerebral warts on the orbitofrontal surface of a manatee (*Trichechus manatus*). As in many human cases, this *verrucose dysplasia* may be found without other neuroanatomical malformations. These warts were seen in several manatee brains. They look like miniature gyri, having a central myelinated bundle, but they actually are disorganized herniations of layers II and III, with layer I being slightly thinner than normal. In this case, the wart occurs in the fundus of a shallow sulcus on the right orbitofrontal cortex (indicated by arrow on frontal view of the brain). Other warts are visible on the other hemisphere lateral to the olfactory tract. A central blood vessel is typical in this type of simple malformation. Horizontal section 881 is stained with hematoxylin and 882 with thionin.

Studies of experimental teratology have produced a variety of developmental neuropathologies, many involving cerebral cortex (Kalter, 1968). Ionizing radiation and genetic manipulation have also been successfully used to induce cerebral malformations. Animal models of various human neuropathologies have been induced by many of the causative agents mentioned above. An advantage of some of these experiments is that they allow some degree of parametric control of the agent as well as the timetable of its effect in relation to different stages of embryonic and fetal development. Because of their invasive generalized effects on the brain, however, most such studies do not provide direct or conclusive evidence regarding the normal development of specific features of cerebral convolutions. Nevertheless, such studies may provide invaluable information that is relevant to understanding and preventing the various devastating human neuropathologies.

4. Neuroanatomical Features of Convoluted Cortex: Architecture and Connectivity

Since the beginning of microscopic study of cerebral cortex, many investigators have observed that cytoarchitecture and myeloarchitecture differ in the cortex of gyral crowns, sulcal walls, and fundi (Figs. 28, 19; Table VI). Many of these differences are found in all regions of convoluted cerebral cortex in all mammals that have been examined. As previously mentioned, some early observers believed that such differences were secondary to mechanical folding of cortex, whereas others believed that such easily-seen differences indicated functional differences. Yet, only a few investigators have found these differences of sufficient interest to merit systematic study. Most published work is many years old. Only occasionally have modern techniques provided pertinent information regarding the significance of these architectural differences between gyri and sulci, and, even then, only incidentally to data obtained for other purposes.

Table VI.   Literature of Neuroanatomical Features of Cortex

Historical
Brazier (1978)	Lashley and Clark (1946)
Cunningham (1890a–c)	Meyer (1971)
Flechsig (1898)	Polyak (1957)
Fleischhauer (1978)	Rasmussen (1947)
Jones (1984a)	Sanides (1962)
Landau (1911, 1923)	Vogt 1943

General architecture
Bok (1929, 1959, 1960)	Reep and Goodwin (1988)
Braitenberg (1974)	J. Rose (1949)
Chow and Leiman (1970)	Sholl (1956, 1960)
Colonnier (1966)	Szentágothai (1969)
Colonnier and Rossignol (1969)	Tömböl (1984)
Ferrer *et al.* (1986a,b)	Tower and Schadé (1960)
Fleischhauer and Detzer (1975)	B. Vogt (1985)
Harman (1947a)	Wong (1967)

Table VI. (*Continued*)

43

DETERMINANTS OF
GYRI AND SULCI

Jones (1984a)
Peters and Jones (1984)

Architectonic areas
  Bailey and Bonin (1951)
  Bailey *et al.* (1950)
  Bok (1959)
  Bonin (1944)
  Braak (1978, 1984)
  Braitenberg (1962, 1978)
  Brazier and Petsche (1978)
  Campbell (1905)
  Eccles (1984)
  Economo (1927, 1930)
  Economo and Koskinas (1925)
  Fleischhauer *et al.* (1980)
  Galaburda and Pandya (1982)
  Gerhardt (1940)
  Hassler and Muhs-Clement (1964)
  Hopf (1954, 1964)
  Jones and Burton (1974, 1976)

Connectivity
  Akert (1964)
  Asanuma and Fernandez (1974)
  Avendaño and Llamas (1984)
  Berson and Graybiel (1983)
  Burton and Jones (1976)
  Constantine-Paton (1983)
  Ebner and Myers (1962, 1965)
  Foster *et al.* (1981)
  Friedman (1983)
  Friedman and Jones (1981)
  Giguere and Goldman-Rakic (1988)
  Goldman and Nauta (1977)
  Goldman-Rakic and Schwartz (1982)
  Graybiel (1972)
  Graybiel and Berson (1981, 1982)
  Haight and Neylon (1978b)
  Harting and Noback (1970)
  Herron (1983)
  Herron and Johnson (1987)
  Innocenti (1986)
  Jones (1976, 1984b,c, 1985, 1986)
  Jones and Powell (1969a,b, 1970)
  Jones and Wise (1977)
  Jones *et al.* (1975, 1977, 1978, 1979)
  Kawamura (1973a–c)
  Kawamura and Naito (1976)
  Kawamura and Otani (1970)
  Killackey (1973)
  Killackey and Ebner (1972, 1973)

General and evolution
  Armstrong (1982a,b)
  Creutzfeldt (1976a,b)
  Hershkovitz (1970)
  R. Martin (1982)
  Martin and Harvey (1985)

Zurabashvili (1964)

Kemper *et al.* (1984)
Kreiner (1960, 1961a,b, 1962, 1964a–c, 1971,
  1973)
Mesulam and Mufson (1985)
Ngowyang (1934)
Pandya and Sanides (1973)
Pandya and Yeterian (1985)
Powell and Mountcastle (1959b)
M. Rose (1928)
Sanides (1962, 1964, 1969b)
Sanides and Krishnamurti (1967)
Sarkissov *et al.* (1955)
Strasburger (1937)
O. Vogt (1910, 1923)
Wree *et al.* (1981, 1983)

Krieg (1952, 1963, 1966)
Künzle (1978)
Kuypers (1981)
Kuypers *et al.* (1984)
Leichnetz (1980)
Lin *et al.* (1982)
Lorente de Nó (1938)
Macchi and Bentivoglio (1986)
Martin (1984)
Miodoński (1974)
Mizuno *et al.* (1975)
Montero (1981, 1982)
Rakic (1975a)
Reinoso-Suárez (1984)
Reinoso-Suárez and Ajmone-Marsan (1984)
Roberts and Akert (1963)
Rose and Woolsey (1949)
Rosenquist (1985)
Sakai (1982)
Scollo-Lavizzari and Akert (1963)
Seltzer and Pandya (1978)
Shanks *et al.* (1975)
Sherk (1986)
Strick and Sterling (1974)
Symonds and Rosenquist (1984a,b)
Warren and Pubols (1984)
Welker and Lende (1980)
Weller and Kaas (1983, 1985)

Rockel *et al.* (1980)
Sanides (1964)
Schmitt *et al.* (1981)
Thompson and Green (1982)

4.1. Architectural Differences between Crowns, Walls, and Fundi

When compared to cortex found in fundi, crown cortex is thicker, and its cell bodies are farther apart vertically and horizontally, being interspersed with a dense neuropil and clusters of myelinated fibers (Figs. 28–30). Crown cortex also has more pronounced cell columns (Figs. 28, 29) and cellular and fibrous laminae (Fig. 30), with most laminae being thicker than those in fundic cortex. Individual cortical layers are more prominent in crown than in fundic cortex (Figs. 28, 29). The outer laminae (I and II) are somewhat thinner and the deeper laminae (V and VI) are generally thicker in crowns than in fundi (Figs. 28, 29). In addition, myelinated fibers are more conspicuous, vertically oriented to the surface, and their terminal arbors are more dense and prominently laminar in crown cortex (Fig. 28), whereas in fundi, such fibers are sparse (with poorly elaborated arbors), tend to enter cortex obliquely to the cortical surface in sulcal

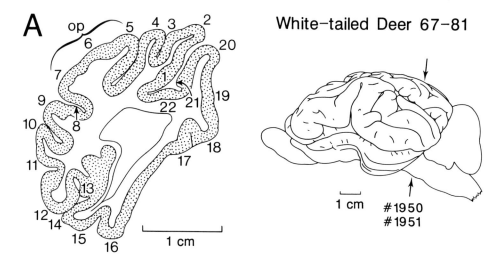

Figure 28. Gyral and sulcal architecture in convoluted cerebral cortex of the white-tailed deer (*Odocoileus virginianus*). (A) Coronal selection through left hemisphere at location indicated by arrows in brain drawing at right. Gyral crowns indicated by numbers and fundi by arrows in photomicrographs (B–I) on the following pages. Photomicrographs of thionin-stained cells are from section #1950, and those of hematoxylin-stained myelinated fibers are from the adjacent section #1951. (A) Gyral crowns or eminences in this and subsequent figures (B–I) are numbered 1–22. Most crowns are at the surface of the brain, but some are buried in sulci.

(B–I) In this and all subsequent photomicrographs it can be seen that cortex in gyral crowns is generally thicker and cell columns and cell layers are more sharply demarcated from one another than they are in sulcal walls and fundi. Fundic cortex (indicated by short arrows), on the other hand, is not only thinner and less clearly laminated, but its cell bodies are more densely packed and not as clearly oriented in cell columns vertical to the cortical surface. Moreover, myelinated fibers are not as vertically oriented or as dense in fundi, nor do they penetrate as far toward the surface as they do in gyral crowns. Although fundic cortex is thinner, its lamina I is thicker (possibly due to a greater number of dendrites arising from the more densely packed neurons in the fundus). Asterisks mark locations where fundic cortex is thicker than cortex in adjacent gyral crowns. This occurs where a sulcus or dimple is ascending to the surface and has been sectioned tangentially. Small regions of operculated cortex occur in several locations (e.g., designated "op" in A). Buried gyri are common (1, 8, 13, 21, 22). Note that, in many cases, fiber stalks (designated by a star) subserving a gyrus, operculum, or effloresced lobule are smaller in cross section than is the white matter contained within the opercula and lobules themselves.

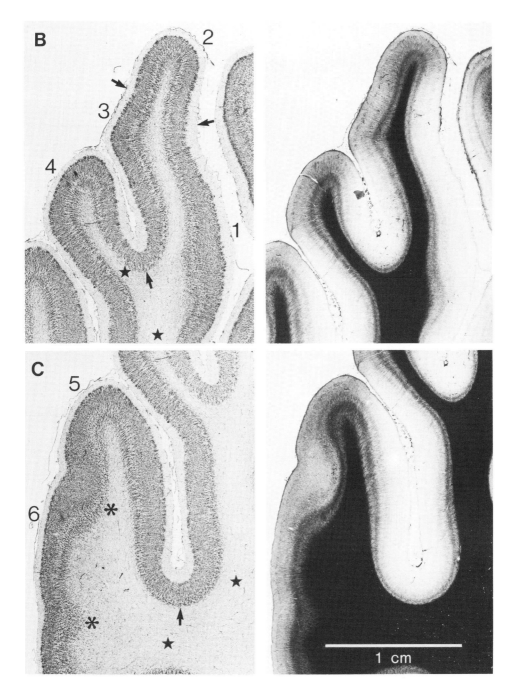

Figure 28. (*Continued*)

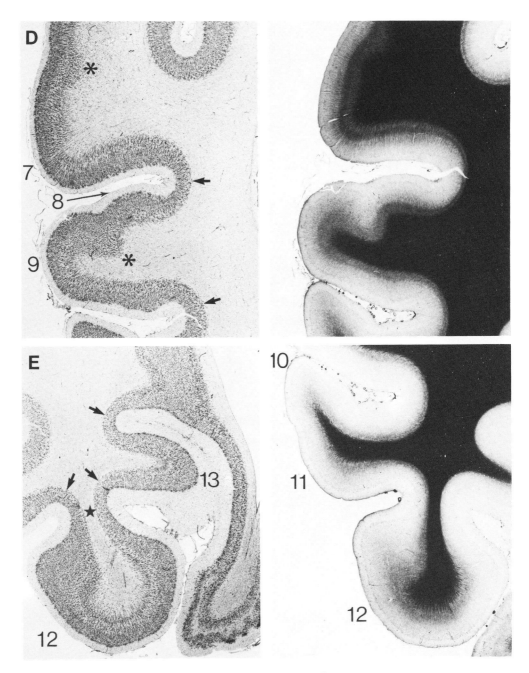

Figure 28. (*Continued*)

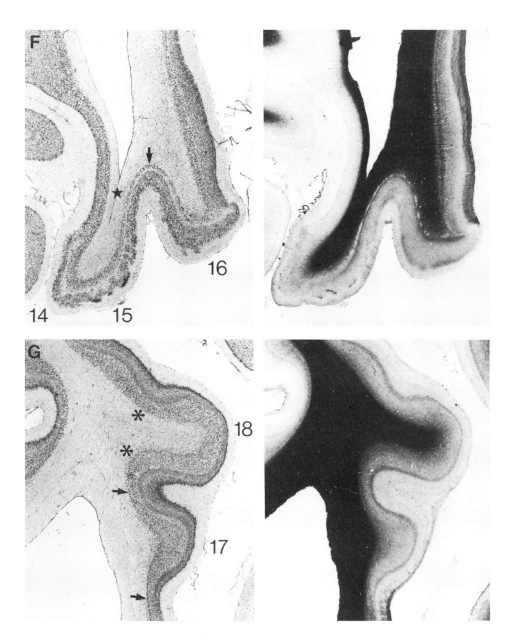

Figure 28. (*Continued*)

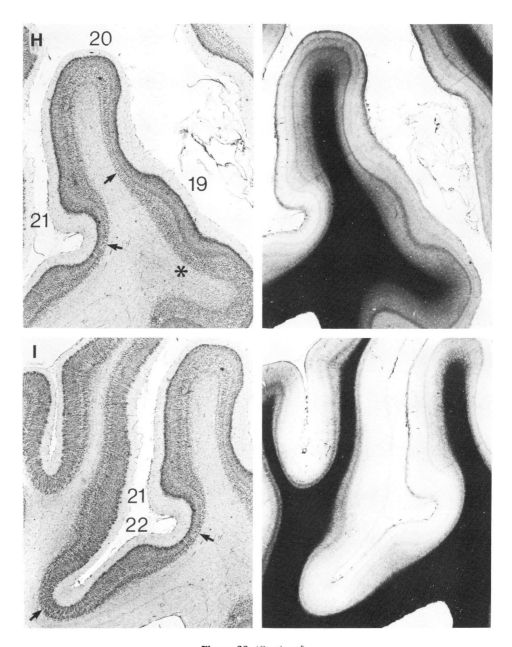

Figure 28. (*Continued*)

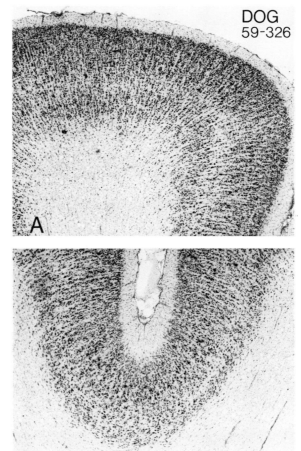

Figure 29. Photomicrographs of gyral crown (A) and fundus and parasulcal cortex (B) in a beagle dog. Note radial orientation of cell columns in gyral crown, progressive bending of radial columns at the angulus and into the walls of the sulcus. In parafundic cortex (B), cell columns appear more bent deeper near the white matter. Cell columns are not distinct in fundic cortex. Thionin stain.

walls, and pass tangentially in fundi (Figs. 31, 32). Moreover, the boundary between deep cellular layers and underlying fibers is more diffuse in crown cortex, whereas in fundi, the boundary between the deepest cell lamina and the underlying white matter is sharply demarcated by the underlying arcuate fibers (Figs. 28–31, 35). In addition, pyramidal cells of crown cortex have longer and more elaborately branched apical and basal dendritic arbors (Fig. 34). In layer VI, cells and their dendrites are more vertically oriented in crown cortex than they are in fundic cortex, where they often lie tangential to the fundic cortex, in parallel with the underlying "U" fibers (Fig 33). Cortex on the walls of sulci (sides of gyri) is intermediate in many of the above-mentioned characters. All these observations support the view that cortical crowns, sulcal walls, and fundi are structurally, connectionally, and, therefore, functionally different from one another. Some of the differences between crowns, walls, and fundi mentioned above also characterize convoluted cerebellar cortex (Fig. 6). I will discuss determinants of foliation of cerebellar cortex elsewhere (Welker, 1990).

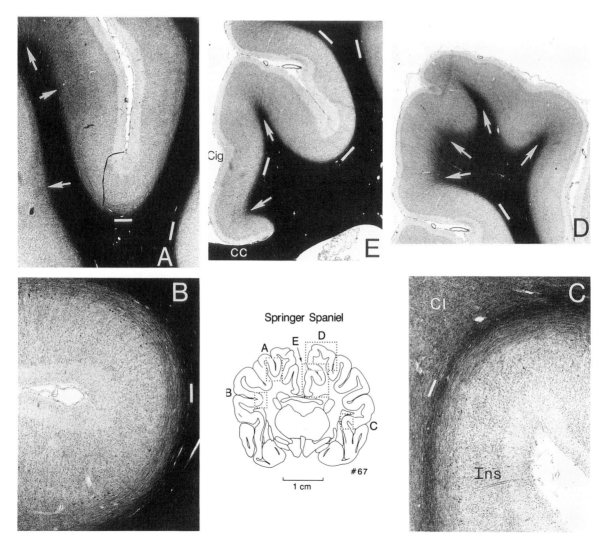

Figure 30. Myeloarchitectural features of gyral crowns, walls, and fundi in cerebral cortex of a springer spaniel (*Canis familiaris*). Location of photomicrographs (A–E) indicated by dashed rectangles on coronal section #67. In A–E, arrows indicate radially oriented fibers innervating gyral crowns or protuberances. White bars beneath fundi indicate locations where fibers course tangentially beneath the cortex and ascend into gyral cortex on both sides of the sulcus. A narrowed fiber stalk of fibers subserving an efflorescence of gyral crowns occurs in several places. CC, corpus callosum; Cig, cingulate gyrus; Cl, claustrum; Ins, insula.

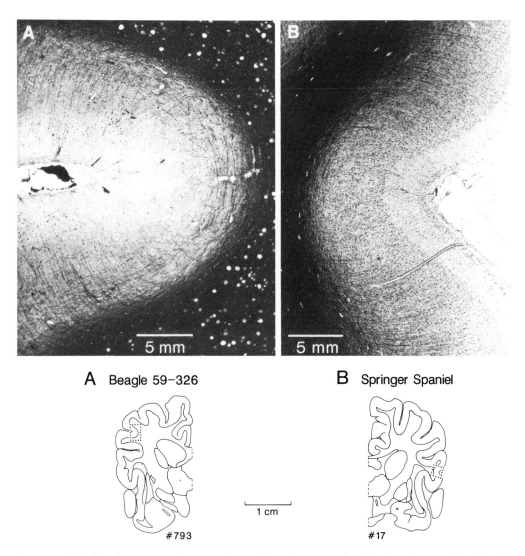

Figure 31. Myeloarchitecture of fundus and parasulcus of a sulcus (A) and a dimple (B) in dogs. Note tangentially coursing fibers in fundus in both cases, and the beginning of radially oriented fibers on either side of the fundus in parasulcal cortex.

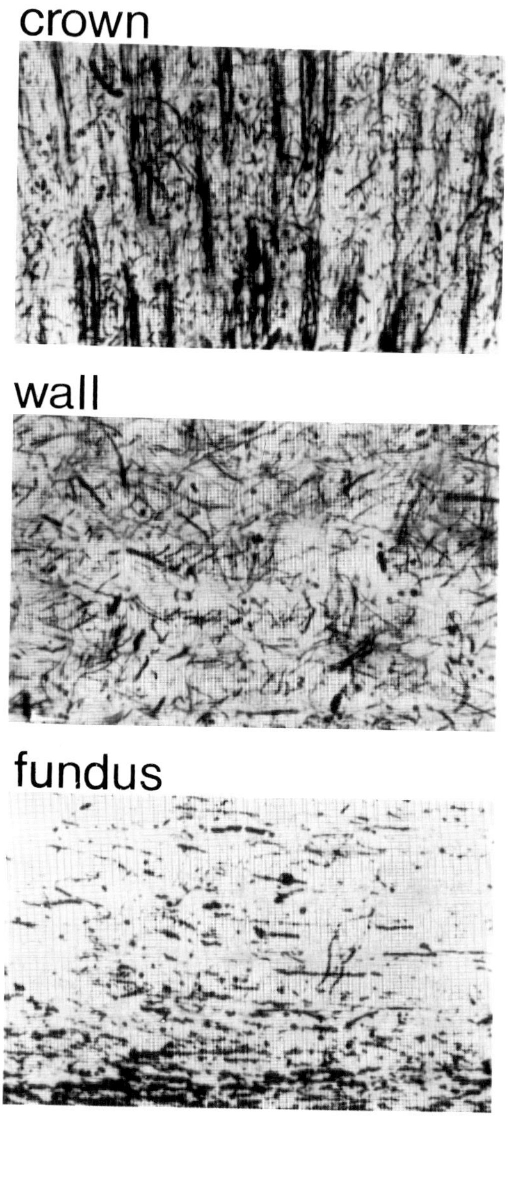

Figure 32. Pattern of myelinated fibers in layer VI and part of layer V of gyral crown (top), sulcal wall (middle), and fundus (bottom) of human cerebral cortex. Cortical surface is at the top of each photomicrograph. Most fiber bundles are oriented vertically in gyral crowns, whereas they are multidirectional and scattered in the sulcal wall, and predominantly horizontal in the fundus. Weigert–Pal–Kultschilzki staining procedure. (Reproduced with permission from Bok, 1959, Fig. 16.)

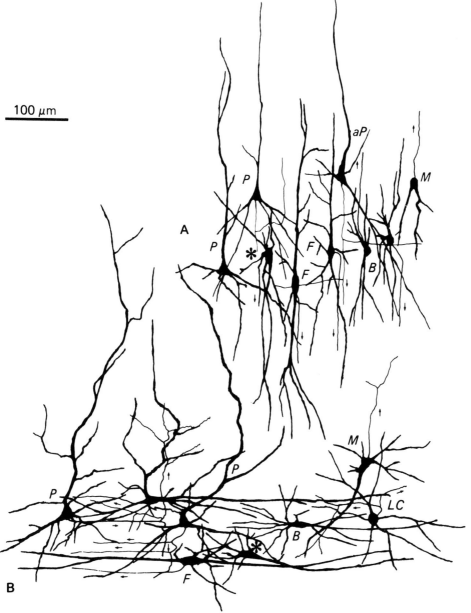

100 μm

Figure 33. Composite drawings of Golgi-stained neurons of the sixth layer in cat's cerebral cortex typically found in gyral crowns (A), and fundic (B) regions. P, pyramidal neuron; aP, atypical pyramidal neuron; M, Martinotti cell; F, fusiform neurons; B, bipolar cells; LC, local circuit neuron. Asterisks indicate an inverted pyramidal cell in the gyral crown and a horizontal pyramidal cell in the sulcal region. Small arrows point to the course of the axons and collaterals. Dendritic fields are arranged vertically in gyral crowns, but are more horizontal in sulcal regions. Fundic dendrites extend much farther tangentially than the width of columnar modules. Axons of horizontal neurons in sulcal regions are more extensive than they are in gyral crowns. (Reproduced with permission from Ferrer *et al.*, 1986b, Fig. 7a.)

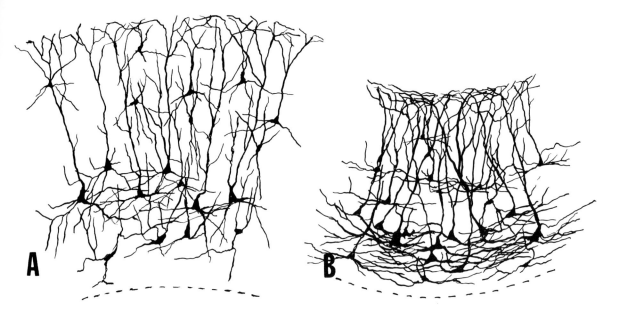

Figure 34. Drawings of Golgi-stained neurons in cerebral cortex of gyral crown of the middle temporal gyrus (A), and the fundus (B) of the superior temporal sulcus in a human brain. Note more extensive horizontal ramifications of basal dendrites in fundus than in crown. (These drawings were produced and generously provided by Arnold Scheibel, unpublished data.)

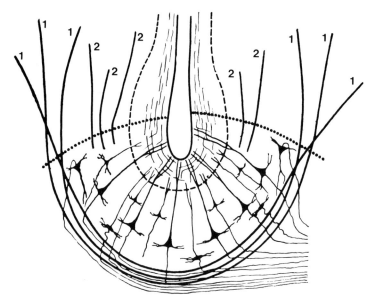

Figure 35. Composite schematic conception of cortex of fundi in prefrontal cortex of the dog, showing location and suspected trajectories of the "U" fibers that are prominent beneath fundic cortex. Radial orientation and layer I penetration of dendrites of pyramidal neurons are depicted, as is the relatively thicker layer I (demarcated by a dashed line), and the tangential axons within layer I. Lines labeled "1" represent U fibers interconnecting gyral crown cortex, and those labeled "2" represent interconnections of parasulcal cortex. (Reproduced with permission from Miodoński, 1974, Fig. 36.)

4.2. Architectonic Areas and Their Relation to Gyral Crowns, Sulcal Walls, and Fundi

The parcellation of neocortex into structurally different cytoarchitectonic or myeloarchitectonic areas has a long history, and has been the subject of numerous reviews (Table VI). Efforts to distinguish different cortical areas continues up to the present day. The difficulties and usefulness of architectural parcellation have been discussed often and at great length elsewhere (Table VI). The criteria used to differentiate one cortical area from another (Fig. 36) are numerous and have varied from one author to another. Variability in cortical architecture in different specimens has undoubtedly been one source of disagreement, as have differences in experience, training, and perceptual–conceptual capability in discerning and characterizing architectural differences. It is sufficient here to mention that it is now generally accepted that, despite their validity, architectonic distinctions alone do not provide an adequate or accurate view of areal differences in cortical organization. My goal here is simply to briefly cite a few of the well-known examples in which correlations have been made between certain architectonic areas and specific gyri and sulci (Fig. 36).

4.2.1. Differences between Two Adjacent Gyri

Different architectonic fields often occupy different, but adjacent, gyri. The borders or transitional zones between them commonly lie either near the angulus, within the wall, or, more commonly, at the fundus of the interposed sulcus or dimple. Such sulci have been called *limiting sulci*. Common examples are the arcuate, central (Fig. 37), and lunate sulci in primates, the ansate, lateral, suprasylvian, postcruciate, and cruciate sulci in carnivores, and the cingulate, rhinal, and Sylvian sulci in most mammals.

4.2.2. Similarities between Two Adjacent Gyri

However, many sulci lie within a single architectonic field, despite the fact that the architecture of such a field is modified within the fundus of the sulcus in ways mentioned in previous paragraphs. Within-field sulci are called *axial sulci*. Examples of such sulci are the superior and inferior precentral sulci and calcarine sulcus in primates (Fig. 38), the triradiate sulcus in raccoons (Fig. 44), and the caudal portions of the coronal sulcus in carnivores (Figs. 48, 54). Despite the fact of architectural similarity between gyral cortex on the two sides of axial sulci, such gyri are now known to receive afferents from different thalamic and cortical sources.

4.2.3. Differences within a Single Gyrus

In some instances a single gyrus contains two or more architectonic fields, either on its crown or along its walls and at the fundus. Examples are found in subareas 3a,b, 1, and 2 of the postcentral gyrus of primates. In this gyrus, these different subareas have different modality, topographic pattern, and subnuclear, as well as cortical, sources of their projections.

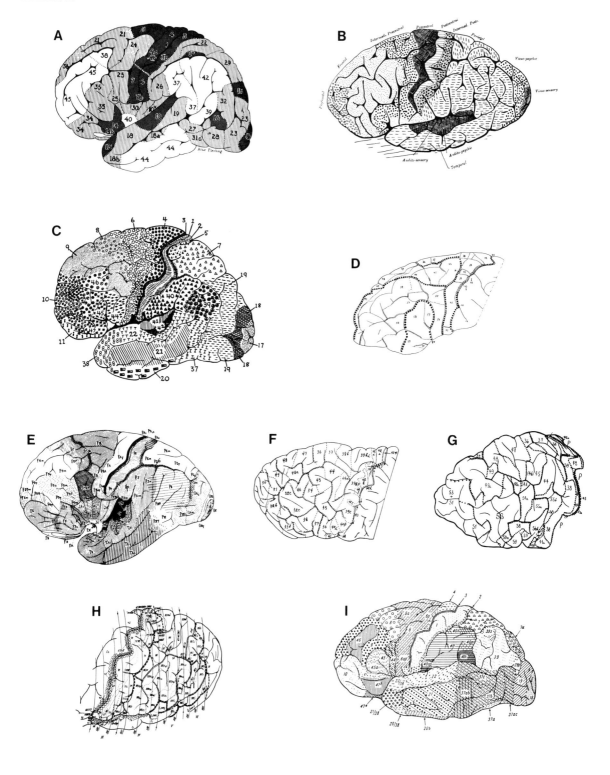

It is now a well-established principle that different cortical architectonic fields receive projections from different neuron types, nuclei, subnuclei, or nuclei complexes of the thalamus (Jones, 1985; Table VI). Another general principle is that a specific cortical field or gyrus that receives projections from specific thalamic sources sends efferents reciprocally to these same thalamic entities (Jones, 1985). Thus, different gyri, as well as architectonic fields differ in both their afferent and efferent thalamic projections. Examples are found in the connections between the postcentral gyrus and ventroposterior thalamic complex (VP), and between the precentral gyrus and the ventrolateral complex in primates; between the coronal gyrus and the arcuate subnucleus of VP in carnivores; and between the mediofrontal gyrus and the ventrolateral (VL) nuclear complex in larger rodents.

Limiting sulci which lie at the borders of cortical areas receive projections from different thalamic nuclei or nuclear complexes. However, there are also cases where adjacent gyri separated by *axial sulci* within a single cortical field are interconnected with different but adjacent thalamic *sub*nuclei. A well-studied example of this is found in the connections of the subnuclei of the raccoon's ventrobasal complex (Vb) with the several cortical subgyri within somatosensory cortex (Welker and Johnson, 1965). Table VI lists a number of examples of such mutual links between adjacent thalamic nuclear entities and adjacent cortical gyri.

In summary, different, large well-organized thalamic nuclei send projections to (and receive reciprocal connections from) different specific cortical gyri or gyral groups.

On the other hand, smaller thalamic nuclear regions tend to have either diffuse cortical projections, or they project predominantly to cortex within the walls or fundi of sulci. Examples of the latter are found in the projections of the thalamic lateral posterior nuclear complex (LP) to the walls and fundus of the coronal, suprasylvian, and lateral sulci in cats (Fig. 39), the projections of VP oralis to area 3a at the fundus of the central sulcus in primates, or the projections of the rostrodorsal rim of cells surrounding the ventrobasal complex (Vb) to the walls and fundus of the sulci that lie between somatosensory and motor cortex in raccoons (Feldman and Johnson, 1988; Johnson *et al.*, 1982; Wiener *et al.*, 1987a,b).

Figure 36. Schematic diagram of cyto- and myeloarchitectonic maps of the lateral aspect of the human brain that have been prepared by nine different neuroanatomists over a period of half a century. Different anatomists use different methods and criteria to demarcate one area from another. Systems of nomenclature also varied considerably. Most authors agree as to the location and boundaries of certain areas such as the primary motor, somatosensory, visual, and auditory fields. Many of the different architectonic fields were found to be associated with specific but different gyri or lobules, and many sulci reliably demarcated one such field from another. However, other sulci showed little or no apparent association with specific architectonic fields. (A) Myeloarchitectonic map of Flechsig (1898); (B) cytoarchitectonic map of A. Campbell (1905); (C) cytoarchitectonic map of Brodmann (1909); (D) partial myeloarchitectonic map of O. Vogt (1910); (E) cytoarchitectonic map of Economo and Koskinas (1925); (F) cytoarchitectonic map of Ngowyang (1934); (G) myeloarchitectonic map of Strasburger (1937); (H) cytoarchitectonic map of Sarkissov *et al.* (1955); (I) cytoarchitectonic map of Gerhardt (1940). A–H are left lateral or left dorsolateral views, but I is a right dorsolateral view.

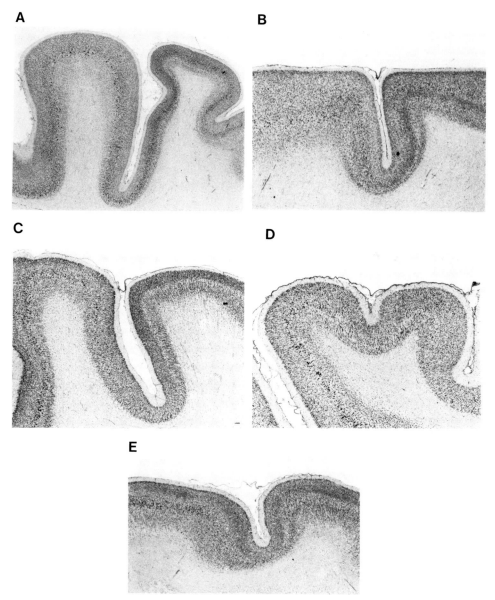

A

B

C

D

E

Figure 37. Examples of the limiting sulcus that lies between two different cytoarchitectonic areas: agranular motor (MI) cortex and granular somatosensory (SI) cortex, in chimpanzee (A, #63-387, section #1075), squirrel monkey (B, #55-11, section #146), raccoon (C, #57-115, section #258), domestic cat (D, #59-37, section #170), and capybara (E, #61-248, section #612). Motor cortex is to the left in all cases. The sulcus that divides MI and SI is called the *central sulcus* in primates, the *postcruciate sulcus* in carnivores, and the *frontolateral sulcus* in rodents.

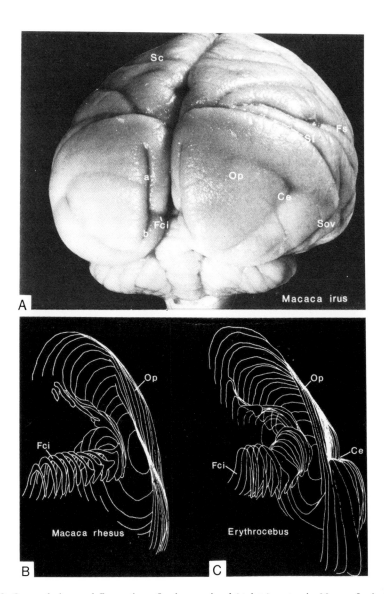

Figure 38. Operculation and fissuration of primary visual (striate) cortex in *Macaca fascicularis*. (A) Posterior view showing operculum (Op), external or lateral calcarine sulcus (Ce), internal calcarine fissure (Fci) with its ascending (a) and descending (b) rami, and the lunate sulcus (Sl). Central sulcus (Sc), Sylvian fissure (Fs), and ventral occipital sulcus (Sov) are also identified. (B, C) Computer perspective reconstructions of the primary visual cortex in rhesus monkey (*Macaca mulatta*) and *Erythrocebus* (patas guenon) drawn as if viewed from inside the brain near the temporal pole. Reconstructions made from outlines of layer IV in thionin-stained serial sections. Striate cortex extends over the entire operculated occipital pole (on both walls of the external calcarine sulcus in C), and rostrally to the lunate sulcus (beyond which are the parietal and temporal lobes), as well as laterally to the sulcus occipitalis ventralis (Sov). On the medial surface, the striate cortex curves into the depths of the internal calcarine sulcus. (Reproduced with permission from Valverde, 1985, Fig. 2.)

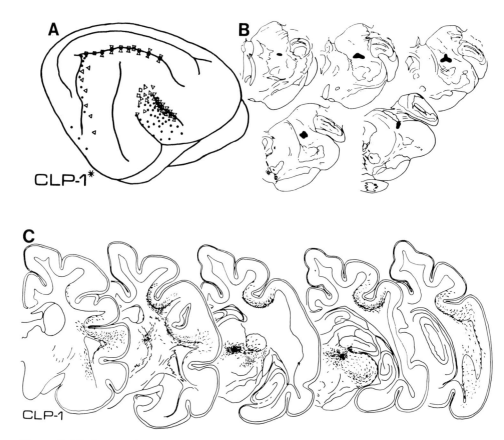

Figure 39. Thalamocortical anterograde degeneration (silver methods) following a lesion centered in the ventral and medial region of the lateroposterior nucleus (LP) in the cat (#CLP-1). This lesion produced fiber degeneration along the banks and fundus of the anterior ectosylvian sulcus and along the middle, and to a lesser extent, the posterior cortex of the suprasylvian sulcus (A and C). The thalamic lesion is shown in solid black in selected transverse sections (B and C), degenerating axons by dotted lines, and preterminal degeneration by smaller, irregularly spaced dots (C). In reconstructions of the right hemisphere (A), the resultant degeneration in gyral crowns is represented by solid black circles, and degeneration buried in sulcal cortex is represented by outline symbols: squares in the case of sulcal fundi, and triangles in the case of sulcal walls. Differential density of degeneration indicated by spacing of the symbols. (Reproduced with permission from Graybiel, 1972, Figs. 2C and 3A,B.)

4.4. Intergyral Connections

Within each cerebral hemisphere there are many well-known interlobar, intergyral, and interareal connections. In human neuroanatomy, the superior and inferior longitudinal fasciculi, the uncinate fasciculus, and the cingulum are the large fiber bundles which interconnect major lobes of the cerebral hemisphere and are easily seen macroscopically (Clemente, 1985). Histological sections that cut across a sulcus and are stained for myelin sheaths reveal arcuate fibers which pass beneath fundic cortex and course vertically into the cortical gyri on either side of the sulcus (Figs. 30, 35). Such intergyral "U" fiber connections are demonstrated by techniques designed to reveal retrograde and anterograde degeneration (Krieg, 1952, 1963, 1966), as well as by axonal transport studies. They show that adjacent gyral crowns are richly interconnected, whereas

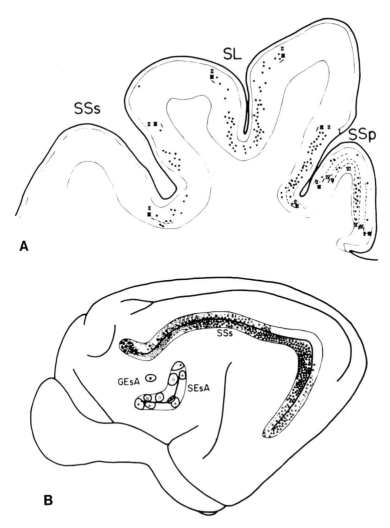

Figure 40. Distributed, but focalized, interareal projections in cat cerebral cortex. (A) After HRP injections in the ventral posterior suprasylvian area (area 20; see Fig. 41B), neurons were labeled retrogradely in visual and cingulate cortex. Labeling was heavy in the fundus and medial wall of the suprasylvian sulcus (SSs), in the fundus and both walls of the lateral sulcus (SL), and in both walls and fundus of the splenial sulcus (SSp), as well as the posterior cingulate gyrus. The largest number of neurons was found in superficial cortical layers, except for the cingulate gyrus, in which labeling was primarily in the deeper layers. (B) Systematic topographic distribution of projections (indicated by open or closed triangles or circles) to buried cortex of the different portions of the suprasylvian sulcus (SSs) from different loci in the buried cortex of both walls and fundus of the anterior ectosylvian sulcus (SEsA), as well as the anterior ectosylvian gyrus (GEsA). Composite results from several HRP injection experiments. (Reproduced with permission from Reinoso-Suárez, 1984, Figs. 7 and 8.)

fundic cortex is sparsely interconnected. There are other examples where walls of one sulcus send projections to the fundus and walls of another sulcus (Fig. 40). Moreover, the gyral crowns of some cortical areas send projections to the walls or fundi of adjacent, as well as distant, sulci (Fig. 41). No study has been undertaken to define the specific spatial and laminar pattern of cortical projections between gyral crowns, sulcal walls, and fundi of either adjacent or distant gyri.

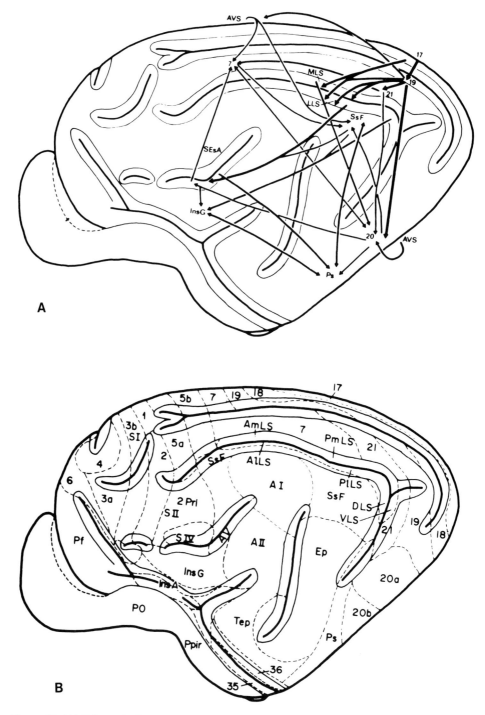

Figure 41. (A). Schematic diagram showing several transcortical routes through which visual inputs may reach other cortical areas that are more or less intimately related to the visual system in the cat. (B) Areal distribution of anatomically and physiologically defined cortical areas in the cat. (Reproduced with permission from Reinoso-Suárez, 1984, Figs. 9 and 1.)

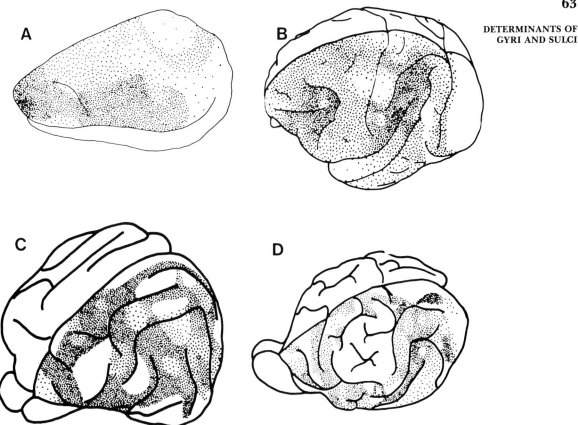

Figure 42. Comparison of total pattern of commissural termination in opossum (A), and monkey (B), cat (C), and raccoon (D). Relative density of dots indicates the approximate density of degenerating commissural fibers in each cortical region. Results obtained by section of corpus callosum and plotting subsequent degeneration of axon terminals (Nauta silver-stained preparations). In opossum (A), there are no neocortical areas absolutely free of commissural terminals, while in more specialized mammals, parts of visual and somatic sensory cortex remain free of interhemispheric connections. Some of these unconnected areas are confined to specific gyri or lobules that are delimited by sulci. In all these animals there are small focalized patches of denser as well as sparser connectivity, many of which occur in buried cortex, and which exhibit complex patterns of distribution suggesting even greater heterogeneity of gyral, sulcal, and fundic callosal connectivity. (Reproduced with permission from Ebner, 1969, Fig. 4.)

4.5. Interhemispheric Connections

Experimental studies of anterograde and retrograde degeneration or transport reveal that most topographically homologous gyri of the two hemispheres have reciprocal connections that are symmetric (Innocenti, 1986). Many gyral crowns project to gyral crowns, and sulcal walls to sulcal walls (Goldman and Nauta, 1977; Goldman-Rakic and Schwartz, 1982). On the other hand, some cortical gyri send projections primarily to the walls and fundi of certain sulci in the opposite hemisphere (Table VI). In several mammals, gyri that contain specialized sensory or motor representations are *devoid* of reciprocal interhemispheric connections. This is strikingly seen, for example, in somatosensory hand cortex, in visual foveal cortex, and in primary auditory cortex in some mammals (Fig. 42). Major studies of interhemispheric connections that are relevant to gyri and sulci are listed in Table VI.

4.6. Other Efferent Connections

There are many examples in which cortical efferents from specific gyral regions send descending projections not only to specific thalamic nuclei, but also to specific basal ganglia, or brain-stem, cerebellar, medullary, and spinal cord nuclei (Fig. 43).

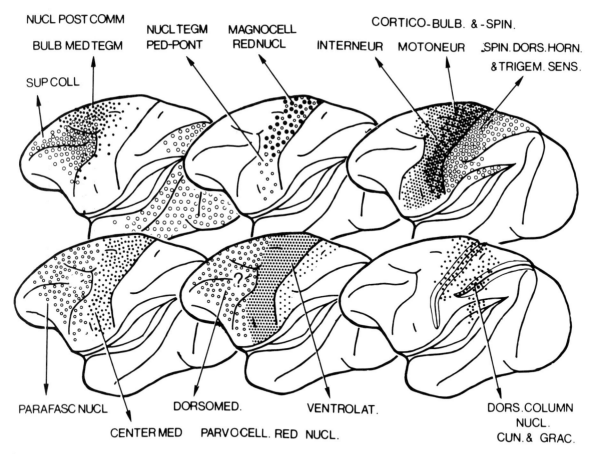

Figure 43. Composite schematic portrayal of origin of cortical projections to different cell groups in the thalamus, brain stem, and spinal cord in the monkey. Note that many of these projections are confined to specific gyri or lobules, as well as being bounded by specific sulci. Such source-specificity is revealed despite the fact that HRP injections were not selectively confined to specific nuclear entities. (Reproduced with permission from Kuypers, 1981, Fig. 16.)

4.7. Intragyral Connections

There are, of course, numerous local circuit connections between different parts of a single cytoarchitectonic field located on a gyrus, as well as between different adjacent subfields on the same gyrus. Most of the studies of such connections have focused on deciphering details of interlaminar, intracolumnar, interpatch, and interstripe connections. Although such information clarifies the spatial character of information flow within different functional areas, much of this work has not been concerned with the larger gyral crown, sulcal wall, and fundic morphologic entities with which this chapter is concerned.

Table VII. Literature on Neurophysiological Features of Cerebral Cortex

Reviews	
Schaltenbrand and Woolsey (1964)	Zulch et al. (1975)
Woolsey (1960b, 1964))	
Somatosensory	
Barker and Welker (1969)	Meulders et al. (1966)
Bohringer and Rowe (1977)	Nelson et al. (1979)
Burton (1968)	Paul et al. (1972)
Campos and Welker (1976)	Pimentel-Souza et al. (1980)
Carlson and Welker (1976)	Pinto Hamuy et al. (1956)
Carlson and Welt (1981)	Powell and Mountcastle (1959a)
Feldman and Johnson (1988)	Pubols et al. (1976)
Friedman et al. (1980)	Rubel (1971)
Herron (1978)	Welker and Campos (1963)
Johnson (1985)	Welker and Carlson (1976)
Johnson et al. (1973, 1974, 1982)	Welker and Seidenstein (1959)
Krishnamurti et al. (1976)	Welker et al. (1964, 1976)
Magalhães-Castro and Saraiva (1971)	Woolsey (1981a, 1984)
Merzenich (1982)	Woolsey and Fairman (1946)
Auditory	
Alderson et al. (1960)	Fitzpatrick and Imig (1982)
Brugge and Reale (1985)	Imig et al. (1982)
Downman et al. (1960)	Woolsey (1960a, 1981c)
Visual	
Allman and Kaas (1971)	Tusa et al. (1982)
Cowey (1981)	Valverde (1985)
Crawford (1985)	Van Essen (1985)
Diamond et al. (1985)	Van Essen and Maunsell (1980)
Gross et al. (1984)	Van Essen et al. (1981)
Olson and Graybiel (1987)	Woolsey (1981b)
Motor	
Bagley (1922)	Vicario et al. (1983)
Hardin et al. (1968)	Wiesendanger (1981)
Jameson et al. (1968)	Wise (1985)
Saraiva and Magalhães-Castro (1975)	Woolsey (1963)
Sessle and Wiesendanger (1982)	

5. Electrophysiological Correlates of Gyri and Sulci

There is an enormous literature to choose from if one were to thoroughly review those electrophysiological studies that have attempted to localize sensory or motor areas of cerebral neocortex (Table VII). The earliest careful experimental studies were those of Sherrington and his colleagues (Clarke and O'Malley, 1968), but it was Clinton Woolsey's pioneering studies which ushered in the

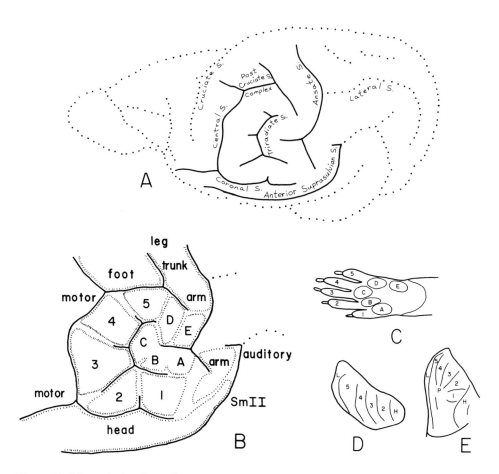

Figure 44. Schematic drawings of raccoon cerebral cortex (A) showing that cortical sulci delimit somatosensory representations of different body structures (B), particularly from the contralateral forepaw (C). The subgyri within the large hand lobule in panel B reveal topographic similarity of the central representations of the glabrous forepaw with the actual peripheral relationshps shown in panel C. Cortical projections from each digit project to separate gyri demarcated by sulci. Each of these projection-specific gyri receives afferents from a specific subnucleus within the ipsilateral ventrobasal complex shown in coronal (D) and horizontal (E) sections. Each of these thalamic subnuclei receives projections from an individual digit. And each thalamic subnucleus projects to the cortical subgyrus having the same peripheral digital projections. Major delimiting sulci within and surrounding somatosensory cortex are identified in A. Abbreviations in B–E: 1–5, forepaw digits 1–5; A–E, palm pads A–E. (Reproduced with permission from Welker and Seidenstein, 1959, Fig. 9; Welker and Johnson, 1965, Fig. 10; and Welker *et al.*, 1964, Fig. 15.)

modern era of electrophysiological mapping of sensory and motor areas (Welker, 1976). The early macroelectrode surface recording and stimulating studies rapidly led to improvements and refinements in techniques and experimental design that are required to define differences in function and connectivity between gyral crowns, sulcal walls, and fundi. Now, nearly all studies aimed at localizing functional areas within cerebral neocortex utilize systematic in-depth microelectrode mapping methods, as well as focalized, threshold natural peripheral stimulation of sensory receptors, and threshold electrical activation of cortex or subcortical structures.

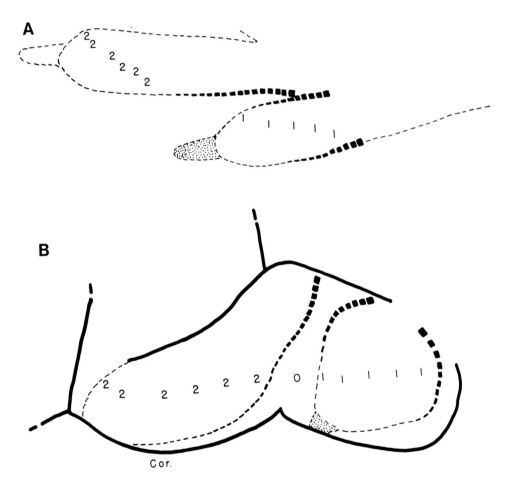

Figure 45. Diagram of lower portion of a raccoon's cortical hand gyrus (B) of the left hemisphere showing the relationships between various portions of digits 1 and 2 (A) and their corresponding cortical representations. The representation of the more highly innervated glabrous ventral distal portions of each digit is located on the crown of a different subgyrus which, in turn, may be bounded by sulci or sulcal spurs. The line of numbers in B indicates a single line of cortical recording points. The sequence of peripheral representations along this row of recording points is the same as indicated by numbers on the drawing of the digits themselves (A). The "O" between the two representations denotes a cortical zone unresponsive to stimulation of ventral glabrous skin. Cor., coronal sulcus. (Reproduced with permission from Welker and Seidenstein, 1959, Fig. 6.)

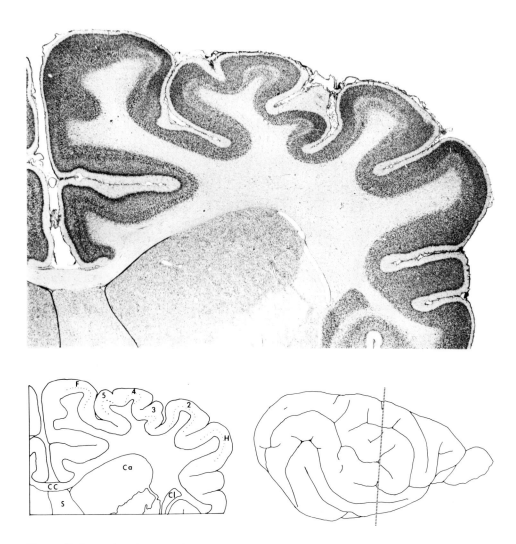

Figure 46. Coronal section (top) through somatosensory cortex of raccoon (#58-133, section #622). Drawing of this same section at lower left indicates how cortical representations of different body parts are distributed within the different cortical gyri indicated at lower left (H, head; 2–5, forepaw digits 2–5; F, foot; dotted line, accentuated layer IV in gyral crowns). Plane of section indicated on brain diagram at lower right. (Reproduced with permission from Welker *et al.,* 1964, Fig. 19.)

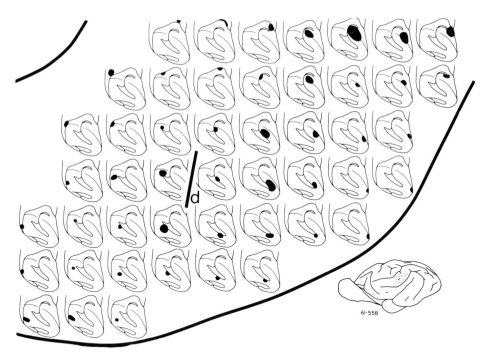

Figure 47. Map of the relatively large somatosensory representation of the contralateral rhinarium on the crown of the coronal gyrus in the coatimundi (*Nasua narica*). A small dimple (solid line: d) commonly appears within the coati's rhinarial representation at a location (indicated in brain diagram at lower right) that is surrounded by a slightly elevated gyral formation which contains peripheral projections from the ring of highly innervated rhinarium that surrounds the nostril. (Reproduced with permission from Welker and Campos, 1963, Fig. 7.)

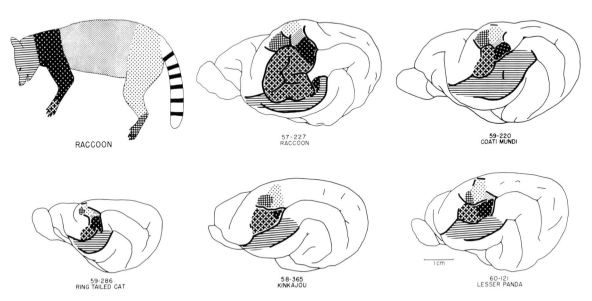

Figure 48. Different body parts send somatosensory projections to different gyri that are separated by sulci. Drawings of left dorsolateral views of brains of five procyonids. Different geometric patterns on cortex are keyed to the body parts on the diagram of the raccoon at upper left. Note that, although the different animals exhibit different gyral and sulcal patterns, in all cases the major representations occupy gyri that are separated from different representations by sulci, spurs, or dimples, wherever they occur. (Reproduced with permission from Welker and Campos, 1963, Figs. 2–5.)

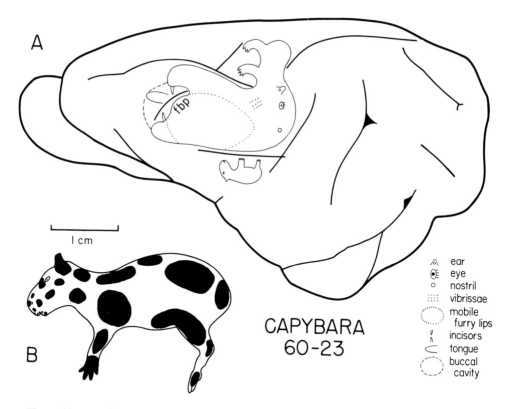

Figure 49. (A) Schematic brain diagrams of the capybara showing the occurrence of several sulci which delimit different cortical gyri containing somatosensory representations from different body parts. Note sulcus occurs between representations of upper and lower lip in SI and between SI and SII. Key to symbols of body parts in the somatosensory cortex at lower right. (B) Drawing of lateral view of capybara (black patches indicate relative sizes of multiple unit receptive fields on different parts of the body). (Reproduced with permission from Campos and Welker, 1976, Fig. 4.)

The most striking early evidence for a precise correlation of functional areas with gyral and sulcal features came from mapping studies of somatosensory cerebral cortex in raccoons (Welker and Seidenstein, 1959; Fig. 44). The heightened repertoire of forepaw behavior of this mammal indicated an unusual responsiveness and tactile perception involving the glabrous forepaws. The initial study revealed that this animal had an enormously enlarged cortical forepaw projection lobule, within which each small subgyrus received information from a different single glabrous digit of the contralateral hand (Figs. 44, 46). Moreover, receptive fields (RFs) at the center of each glabrous digit were represented near the center of a gyral crown (Fig. 45), and the RFs of crown cortex were tiny, having low mechanical thresholds. As the mapping electrode moved into the walls of the adjacent sulci, the activating RFs moved to the lateral digital surfaces. Then, in the fundus, the activating RFs moved to the hairy dorsal surfaces of the digits. In addition, the evoked multiple unit responses were more robust on the gyral crowns in ways which indicated a larger or more densely activated neuronal population there, whereas the neuroelectric activity evoked within gyral walls and fundi became progressively weaker as the peripheral RF moved to the sides and dorsum of the digit. Pertinent is the fact that the ventral glabrous hand surfaces are more densely innervated than are the sides and dorsum (see Welker *et al.*, 1964, for references). In addition, other sulci in and around the somatosensory area are situated either between projections from different body parts, between the first and second somatosensory areas, or between somatosensory (SI) and motor (MI) areas (Fig. 48). Additional studies of the raccoon found that not only the ventrobasal thalamus, but also the dorsal column nuclei, were subdivided into as many subnuclei as there were gyral crowns in somatosensory cortex (Fig. 44; Johnson *et al.*, 1968; Welker and Johnson, 1965). Moreover, each different thalamic subnucleus was linked with a different cortical gyrus. Johnson and his colleagues later found that somatosensory projections to the walls and fundi of sulci between somatosensory and motor cortex had broad multidigit

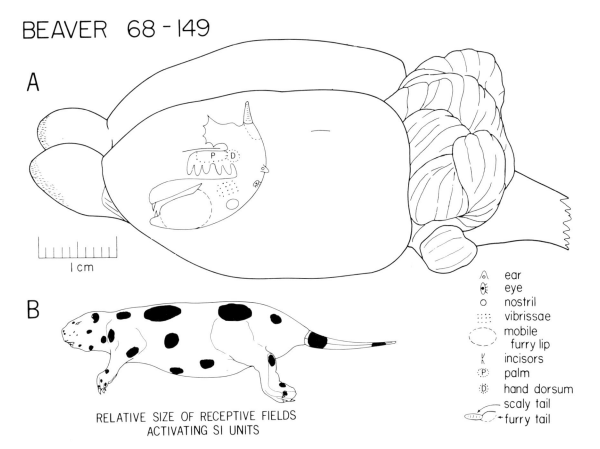

Figure 50. (A) Schematic brain diagram of the North American beaver (*Castor canadensis*) showing the occurrence of a small sulcus between the forelimb and hindlimb representations. The meaning of the symbols at lower right are similar to those in Fig. 49. (B) Relative size of receptive fields depicted by black patches on drawing of the beaver's body. Note sulcus between hindlimb and forelimb representations. (Reproduced with permission from Carlson and Welker, 1976, Fig. 9.)

RFs, or RFs from higher threshold noncutaneous sources (Feldman and Johnson, 1988; Johnson, 1985; Johnson *et al.*, 1982). Such RFs are in contrast to the relatively small, single digit RFs that project to the angulis and summits of adjacent hand subgyri. Moreover, Warren and Pubols (1984) found that ventrobasal thalamic sources of projections to a fundus were more diffuse, whereas those to a gyral crown originated from only a specific thalamic subnucleus.

Studies of somatosensory cortex in other mammals also revealed that different gyri received projections from different body parts, and that both walls and fundi of an axial sulcus contained representations of RFs on tissues between the

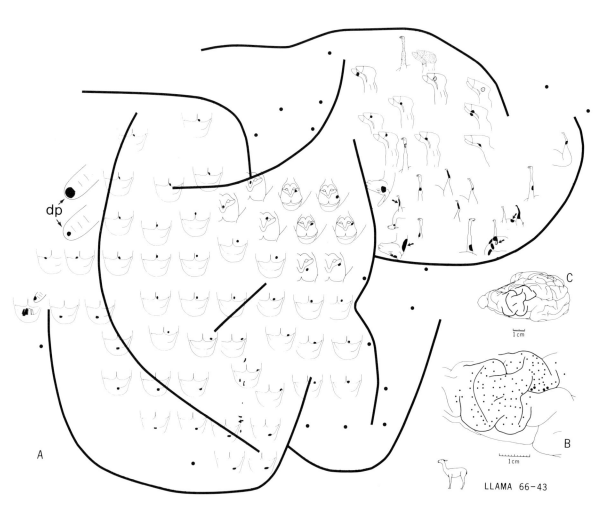

Figure 51. Map of the relatively large somatosensory representation of the contralateral lips on a convoluted lobule of the cortex of the llama (*Lama glama*). A large curved sulcus separates the large upper lip gyral region from the rostrally situated lower lip, maxillary dental pad (dp), and all the ipsilateral representations. Another sulcus demarcates the caudal boundary of the face representation. The representation of the SII region is bounded rostrally, medially, laterally, and to some extent caudally by sulci. Because of the large size of this somatic sensory region and constraints on animal availability and duration of each experiment, the finer details of these representations were not explored in these experiments. (Reproduced with permission from Welker *et al.*, 1976, Fig. 2.)

body parts (Fig. 48). Fundi were often so weakly activated by peripheral stimulation that activating RFs were not found in the fundus. Moreover, only the inside walls of limiting sulci at the boundary of somatosensory cortex were activated by low-threshold mechanoreceptors. These electrophysiological projectional differences between gyri, sulcal walls, and fundi were found in and around somatosensory cortex of different mammals having gyri and sulci of varied sizes, shapes, orientations, and patterns (Figs. 47–53; Campos and Welker, 1975; Carlson and Welker, 1976; Krishnamurti *et al.*, 1976; Pimentel-Souza *et al.*, 1980; Ray and Craner, 1988; Welker and Campos, 1963; Welker and Carlson, 1976).

In mammals, motor and somatosensory cortical regions always lie adjacent to one another, and are often separated from one another by one or more limiting sulci (Figs. 37, 54; Table VII). Axial sulci also occur within motor cortex, and separate projections from hand and head, forelimb and hindlimb, or from hindlimb and tail. In raccoons, it appears that the cruciate sulcus (which is a

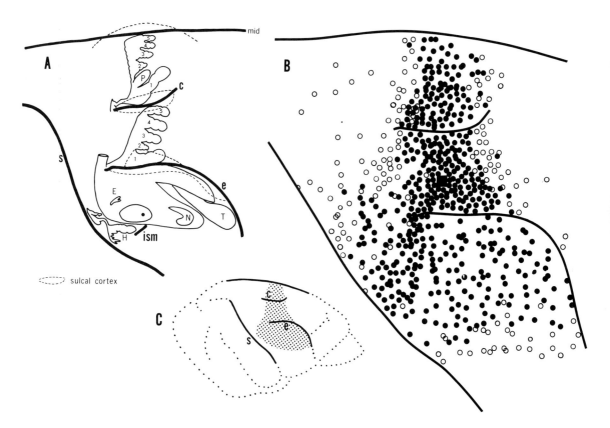

Figure 52. Schematic brain diagram (C) of cortical somatosensory representation of slow loris (*Nycticebus coucang*), an enlarged portion of which (A) shows a sulcus (c) between the foot and hand representations, and a curved sulcus (e) whose caudomedial portion lies between the hand and caudal head representation, and whose rostrolateral portion lies between somatosensory and motor cortex. A small dimple (ism) often was situated at the rostral juncture of SII and SI. (B) Scatter plot of all active (dots) and unresponsive (circles) puncture locations recorded from in 17 animals. (Reproduced with permission from Krishnamurti *et al.*, 1976, Fig. 4.)

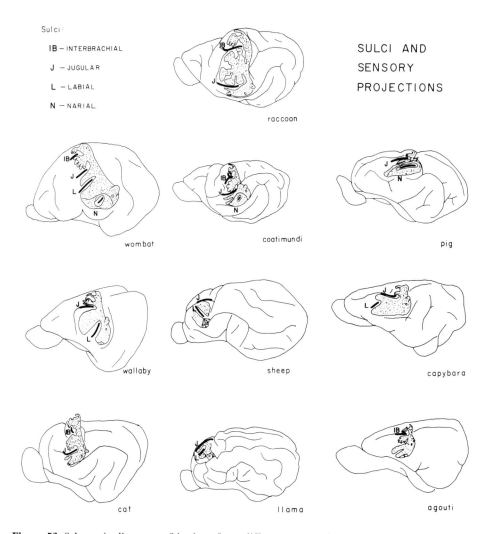

Figure 53. Schematic diagrams of brains of ten different mammals showing Johnson's suggested nomenclatural scheme in which limiting sulci in somatosensory cortex are named on the basis of the body parts whose representations they separated. In this scheme, the interbrachial sulcus (IB) is situated between the fore- and hindlimbs, the jugular (J) at the neck between the arm and head, the labial (L) between the upper and lower lips, and the narial (N) within the rhinarial representation. (Reproduced with permission from Johnson, 1980, Fig. 7.) Sources of data: wombats (Johnson *et al.,* 1973), wallaby (Lende, 1963a), cat (Rubel, 1971), raccoon (Welker and Seidenstein, 1959), coatimundi (Welker and Campos, 1963), sheep (Johnson *et al.,* 1974), llama (Welker *et al.,* 1976), pig (Woolsey and Fairman, 1946), capybara (Campos and Welker, 1976), and agouti (Pimentel-Souza *et al.,* 1980).

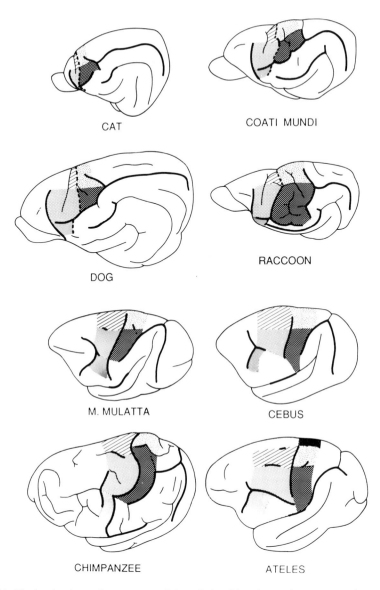

Figure 54. Woolsey's schematic summary of the relationship of somatic sensory and motor cortical areas to cortical fissures. Depicted are brains of four carnivores (above) and four primates (below) showing musculo- and somatotopically similar subdivisions (leg, arm, face) of motor ("precentral") and somatosensory ("postcentral") areas. In the carnivores, motor cortex is to the left of the dotted line. In the primates, motor cortex is to the left of the central sulcus. Heavy lines in carnivores and in primates indicate topographically similar sulci. Hindlimb, forelimb, and head representations are indicated by different shaded symbols for both somatosensory and motor cortex. Many sulci, indicated by heavy lines, lie between sensory and motor cortex. Different representations within each region are also occasionally separated by sulci. Most of the studies from which these data were abstracted utilized macroelectrode surface electrical stimulating and evoked potential recording techniques. (Reproduced with permission from Woolsey, 1960b, Figs. 2 and 4.)

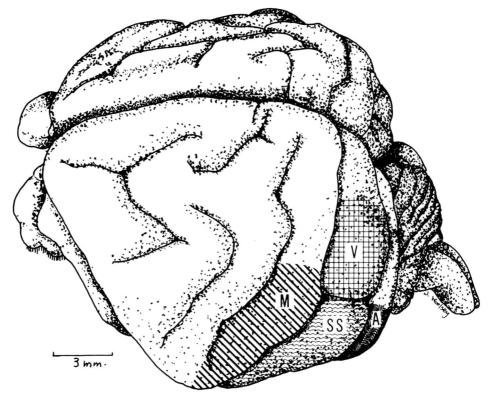

Figure 55. Diagram of brain of the echidna (*Tachyglossus aculeatus*) showing that sulci delimit motor (M), somatosensory (SS), visual (V), and auditory (A) areas. (Reproduced with permission from Lende, 1969, Fig. 9.)

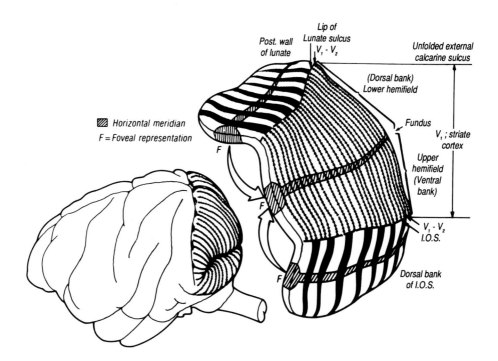

major cortical feature of all carnivores) lies between the medial part of the primary motor cortex on the posterior sigmoid gyrus (Hardin *et al.*, 1968) and the supplementary motor area which lies on that broad gyrus which lies beneath the posterior sigmoid gyrus and protrudes onto the medial wall of the hemisphere (Jameson *et al.*, 1968). The gyral bulge at the lateral edge of the cruciate sulcus contains the motor representation of the head musculature.

The boundary relation of sulci to different specific somatosensory cortical areas is seen in most mammals. It is evident in several marsupials studied (Fig. 53; Haight and Murray, 1981; Haight and Neylon, 1978a,b; Johnson, 1977, 1980; Johnson *et al.*, 1973; Pubols *et al.*, 1976), including the North American opossum, where the small orbital sulcus lies rostral to the sensorimotor amalgam area (Ebner, 1967; Lende, 1963a,b). Cortex rostral to this sulcus receives a distinct set of projections from the mediodorsal thalamic nucleus. Other thalamic nuclei send projections to the cortex caudal to this sulcus (Killackey and Ebner, 1972, 1973). The echidna, a monotreme with a relatively large highly convoluted brain, has portions of separate gyri devoted to motor, somatosensory, auditory, and visual areas, and sulci reliably lie between these functionally different gyri (Lende, 1969; Welker and Lende, 1980; Fig. 55).

Studies of visual cortex in primates reveal several aspects of gyral-specific projections. In V1, the upper and lower hemifields send projections to the lower and upper gyral folds which create the calcarine sulcus (Polyak, 1957; Crawford, 1985; Fig. 56). RFs from the far periphery project to the gyral crowns, and the horizontal meridian is represented along the fundus of the external calcarine. V1 also extends dorsally to the angulus of the lunate sulcus, and caudally to the angulus of the inferior occipital sulcus (Fig. 56; Crawford, 1985). In V2, the hemiretina projects along the caudal wall of the lunate sulcus as well as onto the upper wall of the inferior occipital sulcus (Crawford, 1985).

The complex convolutional pattern of visual cortex, especially in primates, has been studied extensively and a large number of visually related areas have been identified by diverse methods and criteria. In the few cases mentioned above, there are several well-established correlations between gyral crowns, walls, and fundi. Van Essen's (1985) review reveals the great complexity in the varieties of interconnected areas. For the cat, Rosenquist (1985) has also summarized available evidence, and his summary, partially portrayed in Fig. 57, reveals several correlations of features of different visual areas and specific gyral crowns, walls, and fundi.

The relatively large convoluted auditory region found in many carnivores

---

Figure 56. Summary diagram of distribution and orientation of visually activated [^{14}C]-2-deoxyglucose patterns in both striate (area V1) and prestriate (V2) in relation to the calcarine, lunate, and inferior occipital sulci. Monocular chromatic visual stimulation produced narrow columns of increased radioactivity in the contralateral striate cortex extending from the lip of the lunate sulcus into the external calcarine and ventrolaterally to the lip of the inferior occipital sulcus. The horizontal meridian is located along the fundus of the external calcarine sulcus and the fovea is represented at the lateral fundic margin of this sulcus. In striate cortex, separate fiber bundles from the lateral geniculate nucleus distribute projections from the lower hemifield (upper retina) to the upper bank of the calcarine sulcus, and from the upper hemifield (lower retina) to the lower bank of the calcarine sulcus. In prestriate cortex, monocular visual stimulation produces broader patterns of increased radioactivity on the posterior bank of the lunate sulcus, as well as on the upper bank and into the fundus of the inferior occipital sulcus. (Reproduced with permission from Crawford, 1985, Fig. 4.)

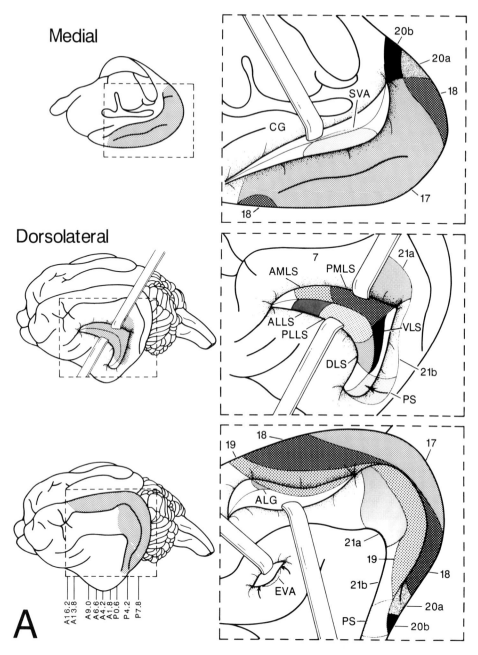

Figure 57. (A) Schematic diagrams of the many visual areas that have been identified in the cat's cerebral cortex by a number of researchers using a variety of methods (modified from John Woolsey's original drawings, and reproduced with permission from Rosenquist, 1985, Fig. 2). These diagrams show the association of numerous specific visual areas with specific gyri and sulcal walls (depicted artistically by retraction of sulcal walls). These several visual areas are interconnected by many specific pathways to form families of networks. (B) Nine coronal sections through the several visual areas of the cat's cerebrum at coronal planes indicated in lower left brain diagram in A. Inspection of these sections provides additional perspective on the relation of different visual areas to specific gyral crowns, within sulcal walls, or at the parafundic regions. Omitted from these drawings are the locations of horizontal and vertical meridians, as well as the azimuth or degrees distal to the vertical meridian, and elevation above or below the horizontal meridian. Such details are often associated with specific walls and fundi of sulci within the cat's visual cortex and are shown in Rosenquist's original drawings.

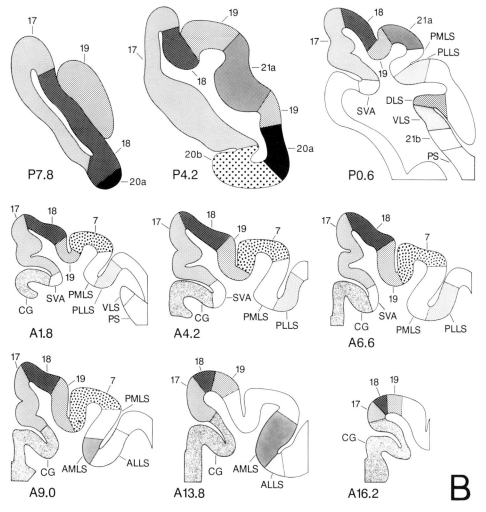

Figure 57. (*Continued*)

has been found in cats to exhibit specific gyral morphological–functional correlates. In carnivores, the middle, anterior, and posterior ectosylvian gyri contain an assemblage of interconnected auditory areas (Fig. 58; Downman *et al.*, 1960). The distribution and interconnections of all these areas has not been as thoroughly worked out as it has in visual cortex, partly because of greater methodological difficulties.

Although the several examples cited above of neurophysiological correlates with gyral crowns, sulcal walls, and fundi reveal numerous functional and connectional differences between these structures, few experiments have been specifically designed to delineate and define gyral–sulcal differences in functional connections. Since functional correlates of convolutions have been examined in detail in only a few cases, we clearly have a long way to go in exploring this question. Most of the gyral–sulcal complexes of convoluted brains of the majority of mammals remain to be studied.

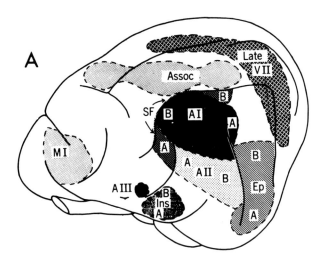

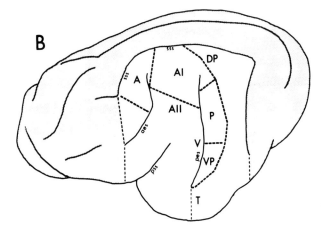

Figure 58. Auditory cortical fields in the cat. (A) Woolsey's (1960a) summary diagram showing four central auditory areas, with the cochlea represented anteroposteriorly from apex, A, to base, B, in the suprasylvian fringe (SF) sector as well as in AI, AII, and Ep (posterior ectosylvian area), and insular area. AIII is Tunturi's third auditory area. Late responding auditory response areas were located in motor (MI) cortex, "association" cortex (Assoc), and visual area II (VII). (B) Imig, Reale, and Brugge's portrayal of auditory cortex showing fields A, AI, AII, P, VP, DP, and T. Heavy dotted lines delimit four tonotopically organized fields (A, AI, P, and VP). Surrounding these fields is a belt of cortex that also is responsive to acoustic stimulation: dorsal posterior (DP), posterior (P, temporal (T), and ventral (V) regions. In all carnivores studied the major collection of interconnected auditory areas is circumscribed rostrally, dorsally, and caudally by the different limbs of the suprasylvian sulcus. The ectosylvian sulci also appear to be limiting sulci. (Reproduced with permission from Imig *et al.*, 1982, Fig. 1.1, and from Woolsey, 1960a, Fig. 128.)

6. Comparative Studies of Gyri and Sulci (Table VIII)

6.1. Phylogeny Evaluated by Paleoneurology

Brain phylogeny can only be assessed directly by comparing the brains of living mammals with those of endocranial casts of a series of related mammals of dated and identified ancestry. This is the field of paleoneurology (Table VIII). Although the brains of some lineages do not produce gyral impressions on the endocranial surfaces, many do, and studies of such cranial endocasts have provided valuable information regarding brain size and gyral and sulcal patterns. Outstanding have been the studies carried out by T. Edinger (1948, 1967, 1975), Jerison and Jerison (1970–1988), and Radinsky (1968–1981). In many lineages the brain and body sizes became progressively larger over time (Cope's law; see Jerison, 1973), and the larger brains tended to be more convoluted (Figs. 59, 60).

Historical
  Beddard (1899)
  Bolk *et al.* (1934)
  Bradley (1899)
  Brandt (1867)
  Broca (1878a)
  Brodmann (1909)
  Clarke and Dewhurst (1972)
  Cole (1944)
  Connolly (1950)
  Count (1947)
  Edinger (1899)

  Galaburda *et al.* (1985)
  Gould (1977)
  Hodos and Campbell (1969)
  Jerison (1973, 1977a)
  Noback (1959)
  Oboussier (1949, 1950)
  Owen (1868)
  Pearson and Pearson (1976)
  Petras and Noback (1969)
  Smith (1931)
  Turner (1890)

Paleoneurology
  Edinger (1984, 1967, 1975)
  Falk (1980, 1981, 1982)
  Haight and Murray (1981)
  Holloway (1976)
  Jerison (1970b, 1979a,c, Volume 8B)
  Kruska (1970, 1973, 1982)
  Moodie (1922)

  Packer (1949)
  Radinsky (1968a-c, 1969, 1970, 1971, 1972,
    1973a–c, 1974, 1975a–c, 1976a–d, 1977a,b,
    1978, 1979, 1980, 1981, 1982)
  Romer and Edinger (1942)
  Steudel (1985)
  Symington (1915, 1916)

Comparative
  Black (1915a,b)
  Bonin (1941b)
  Bradley (1899)
  Brauer Schober (1970)
  Chi and Chang (1941)
  Clark *et al.* (1936)
  Connolly (1936, 1950)
  Darlington (1957)
  Diamond and Hall (1969)
  Dillon (1963)
  Dimond and Blizard (1977)
  England and Dillon (1972)
  Gould (1975)
  Haug (1976, 1987)
  Jacobs *et al.* (1984)
  Johnson (1977, 1980)
  Kaas (1982, 1987)
  Krueg (1878)
  Landacre (1930)
  Lende (1963a,b, 1969)
  Lende and Sadler (1967)
  Lende and Woolsey (1956)
  Mann (1896)
  Mann *et al.* (1988)
  Merzenich (1985)
  Mettler (1933)
  Morgane and Jacobs (1973)
  Morgane *et al.* (1985, 1986)

  Noback and Montagna (1970)
  Papez (1929)
  Papez and Hunter (1929)
  Pilleri (1959)
  Ridgway (1986)
  Sacher (1970)
  Sanides (1969a)
  Santee (1914)
  Shariff (1953)
  Shellshear (1927)
  Smith (1902a,c)
  Stephan (1960)
  Stephan *et al.* (1970, 1982, 1986)
  Tobias (1968, 1971)
  Tower (1954)
  Turner (1890)
  Valverde (1986)
  Weinberg (1902)
  Welker and Campos (1963)
  Welker and Carlson (1976)
  Welker and Johnson (1965)
  Welker and Seidenstein (1959)
  Welker *et al.* (1964, 1976)
  Wirz (1950)
  Woolsey (1984)
  Ziehen (1896)
  Zilles *et al.* (1982, 1986, 1989a,b)

Taxonomy, domestication
  Frick and Nord (1963)
  Klatt (1921)
  Klatt and Oboussier (1951)
  Kruska (1982, 1988)

  Pirlot (1986)
  Stephan (1954)
  Whitney (1976)

(continued)

Table VIII. (*Continued*)

General, theory, reviews

Armstrong and Falk (1982)	Holloway (1970)
Bauchot (1978, 1982)	Jerison (1970a, 1973, 1976, 1977b, 1979a,b)
Bonin (1963)	Kruska (1987)
Bullock (1983)	MacPhail (1982)
Calder (1984)	Northcutt (1981, 1984)
Campbell and Hodos (1970)	Oboussier (1972)
Cohen and Strumwasser (1985)	Olson (1976)
Ebner (1969)	Passingham (1985)
Edelman (1987)	Pearson and Pearson (1976)
Finlay *et al.* (1987)	Peters (1983)
Galaburda and Pandya (1982)	Pilbeam and Gould (1974)
Gould (1977)	Rensch (1948)
Gurche (1982)	Sacher (1982)
Hahn *et al.* (1979)	Sanides (1970a,b, 1975)
Herre (1967)	Schmidt-Nielsen (1984)
Hodos (1982, 1986, 1988)	R. Smith (1985)
Hofer (1969)	Webster (1976)
Hofman (1984, 1985a,b, 1989)	

Homology

Bock (1969)	Ghiselin (1976)
Campbell (1976a,b, 1982)	Hodos (1976)
Connolly (1950)	Kreiner (1968)
Filimonoff (1964)	Smith (1902b)

Laterality and symmetry

Bay (1964)	Harnad *et al.* (1977)
de Lacoste *et al.* (1988)	LeMay (1976, 1984, 1985)
Dimond and Blizard (1977)	LeMay *et al.* (1982)
Falzi *et al.* (1982)	Myers (1976)
Galaburda (1979)	Rubens (1977)
Galaburda *et al.* (1978, 1985)	Tan and Çalişkan (1987)
Geschwind and Galaburda (1984, 1985, 1987)	Webster (1977)
Geschwind and Levitsky (1968)	Whitaker and Selnes (1976)
Glick (1985)	Yeni-Komshian and Benson (1976)

Variability

Connolly (1950)	Jefferson (1913)
Donaldson (1928)	Kawamura (1971)
Filimonoff (1928)	Pubols and Pubols (1979)
Haight and Neylon (1978a)	Smith (1929)
Haug (1987)	Whitaker and Selnes (1976)

Because of the common correlation of certain structurally and functionally distinct cortical areas with specific gyri and sulci, several hypotheses regarding the adaptive and functional significance of some evolutionary trends have been put forward. In some instances such hypotheses are not altogether unreasonable (Jerison, 1973, 1976, 1977b, 1978, 1979c; Jerison and Jerison, 1988; Radinsky, 1968a, 1974, 1975b, 1982). Outstanding of all the reviews on such topics have been those articulated in depth by Jerison, who has assembled an impressive variety of paleoneurological, quantitative neuroanatomical, paleogeographical, and psychobiological evidence in support of several specific hypotheses regarding the evolution of the brain and intelligence. Jerison's work has generated renewed interest in such issues by many investigators.

However, brain size and external morphology do not provide information regarding cortical architecture, areal differentiation, connectivity, presence of buried gyri, or functional organization within cerebral cortex, all of which are known to reflect the degree of complexity of cortical circuit functions in living mammals. In addition, paleoneurological evidence does not yield information that is relevant to understanding the underlying mechanisms of gyrification with which this chapter is primarily concerned. Therefore, the bulk of this literature is only of ancillary relevance to questions regarding causes and correlates of cortical convolutions.

6.2. Evolution of Gyri and Sulci Inferred from Comparative Neurobiology

I began this chapter with a few examples of the wide diversity in brain size and convolutional developmental of several different living mammals (Fig. 1). It was such variety, as well as taxon-specific similarities, for which comparative neuroanatomists and evolutionists, from the middle to late 1800s up to the

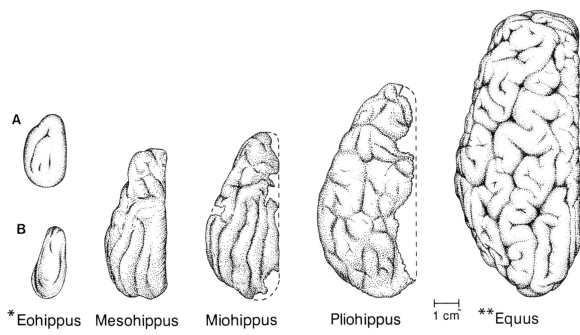

Figure 59. Evolution of the horse brain. (a) *Eohippus* (*Hyracotherium*), left dorsal view as reconstructed by Radinsky (1976d) based on AMNH specimen Nos. 55266, 55267, and 55268, early Eocene. (Reproduced with permission from Radinsky, 1976d, Fig. 1A.) (b) *Eohippus*, dorsal view of right hemisphere (reversed to appear as left). Reconstructed by T. Edinger (1948) from Yale Peabody Museum specimen No. VP-11624 (Fig. 2A, p. 21), Lower Eocene. This and subsequent endocasts reproduced with permission from Edinger (1948). Radinsky's reconstruction of *Eohippus* is judged more valid since it was based on specimens that were unequivocally identified as *Hyracotherium*. *Mesohippus*, left dorsal view; Edinger's reconstruction of AMNH specimen No. 39408 (Fig. 10A, p. 47), Middle Oligocene. *Miohippus*, left dorsal view; Edinger's reconstruction of specimen PU 11127 (Fig. 12A, p. 64), Upper Oligocene. *Pliohippus*, left dorsal view; Edinger's reconstruction of AMNH specimen No. 10844 (Fig. 16A, p. 80), Lower Pliocene. *Equus*, left dorsal view of modern horse (reproduced with permission from Dellmann and McClure, 1975, Fig. 24-9.) All specimens reproduced to the same scale.

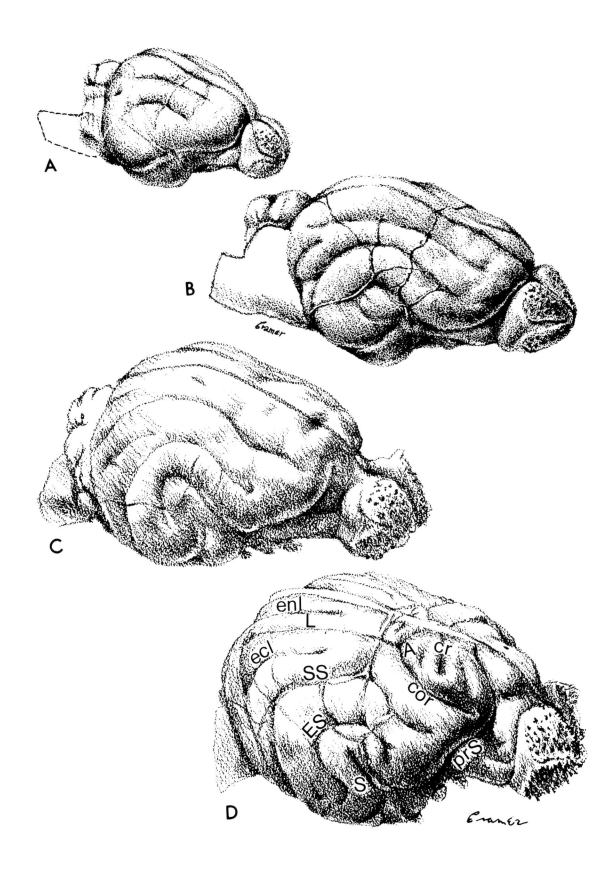

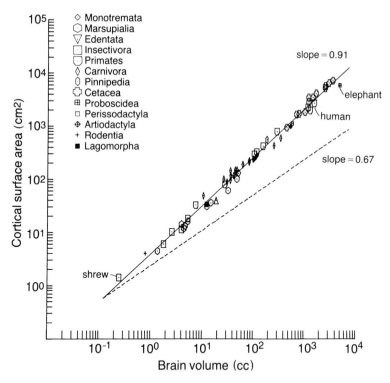

Figure 61. Relation between total cortical surface area and brain volume in representatives of 13 orders of mammals. The slope of the regression line through these data is 0.91, plus or minus 0.01. The dashed line represents the scaling of cortical surface area according to a two-thirds power relation. The larger brains are more convoluted and the presumption is that gyral folding "permits" cortical surface area to increase faster than the two-thirds power with brain weight. Both scales are logarithmic. (Reproduced with permission from Prothero and Sundsten, 1984, Fig. 1.)

present time, have tried to find explanations by studying a broad assemblage of living mammals (Table VIII). Several general concepts grew out of such studies. (1) A common evolutionary trend involved an increase in body size. (2) In such lineages, increased body size was associated with increases in brain size. In comparative studies of living mammals, other changes in the brain are commonly

Figure 60. Canid endocasts viewed from anterodorsolateral aspect revealing progressive increases in gyral and sulcal number and changes in orientation and shape of several gyri and sulci that are proposed as being homologous, or at least topographically similar. (A) *Hesperocyon gregarius* [AMNH No. 39475, Middle Oligocene, 30 million years ago (mya)] exhibits only two well-developed neocortical sulci: the coronal-lateral (cor) (L), and suprasylvian (SS), which are less arched than in later canids. (B) *Mesocyon* sp. (AMNH No. 6946, early Miocene) has a well-developed ectolateral sulcus (ecl), a longer more arcuate suprasylvian sulcus, and an arched ectosylvian sulcus. (C) *Tomarctus* cf. *euthos* (F:AMNH No. 61074, late Miocene and early Pliocene, 10–15 mya) exhibits the presence of entolateral (enl), pseudosylvian (S), presylvian (prS), and cruciate (cr) sulci (cruciate area restored from F:AMNH No. 27534). Expansion of cortex around the cruciate sulcus in this specimen marks the first appearance of a sigmoid gyrus. Cortex in this specimen is sufficiently expansive to make the rhinal sulcus appear lower. Occipital cortex also protrudes over the cerebellum more extensively. (D) *Canis mesomelas*, the modern jackal, exhibits a relatively greater amount of neocortex (as seen by the lower posterior rhinal sulcus, more overlapped cerebellum, better developed pseudosylvian and cruciate sulci, and appearance of postcruciate and ansate sulci). All drawn to about natural size. (Reproduced with permission from Radinsky, 1969, Fig. 1.)

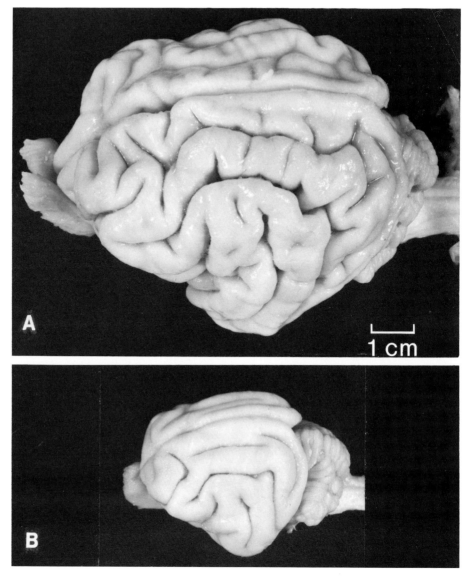

Figure 62. Association of brain size and gyrification in a large and small felid. (A) African lion (*Panthera leo*) shows similar pattern of major gyri and sulci as does the domestic cat (*Felis domesticus*, B). However, the lion brain exhibits numerous additional small gyri and eminences separated by small sulci, spurs, and dimples. Brain weights: lion, 177 g (#62-566, female, 1 year old); cat, 29 g (#62-184, female, adult).

associated with increased brain size: (3) Larger brains have greater surface areas of cerebral cortex. (4) Larger brains also are usually more convoluted, (5) exhibit new cortical areas, and (6) a larger number of differentiated cortical areas, (7) which have more numerous and complex interconnections. Moreover, (8) some taxa exhibit differential enlargement or specialization of certain cortical areas or regions. (9) An overriding common theme has been that mammals having larger brains with more convoluted and differentiated cerebral cortex are cognitively, perceptually, and behaviorally more complex. In most of the studies devoted to these topics over the last century, there has been a persistent search for neural correlates of intelligence (Jerison, 1973; Jerison and Jerison, 1988). Most of the

literature on the several interrelated themes mentioned above will not be discussed here because it does not provide direct evidence regarding the underlying determinants of gyrogenesis and fissuration. Those ideas that do have some
ancillary bearing on the formation of gyri are discussed briefly below.

87

DETERMINANTS OF
GYRI AND SULCI

6.2.1. Body Size, Brain Size, Cortical Surface Area, and Convolutedness

A common finding in comparative neurology is that animals with larger
brains also have greater areal extents of cortex (Fig. 61). This relationship holds
for a wide variety of mammals, both within and across taxa. It is still seen when
one factors out those animals that are not only just larger, but also more encephalized (Jerison, 1973, 1982, this volume). Usually, cerebral cortex of larger brains
is also more convoluted.

In closely related mammals that differ markedly in body size, such as lions
and domestic cats, but which seem to have similar general perceptual–behavioral
repertoires, the larger African lion has a larger brain with a more convoluted
cortex (Fig. 62). Yet, on the very little evidence available, the brains of these two
felids otherwise appear to exhibit similar degrees of architectonic complexity.
The reasons why larger animals have larger brains is not clear. It has been
hypothesized that larger animals require larger brains (containing greater numbers of neurons) in order to contain the representations of larger peripheral
sensory surfaces and motor apparatus, process information from larger sensory
surfaces, or to activate and control the contractions and relaxations of larger
muscles which move heavier body parts. Moreover, it is possible that larger
bodies require larger numbers of neurons to produce motor responses that are
precise, careful, and strong, but also are graded in velocity, acceleration, and
amplitude. However plausible they sound, such conjectures are too general to be
amenable to test by experiment. As a result, the overall correlations between
body size, brain size, and degree of gyrification remain unexplained. However,
the data do suggest specific questions that are not only pertinent, but answera-
ble. For example: are there greater numbers of sensory neurons in the first-
order sensory ganglia of different sensory modalities in lions than in domestic
cats? Similarly, are there greater numbers of motor neurons for homologous
muscles in the bigger versus smaller cats? Is peripheral innervation density
greater in homologous body parts of the larger animals? It is, of course, possible
that larger felids actually have greater numbers and varieties of cortical circuits
than do the smaller cats. Increased cortical differentiation and interconnectivity
would be expected to be reflected in a greater number and complexity of gyri
and sulci. Moreover, closer examination of their perceptual, cognitive, and behavioral repertoires might reveal greater behavioral complexity in the larger
animals. However, too little is known at present regarding the relevant anatomical, functional, or behavioral characters to firmly support most hypotheses
about the underlying factors that determine the greater convolutional complexity in larger animals within closely related taxa.

6.2.2. Encephalization, Corticalization, and Increased Gyral–Sulcal Complexity

Another major conclusion of comparative neuroscientists has been that
mammals which have larger, more differentiated cerebral cortex also have brains
that are more convoluted (Table VIII). Studies of architecture of cerebral cortex

in a variety of species within different orders of mammals have revealed increased architectonic diversity in the more convoluted, larger brains. The evidence is most extensive within the Primate order. Evidence also indicates increased cortical architectural diversity (correlated with increased gyrification) in mammals of increasing perceptual–behavioral complexity, regardless of taxonomic group. However, only a beginning has been made in defining and delineating differences in areal diversity in the cerebral cortex, as well as adequately characterizing level of behavioral complexity, in most living mammals.

6.2.3. Differential Enlargements and Specializations

Relatively larger amounts of localized areas of convoluted cortex are found also in mammals that have increased innervation of specialized sensory surfaces (Figs. 44–53). The relatively large cortical somatosensory hand area in raccoons (Welker and Campos, 1963), rhinarial area in pigs (Ray and Craner, 1988; Woolsey and Fairman, 1946) and coatis (Welker and Campos, 1963), lip area in llamas (Welker *et al.*, 1976), and tail area in spider monkeys (Pubols and Pubols, 1979; Woolsey, 1964) all exhibit increased gyrification of these relatively enlarged cortical regions. Areal assemblies of auditory cortex occupy relatively larger, more differentiated, and more convoluted regions of cortex in some mammalian groups, especially in predatory carnivores, and particularly in felids (Fig. 58) and canids, in which auditory perceptuomotor capabilities are relatively enhanced (Brugge and Reale, 1985; Imig *et al.*, 1982; Woolsey, 1960a, 1981c). Likewise, families of visual cortical areas are more numerous and occupy relatively larger amounts of convoluted cortex in mammals that have enhanced visual capabilities (Figs. 56, 57). The frontal lobes, the temporal pole, and parietal cortex appear to be larger and more convoluted in adaptively more complex primate groups (Table VIII; Connolly, 1950). The architecture, connectivity, and functions of cortical fields in such enlarged regions of cortex are only recently being defined with precise methods, but only in a few mammals (Table VIII). The needed comparative study of species differences in differential enlargement of most cortical regions has only just begun. Consequently, evidence for structural–functional correlates of gyral–sulcal entities, particularly in nonsensory cortex is meager at present.

6.2.4. Development of New Areas and Gyri

There is some evidence from comparative electrophysiological studies which suggests that there are a greater number and variety of cortical visual, auditory, and somatosensory areas in mammals which have more sophisticated visual, auditory, and somatosensory capabilities. Concepts of subdivision, duplication, or multiplication are now more widely used to suggest ways by which new cortical areas and circuits might be added during evolution, thereby resulting in greater neurobehavioral complexity (Carlson, 1985; Edelman, 1987; Kaas, 1982). Adding circuits by increased differentiation and duplication of existing cortical areas could result in increased gyral–sulcal development. Such duplications are hypothesized to take place by additional cell divisions of ependymal stem cells before they begin their migration to the cortical mantle (Rakic, 1988).

6.2.5. Gyrification Not Associated with Brain or Body Size

There are a number of notable exceptions to the general rule that larger brains are more convoluted. The large, relatively lissencephalic brain of the Florida manatee has always been viewed as exceptional (Figs. 1, 7; Smith, 1902a). Another unusual example is seen when comparing the brains of two large rodents. For example, the cerebral cortex of the slightly larger capybara brain is quite fissured, whereas that of the large North American beaver is relatively smooth (Fig. 63; Campos and Welker, 1976). In another example, the least weasel, the smallest living carnivore, has a highly convoluted brain which is somewhat smaller than that of a smooth-brained rodent, such as the larger-bodied muskrat (Fig. 64). The reasons for the convolutional differences in brains of similar size have not been adequately studied. Jerison (1973) has proposed that such cases are aberrant in brain–body relations and, in the case of the least weasel, reflects the existence of selection pressures toward smaller (pygmy) body sizes.

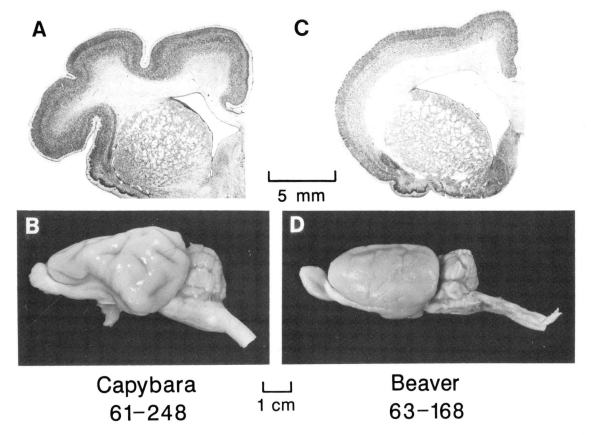

Capybara 61–248 ⊔ 1 cm **Beaver 63–168**

Figure 63. Comparison of convoluted and unconvoluted brains of two large rodents in lateral view (B, D) and cross section (A, C). The capybara (*Hydrochoerus hydrochoerus,* #61-248, young female, 11.6 kg body weight; 54.1 g brain weight; section #612) is the largest living rodent. It also has the largest brain of any rodent, as well as a fissured cerebral cortex. The beaver (*Castor canadensis,* #63-168, adult male, 19.5 kg body weight; 36.5 g brain weight; section #798) also has quite a large brain, but its cortex is essentially smooth except for a dimple or two dorsally. Coronal sections of the two animals are from roughly equivalent rostrocaudal locations. (A reproduced with permission from Campos and Welker, 1976, Fig. 9.)

6.2.6. Cortical Thickness, Brain Size, and Convolutedness

Another general relationship which is well documented is that thickness of cerebral cortex varies relatively little (1–4 mm) among brains of different mammals over a wide range of brain and body sizes, from mouse to elephant. It is generally assumed that whatever processing functions are performed by cell columns in cerebral cortex, such functions require only a small, relatively limited number of vertically arranged and interconnected neurons, regardless of brain size. This general notion has several important (but undocumented) implications. The two major ones are: (1) that the processing operations of cerebral cortex are everywhere basically the same (Braitenberg, 1974, 1978; Fleischhauer, 1978; Lorente de Nó, 1938; Szentágothai, 1969), and (2) that increasing

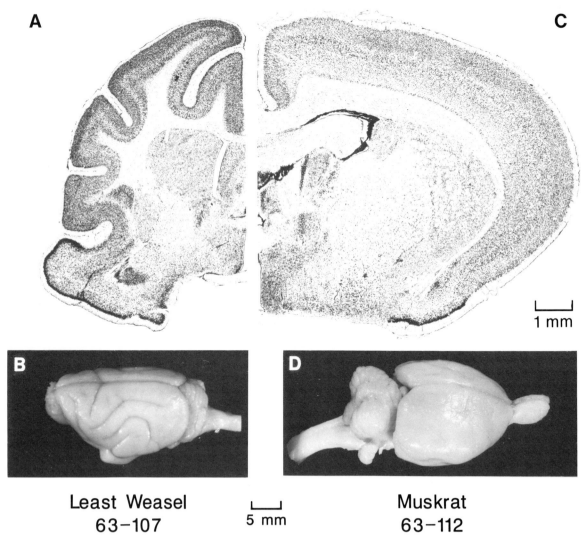

A

C

1 mm

B

D

Least Weasel 63–107

5 mm

Muskrat 63–112

Figure 64. Comparison of convoluted brains of the smallest living carnivore (least weasel, *Mustela nivalis*, A, B; #63-107, section #306) and the slightly larger unconvoluted brain of a rodent (muskrat, *Ondatra zibethicus*, C, D; #63-112, section #506). Note differences in cortical thickness and typical crown, sulcal wall, and fundic differences in cortex of the weasel. Brain weights: weasel, 2.4 g; muskrat, 3.8 g.

the number of processing modules in larger and adaptively more complex mammals is tantamount to increasing cortical surface area (Jerison, 1973). Again, however, there are two notable exceptions to this general rule regarding the relative constancy of cortical thickness, and for these other explanations must be found. One exception, discussed in Section 4, is found in convoluted cortex where cortex is thinner in fundi than in gyral crowns. It is likely that there are fewer neurons and less neuropil in cell columns in fundic cortex than there are in crown cortex. Another type of exception is seen in Fig. 63, where the cortex of a lissencephalic rodent is much thicker than that of the gyral crowns of a gyrencephalic carnivore of somewhat smaller brain size. The reasons for these, and many other, variations are unknown.

6.2.7. Relevance of Other Biological Variables

There are a number of biological variables which show significant correlations with variations in body size and brain size (Armstrong, 1983, 1985; Peters, 1983; Sacher, 1970). For example, there is evidence that larger-bodied mammals with larger and more convoluted brains also have, among other features, higher standard metabolic rates, slower heart rates, longer gestation times, greater longevity, and shorter diurnal sleep periods (Peters, 1983). Certain ecological and

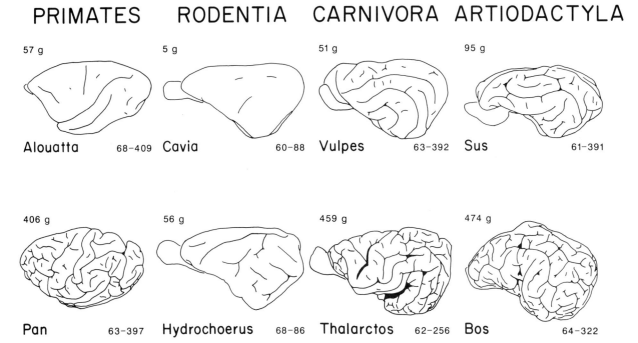

Figure 65. Interorder differences. The brains of members of different orders exhibit several differences, not only in overall shape, but also in the general size, shape, orientation, and pattern of organization of the major gyri and sulci. Primates: *Alouatta* (howler monkey) and *Pan* (chimpanzee). Rodents: *Cavia* (guinea pig) and *Hydrochoerus* (capybara). Carnivores: *Vulpes* (fox) and *Thalarctos* (polar bear). Ar-

tiodactyls: *Sus* (pig) and *Bos* (cow). Animal number of each specimen is listed below each drawing, and total brain weight (including cerebellum, brain stem, medulla, and C1 spinal cord) is listed above each drawing. These brain diagrams are not drawn to the same scale in order to permit direct comparison of shapes and gyral–sulcal patterns for the different specimens.

ethological variables such as predator–prey relationships and patterns of social organization have also been found to associate with brain size and body size variables (Sawaguchi, 1988).

It is not my purpose to explore such issues here since the scope of body size relations is wide (Peters, 1983), and the literature on such topics is extensive. This literature contains a set of theories regarding body size relations which make simple, quantitative, and reasonably accurate predictions of many biological phenomena. Peters (1983) has pointed out that there are no good empirically based explanations of many such body size relations. This is not, of course, a critique of allometric studies, since they indicate important relations between different biological parameters, and they do reflect the operation of physical laws (Schmidt-Nielsen, 1984). It must be realized that selection is based on an optimal balancing of all the biological variables within an organism, and that there are an enormous number of possible interrelations among such variables in living animals. As a result of such considerations, Schmidt-Nielsen (1984) concludes that animal size is a complex subject, and that simple conclusions cannot be drawn from comparison of a few biological parameters. Such a conclusion is also relevant to predictive theories based on relationships between body size and brain size. With respect to questions regarding the determinants of gyri and sulci among mammals, most such theories appear to be too general since they have not generated specific ethologically relevant hypotheses that are testable. It is not because testable hypotheses cannot be made. Rather, I think that it is more likely that the oft-quoted notion that gyrification and fissuration are mechanical solutions to a packaging problem is intuitively so simple and easily understood, that it has been accepted widely as having explanatory value. As a result, further inquiry into the neurobiological correlates or determinants of gyri and sulci has been forestalled.

6.3. Taxon-Specific Gyral–Sulcal Patterns

It was realized early in comparative studies of the nervous system that the brains of mammals within specific taxonomic groups were more similar to one another in gyral–sulcal pattern than they were to those patterns found in brains of different groups (Table VIII). The important conclusion was also reached that convolutions and sulci did not appear randomly in different mammalian groups, but tended to occur in taxon-specific patterns.

In the paragraphs that follow, I will merely illustrate a few of these similarities or constancies for a few of the major mammalian taxonomic groups. Also, I will consider only information about gyral and sulcal *external morphology.* This is the customary approach and, because of its superficiality, limits the significance of conjectures regarding the homology of gyri and sulci in different mammals.

6.3.1. Differences between Orders

The brains of representatives of different orders of mammals differ from one another in a number of conformational, gyral, and sulcal features. Within each order there are greater similarities, despite wide intraorder variations in brain size and gyral and sulcal complexity (Fig. 65). Brains of a large and small species within each order are similar to each other, but differ from large and small brains in the other orders with respect to (1) general shape, (2) location and orientation of frontal, temporal, and occipital lobes, and (3) location, shape, and orientation of the primary sulci. For example, the central sulcus, Sylvian fissure, superior temporal sulcus, calcarine fissure, and several other gyri and sulci (if present) are similarly located on the brains of the two (as well as many other) primates shown in Fig. 65. The result is a typical primate pattern of gyrification, fissuration, and lobation. This pattern is different from the gyral–sulcal patterns typically found in carnivores, among which the cruciate, coronal, suprasylvian, lateral, anterior, and posterior ectosylvian are typically identifiable. The primate and carnivore gyral–sulcal patterns differ, in turn, from those found in both artiodactyls and rodents (Fig. 65). The same generalization holds

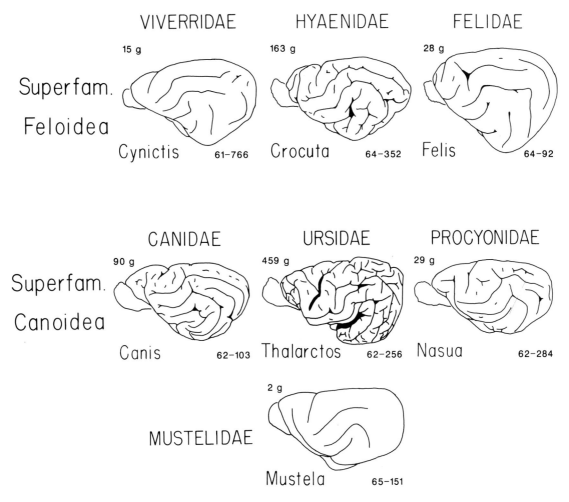

Figure 66. Interfamily differences in carnivores. The members of different families within an order tend to exhibit differences in brain shape, as well as in size, shape, orientation, and pattern of major gyri and sulci. This is not evident from the drawings in this figure since only one specialized member of each family is depicted in order to compactly illustrate a member of each family in each superfamily (Feloidea and Canoidea). The brains depicted are drawn to the same size (not to the same scale) to permit direct comparison of their shapes and gyral–sulcal patterns.

for the major lobes, gyri, and sulci of the brains from members of other orders of mammals such as cetaceans, perissodactyls, sirenians, chiropterans, pinnipeds, insectivores, and edentates.

6.3.2. Differences between Families

The gyral–sulcal patterns of brains of different representatives of each mammalian family within a given order differ from those of other families within that order (Fig. 66 depicts only one member of each family). Within each

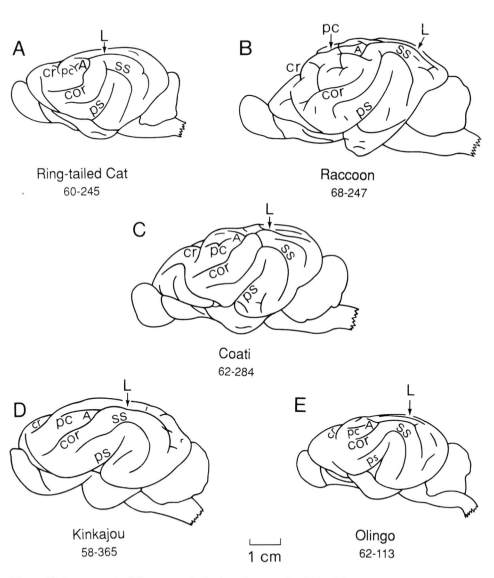

Figure 67. Intergeneric differences. The brains of mammals within different genera within a given family (e.g., Procyonidae) exhibit different gyral and sulcal features that characterize the members of each genus. Several sulci that appear to separate similar gyri in the different animals are indicated: A, ansate; cor, coronal; cr, cruciate; L, lateral; pc, postcruciate; ps, pseudosylvian; ss, suprasylvian. All brains are drawn to the same scale.

family group there are family resemblances. For example, in canids the anterior and posterior ectosylvian sulci are connected by a sulcus that arches over the pseudosylvian sulcus. This does not occur in felids. In addition, in canids the frontal pole protrudes farther rostrally and the cruciate sulcus is oriented more rostrolaterally. In felids, on the other hand, the frontal pole is typically foreshortened and the cruciate sulcus is oriented mediolaterally. In addition, in canids there is a sulcus on the posterior suprasylvian gyrus lateral to, and parallel with, the postero-occipital sulcus. This sulcus does not typically appear in felids. In felids, the postero-occipital sulcus is separate from the lateral sulcus, whereas in canids these two sulci merge with one another. In members of both Ursidae and Procyonidae, the cortical gyri lying beneath the suprasylvian gyrus are relatively small and fewer in number, whereas in canids and felids these gyri are large and more numerous, the entire region being more extensive. Not all families have more than one or a few different representatives, so that generalizations about interfamily differences in patterns in such cases are supported by less data.

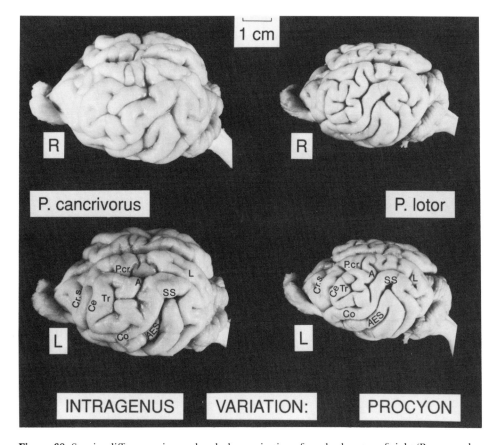

Figure 68. Species differences in gyral–sulcal organization of cerebral cortex of right (R, reversed to appear as left) and left (L) hemispheres of *Procyon cancrivorous* (crab-eating raccoon, #63-312) and *Procyon lotor* (North American raccoon). The larger *P. cancrivorous* brain appears to have a greater number of subgyri and small sulci, dimples, and spurs, and its elliptical somatosensory hand gyrus (see Figs. 44 and 48) also appears relatively larger than in *P. lotor.* Otherwise, the pattern of organization of the gyri and sulci in the two species is similar.

6.3.3. Differences between Genera

The gyral–sulcal patterns of brains of representatives of different genera within a family, such as the Procyonidae (Fig. 67), differ from one another in several relatively minor ways when compared with the differences between procyonids and felids (Fig. 66). Again, the number of living species within many genera is limited, so that generalizations about intergeneric gyral patterns in such cases are less secure.

6.3.4. Species Differences

In the example shown in Fig. 68, the two species of *Procyon* (raccoons) are similar in general shape, gyral location, relative size, and pattern. The brain of the crab-eating raccoon (*Procyon cancrivorous*) differs from that of the North American raccoon (*P. lotor*) in that it is larger, and has numerous added small gyri and sulci. Both species even have a large elliptical gyrus which, in *P. lotor*, has been shown to contain the relatively large representation of the glabrous forepaw (Welker and Seidenstein, 1959).

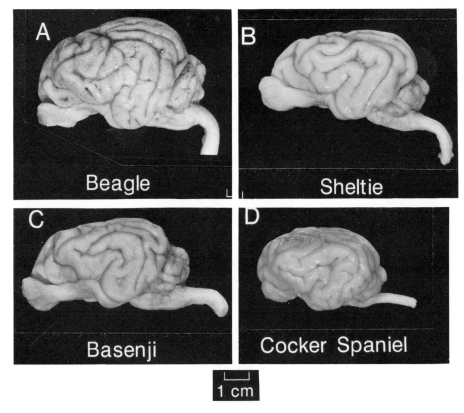

Figure 69. Breed differences in gyri and sulci. Selective breeding has produced an enormous variation in breeds of dogs. The members of each purebred line have brains that are characteristic in size and shape for that breed. Each breed has a distinctive pattern and arrangement of gyri and sulci. Nevertheless, the similarities among dogs are much greater than the similarities between dogs and cats. (All specimens were obtained from The Jackson Laboratory at Bar Harbor, Maine.)

Domestication has produced a variety of breeds of mammal (Kruska, 1987, 1988). These include gyrencephalic breeds of dogs, cats, cows, sheep, goats, pigs, and horses (Klatt, 1921; Klatt and Oboussier, 1951; Kruska, 1973, 1982, 1988). Within each of these groups, selective breeding has yielded specialized breeds or strains having the desired behavioral, anatomical, or physiological features. The brains of the different breeds of a given species, such as of dogs, may differ widely in size, shape, and, to some extent, gyral and sulcal patterns (Fig. 69). Nevertheless, the brains of different breeds within a given species share many features of gyral and sulcal organization (Fig. 69). If they still survive, wild forms can interbreed with related domestic varieties. Where this has been done, a variety of altered brain size and gyral and sulcal patterns result. Kruska (1988)

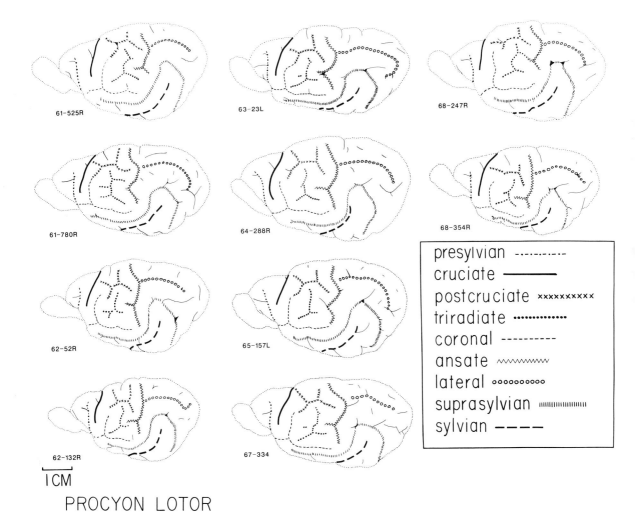

Figure 70. Individual variations in overall arrangement and patterns of gyri, major sulci, lobules, and lobes are revealed in the left hemispheres of ten different raccoons. The animal number and hemisphere (right = R, left = L) depicted are indicated beneath each brain. The different sulci being compared as indicated by different symbols (see key). All brains are drawn to the same scale.

has reviewed available literature regarding the effects of domestication on brain size and gyral–sulcal patterns.

6.3.6. Individual Differences in Gyral and Sulcal Patterns

Interanimal variability in sulcal and gyral patterns has been noted and discussed from the earliest studies up to the present (Table VIII). Most studies have referred only to external morphology where there are obvious interanimal dif-

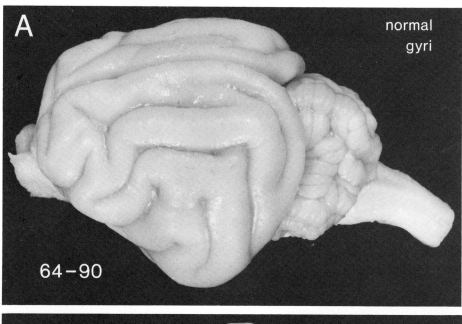

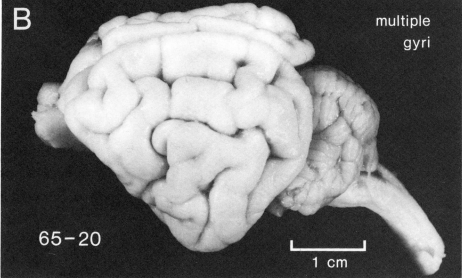

Figure 71. An unusual case of interanimal variability in gyral–sulcal patterns in two domestic cats. Brain A reveals the more usual gyral pattern, whereas B exhibits supernumerary subgyri and hummocks as well as dimples and sulcal spurs, in a cat that otherwise appeared normal. The two hemispheres of each cat were similar to one another in gyral and sulcal pattern and complexity.

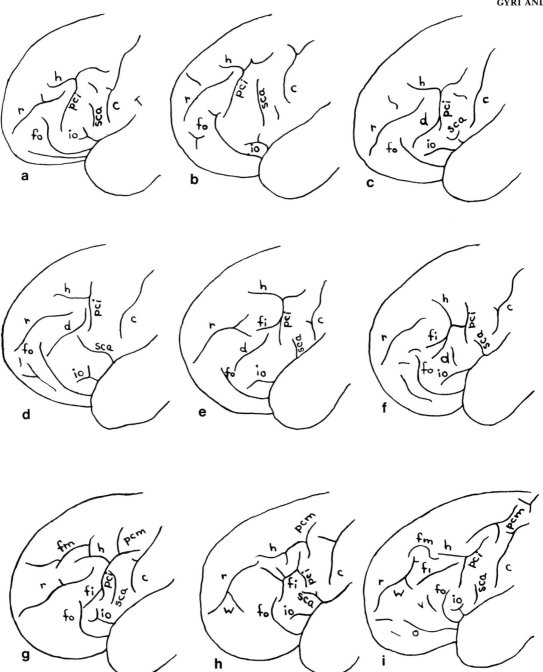

Figure 72. Individual variability in patterns of frontal lobe sulci in nine different orangutan brains. Connoly arranged drawings a–i so as to show progressively increased differentiation of the convolutions. He suggested that such variations reflected differences in underlying cellular organization. (Reproduced with permission from Connolly, 1950, Fig. 59.)

ferences in gyral (and sulcal) length, width, shape, orientation of the brain, and spatial relationships to surrounding gyri (and sulci). Examples of such variability from our own studies of raccoons are shown in Fig. 70. Such variations are very common in secondary and tertiary sulci, despite an overall consistency of the major species-typical primary gyri and sulci (Bailey and Bonin, 1951; Connolly, 1950; Jacobson, 1978). Occasionally, striking divergences are seen from the species-typical pattern. One example is seen in Fig. 71, which depicts the typical cortical gyral configuration of a domestic cat together with another cat brain having supernumerary subgyri, hummocks, and sulci which embellish the simpler basic gyral–sulcal patterns.

Connolly (1950) discussed interanimal variability at some length and Fig. 72 shows his example of variations in frontal lobe sulci in several orangutan brains. He suggested that such graded variations reflect different degrees of increasing complexity of underlying cortical organization. Because of such marked variability, Connolly found it difficult to say whether a particular sulcus on a given brain should be given one name or another. This points up the uncertainty of using external morphological criteria alone (particularly those of sulci) in attempting to identify homologous cortical entities.

6.3.7. Interhemispheric Variations in Gyral–Sulcal Patterns

Interhemispheric variations in gyral–sulcal organization have been commonly observed. Our data for certain sulci in and around somatosensory cortex of raccoons are shown in Fig. 73, which reveals numerous variations, as well as many similarities, between the sulcal patterns on the two hemispheres of 37 raccoons. It is striking that there are a number of cases in this figure (outlined by rectangles) in which cerebral sulci of both hemispheres of a brain are nearly identical in their size, shape, spatial orientation, and degree of complexity.

Hemispheric asymmetry or laterality has been a topic of great interest in the human literature, not only in recent times, but in the early literature as well. There are several instances of increased gyrification and fissuration as well as differential enlargement of cortex in one hemisphere or the other (Table VIII). It has been strongly affirmed that differential development or lateralization of specific functions to specific regions of cortex in one hemisphere or the other is an additional dimension along which evolutionary differentiation has taken place.

6.4. Significance of Taxon-Specific, Individual, and Interhemispheric Differences

Taxon-specific consistency in gyral–sulcal patterns, together with reliable intertaxon differences in such patterns, indicate that basic cortical convolutional patterns are heritable. The data reviewed earlier make clear that the larger primary gyral–sulcal patterns can be used as indicators of the relative size, shape, location, and spatial arrangement of the major sensory, motor, and other related cortical areas in different mammals. An important question is whether

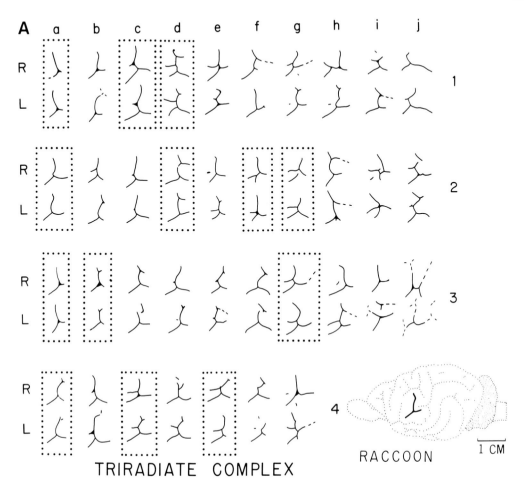

TRIRADIATE COMPLEX

RACCOON

1 CM

Figure 73. Interhemispheric (as well as interanimal) variations in cerebral neocortical sulcal pattern (which reflect convolutional variations) in the brains of 37 North American raccoons. In A–D, the sulci from the right and the left hemispheres are shown as pairs, with the right hemisphere reversed to appear as the left. Dotted lines enclose those pairs of sulci that appear most similar on the two hemispheres. Brain diagram at lower right in each figure shows the sulcal complex being compared for that figure. (A) Triradiate sulcal complex. This complex lies within the relatively large elliptical gyrus containing the hand representation, and its different sulcal parts separate representations of different parts of digits and palm. (B) Coronal–"central" complex. The horizontal limb of this sulcus bounds the medial side of the head gyrus. The vertical limb separates the somatosensory hand from the MI motor cortex. (C) Postcruciate complex. The different limbs of this complex delimit different somatosensory representations from one another, as well as motor from sensory cortex. (D) Ansate complex. This complex lies at the caudal margin of the somatosensory cortex. Laterally, the rostral spur separates the representations of the radial from the ulnar palm pads.

Examination of all these figures reveals that there is considerable interhemispheric variability, as well as interanimal variability, in sulcal (and therefore gyral) patterns. Yet, there are many cases where the sulci are remarkably similar on the two hemispheres of a particular animal. Such symmetry is especially striking in those cases where there are marked deviations in sulcal pattern from the typical pattern. In such cases, the aberrations occur on both hemispheres.

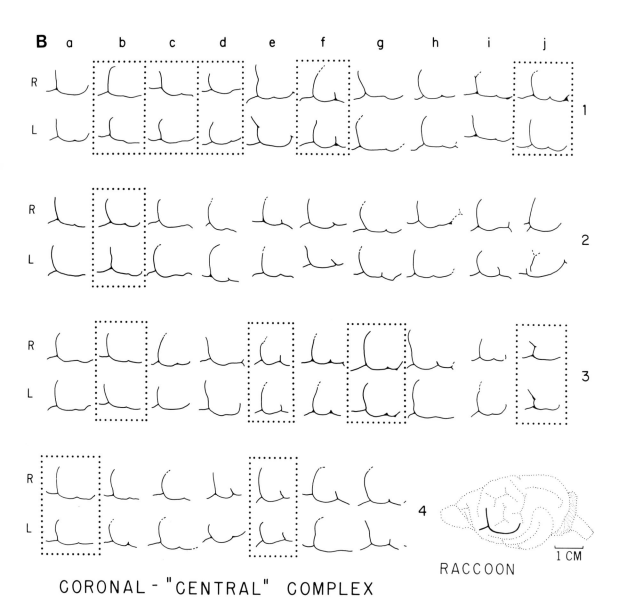

CORONAL - "CENTRAL" COMPLEX

RACCOON

1 CM

Figure 73. (*Continued*)

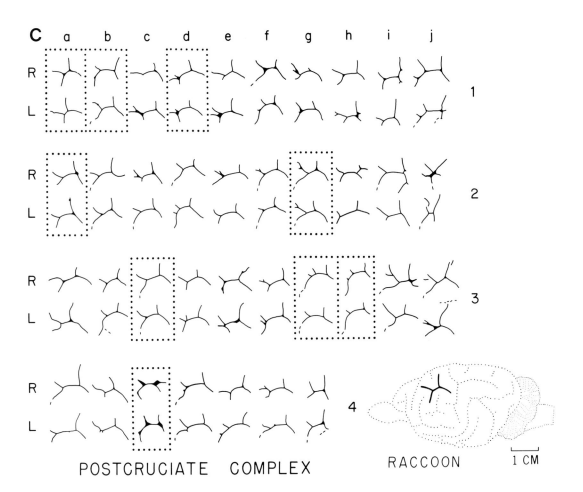

POSTCRUCIATE COMPLEX

RACCOON

1 CM

Figure 73. (*Continued*)

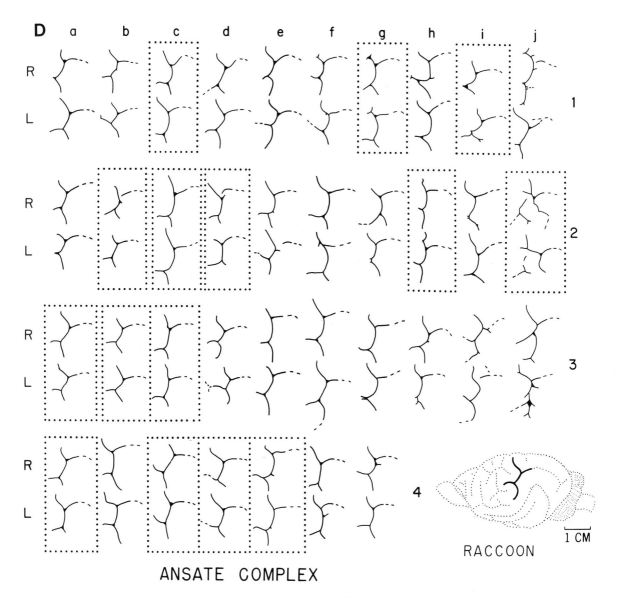

ANSATE COMPLEX

RACCOON

1 CM

Figure 73. (*Continued*)

minor variations of gyral–sulcal features also are significant indicators of structural, connectional, and functional differences within cortex of different individuals within a species or breed. In addressing this question in somatosensory cortex in raccoons, we discovered that such minor interanimal differences were associated with variations in the deployment of specific peripheral somatosensory projections to cerebral cortex (Fig. 74).

The conclusion seems inevitable that intertaxon differences in gyral–sulcal pattern of organization reflect fundamental taxonomic differences in the number, diversity, relative size, spatial organization, and connectivity patterns of cortical areas. These data, together with the fact that such features are relatively similar within each taxon, indicate that gyral–sulcal patterns have genetic–epigenetic determinants. Moreover, individual differences in gyral–sulcal configuration, like fingerprints, very likely reflect genetically dependent differences.

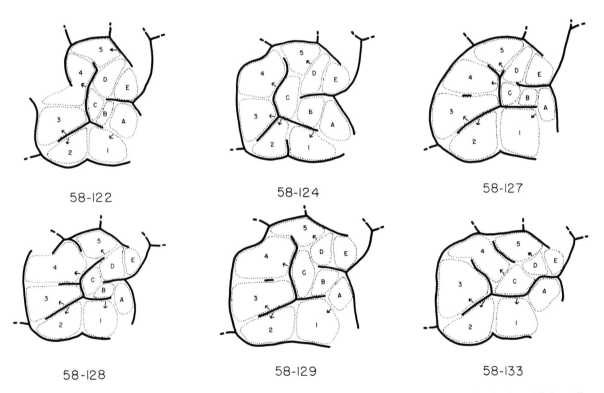

Figure 74. Variability in cortical somatosensory representations of digits 1–5 and palm pads A–E of raccoon's glabrous forepaw. Each numbered drawing represents electrophysiological results obtained from a different animal. The general and detailed topographic relationships are similar in all cases despite variations in size, shape, and relative position of digital and palm pad representations. Note that despite variations in presence, size, orientation, and location of sulcal patterns in the different animals, the sulci always lie between gyri that contain peripherally distinct representations. Such data suggest that interanimal variations in gyral–sulcal arrangement do reflect individual differences in underlying connectional and functional organization. Arrows indicate proximodistal orientation of the digital representations. (Reproduced with permission from Welker and Seidenstein, 1959, Fig. 7.)

6.5. Questions of Evolution and Homology

A phylogenetic perspective is implied in all comparative studies of the brain. Attempts to identify homologous brain structures have been made from the earliest of brain studies right up to the present. Homology refers basically to phylogeny, to commonality of ancestry (Bock, 1969). It has not been easy to use brain characters to assess phyletic relationships (Kirsch and Johnson, 1983). This is due in part to the fact that the brains of different mammals tend to differ with respect to many features, as well as to the fact that only a few of their important neurobiological features have been examined in sufficient detail in too small a sample of relevant mammals. Concepts such as homology, homoplasy, convergence, and parallelism, which are often used in discussions of brain evolution, are sometimes misunderstood or misapplied. Such issues have been discussed in detail by Bock (1969), Campbell (1976a,b), Hodos (1976, 1988), Hodos and Campbell (1969, 1989), Northcutt (1985), and Simpson (1961).

Much has been written about homologies of cortical gyri and sulci, as well as about the evolution of cerebral cortex in general (Table VIII). It has been common in comparative studies of cerebral cortex to identify sulci and gyri in different mammals as homologous on the basis of their similarity in topography, particularly their similarity in size, shape, spatial orientation, and relative position with respect to other sulci and gyri. It should be remembered that although sulci are useful guides to the location of gyri, it is not appropriate to consider sulci as being homologous under any circumstances since sulci are merely gaps between adjacent gyri. Sulci are not functional neuronal entities. The gyri are the entities which should be compared.

In attempting to homologize cortical gyri or their component areas, it is essential to make comparisons of as many neural characters, and their correlated developmental and functional features, as possible. Mere comparison of external morphologic or topographic appearance is inadequate. Gyri are clearly multifaceted entities.

Enough has been said to make it clear that much more needs to be known about gyral structures, their development, architecture, connectivity, and function before conclusions regarding the evolution of cerebral convolutions can be considered well founded. Moreover, it is of little value to discuss such matters further here since they have little direct relevance to the determinants of gyri and sulci.

7. Explanation of Gyrification and Fissuration

I have repeatedly emphasized the fundamental role of gyrogenesis in producing convoluted cerebral cortex. My approach to this topic has employed the traditional reductionist approach for explaining biological phenomena. I believe that many answers to the questions I have raised regarding determinants of the many micro- and macroscopic features of gyral–sulcal cortex can be answered directly by experimentation. This is my personal bias.

Others have employed mechanical, geometric, or mathematical models to account for the phenomena of convolutions (Table IX). Bok (1929, 1959) was one of the first to treat the topic of fissuration in a detailed, extensive, and quantitative manner (Fig. 75B). His model is basically mechanical. Clark (1945)

Table IX. Literature on Explanations of Cortical Folding

Ariëns Kappers (1913)	Holloway (1974, 1975, 1979)
Armstrong (1982a,b, 1983)	Jefferson (1915)
Baillarger (1845)	Jerison (1970a, 1973, 1976, 1977b, 1978,
Bauchot (1978)	1979a–c)
Bok (1929, 1959)	Jerison and Jerison (1988)
Castle (1932)	Kaas (1982, 1987)
Clark (1945)	Lewis (1947)
Clark and Medawar (1945)	Northcutt (1985)
Cole (1911)	Peters (1983)
Count (1947)	Prothero and Sundsten (1984)
Dareste (1852)	Richman *et al.* (1975)
Dubois (1928, 1930)	Seitz (1887)
Ebbesson (1984)	Smith (1907a)
Geschwind and Galaburda (1985, 1987)	Todd (1982)
Glasser (1916)	Wall (1988)
Harde (1957)	Weiss (1967)
Harman (1943, 1947a,b)	Wright (1934)
Hofman (1989)	

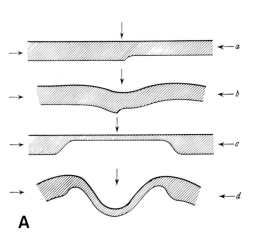

A

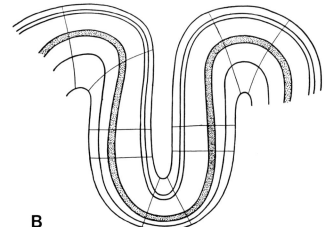

B

Figure 75. Diagrammatic conceptions of cortical folding. (A) Clark's (1945) schematic diagram illustrating how beams off uneven thickness (a and c) are expected to deform by buckling (b and d) by lateral compressive mechanical forces. Clark used physical analogies to suggest why adjacent cortical areas that have different structure, connections, and functions tend to be separated by limiting sulci. He held that the cortex buckles at such locations such that fundi fold inward and gyral crowns pitch outward. (B) Bok's (1959) portrayal of the relative thickness and curvature of cortical layers in a sulcus and in the adjacent walls and gyri within a single architectonic field. In the concave fundic cortex, cortex is thinnest, but the deeper layers are less thick, whereas the outer layers (I and II) are thicker than in the flat cortex of the sulcal walls. The opposite is seen in crown cortex, which is not only thicker overall, but its deeper layers are relatively thicker and the upper layers (I and II) are thinner than in the flat cortex of sulcal walls. Bok attributed these differences between crown and fundic cortex as due to bunching and stretching due simply to the mechanical fold-ing of flat cortex. Bok's thesis was that in crown cortex superficial layers became stretched out and deeper layers bunched up, whereas in concave fundic cortex superficial layers bunched up and deeper layers became stretched. He held that in both crown and fundus, these reverse patterns of stretching and bunching maintained constant volume relationships between superficial and deeper layers, relationships such as exist in the superficial and deep layers of the flat cortex of sulcal walls. Thin lines demarcate such equivalent volume sectors in the crown, wall, and fundus. These lines were drawn aligned with cell columns in human cortex. His quantitative results of cortical and laminar thickness were the same in 17 different architectonic fields. Bok discounted the views of Ariëns Kappers (1913) and others who believed that these laminar differences, as well as the myeloarchitectonic differences (see Fig. 32), reflected functional differences between crown, wall, and fundus. (A reproduced with permission from Clark, 1945, Fig. 6; B reproduced with permission from Bok, 1959, Fig. 1.)

also held a simple mechanical view of cortical folding (Fig. 75A). Other types of models have been proposed (see Hofman, 1989), but the one that I find most interesting is the one by Prothero and Sundsten (1984) depicted in Fig. 76. An important discovery in their model was the concept of a gyral window; that a gyrus must remain sufficiently broad to allow passage of afferent and efferent

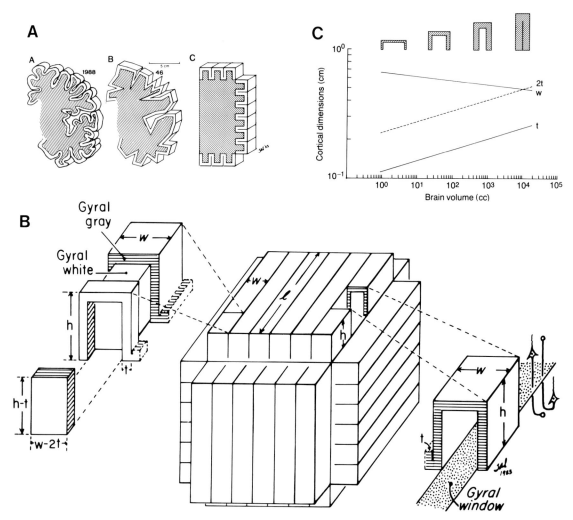

Figure 76. Prothero and Sundsten's illustrations of a model of cortical folding. (A) Macroscopic model showing (A) direct tracing of the cortical surface of a slab of human brain in frontal section; (B) low-resolution representation of A produced from digitized coordinates after omitting 98% of the points; (C) a section of an idealized model of the brain with the gyri represented by close-patterned slabs superimposed on the cut surface of a hemisected cube. (B) Dimensions of the full model. A model gyrus is defined by four parameters: length (l), width (w), height (h), and cortical thickness (t). A gyral "window" is shown in dots. It is the hypothetical plane at the base of each gyrus through which all the cortical fibers leaving and entering a gyrus must pass.

(C) A maximum brain size predicted by the model. Since gyral width decreases (simulated), and cortical thickness increases (empirical) with increases in brain size, there is a hypothetical extrapolated brain size at which gyral width is equal to twice its cortical thickness. The lines in the graph representing cortical thickness (t), twice cortical thickness (2t), and gyral window (w) are shown as a function of brain size. The reduction in gyral width with increasing brain size is illustrated in the cartoons at the top. This scheme reveals that a gyrus must remain sufficiently broad to allow passage of afferent and efferent fibers to its cortex. (Reproduced with permission from Prothero and Sundsten, 1984, Figs. 5 (A), 6 (B), and 7 (C) above.)

fibers to its cortex. Mechanical folding models never seemed to take this inherent limitation seriously. It was as if a slab of cortex, with all its afferents and efferents intact, could simply fold without crimping these subjacent fibers, or by reducing their number or diameter. Developmental studies make it clear that cortex does not fold in this way. Moreover, architectural studies make it clear that gyral crowns have greater innervation than walls and fundi. I conclude, therefore, that models which do not take into account the facts revealed by developmental, neuroanatomical, and neurophysiological studies are not sufficiently realistic to be useful accounts of gyrification and fissuration. The explanatory concepts developed in this chapter were presented early on in Tables IV and V. The explanatory arguments which I have presented are to be viewed as suggestions or hypotheses, even when they are stated in what seems as categorical tone.

8. Methodological Issues

Clearly, only a beginning has been made in assessing the detailed determinants of all features of convoluted cortex mentioned in this chapter. Numerous methods have already been used in examining convoluted cortex (Table X). Only a few of them have been directly applied to the study of the morphological entities of the gyri themselves. What is needed is a redirection of focus. A major boost to understanding gyral formation would occur with the use of autoradiographic techniques to examine whether timetable differences in migration, differentiation, lamination, innervation, synaptogensis, cell death, and so on

Table X. Literature on Methods

Aherne and Dunhill (1982)	Holloway and Post (1982)
Armstrong (1982a, 1985)	Hopf (1954)
Bauchot (1978)	Jerison (1973, 1979a, 1982)
Bok (1959, 1960)	Jungers (1985)
Bok and van erp Taalman Kip (1939)	Kraus *et al.* (1928)
Bonin (1941a)	Mitra (1956)
Braendgaard and Gundersen (1986)	Peters (1983)
Braitenberg (1962, 1978)	Pilbeam and Gould (1974)
Brandt (1867)	Prothero (1986)
de Beer (1948)	Radinsky (1967)
de Groot and Bierman (1986)	Rubinstein (1934)
Dubois (1920)	Sacher (1970)
Elias and Schwartz (1969, 1971)	Schmidt-Nielsen (1984)
Elias *et al.* (1967a,b, 1969, 1983)	Shariff (1953)
Fleischhauer (1978)	Sholl (1948)
Fox and Wilczynski (1986)	Siuta (1967)
Galaburda and Pandya (1982)	Snell (1891)
Gould (1975)	Stephan (1960)
Haug (1956, 1970, 1979, 1982, 1986, 1987)	Uylings *et al.* (1986)
Henneberg-Neubabelsberg (1900)	Webster (1976)
Hennig (1958)	Weibel (1979)
Hofman (1985a, 1989)	Welker (1976)
Hofman *et al.* (1986)	Wree *et al.* (1981)
Holloway (1979)	

occur between gyral crowns, walls, and fundi, or between different gyri or portions of gyri that might explain many of the unique morphological features of different gyri. Connectivity studies could be designed specifically to examine connections between specific gyri, walls, and fundi.

Species differences in gyral–sulcal patterns can be addressed best by experimental study of developmental sequences of species-typical cortical gyrogenesis. Another approach would involve genetic techniques in which selective breeding would be employed to produce lineages that exhibited specific gyral–sulcal features. One could select for differential gyral enlargement, changes in gyral width, length, shape, or number.

9. Structural–Functional Significance of Gyrification

This chapter has been an essay aimed at exploring the idea that gyri of the cerebral cortex are structural–functional entities. There is much evidence that all gyral crowns, whether at the surface or buried in depth, have enriched, hypertrophied, or specialized organization and connectivity. Every gyrus has unique families of connections, and all gyri differ from one another in such connectivities. Sulcal walls and fundi have lesser elaboration of organization and connectivity, but they too have sets of specialized connections which are different in specific ways from those of gyral crowns. Such a view of gyrification implies that different gyri have different functions, and that each one is functionally unique. In many cases, we know this to be true.

This viewpoint also implies that lissencephalic mammals have the same *basic* cortical circuits as do gyrencephalic mammals, but that their cortical areas are fewer in number, less elaborated, and interconnected in fewer or different ways with other areas.

In the various sections of this chapter, I have stated or suggested numerous testable hypotheses regarding the viewpoints expressed above. Clearly, only a smattering of evidence directly bears on many of the issues which are the main concern of this essay. It has been my aim to assemble data which seemed to me to be reasonably relevant to these issues. For my readers, I hope that this essay has raised legitimate questions that might stimulate the design of experiments which could provide more definitive answers than are now available regarding the determinants of gyri and sulci.

ACKNOWLEDGMENTS. This study received generous support over a period of 35 years from numerous sources: a Postdoctoral Fellowship from NIH (1954–1956), and Grants B-732, B-3249, B-6225, NS-14748, and K3-NB-4892 from NIH, Grant M-2786 from NIMH, and Grants BNS-08124, BNS-16230, BNS-08995, BNS-08866, BNS-42805, BSR-85036, and BSR-03687 from NSF. Further support was obtained from The Jackson Laboratory, Bar Harbor, Maine, Marineland Studios of Marineland, Florida, The Henry Vilas Park Zoological Society of Madison, Wisconsin, the State Game Farm of the (formerly) Wisconsin Conservation Department, The Alaska Fish and Game Department, The Florida Game and Fresh Water Fish Commission, The California Department of Fish and Game, the United States Fish and Wildlife Service of the Department of the Interior, and the Wisconsin Alumni Research Foundation and the University of Wisconsin Graduate School Research Committee.

The author gives special thanks to Dr. Clinton N. Woolsey, who, over the years, has given patient, kind, and generous tutelage and continuing support to the research reported here. Dr. Jerzy E. Rose also markedly influenced the points of view that I have expressed in this chapter by sharing his knowledge and wisdom about the organization of cerebral cortex. To both these great gentlemen, I am profoundly grateful.

I also thank the many coauthors (listed in the published papers from my laboratory) who made essential contributions to the conduct of experiments and data analysis, as well as to the conceptualization and written description of the research results which are summarized here. Particularly important was the continuing collaboration of my friend and colleague John I. Johnson, Jr., with whom I shared many interesting and fruitful discussions. Harry Jerison, Lenny Radinsky, Ted Bullock, Mary Carlson, Este Armstrong, Roger Reep, and many other friends and colleagues have influenced my thought, and to them I am grateful. Thanks also go to Carol Welt, who gave valuable assistance in the developmental studies that involved cortical ablations in infant kittens and raccoons. I was fortunate to have the considerable help of my colleague Tom Parker in finding, copying, and assembling the extensive bibliographic source material used in this chapter, as well as in helping me keep a balanced perspective throughout its long preparation.

I am also thankful to the many other staff members who have contributed to this work over the years. Most of them are acknowledged in our previously published comparative studies. For their contributions to the current work, I gratefully acknowledge the expert, patient, and elegant histological preparations of brain specimens by Inge Siggelkow, Jo Ann Ekleberry, and Joan Meister. I am especially grateful to Carol Lee Dizack for her artistic skill and careful concern that the illustrations which she prepared for this chapter should meet high professional standards of excellence. Her talented hand is particularly evident in the design and composition of most of the figures. I also am grateful to Terrill P. Stewart, who gave generously of his photographic talent to ensure that the illustrations and drawings included herein were of highest quality. I also give special thanks to Paul Luther, whose machinist, mechanical, woodworking, and all-around laboratory skills provided numerous ingenious customized means to make possible the necessary laboratory operations involved in our research. Also, thanks go to Iola Babcock who, throughout the years, gave abiding, efficient, and generous assistance in the preparation and conduct of sterile neurosurgical operations. Finally, I want to thank Becky Sorensen for her determined, attentive, and congenial secretarial and typing assistance, and Robert Klipstein for his friendly and efficient fiscal and office management skills, all of which facilitated the conduct of our research.

I apologize to those authors whose particularly relevant reports are cited only in tabular form, or who were not specifically cited because they were included in edited volumes which were cited instead. This was often necessary to keep the bibliography to an acceptable length, and because of a too hasty preparation of the final draft as the publishing deadline drew near and passed.

10. References

Abbie, A. A., 1947, Headform and human evolution, *J. Anat.* **81:**233–259.

Ackerknecht, E. H., and Vallois, H. V., 1956, *Franz Joseph Gall, Inventor of Phrenology and His Collection*, University of Wisconsin Medical School, Madison.

Adams, J. H., Corsellis, J. A. N., and Duchen, L. W. (eds.), 1984, *Greenfield's Neuropathology*, 4th ed., Wiley, New York.

Aherne, W. A., and Dunhill, M. S. 1982, *Morphometry*, Arnold, London.

Akert, K., 1964, Comparative anatomy of frontal cortex and thalamocortical connections, in: *The Frontal Granular Cortex and Behavior* (J. M. Warren and K. Akert, eds.), McGraw–Hill, New York, pp. 372–396.

Alderson, A. M., Diamantopoulos, E., and Downman, C. B. B., 1960, Auditory cortex of the seal (*Phoca vitulina*), *J. Anat.* **94:**506–511.

Allman, J. M., and Kaas, J. H., 1971, Representation of the visual field in striate and adjoining cortex of the owl monkey (*Aotus trivirgatus*), *Brain Res.* **35:**89–106.

Anker, M. V., Millsap, M., and Magoun, H. W., 1987, Felice Fontana's wax figures of the cortical convolutions, *FASEB J.* **1:**506.

Ariëns Kappers, C. U., 1913, Cerebral localisation and the significance of sulci, *Anat. Embryol. (XVIIth Int. Congr. Med. London Sect. I)* 273–392.

Ariëns Kappers, C. U., 1932, On some correlations between skull and brain, *Philos. Trans. R. Soc. London* **221:**391–429.

Ariëns Kappers, C. U., Huber, G. C., and Crosby, E. C., 1936, *The Comparative Anatomy of the Nervous System of Vertebrates Including man,* Macmillan Co., New York.

Armstrong, E., 1982a, A look at relative brain size in mammals, *Neurosci. Lett.* **34:**101–104.

Armstrong, E., 1982b, Mosaic evolution in the primate brain: Differences and similarities in the hominoid thalamus, in: *Primate Brain Evolution: Methods and Concepts* (E. Armstrong and D. Falk, eds.), Plenum Press, New York, pp. 131–161.

Armstrong, E., 1983, Relative brain size and metabolism in mammals, *Science* **220:**1302–1304.

Armstrong, E., 1985, Allometric considerations of the adult mammalian brain, with special emphasis on primates, in: *Size and Scaling in Primate Biology* (W. L. Jungers, ed.), Plenum Press, New York, pp. 115–146.

Armstrong, E., and Falk, D. (eds.), 1982, *Primate Brain Evolution: Methods and Concepts,* Plenum Press, New York.

Armstrong-James, M., and Fox, K., 1988, The physiology of developing cortical neurons, in: *Cerebral Cortex,* Volume 7 (A. Peters and E. G. Jones, eds.), Plenum Press, New York, pp. 237–272.

Asanuma, H., and Fernandez, J., 1974, Characteristics of projections from the nucleus ventralis lateralis to the motor cortex in the cats: An anatomical and physiological study, *Exp. Brain Res.* **20:**315–330.

Avendaño, C., and Llamas, A., 1984, Thalamic and nonthalamic direct subcortical projections to association areas of the cat's cerebral cortex, in: *Cortical Integration* (F. Reinosa-Suárez and C. Ajmone-Marsan, eds.), Raven Press, New York, pp. 195–221.

Bagley, C., Jr., 1922, Cortical motor mechanism of sheep brain, *Arch. Neurol. Psychiatry* **7:**417–453.

Bailey, P., and Bonin, G. von, 1951, *The Isocortex of Man,* University of Illinois Press, Urbana.

Bailey, P., Bonin, G. von, and McCulloch, W. S., 1950, *The Isocortex of the Chimpanzee,* University of Illinois Press, Urbana.

Baillarger, J. G. F., 1853, De l'etendue de la surface du cerveau et de ses rapports avec le développement de l'intelligence, *Ann. Med. Psych.* (Ser. 2) **5:**1–9.

Barker, D. J., and Welker, W. I., 1969, Receptive fields of first-order somatic sensory neurons innervating rhinarium in coati and raccoon, *Brain Res.* **14:**367–386.

Barron, D. H., 1950, An experimental analysis of some factors involved in the development of the fissure pattern of the cerebral cortex, *J. Exp. Zool.* **113:**553–573.

Bauchot, R., 1978, Encephalization in vertebrates. A new mode of calculation for allometry coefficients and isoponderal indices, *Brain Behav. Evol.* **15:**1–18.

Bauchot, R., 1982, Brain organization and taxonomic relationships in Insectivora and primates, in: *Primate Brain Evolution: Methods and Concepts* (E. Armstrong and D. Falk, eds.), Plenum Press, New York, pp. 163–175.

Bay, E., 1964, The history of aphasia and the principles of cerebral localization, in: *Cerebral Localization and Organization* (G. Schaltenbrand and C. N. Woolsey, eds.), University of Wisconsin Press, Madison, pp. 43–65.

Beddard, F. E., 1899, A contribution to our knowledge of the cerebral convolutions of the gorilla, *Proc. Zool. Soc. London* **5:**65–76.

Berson, D. M., and Graybiel, A. M. 1983, Subsystems within the visual association cortex as delineated by their thalamic and transcortical affiliations, in: *Molecular and Cellular Interactions Underlying Brain Functions* (J.-P Changeux, J. Glowinski, M. Imbert, and F. E. Bloom, eds.), Elsevier, Amsterdam, pp. 229–238.

Biegert, J., 1957, Der Formvandel des Primatenschädels und seine Beziehungen zur ontogenetischen

Entwicklung und den phylogenetischen Spezialisation der Kopforgane, *Gegenbauers Morphol. Jahrb.* **98**:77–199.

Bielschowsky, M., 1915, Über Mikrogyrie, *J. Psychol. Neurol.* **22**:1–83.

Bielschowsky, M., 1923, Über die oberflächengastaltung des Grosshirnmantels bei Pachygyrie, Mikrogyrie und bei normaler Entwicklung, *J. Psychol. Neurol.* **30**:29–76.

Bischoff, T. L. W., 1870, Die Grosshirnwindungen des Menschen mit Berücksichtigung ihrer Entwicklung bei dem Foetus und ihrer Anordnung bei den Affen, *Abh. Math. Phys. Kl. Bayer. Akad. Wiss.* **2**:389–499.

Black, D., 1913, The study of an atypical cerebral cortex, *J. Comp. Neurol.* **23**:351–369.

Black, D., 1915a, A note on the sulcus lunatus in man, *J. Comp. Neurol.* **25**:129–134.

Black, D., 1915b, A study of the endocranial casts of Ocapia, Giraffa and Samotherium, with special reference to the convolutional pattern in the family of Giraffidae, *J. Comp. Neurol.* **25**:329–360.

Blackwood, W., and Corsellis, J. A. N. (eds.), 1976, *Greenfield's Neuropathology*, 3rd ed., Arnold, London.

Bock, W. J., 1969, Discussion: The concept of homology, *Ann. N.Y. Acad. Sci.* **167**:71–73.

Bohringer, R. C., and Rowe, M. J., 1977, The organization of the sensory and motor areas of cerebral cortex in the platypus (*Ornithorhynchus anatinus*), *J. Comp. Neurol.* **174**:1–14.

Bok, S. T., 1929, Der Einfluss der in den Furchen und Windungen auftretenden Krümmungen der Grosshirnrinde auf die Rindenarchitecktur, *Z. Gesamte Neurol. Psychiatr.* **121**:682–750.

Bok, S. T., 1959, *Histonomy of the Cerebral Cortex*, Elsevier, Amsterdam.

Bok, S. T., 1960, Quantitative analysis of the morphological elements of the cerebral cortex, in: *Structure and Function of the Cerebral Cortex* (D. B. Tower and J. P. Schade, eds.), Elsevier, Amsterdam, pp. 7–17.

Bok, S. T., and van Erp Taalman Kip, M. J., 1939, The size of the body and the size and the number of nerve cells in the cerebral cortex, *Acta Neerl. Morphol.* **3**:1–22.

Bolk, L., Goppert, E., Kallius, E., and Lubosch, W., 1934, *Handbuch der Vergleichende Anatomie der Wirbeltiere*, Urban & Schwarzenberg, Munich.

Bonin, G. von, 1934, On the size of man's brain as indicated by skull capacity, *J. Comp. Neurol.* **59**:1–28.

Bonin, G. von, 1941a, On encephalometry, *J. Comp. Neurol.* **75**:287–314.

Bonin, G. von, 1941b, Side lights on cerebral evolution: Brain size of lower vertebrates and degree of cortical folding, *J. Gen. Psychol.* **25**:273–282.

Bonin, G. von, 1944, Architecture of the precentral motor cortex and some adjacent areas, in: *The Precentral Motor Cortex* (P. C. Bucy, ed.), University of Illinois Press, Urbana, pp 7–82.

Bonin, G. von, 1963 (Midway reprint, 1970), *The Evolution of the Human Brain*, University of Chicago Press, Chicago.

Braak, H., 1978, On the pigmentarchitectonics of the human telencephalic cortex, in: *Architectonics of the Cerebral Cortex* (M. A. B. Brazier and H. Petsche, eds.), Raven Press, New York, pp. 137–157.

Braak, H., 1984, Architectonics as seen by lipofuscin stains, in: *Cerebral Cortex*, Volume 1 (A. Peters and E. G. Jones, eds.), Plenum Press, New York, pp. 59–106.

Bradley, O. C., 1899, The convolutions of the cerebrum of the horse. Part I, *J. Anat. Physiol.* **33**:215–227.

Braendgaard, H., and Gundersen, H. J. G., 1986, The impact of recent stereological advances on quantitative studies of the nervous system, *J. Neurosci. Methods* **18**:39–78.

Braitenberg, V., 1962, A note on myeloarchitectonics, *J. Comp. Neurol.* **110**:141–156.

Braitenberg, V., 1974, Thoughts on the cerebral cortex, *J. Theor. Biol.* **46**:421–447.

Braitenberg, V., 1978, Cortical architectonics: General and areal, in: *Architectonics of the Cerebral Cortex* (M. A. B. Brazier and H. Petsche, eds.), Raven Press, New York, pp. 443–466.

Brandt, A., 1867, Sur le rapport du poids du cerveau à celui du corps chez différénts animaux, *Bull. Soc. Imp. Nat. Moscou* **40**:525–543.

Brauer, K., and Schober, W., 1970, *Catalogue of Mammalian Brains*, Fischer, Jena.

Brazier, M. A. B., 1978, Architectonics of the cerebral cortex: Research in the 19th century, in: *Architectonics of the Cerebral Cortex* (M. A. B. Brazier and H. Petsche, eds.), Raven Press, New York, pp. 9–30.

Brazier, M. A. B., and Petsche, H. (Eds.), 1978, *Architectonics of the Cerebral Cortex* Raven Press, New York,

Broca, P., 1878a, Anatomie comparée des circonvolutions cérébrales. Le Grand Lobe Limbique et la scissure limbique dans la serie des Mammiferes, *Rev. Anthropol.* **1**:385–498.

Broca, P., 1878b, Nomenclature cérébrale. Dénomination des divisions et subdivisions des hémisphéres et des anfractuosités de leur surface, *Rev. Anthropol.* **1**:193–236.

Brodmann, K., 1909, *Vergleichende Localizationslehre der Grosshirnrinde*, Barth, Leipzig.

Bruce, A., 1889, On the absence of the corpus callosum in the human brain, with the description of a new case, *Brain* **12:**171–190.

Brugge, J. F., and Reale, R. A., 1985, Auditory cortex, in: *Cerebral Cortex,* Volume 4 (A. Peters and E. G. Jones, eds.), Plenum Press, New York, pp. 229–271.

Brun, A., 1965, The subpial granular layer of the foetal cerebral cortex in man. Its ontogeny and significance in congenital cortical malformations, *Acta Pathol. Microbiol. Scand. Suppl.* **179:**1–88.

Buchwald, N. A., and Brazier, M. A. B. (eds.), 1975, *Brain Mechanisms in Mental Retardation,* Academic Press, New York.

Bullock, T. H., 1983, Epilogue: Neurobiological roots and neuroethological spouts, in: *Neuroethology and Behavioral Physiology* (F. Huber and H. Markl, eds.), Springer, Berlin, pp. 403–412.

Burton, H., 1986, Second somatosensory cortex and related areas, in: *Cerebral Cortex,* Volume 5 (E. G. Jones and A. Peters, eds.), Plenum Press, New York, pp. 31–98.

Burton, H., and Jones, E. G., 1976, The posterior thalamic region and its cortical projection in New World and Old World monkeys, *J. Comp. Neurol.* **168:**249–302.

Calder, W. A., III, 1984, *Size, Function, and Life History,* Harvard University Press, Cambridge, Mass.

Cameron, J., 1907, A brain with complete absence of the corpus callosum, *J. Anat.* **41:**293–301.

Camosso, M. E., Ambrosi, G., and Roncali, L., 1980, Correlations between developmental patterns of CNS vascular and nervous components, in: *Multidisciplinary Approach to Brain Development* (C. Di Benedetta, R. Balázs, G. Gombos, and G. Porcellati, eds.), Elsevier/North-Holland, Amsterdam, pp. 107–108.

Campbell, A. W., 1905, *Histological Studies on the Localisation of Cerebral Function,* Cambridge University Press, London.

Campbell, C. B. G., 1976a, Morphological homology and the nervous system, in: *Evolution, Brain, and Behavior: Persistent Problems* (R. B. Masterton, W. Hodos, and H. Jerison, eds.), Erlbaum, Hillsdale, N.J., pp. 143–151.

Campbell, C. B. G., 1976b, What animals should we compare? in: *Evolution, Brain, and Behavior: Persistent Problems* (R. B. Masterton, W. Hodos, and H. Jerison, eds.), Erlbaum, Hillsdale, N.J., pp. 107–113.

Campbell, C. B. G., 1982, Some questions and problems related to homology, in *Primate Brain Evolution: Methods and Concepts* (E. Armstrong and D. Falk, eds,), Plenum Press, New York, pp.1–11.

Campbell, C. B. G., and Hodos, W., 1970, The concept of homology and the evolution of the nervous system, *Brain Behav. Evol.* **3:**353–367.

Campos, G. B., and Welker, W. I., 1976, Comparisons between brains of a large and a small hystricomorph rodent: capybara, *Hydrochoerus* and guinea pig, *Cavia;* Neocortical projection regions and measurements of brain subdivisions, *Brain Behav. Evol.* **13:**243–266.

Carlson, M., 1985, Significance of single or multiple cortical areas for tactile discrimination in primates, in: *Hand Function and the Neocortex* (A. W. Goodwin and I. Darian-Smith, eds.), Springer, Berlin, pp. 1–16.

Carlson, M., and Welker, W. I., 1976, Some morphological, physiological and behavioral specializations in North American beavers (*Castor canadensis*), *Brain Behav. Evol.* **13:**302–326.

Carlson, M., and Welt, C., 1981, The somatic sensory cortex: Sm I in prosimian primates, in: *Cortical Sensory Organization,* Volume 1 (C. N. Woolsey, ed.), Humana Press, Clifton, N.J., pp. 1–27.

Castle, W. E., 1932, Body size and body proportions in relation to growth rates and natural selection, *Science* **76:**365–366.

Caviness, V. S., Jr., and Williams, R. S., 1979, Cellular pathology of developing human cortex, in: *Congenital and Acquired Cognitive Disorders* (R. Katzman, ed.), Raven Press, New York, pp. 69–89.

Caviness, V. S., Jr., Crandall, J. E., and Edwards, M. A., 1988, The reeler malformation. Implications for neocortical histogenesis, in: *Cerebral Cortex,* Volume 7 (A. Peters and E. G. Jones, eds.), Plenum Press, New York, pp. 59–89.

Chi, J. G., Dooling, E. C., and Gilles, F. H., 1977, Gyral development of the human brain, *Ann. Neurol.* **1:**86–93.

Chi, T. K., and Chang, C., 1941, The sulcal pattern of the Chinese brain, *Am. J. Phys. Anthropol.* **28:**167–211.

Chow, K. L., and Leiman, A. L., 1970, The structural and functional organization of the neocortex. A report based on an NRP work session, *Neurosci. Res. Progr. Bull.* **8:**153–220.

Clark, W. E. L., 1945, Deformation patterns in the cerebral cortex, in: *Essays on Growth and Form: Presented to D. W. Thompson* (W. E. L. Clark and P. B. Medawar, eds.), Oxford University Press (Clarendon), London, pp. 1–23.

Clark, W. E. L., and Medawar, P. B., 1945, *Essays on Growth and Form: Presented to D'Arcy Wentworth Thompson,* Oxford University Press (Clarendon), London.

Clark, W. E. L., Cooper, D. M., and Zuckerman, S. 1936, The endocranial cast of the chimpanzee, *J. R. Anthropol. Inst. Great Britain Ireland* **66:**249–268.

Clarke, E., and Dewhurst, K., 1972, *An Illustrated History of Brain Function*, University of California Press, Los Angeles.

Clarke, E., and O'Malley, C. D., 1968, *The Human Brain and Spinal Cord: A Historical Study Illustrated by Writings from Antiquity to the Twentieth Century*, University of California Press, Berkeley.

Clemente, C. D. (ed.), 1985, *Anatomy of the Human Body by Henry Gray*, 30th Am. ed., Lea & Febiger, Philadelphia.

Clemente, C. D., and Marshall, L. H., 1987, Experimental and clinical studies of the cortical convolutions, *FASEB J. (Abstr.)* **1:**506.

Cohen, M. J., and Strumwasser, F. (eds.), 1985, *Comparative neurobiology: Modes of Communication in the Nervous System*, Wiley, New York.

Cole, F. J., 1944, *A History of Comparative Anatomy*, Macmillan & Co., London.

Cole, F. J., 1911, Remarks on some points in the fissuration of the cerebrum, *J. Anat.* **46:**54–68.

Colonnier, M. L., 1966, The structural design of the neocortex, in: *Brain and Conscious Experience* (J. C. Eccles, ed.), Springer, Berlin, pp. 1–23.

Colonnier, M. L., and Rossignol, S., 1969, Heterogeneity of the cerebral cortex, in: *Basic Mechanisms of the Epilepsies* (H. H. Jasper, A. A. Ward, and A. Pope, eds.), Little, Brown, Boston, pp. 29–40.

Connolly, C. J., 1967, Development of the cerebral sulci, *Am. J. Phys. Anthropol.* **26:**113–149.

Connolly, C. J., 1936, The fissural pattern of the primate brain, *Am. J. Phys. Anthropol.* **21:**301–422.

Connolly, C. J., 1950, *External Morphology of the Primate Brain*, Thomas, Springfield, Ill.

Constantine-Paton, M., 1983, Position and proximity in the development of maps and stripes, *Trends Neurosci.* **6,** 32–36.

Count, E. W., 1947, Brain and body weight in man: Their antecedents in growth and evolution, *Ann. N.Y. Acad. Sci.* **46:**993–1122.

Courville, C. B., 1971, *Birth and Brain Damage: An Investigation into the Problems of Antenatal and Paranatal Anoxia and Allied Disorders and Their Relation to the Many Lesion-Complexes Residual Thereto*, Margaret Farnsworth Courville, Pasadena, Calif.

Cowan, W. M., 1979, The development of the brain, in: *The Brain (A Scientific American Book)*, Freeman, San Francisco, pp. 56–67.

Cowey, A., 1981, Why are there so many visual areas? in: *The Organization of the Cerebral Cortex: Proceedings of a Neurosciences Research Program Colloquium* (F. O. Schmitt, F. G. Worden, G. Adelman, and S. G. Dennis, eds.), MIT Press, Cambridge, Mass., pp. 395–413.

Crawford, M. L. J., 1985, Stimulus-specific columns in monkey visual cortex as revealed by the [^{14}C]-2-deoxyglucose method, in: *Cerebral Cortex*, Volume 3 (A. Peters and E. G. Jones, eds.), Plenum Press, New York, pp. 331–349.

Creutzfeldt, O., 1975, Some problems of cortical organization in the light of ideas of the classical hirnpathologie and of modern neurophysiology. An essay, in: *Cerebral Localization: An Otfrid Foerster Symposium* (K. J. Zulch, O. Creutzfeldt, and G. C. Galbraith, eds.), Springer, Berlin, pp. 217–226.

Creutzfeldt, O., 1976a, Thematic introduction: Definition and comparison of principles of functional organization of laminated structures in the brain, in: *Afferent and Intrinsic Organization of Laminated Structures in the Brain* (O. Creutzfeldt, ed.), Springer, Berlin, pp. xii–xxiii.

Creutzfeldt, O. (ed), 1976b, *Afferent and Intrinsic Organization of Laminated Structures in the Brain, Exp. Brain Res. Suppl.* **1.**

Cunningham, D. J., 1890a, The complete fissures of the human cerebrum, and their significance in connection with the growth of the hemisphere and the appearance of the occipital lobe, *J. Anat. Physiol.* **24:**309–345.

Cunningham, D. J., 1890c, On cerebral anatomy, *Br. Med. J. (Clin. Res.)* **2:**277–283.

Cunningham, D. J., 1892, Contribution to the surface anatomy of the cerebral hemispheres, *R. Ir. Acad. Sci. (Cunningham Mem.)* **7.**

Dareste, C., 1852, Memoire sur les circonvolutions du Cerveau chez les mammiferes, *Ann. Sci. Nat. 3 eme Ser. Zool.* **17:**34–54.

Darlington, D., 1957, The convolutional pattern of the brain and endocranial cast in the ferret (*Mustela furo* L.), *J. Anat.* **91:**52–60.

de Beer, G. R., 1937, *The Development of the Vertebrate Skull*, Oxford University Press, London.

de Beer, G. R., 1948, The quantitative investigation of the vertebrate brain and the applicability of allometric formulae to its study, *Proc. R. Soc. London (Biol.)* **135:**342–258.

de Groot, D. M. G., and Bierman, E. P. B., 1986, A critical evaluation of methods for estimating the numerical density of synapses, *J. Neurosci. Methods* **18:**79–103.

de Lacoste, M.-C., Horvath, D. S., and Woodward, D. J., 1988, Prosencephalic asymmetries in Lemuridae, *Brain Behav. Evol.* **31:**296–311.

Dellmann, H. D., and McClure, R. C., 1975, Nervous system. Central, in: *Sisson and Grossman's The Anatomy of the Domestic Animal*, 5th ed. (R. Getty, ed.), Saunders, Philadelphia, pp. 633–650.

Diamond, I. T., and Hall, W. C., 1969, Evolution of neocortex, *Science* **164:**251–262.

Diamond, I. T., Fitzpatrick, D., and Sprague, J. M. 1985, The extrastriate visual cortex: A historical approach to the relation between the "visuo-sensory" and "visuo-psychic" areas, in: *Cerebral Cortex*, Volume 4 (A. Peters and E. G. Jones, eds.), Plenum Press, New York, pp. 63–87.

Diamond, M. C., Law, F., Rhodes, H., Lindner, B., Rosenzweig, D. K., and Bennett, E. L., 1966, Increases in cortical depth and glia numbers in rats subjected to enriched environment, *J. Comp. Neurol.* **128:**117–125.

Di Benedetta, C., Balázs, R., Gombos, G., and Porcellati, G., 1980, *Multidisciplinary Approach to Brain Development*, Elsevier/North Holland, Amsterdam.

Dillon, L. S., 1963, Comparative studies of the brain in the Macropodidae. Contributions to the phylogeny of the mammalian brain. II, *J. Comp. Neurol.* **120:**43–51.

Dimond, S. J., and Blizard, D. A. (eds.), 1977, *Evolution and Lateralization of the Brain*, Ann. N.Y. Acad. Sci. **299.**

Dodgson, M. C. H., 1962, *The Growing Brain: An Essay in Developmental Neurology*, Williams & Wilkins, Baltimore.

Donaldson, H. H., 1895, *The Growth of the Brain*, Scribner's, New York.

Donaldson, H. H., 1928, A study of the brains of three scholars: Granville Stanley Hall, Sir William Osler, Edward Sylvester Morse, *J. Comp. Neurol.* **46:**1–95.

Douglas-Crawford, D., 1906, A case of absence of the corpus callosum, *J. Anat. Physiol.* **40:**57–64.

Downman, C. B. B., Woolsey, C. N., and Lende, R. A., 1960, Auditory areas I, II and Ep: Cochlear representation, afferent paths and interconnections, *Bull. Johns Hopkins Hosp.* **106:**127–142.

Dubois, E., 1920, The quantitative relations of the nervous system determined by the mechanism of the neuron, *Proc. K. Ned. Akad. Wet.* **22:**665–680.

Dubois, E., 1928, The law of necessary phylogenetic perfection of the psychencephalon, *Proc. K. Ned. Akad. Wet.* **31:**304–314.

Dubois, E., 1930, Die phylogenetische Grosshirnzunahme autonome Vervollkommnung der animalen Functionen, *Biol. Gen.* **6:**247–292.

DuBrul, E. L., 1958, *Evolution of the Speech Apparatus*, Thomas, Springfield, Ill.

DuBrul, E. L., and Laskin, D. M., 1961, Preadaptive potentialities of the mammalian skull: An experiment in growth and form, *Am. J. Anat.* **109:**117–132.

Dvořák, K., Feit, J., and Juránková, Z., 1978, Experimentally induced focal microgyria and status verrucosus deformis in rats—Pathogenesis and interrelation. Histological and autoradiographical study, *Acta Neuropathol.* **44:**121–129.

Ebbesson, S. O. E., 1984, Evolution and ontogeny of neural circuits, *Behav. Brain Sci.* **7:**321–366.

Ebner, F. F., 1967, Afferent connections to neocortex in the opossum (*Didelphis virginiana*), *J. Comp. Neurol.* **129:**241–268.

Ebner, F. F., 1969, A comparison of primate forebrain organization in metatherian and eutherian mammals, *Ann. N.Y. Acad. Sci.* **167:**241–257.

Ebner, F. F., and Myers, R. E., 1962, Commissural connections in the neocortex of monkey, *Anat. Rec.* **142:**299.

Ebner, F. F., and Myers, R. E., 1965, Distribution of corpus callosum and anterior commissure in cat and raccoon, *J. Comp. Neurol.* **124:**353–365.

Eccles, J. C., 1984, The cerebral neocortex: A theory of its operation, in: *Cerebral Cortex*, Volume 2 (E. G. Jones and A. Peters, eds.), Plenum Press, New York, pp. 1–36.

Ecker, A., 1873, *The Convolutions of the Human Brain* (translated from German 1869 text), Galton, London.

Economo, C. von, 1927, *L'Architecture Cellulaire Normale de L'Écorce Cérébrale* (French edition translated by L. van Bogasert), Masson, Paris.

Economo, C. von, 1930, Cytoarchitectony and progressive cerebration, *Psychiatr. Q.* **4:**142–150.

Economo, C. von, and Koskinas, G. N., 1925, *Die Cytoarchitektonik der Hirnrinde des erwachsenen Menschen,* Springer, Berlin.

Edelman, G. M., 1986, Cell adhesion molecules in the regulation of animal form and tissue pattern, *Annu. Rev. Cell Biol.* **2:**81–116.

Edelman, G. M., 1987, *Neural Darwinism: The Theory of Neuronal Group Selection*, Basic Books, New York.

Edelman, G. M., and Thiery, J.-P. (eds.), 1985, *The Cell in Contact: Adhesions and Junctions as Morphogenetic Determinants.* Wiley, New York.

Edelman, G. M., Gall, W. E., and Cowan, W. M. (eds.), 1985, *Molecular Bases of Neural Development,* Wiley, New York.

Edinger, L., 1899, *The Anatomy of the Central Nervous System of Man and of Vertebrates in General,* Davis, Philadelphia.

Edinger, T., 1948, Evolution of the horse brain, *Memoir Series of the Geological Society of America (Memoir 25),* Waverly Press, Baltimore.

Edinger, T., 1967, Brains from 40 million years of camelid history, in: *Evolution of the Forebrain: Phylogenesis and Ontogenesis of the Forebrain* (R. Hassler and H. Stephan, eds.), Plenum Press, New York, pp. 153–161.

Edinger, T., 1975, Paleoneurology 1804–1966. An annotated bibliography, *Adv. Anat. Embryol. Cell Biol.* **49.**

Elias, H., and Schwartz, D., 1969, Surface areas of the cerebral cortex of mammals determined by stereological methods, *Science* **166:**111–113.

Elias, H., and Schwartz, D., 1971, Cerebro-cortical surface areas, volumes, lengths of gyri and their interdependence in mammals, including man, *Z. Saeugetierkd.* **36:**147–163.

Elias, H., Haug, H., Lange, W., and Schwartz, D., 1967a, Cerebro-cortical surface areas of some mammals, *Am. Zool.* **7:**291.

Elias, H., Kolodny, S., and Schwartz, D., 1967b, Oberflächenmessungen der Grosshirnrinde von Säugern mit besonderer Berücksichtigung des Menschen, der Cetacea, des Elefanten und der Marsupalia, in: *Stereology: Proceedings of the Second International Congress for Stereology* (H. Elias, ed.), Springer, Berlin, pp. 77–78.

Elias, H., Haug, H., Lange, W., Schlenska, G., and Schwartz, D., 1969, Oberflächenmessungen der Grosshirnrinde von Säugern mit besonderer Berücksichtigung des Menschen, der Cetacea, des Elephanten und der Marsupiala, *Anat. Anz.* **124:**461–463.

Elias, H., Hyde, D. M., and Scheaffer, R. L. (eds.), 1983, *A Guide to Practical Stereology,* Karger, Basel.

England, D. R., and Dillon, L. S., 1972, Cerebrum of the sea otter, *Tex. J. Sci.* **24:**221–232.

Evrard, P., Caviness, V. S., Jr., Prats-Vinas, J., and Lyon, G., 1978, The mechanisms of arrest of neuronal migration in the Zellweger malformation: An hypothesis based upon cytoarchitectonic analysis, *Acta Neuropathol.* **41:**109–117.

Falk, D., 1980, Hominid brain evolution: The approach from paleoneurology, *Yearb. Phys. Anthropol.* **23:**93–107.

Falk, D., 1981, Sulcal patterns of fossil *Theropithecus* baboons: Phylogenetic and functional implications, *Int. J. Primatol.* **2:**57–69.

Falk, D., 1982, Mapping fossil endocasts, in: *Primate Brain Evolution: Methods and Concepts* (E. Armstrong and D. Falk, eds.), Plenum Press, New York, pp. 217–226.

Falzi, G., Perrone, P., and Vignolo, L. A., 1982, Right–left asymmetry in anterior speech region, *Arch. Neurol.* **39:**239–240.

Farkas-Bargeton, E., and Diebler, M. F., 1978, A topographical study of enzyme maturation in human cerebral neocortex: A histochemical and biochemical study, in: *Architectonics of the Cerebral Cortex* (M. A. B. Brazier and H. Petsche, eds.), Raven Press, New York, pp. 175–190.

Feldman, S. H., and Johnson, J. I., Jr., 1988, Kinesthetic cortical area anterior to primary somatic sensory cortex in the raccoon (*Procyon lotor*), *J. Comp. Neurol.* **277:**80–95.

Ferrer, I., 1984, A Golgi analysis of unlayered polymicrogyria, *Acta Neuropathol.* **65:**69–76.

Ferrer, I., Fábregues, I., and Condom, E., 1986a, A Golgi study of the sixth layer of the cerebral cortex. I. The lissencephalic brain of Rodentia, Lagomorpha, Insectivora and Chiroptera, *J. Anat.* **145:**217–234.

Ferrer, I., Fábregues, I., and Condom, E., 1986b, A Golgi study of the sixth layer of the cerebral cortex. II. The gyrencephalic brain of Carnivora, Artiodactyla and Primates, *J. Anat.* **146:**87–104.

Ferrer, I., Fábregues, I., and Condom, E., 1987, A Golgi study of the sixth layer of the cerebral cortex. III. Neuronal changes during normal and abnormal cortical folding, *J. Anat.* **152:**71–82.

Filimonoff, I. N., 1928, Über die Varianten der Hirnfurchen des Hundes, *J. Psychol. Neurol.* **36:**22–43.

Filimonoff, I. N., 1964, Homologies of the cerebral formations of mammals and reptiles, *J. Hirnforsch.* **7:**229–251.

Finlay, B. L., Wikler, K. C., and Sengelaub, D. R., 1987, Regressive events in brain development and scenarios for vertebrate brain evolution, *Brain Behav. Evol.* **30:**102–117.

Fitzpatrick, K. A., and Imig, T. J., 1982, Organization of auditory connections. The primate auditory cortex, in: *Cortical Sensory Organization,* Volume 3 (C. N. Woolsey, ed.), Humana Press, Clifton, N.J., pp. 71–109.

Flechsig, P., 1898, Neue Untersuchungen über die Markbildung in den menschlichen Grosshirnlappen, *Neurol. Centralbl.* **17**:977–996.

Fleischhauer, K., 1978, Cortical architectonics: The last 50 years and some problems of today, in: *Architectonics of the Cerebral Cortex* (M. A. B. Brazier and H. Petsche, eds.), Raven Press, New York, pp. 99–118.

Fleischhauer, K., and Detzer, K., 1975, Dendritic bundling in the cerebral cortex, in: *Physiology and Pathology of Dendrites* (G. W. Kreutzberg, ed.), Raven Press, New York, pp. 71–77.

Fleischhauer, K., Zilles, K., and Schleicher, A., 1980, A revised cytoarchitectonic map of the neocortex of the rabbit *(Oryctolagus cuniculus), Anat. Embryol.* **161**:121–143.

Foster, R. E., Donoghue, J. P., and Ebner, F. F., 1981, Laminar organization of efferent cells in the parietal cortex of the Virginia opossum, *Exp. Brain Res.* **43**:330–336.

Fox, J. H., and Wilczynski, W., 1986, Allometry of major CNS divisions: Towards a reevaluation of somatic brain–body scaling, *Brain Behav. Evol.* **28**:157–169.

Fox, J. L., Kurtzke, J. F., Masucci, E. F., and Ferrero, A. A., 1965, Cerebral midline displacement with a cerebellar lesion, *Acta Neurol. Latinoam.* **11**:174–184.

Frick, H., and Nord, H. J., 1963, Domestikation und Hirngewicht, *Anat. Anz.* **113**:307–316.

Friede, R., 1954, Der quantitative Anteil der Glia an der Cortexentwicklung, *Acta Anat.* **20**:290–296.

Friede, R. L., 1975, *Developmental Neuropathology,* Springer-Verlag, Berlin.

Friedman, D. P., 1983, Laminar patterns of termination of cortico-cortical afferents in the somatosensory system, *Brain Res.* 273:247–151.

Friedman, D. P., and Jones, E. G., 1981, Thalamic input to areas 3a and 2 in monkeys, *J. Neurophysiol.* **45**:59–85.

Friedman, D. P., Jones, E. G., and Burton, H., 1980, Representation pattern in the second somatic sensory area of the monkey cerebral cortex, *J. Comp. Neurol.* **192**:21–41.

Galaburda, A. M., 1979, Anatomical asymmetries, in: *Neural Growth and Differentiation* (E. Meisami and M. A. B. Brazier, eds.), Raven Press, New York, pp. 11–25.

Galaburda, A. M., and Pandya, D. N., 1982, Role of architectonics and connections in the study of primate brain evolution, in: *Primate Brain Evolution: Methods and Concepts* (E. Armstrong and D. Falk, eds.), Plenum Press, New York, pp. 203–216.

Galaburda, A. M., LeMay, M., Kemper, T. L., and Geschwind, N., 1978, Right–left asymmetries in the brain. Structural differences between the hemispheres may underlie cerebral dominance, *Science* **199**:852–856.

Galaburda, A., Sherman, G., and Geschwind, N., 1985, Cerebral lateralization: Historical notes on animal studies, in: *Cerebral Lateralization in Nonhuman Species* (S. D. Glick, ed.), Academic Press, New York, pp. 1–10.

Gerhardt, E., 1940, Die cytoarchitektonik des Isocortex parietalis beim Menschen, *J. Psychol. Neurol.* **49**:367–419.

Geschwind, N., and Galaburda, A. M. (eds.), 1984, *Cerebral Dominance: The Biological Foundations,* Harvard University Press, Cambridge, Mass.

Geschwind, N., and Galaburda, A. M., 1985, Cerebral lateralization. Biological mechanisms, associations, and pathology: I. A hypothesis and a program for research, *Arch. Neurol.* **42**:428–459.

Geschwind, N., and Galaburda, A. M., 1987, *Cerebral Lateralization: Biological Mechanisms, Associations, and Pathology,* MIT Press, Cambridge, Mass.

Geschwind, N., and Levitsky, W., 1968, Human brain: Left–right asymmetries in temporal speech region, *Science* **161**:186–187.

Ghiselin, M. T., 1976, The nomenclature of correspondence: A new look at "homology" and "analogy," in: *Evolution, Brain, and Behavior: Persistent Problems* (R. B. Masterton, W. Hodos, and H. Jerison, eds.), Erlbaum, Hillsdale, N.J., pp. 129–142.

Giguere, M., and Goldman-Rakic, P. S., 1988, Mediodorsal nucleus: Areal, laminar, and tangential distribution of afferents and efferents in the frontal lobe of rhesus monkeys, *J. Comp. Neurol.* **277**:195–213.

Glasser, O. C., 1916, The theory of autonomous folding in embryogenesis, *Science* **44**:505–509.

Glick, S. D. (ed.), 1985, *Cerebral Lateralization in Nonhuman Species,* Academic Press, New York.

Goldman, P. S., and Galkin, T. W., 1978, Prenatal removal of frontal association cortex in the fetal rhesus monkey: Anatomical and functional consequences in postnatal life, *Brain Res.* **152**:451–485.

Goldman, P. S., and Nauta, W. J. H., 1977, Columnar distribution of cortico-cortico fibers in the frontal association, limbic, and motor cortex of the developing rhesus monkey, *Brain Res.* **122**:393–413.

Goldman-Rakic, P. S., 1980, Morphological consequences of prenatal injury to the primate brain, *Prog. Brain Res.* **53**:3–19.

Goldman-Rakic, P. S., 1981, Development and plasticity of primate frontal association cortex, in: *The Organization of the Cerebral Cortex: Proceedings of a Neurosciences Research Program Colloquium* (F. O. Schmitt, F. G. Worden, G. Adelman, and S. G. Dennis, eds.), MIT Press, Cambridge, Mass. pp. 69–97.

Goldman-Rakic, P. S., and Rakic, P., 1979, Experimental modification of gyral patterns, in: *Neural Growth and Differentiation* (E. Meisami and M. A. B. Brazier, eds.), Raven Press, New York, pp. 179–192.

Goldman-Rakic, P. S., and Schwartz, M. L., 1982, Interdigitation of contralateral and ipsilateral columnar projections to frontal association cortex in primates, *Science* **216**:755–757.

Gould, S. J., 1975, Allometry in primates, with emphasis on scaling and the evolution of the brain, in: *Approaches to Primate Paleobiology* (F. S. Szalay, ed.), Karger, Basel, pp. 244–292.

Gould, S. J., 1977, *Ontogeny and Phylogeny,* Harvard University Press, Cambridge, Mass.

Graybiel, A. M., 1972, Some ascending connections of the pulvinar and nucleus lateralis posterior of the thalamus in the cat, *Brain Res.* **44**:99–125.

Graybiel, A. M., and Berson, D. M., 1981, On the relation between transthalamic and transcortical pathways in the visual system, in: *The Organization of the Cerebral Cortex: Proceedings of a Neurosciences Research Program Colloquium* (F. O. Schmitt, F. G. Worden, G. Adelman, and S. G. Dennis, eds.), MIT Press, Cambridge, Mass., pp. 285–319.

Graybiel, A. M., and Berson, D. M., 1982, Families of related cortical areas in the extrastriate visual system. Summary of an hypothesis, in: *Cortical Sensory Organization,* Volume 2 (C. N. Woolsey, ed.), Humana Press, Clifton, N.J., pp. 103–120.

Greenfield, J. G., and Wolfsohn, J. M., 1935, Microcephalia vera. A study of two brains illustrating the agyric form and the complex microgyric form, *Arch. Neurol. Psychiatr.* **33**:1296–1316.

Greenough, W. T., and Chang, F.-L. F., 1988, Plasticity of synapse structure and pattern in the cerebral cortex, in: *Cerebral Cortex,* Volume 7 (A. Peters and E. G. Jones, eds.), Plenum Press, New York, pp. 391–440.

Gross, C. G., Desimone, R., Albright, T. D., and Schwartz, E. L., 1984, Inferior temporal cortex as a visual integration area. in: *Cortical Integration* (F. Reinoso-Suárez and C. Ajmone-Marsan, eds.), Raven Press, New York, pp. 291–315.

Gurche, J. A., 1982, Early primate brain evolution, in: *Primate Brain Evolution: Methods and Concepts* (E. Armstrong and D. Falk, eds.), Plenum Press, New York, pp. 227–246.

Hahn, M. E., Jensen, C., and Dudek, B. C., (eds.), 1979, *Development and Evolution of Brain Size: Behavioral Implications,* Academic Press, New York.

Haight, J. R., and Murray, P. F., 1981, The cranial endocast of the early Miocene marsupial, *Wynyardia bassiana.* An assessment of taxonomic relationships based upon comparisons of recent forms, *Brain Behav. Evol.* **19**:17–36.

Haight, J. R., and Neylon, L., 1978a, Morphological variation in the brain of the marsupial brush-tailed possum, *Trichosurus vulpecula, Brain Behav. Evol.* **15**:415–445.

Haight, J. R., and Neylon, L., 1987b, The organization of neocortical projections from the ventroposterior thalamic complex in the marsupial brush-tailed possum, *Trichosurus vulpecula:* A horseradish peroxidase study, *J. Anat.* **126**:459–485.

Hamburger, V., and Oppenheim, R. W., 1982, Naturally occurring neuronal death in vertebrates, *Neurosci. Comment.* **1**:39–55.

Hanaway, J., Lee, S. I., and Netsky, K. G., 1968, Pachygyria: Relation of findings to modern embryological concepts, *Neurology (Minneapolis)* **18**:791–799.

Harde, K. W., 1957, Das problem der Furchenbildung in Vorderhirn, untersucht an indischen Sciuriden, *Zool. Jahrb. Abt. Allg. Zool. Physiol. Tiere* **67**:207–228.

Harden, W. B., Jr., Arumugasamy, N., and Jameson, H. D., 1968, Pattern of localization in 'precentral' motor cortex of raccoon, *Brain Res.* **11**:611–627.

Harman, P. J., 1943, Volumes of basal ganglia and cortex in mammals, *Proc. Soc. Exp. Biol. Med.* **54**:297–298.

Harman, P. J., 1947a, On the significance of fissuration of the isocortex, *J. Comp. Neurol.* **87**:161–168.

Harman, P. J., 1947b, Quantitative analysis of the brain–isocortex relationship in mammals, *Anat. Rec.* **97**:342.

Harnad, S., Doty, R. W., Goldstein, L., Jaynes, J., and Krauthamer, G. (eds.), 1977, *Lateralization in the Nervous System,* Academic Press, New York.

Harting, J. K., and Noback, C. R., 1970, Corticospinal projections from the pre- and postcentral gyri in the squirrel monkey *(Saimiri sciureus), Brain Res.* **24:**322–328.

Hassler, R., and Muhs-Clement, K., 1964, Architektonischer Aufbau des sensorimotorischen und parietalen Kortex der Katze, *J. Hirnforsch.* **6:**377–420.

Haug, H., 1956, Remarks on the determination and significance of the gray cell coefficient, *J. Comp. Neurol.* **104:**473–492.

Haug, H., 1970, Quantitative data in neuroanatomy, *Prog. Brain Res.* **33:**113–127.

Haug, H., 1976, Die Zelldichte im Cortex der Primaten und ihre Bedeutung für die Phylogenese der Schaltzellen, *Verh. Anat. Ges.* **70:**253–258.

Haug, H., 1979, The evaluation of cell-densities and of nerve-cell size distribution by stereological procedures in a layered tissue (cortex cerebri), *Microsc. Acta* **82:**147–161.

Haug, H., 1982, The location and size distribution of neurons in the layered cortex, *Acta Stereol.* **1:**259–267.

Haug, H., 1986, History of neuromorphometry, *J. Neurosci. Methods* **18:**1–17.

Haug, H., 1987, Brain sizes, surfaces, and neuronal sizes of the cortex cerebri: A stereological investigation of man and his variability and a comparison with some mammals (primates, whales, marsupials, insectivores and one elephant), *Am. J. Anat.* **180:**126–142.

Haymaker, W., and Adams, R. D. (eds.), 1982, *Histology and Histopathology of the Nervous System,* Thomas, Springfield, Ill.

Haymaker, W., and Schiller, F., 1970, *The Founders of Neurology,* 2nd ed., Thomas, Springfield, Ill.

Hefftler, F., 1878, Die Grosshirnwindungen des Menschen und deren Beziehungen zum Schädeldach, *Arch. Anthropol.* **10:**243–252.

Henneberg-Neubabelsberg, R., 1900, Messung der Oberflächenausdehnung der Grosshirnrinde, *J. Psychol. Neurol.* **17:**144–158.

Hennig, A., 1958, Kritische Betrachtungen zur Volumen- und Oberflächenmessungen in der Mikroskopie, *Zeiss-Werkzeitschrift* **30:**3–12.

Herre, v. W., 1967, Einige Bemerkungen zur Modifikabilität, Vererbung und Evolution von Merkmalen des Vorderhirns bei Säugetieren, in: *Evolution of the Forebrain. Phylogenesis and Ontogenesis of the Forebrain* (R. Hassler and H. Stephan, eds.), Plenum Press, New York, pp 162–174.

Herron, P., 1978, Somatotopic organization of mechanosensory projections to SII cerebral neocortex in the raccoon *(Procyon lotor) J. Comp. Neurol.* **181:**717–728.

Herron, P., 1983, The connections of cortical somatosensory areas I and II with separate nuclei in the ventroposterior thalamus in the raccoon, *Neuroscience* **8:**243–257.

Herron, P., and Johnson, J. I., 1987, The organization of intracortical and commissural connections in somatosensory cortical areas I and II in the raccoon, *J. Comp. Neurol.* **257:**359–371.

Hershkovitz, P., 1970, Cerebral fissural patterns in platyrrhine monkeys, *Folia. Primatol.* **13:**213–240.

Hochstetter, F., 1924, Ueber die Entwicklung des Gehirns, *Verh. Anat. Ges.* **33:**4–23.

Hodos, W., 1976, The concept of homology and the evolution of behavior, in: *Evolution, Brain, and Behavior: Persistent Problems* (R. B. Masterton, W. Hodos, and H. Jerison, eds.), Erlbaum, Hillsdale, N.J., pp. 153–167.

Hodos, W., 1982, Some perspectives on the evolution of intelligence and the brain, in: *Animal Mind–Human Mind* (D. R. Griffin, ed.), Springer-Verlag, Berlin, pp. 44–53.

Hodos, W., 1986, The evolution of the brain and the nature of animal intelligence, in: *Animal Intelligence: Insights into the Animal Mind* (R. J. Hoage and L. Goldman, eds.), Smithsonian Museum, Washington, D.C.

Hodos, W., 1988, Comparative neuroanatomy and the evolution of intelligence, in: *Intelligence and Evolutionary Biology* (H. J. Jerison and I. Jerison, eds.), Springer-Verlag, Berlin, pp. 93–108.

Hodos, W., and Campbell, C. B. G., 1969, *Scala Naturae:* Why there is no theory in comparative psychology, *Psychol. Rev.* **76:**337–350.

Hodos, W., and Campbell, C. B. G., 1989, Evolutionary scales and comparative studies of animal cognition, in: *The Neurobiology of Comparative Cognition* (R. P. Kesner and D. S. Olton, eds.), Erlbaum, Hillsdale, N.J.

Hofer, H., 1952, Der Gestaltwandel des Schädels der Saugetierer und Vogel, mit besonderer Berücksichtigung der Knickungstypen und der Schädelbasis, *Verh. Anat. Ges.* (Suppl. Anat. Anz.) **50:**102–113.

Hofer, H. O., 1969, The evolution of the brain of primates. Its influence on the form of the skull, *Ann. N.Y. Acad. Sci.* **167:**341–356.

Hofman, M. A., 1984, *Towards a General Theory of Encephalization. An Allometric Study of the Evolution and Morphogenesis of the Mammalian Brain,* Academisch Proefschrift, Amsterdam.

Hofman, M. A., 1985a, Size and shape of the cerebral cortex in mammals. I. The cortical surface, *Brain Behav. Evol.* **27**:28–40.

Hofman, M. A., 1985b, Neuronal correlates of corticalization in mammals: A theory, *J. Theor. Biol.* **112**:77–95.

Hofman, M. A., 1989, On the evolution and geometry of the brain in mammals, *Prog. Neurobiol.* **32**:137–158.

Hofman, M. A., Laan, A. C., and Uylings, H. B. M., 1986, Bivariate linear models in neurobiology: Problems of concept and methodology, *J. Neurosci. Methods* **18**:103–114.

Hogben, L., 1971, *The Vocabulary of Science*, Stein & Day, New York.

Holloway, R. L., 1970, Neural parameters, hunting and the evolution of the human brain, in: *The Primate Brain* (C. R. Noback and W. Montagna, eds.), Appleton–Century–Crofts, New York, pp. 299–310.

Holloway, R. L., 1974, On the meaning of brain size, *Science* **184**:677–679.

Holloway, R. L., 1975, The role of human social behavior in the evolution of the brain (Forty-third James Arthur lecture on the evolution of the human brain, 1973), The American Museum of Natural History, New York.

Holloway, R. L., 1976, Paleoneurological evidence for language origins, *Ann. N.Y. Acad. Sci.* **280**:330–348.

Holloway, R. L., 1979, Brain size, allometry, and reorganization: Toward a synthesis, in: *Development and Evolution of Brain Size: Behavioral Implications* (M. E. Hahn, C. Jensen, and B. C. Dudek, eds.) Academic Press, New York, pp. 59–88.

Holloway, R. L., and Post, D. G., 1982, The relative brain measures and hominid mosaic evolution, in: *Primate Brain Evolution: Methods and Concepts* (E. Armstrong and D. Falk, eds.), Plenum Press, New York, pp. 57–76.

Hopf, A., 1954, Zur architektonischen Gliederung der menschlichen Hirnrinde: Kritische Bemerkungen zu modernen Strömungen in der Architektonik, *J. Hirnforsch* **1**:442–496.

Hopf, A., 1964, Localization in the cerebral cortex from the anatomical point of view, in: *Cerebral Localization and Organization* (G. Schaltenbrand and C. N. Woolsey, eds.), University of Wisconsin Press, Madison, pp. 5–16.

Hubel, D. H., and Wiesel, T. N., 1965, Receptive fields and functional architecture in two nonstriate visual areas (18 and 19) of the cat, *J. Neurophysiol.* **28**:229–289.

Huxley, J. S., 1932, *Problems of Relative Growth*, Dial Press, New York.

Huxley, J. S., Needham, J., and Lerner, I. M., 1941, Terminology of relative growth-rates, *Nature* **148**:225.

Imig, T. J., Reale, R. A., and Brugge, J. F., 1982, The auditory cortex. Patterns of corticocortical projections related to physiological maps in the cat, in: *Cortical Sensory Organization*, Volume 3 (C. N. Woolsey, ed.), Humana Press, Clifton, N.J., pp. 1–41.

Innocenti, G. M., 1986, General organization of callosal connections in the cerebral cortex, in: *Cerebral Cortex*, Volume 5 (E. G. Jones and A. Peters, eds.), Plenum Press, New York, pp. 291–353.

Jacob, H., 1936a, Eine Gruppe familiärer Mikro- und Mikrencephalie, *Z. Gesamte Neurol. Psychiatr.* **156**:633–645.

Jacob, H., 1936b, Faktoren bei der Entstehung der normalen und der entwicklungsgestörten Hirnrinde, *Z. Gesamte Neurol. Psychiatr.* **55**:1–39.

Jacob, H., 1940, Die feinere Oberflächengestaltung der Hirnwindungen, die Hirnwarzenbildung und die Mikrogyrie. Ein Beitrag zum problem der Furchen- und Windungsbildung des menschlichen Gehirns, *Z. Gesamte Neurol. Psychiatr.* **170**:64–84.

Jacobs, M. S., Galaburda, A. M., McFarland, W. L., and Morgane, P. J., 1984, The insular formations of the dolphin brain: Quantitative cytoarchitectonic studies of the insular component of the limbic lobe, *J. Comp. Neurol.* **225**:396–432.

Jacobson, M., 1978, *Developmental Neurobiology*, 2nd ed., Plenum Press, New York.

Jameson, H. D., Arumugasamy, N., and Hardin, W. B., Jr., 1968, The supplementary motor area of the raccoon, *Brain Res.* **11**:628–637.

Jefferson, G., 1913, The morphology of the sulcus interparietalis (*B.N.A.*), J. Anat. Physiol. **47**:365–380.

Jefferson, G., 1915, Cortical localisation and furrow formation, *J. Comp. Neurol.* **25**:291–300.

Jellinger, K., and Rett, A., 1976, Agyria–pachygyria (lissencephaly syndrome), *Neuropaediatrie* **7**:66–91.

Jerison, H. J., 1970a, Brain evolution: New light on old principles, *Science* **170**:1224–1225.

Jerison, H. J., 1970b, Gross brain indices and the analysis of fossil endocasts, in: *The Primate Brain* (C. R. Noback, and W. Montagna, eds.), Appleton–Century–Crofts, New York, pp. 225–244.

Jerison, H. J., 1973, *Evolution of the Brain and Intelligence,* Academic Press, New York.

Jerison, H. J., 1976, Principles of the evolution of the brain and behavior, in: *Evolution, Brain, and Behavior: Persistent Problems* (R. B. Masterton, W. Hodos, and H. Jerison, eds.), Erlbaum, Hillsdale, N.J., pp. 23–45.

Jerison, H. J., 1977a, Should phrenology be rediscovered? *Curr. Anthropol.* **18:**744–746.

Jerison, H. J., 1977b, The theory of encephalization, *Ann. N.Y. Acad. Sci.* **299:**146–160.

Jerison, H. J., 1978, Brain and intelligence in whales, in: *Whales and Whaling* (Sir S. Frost, ed.), Government Publishing Service, Canberra, Australia, pp. 159–197.

Jerison, H. J., 1979a, Brain, body and encephalization in early primates, *J. Hum. Evol.* **8:**615–635.

Jerison, H. J., 1979b, The evolution of diversity in brain size, in: *Development and Evolution of Brain Size* (M. E. Hahn, C. Jensen, and B. Dudek, eds.), Academic Press, New York, pp. 29–57.

Jerison, H. J., 1979c, On the evolution of neurolinguistic variability: Fossil brains speak, in: *Individual Differences in Language Ability and Language Behavior* (C. J. Fillmore, D. Kempler, and S.-Y. Wang, eds.), Academic Press, New York, pp. 277–287.

Jerison, H. J., 1982, Allometry, brain size, cortical surface, and convolutedness, in: *Primate Brain Evolution: Methods and Concepts* (E. Armstrong and D. Falk, eds.), Plenum Press, New York, pp. 77–84.

Jerison, H. J., and Jerison, I. (eds.), 1988, *Intelligence and Evolutionary Biology,* Springer-Verlag, Berlin.

Johnson, J. I., 1977, Central nervous system of marsupials, in: *The Biology of Marsupials* (Hunsaker, D., II, ed.), Academic Press, New York, pp. 157–278.

Johnson, J. I., 1980, Morphological correlates of specialized elaborations in somatic sensory cerebral neocortex, in: *Comparative Neurology of the Telencephalon* (S. O. E. Ebbesson, ed.), Plenum Press, New York, pp. 423–447.

Johnson, J. I., 1985, Thalamocortical organization in the raccoon: Comparison with the primate, in: *Hand Function and the Neocortex* (A. W. Goodwin and I. Darian-Smith, eds.), Springer, Berlin, pp. 294–312.

Johnson, J. I., Welker, W. I., and Pubols, B. H., Jr., 1968, Somatotopic organization of raccoon dorsal column nuclei, *J. Comp. Neurol.* **132:**1–44.

Johnson, J. I., Haight, J. R., and Megirian, D., 1973, Convolutions related to sensory projections in cerebral neocortex of marsupial wombats, *J. Anat.* **114:**153 (abstract).

Johnson, J. I., Rubel, E. W., and Hatton, G. E., 1974, Mechanosensory projections to cerebral cortex of sheep, *J. Comp. Neurol.* **158:**81–108.

Johnson, J. I., Ostapoff, E. M., and Warach, S., 1982, The anterior border zones of primary somatic sensory (S1) neocortex and their relation to cerebral convolutions, shown by micromapping of peripheral projections to the region of the fourth forepaw digit representations in raccoons, *Neuroscience* **7:**915–936.

Johnston, M. V., 1988, Biochemistry of neurotransmitters in cortical development, in: *Cerebral Cortex,* Volume 7 (A. Peters and E. G. Jones, eds.), Plenum Press, New York, pp. 211–236.

Jones, E. G., 1976, Commissural, cortico-cortical and thalamic "columns" in the somatic sensory cortex of primates, in: *Afferent and Intrinsic Organization of Laminated Structures in the Brain* (O. Creutzfeldt, ed.), Springer, Berlin, pp. 309–316.

Jones, E. G., 1984a, History of cortical cytology, in: *Cerebral Cortex,* Volume 1 (A. Peters and E. G. Jones, eds.), Plenum Press, New York, pp. 1–32.

Jones, E. G., 1984b, Laminar distribution of cortical efferent cells, in: *Cerebral Cortex,* Volume 1 (A. Peters and E. G. Jones, eds.), Plenum Press, New York, pp. 521–553.

Jones, E. G., 1984c, Organization of the thalamocortical complex and its relation to sensory processes, in: *Handbook of Physiology,* Section 1, Volume III, Part I (J. M. Brookhart and V. B. Mountcastle, eds.), American Physiological Society, Bethesda, pp. 149–212.

Jones, E. G., 1985, *The Thalamus,* Plenum Press, New York.

Jones, E. G., 1986, Connectivity of the primate sensory–motor cortex, in: *Cerebral Cortex,* Volume 5 (E. G. Jones and A. Peters, eds.), Plenum Press, New York, pp. 113–183.

Jones, E. G., and Burton, H., 1974, Cytoarchitecture and somatic sensory connectivity of thalamic nuclei other than the ventrobasal complex in the cat, *J. Comp. Neurol.* **154:**395–432.

Jones, E. G., and Burton, H., 1976, Areal differences in the laminar distribution of thalamic afferents in cortical fields of the insular, parietal and temporal regions of primates, *J. Comp. Neurol.* **168:**197–248.

Jones, E. G, and Powell, T. P. S., 1969a, Connexions of the somatic sensory cortex of the rhesus monkey. I. Ipsilateral cortical connexions, *Brain* **92:**477–502.

Jones, E. G., and Powell, T. P. S., 1969b, Connexions of the somatic sensory cortex of the rhesus monkey. II. Contralateral cortical connexions, *Brain* **92**:717–730.

Jones, E. G., and Powell, T. P. S., 1970, Connexions of the somatic sensory cortex of the rhesus monkey. III. Thalamic connexions, *Brain* **93**:37–56.

Jones, E. G., and Wise, S. P., 1977, Size, laminar and columnar distribution of efferent cells in the sensory-cortex of monkeys, *J. Comp. Neurol.* **175**:391–438.

Jones, E. G., Burton, H., and Porter, R., 1975, Commissural and cortico-cortical "columns" in the somatic sensory cortex of primates, *Science* **190**:572–574.

Jones, E. G., Coulter, J. D., Burton, H., and Porter, R., 1977, Cells of origin and terminal distribution of corticostriatal fibers arising in the sensory–motor cortex of monkeys, *J. Comp. Neurol.* **173**:53–80.

Jones, E. G., Coulter, J. D., and Hendry, S. H. C., 1978, Intracortical connectivity of architectonic fields in the somatic sensory, motor and parietal cortex of monkeys, *J. Comp. Neurol.* **181**:291–348.

Jones, E. G., Wise, S. P., and Coulter, J. D., 1979, Differential thalamic relationships of sensory–motor and parietal cortical fields in monkeys, *J. Comp. Neurol.* **183**:833–882.

Jungers, W. L. (ed.), 1985, *Size and Scaling in Primate Biology,* Plenum Press, New York.

Kaas, J. H., 1982, The segregation of function in the nervous system: Why do sensory systems have so many subdivisions? in: *Contributions to Sensory Physiology* (D. Neff, ed.), Academic Press, New York, pp. 201–240.

Kaas, J. H., 1987, The organization of neocortex in mammals: Implications for theories of brain function, *Annu. Rev. Psychol.* **38**:129–151.

Kalter, H., 1968, *Teratology of the Central Nervous System,* University of Chicago Press, Chicago.

Kandel, E. R., and Schwartz, J. H. (eds.), 1985, *Principles of Neural Science,* 2nd ed., Elsevier, Amsterdam.

Karplus, J. P., 1905, Ueber Familienähnlichkeiten an den Grosshirnfurchen des Menschen, *Arb. Neurol. Inst. Wein* **12**:1–58 (with 20 plates).

Kawamura, K., 1971, Variations of the cerebral sulci in the cat, *Acta Anat.* **80**204–221.

Kawamura, K., 1973a, Corticocortical fiber connections of the cat cerebrum. I. The temporal region, *Brain Res.* **51**:1–21.

Kawamura, K., 1973b, Corticocortical fiber connections of the cat cerebrum. II. The parietal region, *Brain Res.* **51**:23–40.

Kawamura, K., 1973c, Corticocortical fiber connections of the cat cerebrum. III. The occipital region, *Brain Res.* **51**:41–60.

Kawamura, K., and Naito, J., 1976, Corticocortical afferents to the cortex of the middle suprasylvian sulcus area in the cat, in: *Afferent and Intrinsic Organization of Laminated Structures in the Brain* (O. Creutzfeldt, ed.), Springer-Verlag, Berlin, pp. 323–328.

Kawamura, K., and Otani, K., 1970, Corticocortical fiber connections in the cat cerebrum: The frontal region, *J. Comp. Neurol.* **139**:423–448.

Kemper, T. L., and Galaburda, A. M., 1984, Principles of cytoarchitectonics, in: *Cerebral Cortex,* Volume 1 (A. Peters and E. G. Jones, eds.), Plenum Press, New York, pp. 35–58.

Kier, L. E., 1977, The cerebral ventricles: A phylogenetic and ontogenetic study, in: *Radiology of the Skull and Brain: Anatomy and Pathology* (T. H. Newton and D. G. Potts, eds.), Mosby, St. Louis, pp. 2787–2914.

Killackey, H. P., 1973, Anatomical evidence for cortical subdivisions based on vertically discrete thalamic projections from the ventral posterior nucleus to cortical barrels in the rat, *Brain Res.* **51**:326–331.

Killackey, H. P., and Ebner, F. F., 1972, Two different types of thalamocortical projections to a single cortical area in mammals, *Brain Behav. Evol.* **6**:141–169.

Killackey, H. P., and Ebner, F. F., 1973, Convergent projections of three separate thalamic nuclei on to a single cortical area, *Science* **179**:283–285.

Kirsch, J. A. W., and Johnson, J. I., 1983, Phylogeny through brain traits: Trees generated by neural characters, *Brain Behav. Evol.* **22**:60–69.

Klatt, B., 1921, Studien zum Domestikationsproblem. Untersuchungen am Hirn, *Bibl. Genet.* **11**:1–180.

Klatt, B., 1949, Die theoretische Biologie und die Problematik der Schädelform, *Biol. Gen.* **19**:51–89.

Klatt, B., and Oboussier, H., 1951, Weitere Untersuchungen zur Frage der quantitäiven Verschiedenheiten gegensätzlicher Wuchsformtypen beim Hund, *Zool. Anz.* **146**:223–240.

König, N., and Marty, R., 1981, Early neurogenesis and synaptogenesis in cerebral cortex, in: *Studies of Normal and Abnormal Development of the Nervous System* (W. Lierse and F. Beck, eds.), Karger, Basel, pp. 152–160.

Kraus, W. M., Davison, C., and Weil, A., 1928, The measurement of cerebral and cerebellar surfaces. III. Problems encountered in measuring the cerebral cortex surface in man, *Arch. Neurol. Psychiatr.* **19**:454–477.

Kreiner, J., 1960, Myeloarchitectonics of the orbital gyrus of cerebral cortex, *Bull. Acad. Pol. Sci.* **8**:159–162.

Kreiner, J., 1961a, Myeloarchitectonics of the central sulcus in the dog's brain, *Bull. Acad. Pol. Sci.* **9**:481–484.

Kreiner, J., 1961b, The myeloarchitectonics of the frontal cortex in the dog, *J. Comp. Neurol.* **116**:117–133.

Kreiner, J., 1962, Myeloarchitectonics of the cingular cortex in dog, *J. Comp. Neurol.* **119**:255–267.

Kreiner, J., 1964a, Myeloarchitectonics of the sensori-motor cortex in dog, *J. Comp. Neurol.* **122**:181–200.

Kreiner, J., 1964b, Myeloarchitectonics of the parietal cortex in dog, *Acta Biol. Exp. (Warsaw)* **24**:195–212.

Kreiner, J., 1964c, Myeloarchitectonics of the perisylvian cortex in dog, *J. Comp. Neurol.* **123**:231–242.

Kreiner, J., 1968, Homologies of the fissural and gyral pattern of the hemispheres of the dog and monkey, *Acta Anat.* **70**:137–167.

Kreiner, J., 1971, The neocortex of the cat, *Acta Neurobiol. Exp.* **31**:151–201.

Kreiner, J., 1973, Fissural cortex in the brain of the mouse, *Acta Anat.* **86**:23–33.

Krieg, W. J. S., 1952, Differences of connections of gyral, sulcal and fundic cortex within the same cortical area, *Anat. Rec.* **112**:354.

Krieg, W. J. S., 1963, *Connections of the Cerebral Cortex*, Brain Books, Evanston, Ill.

Krieg, W. J. S., 1966, *Functional Neuroanatomy*, 3rd ed., Brain Books, Evanston, Ill.

Krishnamurti, A., Welker, W. I., and Sanides, F., 1976, Microelectrode mapping of modality-specific somatic sensory cerebral neocortex in slow loris, *Brain Behav. Evol.* **13**:267–283.

Krueg, J., 1878, Ueber die Furchung der Grosshirnrinde der Ungulaten, *Z. Wiss. Zool.* **31**:297–345.

Kruska, D., 1970, Über die Evolution des Gehirns in der Ordnung Artiodactyla, Owen, 1848, insbesondere der Teilordnung Suina Gray, 1868, *Z. Saeugetierkd.* **35**:214–238.

Kruska, D., 1973, Cerebralisation, Hirnevolution und domestikationsbedingte Hirngrössenänderungen innerhalb der Ordnung Perrissodactyla, Owen, 1848, und ein Vergleich mit der Ordnung Artiodactyla, Owen, 1848, *Z. Zool. Syst. Evolutionsforsch.* **11**:81–103.

Kruska, D., 1975, Über die postnatale Hirnentwicklung beim *Procyon cancrivorus cancrivorus (Procyonidae; Mammalia)*, *Z. Saeugetierkd.* **40**:243–256.

Kruska, D., 1982, Hirngrösenänderungen bei Tylopoden während der Stammesgeschichte und in der Domestikation, *Verh. Dtsch. Zool. Ges.* **75**:173–183.

Kruska, D., 1987, How fast can total brain size change in mammals? *J. Hirnforsch.* **28**:59–70.

Kruska, D., 1988, Mammalian domestication and its effect on brain structure and behavior, in: *Intelligence and Evolutionary Biology* (H. J. Jerison and I. Jerison, eds.), Springer-Verlag, Berlin, pp. 211–250.

Künzle, H., 1978, Cortico-cortical efferents of primary motor and somatosensory regions of the cerebral cortex in *Macaca fascicularis, Neuroscience* **3**:25–39.

Kuypers, H. G. J. M., 1981, Anatomy of the descending pathways, in: *Handbook of Physiology*, Section I, Volume II, Part I (J. M. Brookhart and V. B. Mountcastle, eds.), American Physiological Society, Bethesda, pp. 597–666.

Kuypers, H. G. J. M., and Catsman-Berrevoets, C. E., 1984, Frontal corticosubcortical projections and their cells of origin, in: *Cortical Integration* (F., Reinoso-Suárez and C. Ajmone-Marsan, eds.), Raven Press, New York, pp. 171–192.

Landacre, F. L., 1930, The major and minor sulci of the brain of the sheep, *Ohio J. Sci.* **30**:36–51.

Landau, E., 1911, Über individuelle, durch mechanischen Druck benachbarter Windungen verursachte Wachstumshemmungen an der Gehirnoberflache, *Morphol. Jahrb. Gegenbauer* **43**:441–448.

Landau, E., 1923, *Anatomie des Grosshirns. Formanalytische Untersuchungen*, Bircher, Bern.

Larroche, J.-C., 1977, Development of the central nervous system, in: *Developmental Pathology of the Neonate* (J.-C. Larroche, ed.), Exerpta Medica, Amsterdam, pp. 319–352.

Larsell, O., and Jansen, J., 1970, *The Comparative Anatomy and Histology of the Cerebellum from Monotremes through Apes*, University of Minnesota Press, Minneapolis.

Lashley, K., and Clark, G., 1946, The cytoarchitecture of the cerebral cortex of Ateles. A critical examination of cytoarchitectural studies, *J. Comp. Neurol.* **85**:223–305.

Leavitt, P., Rakic, P., and Goldman-Rakic, P. S., 1981, Region-specific catecholamine innervation of primate cerebral cortex, *Soc. Neurosci. Abstr.* **7**:801.

Leichnetz, G. R., 1980, An intrahemispheric columnar projection between two cortical multisensory convergence areas (inferior parietal lobule and prefrontal cortex): An anterograde study in macaque using HRP gel, *Neurosci. Lett.* **18**:119–124.

LeMay, M., 1976, Morphological cerebral asymmetries of modern man, fossil man, and nonhuman primate, in: *Origins and Evolution of Language and Speech* (S. R. Harnad, H. D. Steklis, and J. Lancaster, eds.), New York Academy of Sciences, New York, pp. 349–366.

LeMay, M., 1984, Radiological, developmental and fossil asymmetries, in: *Cerebral Dominance: The Biological Foundations* (N. Geschwind and A. M. Galaburda, eds.), Harvard University Press, Cambridge, Mass., pp. 26–42.

LeMay, M., 1985, Asymmetries of the brains and skulls of nonhuman primates, in: *Cerebral Lateralization in Nonhuman Species* (S. D. Glick, ed.), Academic Press, New York, pp. 233–245.

LeMay, M., Billig, M. S., and Geschwind, N., 1982, Asymmetries of the brains and skulls of nonhuman primates, in: *Primate Brain Evolution: Methods and Concepts* (E. Armstrong and D. Falk, eds.), Plenum Press, New York, pp. 263–277.

Lende, R. A., 1963a, Cerebral cortex: A sensorimotor amalgam in the Marsupalia, *Science* **141**:730–732.

Lende, R. A., 1963b, Sensory representation in the cerebral cortex of the opossum (*Didelphis virginiana*), *J. Comp. Neurol.* **121**:395–403.

Lende, R. A., 1969, A comparative approach to the neocortex: Localization in monotremes, marsupials and insectivores, in: *Comparative and Evolutionary Aspects of the Vertebrate Nervous System* (J. M. Petras and C. R. Noback, eds.), New York Academy of Sciences, New York, pp. 262–276.

Lende, R. A., and Sadler, K. M., 1967, Sensory and motor areas in neocortex of hedgehog (*Erinaceus*), *Brain Res.* **5**:390–405.

Lende, R. A., and Woolsey, C. N., 1956, Sensory and motor localization in cerebral cortex of porcupine (*Erethizon dorsatum*), *J. Neurophysiol.* **19**:544–563.

Lewis, W. H., 1947, Mechanics of invagination, *Anat. Rec.* **97**:139–156.

Lierse, W., and Beck, F., 1981, *Studies of Normal and Abnormal Development of the Nervous System*, Karger, Basel.

Lin, C. S., Weller, R. E., and Kaas, J. H., 1982, Cortical connections of striate cortex in the owl monkey, *J. Comp. Neurol.* **211**:165–176.

Loeser, J. D., and Alvord, C. E., 1968, Agenesis of the corpus callosum, *Brain* **91**:553–570.

Lorente de Nó, R., 1938, The cerebral cortex: Architecture, intracortical connections and motor projections, in: *Physiology of the Nervous System* (J. F. Fulton, ed.), Oxford University Press, London, pp. 291–339.

Macchi, G., and Bentivoglio, M., 1986, The thalamic intralaminar nuclei and the cerebral cortex, in: *Cerebral Cortex*, Volume 5 (E. G. Jones and A. Peters, eds.), Plenum Press, New York, pp. 355–401.

Macphail, E. M., 1982, *Brain and Intelligence in Vertebrates*, Oxford University Press, (Clarendon), London.

Magalhães-Castro, B., and Saraiva, P. E. S., 1971, Sensory and motor representation in the cerebral cortex of the marsupial *Didelphis azarae azarae*, *Brain Res.* **34**:291–299.

Magoun, H. W., and Anker, M. V., 1987, Francois Leuret's studies of the cortical convolutions in the mammalian series, *FASEB J. (Abstr.)* **1**:506.

Malamud, N., and Hirano, A., 1974, *Atlas of Neuropathology*, 2nd rev. ed., University of California Press, Berkeley.

Mangold-Wirz, K., 1966, Cerebralization und Ontogenesemodus bei Eutherian, *Acta Anat.* **63**:449–508.

Mann, G., 1896, On the homoplasty of the brain of rodents, insectivores and carnivores, *J. Anat. Physiol.* **30**:1–35.

Mann, M. D., Glickman, S. E., and Towe, A. L., 1988, Brain/body relations among myomorph rodents, *Brain Behav. Evol.* **31**:111–124.

Marin-Padilla, M., 1971, Early prenatal ontogenesis of the cerebral cortex (neocortex) of the cat (*Felis domestica*). A Golgi study. I. The primordial neocortical organization, *Z. Anat. Entwicklungsgesch.* **134**:117–145.

Marin-Padilla, M., 1972, Prenatal ontogenetic history of the principal neurons of the neocortex of the cat (*Felis domestica*). A Golgi study. II. Development differences and their significances, *Z. Anat. Entwicklungsgesch.* **136**:125–142.

Marin-Padilla, M., 1978, Dual origin of the mammalian neocortex and evolution of the cortical plate, *Anat. Embryol.* **152**:109–126.

Marin-Padilla, M., 1984, Neurons of layer I. A developmental analysis, in: *Cerebral Cortex*, Volume 1 (A. Peters and E. G. Jones, eds.), Plenum Press, New York, pp. 447–478.

Marin-Padilla, M., 1988, Early ontogenesis of the human cerebral cortex, in: *Cerebral Cortex*, Volume 7 (A. Peters and E. G. Jones, eds.), Plenum Press, New York, pp. 1–30.

Martin, K. A. C., 1984, Neuronal circuits in cat striate cortex, in: *Cerebral Cortex*, Volume 2 (E. G. Jones and A. Peters, eds.), Plenum Press, New York, pp. 241–284.

Martin, R. D., 1982, Allometric approaches to the evolution of the primate nervous system, in: *Primate Brain Evolution: Methods and Concepts* (E. Armstrong and D. Falk, eds.), Plenum Press, New York, pp. 39–56.

Martin, R. D., and Harvey, P. H., 1985, Brain size, allometry: Ontogeny and phylogeny, in: *Size and Scaling in Primate Biology* (W. Jungers, ed.), Plenum Press, New York, pp. 147–173.

Meisami, E., and Brazier, M. A. B., 1979, *Neural Growth and Differentiation,* Raven Press, New York.

Merritt, H. H., 1959, Developmental defects, in: *A Textbook of Neurology,* Lea & Febiger, Philadelphia, pp. 390–410.

Merzenich, M. M., 1982, Organization of primate sensory forebrain structures: A new perspective, in: *New Perspectives in Cerebral Localization* (R. A. Thompson and J. R. Green, eds.), Raven Press, New York, pp. 47–62.

Merzenich, M. M., 1985, Sources of intraspecies and interspecies cortical map variability in mammals, in: *Comparative Neurobiology: Modes of Communication in the Nervous System* (M. J. Cohen and F. Strumwasser, eds.), Wiley–Interscience, New York, pp. 105–116.

Merzenich, M. M., Recanzone, G., Jenkins, W. M., Allard, T. T., and Nudo, R. J., 1988, Cortical representational plasticity, in: *Neurobiology of Neocortex* (P. Rakic and W. Singer, eds.), Wiley, New York, pp. 41–67.

Mesulam, M.-M., and Mufson, E. J., 1985, The insula of Reil in man and monkey. Architectonics, connectivity and function, in: *Cerebral Cortex,* Volume 4 (A. Peters and E. G. Jones, eds.), Plenum Press, New York, pp. 179–226.

Mettler, F. A., 1933, Brain of Pithecus Rhesus (M. Rhesus), *Am. J. Phys. Anthropol.* **17:**309–331.

Meulders, M., Gybels, J, Bergmans, J., Gerebtzoff, M. A., and Goffart, M., 1966, Sensory projections of somatic, auditory and visual origin to the cerebral cortex of the sloth (*Choloepus hoffmanni* Peters), *J. Comp. Neurol.* **126:**535–546.

Meyer, A., 1971, *Historical Aspects of Cerebral Anatomy,* Oxford University Press, London.

Meyer, H. H., 1937, Die Massen- und Oberflächen-Entwicklung des fetalen Gehirns, *Virchow Arch. Pathol. Anat. Physiol.* **300:**202–224.

Millen, J. W., and Woollam, D. H. M., 1959, Observations on the experimental production of malformations of the central nervous system, *J. Ment. Defic. Res.* **3:**23–32.

Miller, G. S., Jr., 1923, The telescoping of the cetacean skull, *Smithson. Misc. Collect.* **76:**1–71.

Miller, M. W., 1988, Development of projection and local circuit neurons in neocortex, in: *Cerebral Cortex,* Volume 7 (A. Peters and E. G. Peters, eds.), Plenum Press, New York, pp. 133–175.

Minkowski, A. (ed.), 1967, *Regional Development of the Brain in Early Life,* Blackwell, Oxford.

Miodoński, A., 1974, The angioarchitectonics and cytoarchitectonics (impregnation Modo Golgi–Cox) structure of the fissural frontal neocortex in dog, *Folia Biol.* **22:**237–279.

Mitra, N. L., 1955, Quantitative analysis of cell types in mammalian neo-cortex, *J. Anat.* **89:**467–483.

Mizuno, N., Konishi, A., Sato, M., Kawaguchi, S., Yamamoto, T., Kawamura, S., and Yamawaki, M., 1975, Thalamic afferents to the rostral portions of the middle suprasylvian gyrus in the cat, *Exp. Neurol.* **48:**79–87.

Montero, V. M., 1981, Topography of the cortico-cortical connections from the striate cortex in the cat, *Brain Behav. Evol.* **18:**194–218.

Montero, V. M., 1982, Comparative studies on the visual cortex, in: *Cortical Sensory Organization,* Volume 2 (C. N. Woolsey, ed.), Humana Press, Clifton, N.J., pp. 33–81.

Moodie, R. L., 1922, On the endocranial anatomy of some Oligocene and Pleistocene mammals, *J. Comp. Neurol.* **34:**343–379.

Morel, F., and Wildi, E., 1952, Dysgénésie nodulaire disséminée de l'écorce frontale, *Rev. Neurol.* **87:**251–270.

Morgane, P. J., and Jacobs, M. S., 1973, Comparative anatomy of the cetacean nervous system, in: *Functional Anatomy of Marine Mammals* (R. J. Harrison, ed.), Academic Press, New York, pp. 117–244.

Morgane, P. J., Jacobs, M. S., and Galaburda, A., 1985, Conservative features of neocortical evolution in dolphin brain, *Brain Behav. Evol.* **26:**176–184.

Morgane, P. J., Jacobs, M. S., and Galaburda, A., 1986, Evolutionary morphology of the dolphin brain, in: *Dolphin Cognition and Behavior: A Comparative Approach* (R. J. Schusterman, J. A. Thomas, and F. G. Wood, eds.), Erlbaum, Hillsdale, N.J., pp. 5–29.

Moss, M. L., 1957, Experimental alteration of sutural area morphology, *Anat. Rec.* **127:**569–589.

Moss, M. L., 1960, Inhibition and stimulation of sutural fusion in the rat calvaria, *Anat. Rec.* **136**:457–467.

Moss, M. L., and Young, R. W., 1960, A functional approach to craniology, *Am. J. Phys. Anthropol.* **18**:281–292.

Mountcastle, V. B., 1978, Organizing principle for cerebral function: The unit module and the distributed system, in: *The Mindful Brain* (G. M. Edelman and V. B. Mountcastle, eds.), MIT Press, Cambridge, Mass., pp. 7–50.

Myers, R. E., 1976, Comparative neurology of vocalization and speech: Proof of a dichotomy, in: *Origins and Evolution of Language and Speech* (S. R. Harnad, H. D. Steklis, and J. Lancaster, eds.), New York Academy of Sciences, New York, pp. 745–757.

Myers, R. E., Valerio, M. G., Martin, D. P., and Nelson, K. B., 1973, Perinatal brain damage: Prosencephaly in a cynomolgous monkey, *Biol. Neonate* **22**:253–273.

Nelson, R. J., Sur, M., and Kaas, J. H., 1979, The organization of the second somatosensory area (SmII) of the grey squirrel, *J. Comp. Neurol.* **184**:473–490.

Neubauer, G., 1925, Experimentelle Untersuchungen über die Beeinflussung der Schädelform, *Z. Morphol. Anthropol.* **22**:411–442.

Ngowyang, G., 1934, Cytoarchitektonik des menschlichen stirnhirns. Teil I. Cytoarchitektonische Felderung der Regio granularis and dysgranularis, *Nat. Res. Inst. Psychol. Acad. Sin. Monogr.* **7**:1–54.

Noback, C. R., 1959, The heritage of the human brain (*James Arthur lecture on the evolution of the human brain*), pp. 1–30.

Noback, C. R., and Demarest, R. J., 1975, *The Human Nervous System: Basic Principles of Neurobiology,* McGraw–Hill, New York.

Noback, C. R., and Montagna, W., (eds.), 1970, *The Primate Brain,* Appleton–Century–Crofts, New York.

Noback, C. R., and Moss, M. L., 1956, Differential growth of the human brain, *J. Comp. Neurol.* **105**:539–552.

Nomina Anatomica (5th ed.), 1983, Williams & Wilkins, Baltimore.

Northcutt, R. G., 1981, Evolution of the telencephalon in nonmammals, *Annu. Rev. Neurosci.* **4**:301–351.

Northcutt, R. G., 1984, Evolution of vertebrate central nervous system: Patterns and processes, *Am. Zool.* **24**:701–716.

Northcutt, G. R., 1985, Brain phylogeny. Speculations on pattern and cause, in: *Comparative Neurobiology: Modes of Communication in the Nervous System* (M. J. Cohen and F. Strumwasser, eds.), Wiley, New York, pp. 351–378.

Obersteiner, H., 1890, The fissures and convolutions on the surface of the great brain, in: *The Anatomy of the Central Nervous Organs in Health and Disease,* Griffin, London, pp. 84–106.

Oboussier, H., 1949, Über Unterschiede des Hirnfurchenbildes beim Hunde, *Verh. Dtsch. Zool. Mainz* **8**:109–114.

Oboussier, H., 1950, Zur Frage der Erblichkeit der Hirnfurchen. Untersuchungen an Kreuzungen extremer Rassetypen des Hundes, *Z. Menschl. Vererb. Konstit. lehre* **29**:831–864.

Oboussier, H., 1972, Evolution of the mammalian brain. Some evidence on the phylogeny of the antelope species, *Acta Anat.* **83**:70–80.

Olson, C. R., and Graybiel, A. M., 1987, Ectosylvian visual area of the cat: Location, retinotopic organization, and connections, *J. Comp. Neurol.* **261**:277–294.

Olson, E. C., 1976, Rates of evolution of the nervous system and behavior, in: *Evolution, Brain, and Behavior: Persistent Problems* (R. B. Masterton, W. Hodos, and H. Jerison, eds.), Erlbaum, Hillsdale, N.J., pp. 47–77.

Owen, R., 1868, *On the Anatomy of Vertebrates,* Volume 3, Longmans, Green, London.

Packer, A. D., 1949, A comparison of endocranial cast and brain of an Australian aborigine, *J. Anat.* **83**:195–204.

Palade, G. E., 1985, Differentiated microdomains in cellular membranes: Current status, in: *The Cell in Contact: Adhesions and Junctions as Morphogenetic Determinants* (G. M. Edelman and J.-P. Thiery, eds.), Wiley, New York, pp. 9–24.

Pandya, D. N., and Sanides, F., 1973, Architectonic parcellation of the temporal operculum in rhesus monkey and its projection pattern, *Z. Anat. Entwicklungsgesch.* **139**:127–161.

Pandya, D. N., and Yeterian, E. H., 1985, Architecture and connections of cortical association areas, in: *Cerebral Cortex,* Volume 4 (A. Peters and E. G. Jones, eds.), Plenum Press, New York, pp. 3–61.

Papez, J. W., 1929, *Comparative Neurology: A Manual and Text for the Study of the Nervous System of Vertebrates,* Hafner, New York.

Papez, J. W., and Hunter, R. P., 1929, Formation of a central sulcus in the brain of the raccoon, *Anat. Rec.* **42:**60 (abstract).

Passingham, R. E., 1985, Rates of brain development in mammals including man, *Brain Behav. Evol.* **26:**167–175.

Patten, B. M., 1968, *Human Embryology*, 3rd ed., McGraw–Hill, New York.

Paul, R. L., Merzenich, M., and Goodman, H., 1972, Representation of slowly and rapidly adapting cutaneous mechanoreceptors of the hand in Brodmann's areas 3 and 1 of *Macaca mulatta*, *Brain Res.* **36:**229–249.

Payne, B., Pearson, H., and Cornwell, P., 1988, Development of visual and auditory cortical connections in the cat, in: *Cerebral Cortex*, Volume 7 (A. Peters and E. G. Jones, eds.), Plenum Press, New York, pp. 309–389.

Pearson, R., and Pearson, L., 1976, *The Vertebrate Brain*, Academic Press, New York.

Peters, A., and Jones, E. G., 1984, Classification of cortical neurons, in: *Cerebral Cortex*, Volume 1 (A. Peters and E. G. Jones, eds.), Plenum Press, New York, pp. 107–121.

Peters, R. H., 1983, *The Ecological Implications of Body Size*, Cambridge University Press, London.

Petras, J. M., Noback, C. R., 1969, Comparative and evolutionary aspects of the vertebrate central nervous system, *Ann. N.Y. Acad. Sci.* **167.**

Pickering, S. P., 1930, Correlation of brain and head measurements, and relation of brain shape and size to shape and size of the head, *Am. J. Phys. Anthropol.* **15:**1–52.

Pilbeam, D., and Gould, S. J., 1974, Size and scaling in human evolution, *Science* **186:**892–901.

Pilleri, G., 1959, The brains of *Dolichotis patagona* and *Hydrochoerus hydrochoerus*, with suggestions about endocranial relationships, *Acta Zool.* **40:**43–58.

Pimentel-Souza, F., Cosenza, R. M., Campos, G. B., and Johnson, J. I., 1980, Somatic sensory cortical regions of the agouti *Dasyprocta aguti*, *Brain Behav. Evol.* **17:**218–240.

Pinto Hamuy, T., Bromiley, R. G., and Woolsey, C. N., 1956, Somatic afferent areas I and II of dog's cerebral cortex, *J. Neurophysiol.* **19:**485–499.

Pirlot, P., 1986, Understanding taxa by comparing brains, *Perspect. Biol. Med.* **29:**499–509.

Polyak, S., 1957, *The Vertebrate Visual System* (edited by H. Kluver), University of Chicago Press, Chicago.

Powell, T. P. S., and Mountcastle, V. B., 1959a, Some aspects of the functional organization of the cortex of the postcentral gyrus of the monkey: A correlation of findings obtained in a single unit analysis with cytoarchitecture, *Bull. Johns Hopkins Hosp.* **105:**133–162.

Powell, T. P. S., and Mountcastle, V. B., 1959b, The cytoarchitecture of the postcentral gyrus of the monkey *Macaca mulatta*, *Bull. Johns Hopkins Hosp.* **105:**108–131.

Probst, F. P., 1979, *The Prosencephalies: Morphology, Neuroradiological Appearances and Differential Diagnosis*, Springer-Verlag, Berlin.

Prothero, J., 1986, Methodological aspects of scaling in biology, *J. Theor. Biol.* **118:**259–286.

Prothero, J. W., and Sundsten, J. W., 1984, Folding of the cerebral cortex in mammals. A scaling model, *Brain Behav. Evol.* **24:**152–167.

Pubols, B. H., Jr., and Pubols, L. M., 1979, Variations in the fissural pattern of the cerebral neocortex of the spider monkey (*Ateles*), *Brain Behav. Evol.* **16:**241–252.

Pubols, B. H., Jr., Pubols, L. M., DiPette, D. J., and Sheely, J. C., 1976, Opossum somatic sensory cortex: a microelectrode mapping study, *J. Comp. Neurol.* **165:**229–246.

Purves, D., 1988, *Body and Brain: A Trophic Theory of Neural Connections*, Harvard University Press, Cambridge, Mass.

Purves, D., and Lichtman, J. W., 1985, *Principles of Neural Development*, Sinauer, Sunderland, Mass.

Radinsky, L., 1967, Relative brain size: A new measure, *Science* **155:**836–837.

Radinsky, L., 1968a, Evolution of somatic sensory specialization in otter brains, *J. Comp. Neurol.* **134:**495–506.

Radinsky, L., 1968b, A new approach to mammalian cranial analysis, illustrated by examples of prosimian primates, *J. Morphol.* **124:**167–180.

Radinsky, L. B., 1968c, Otter brains, *J. Comp. Neurol.* **134:**495–506.

Radinsky, L., 1969, Outlines of canid and felid brain evolution, *Ann. N.Y. Acad. Sci.* **167:**277–288.

Radinsky, L., 1970, The fossil evidence of prosimian brain evolution, in: *The Primate Brain* (C. R. Noback and W. Montagna, eds.), Appleton–Century–Crofts, New York, pp. 209–224.

Radinsky, L., 1971, An example of parallelism in carnivore brain evolution, *Evolution* **25:**518–522.

Radinsky, L., 1972, Endocasts and studies of primate brain evolution, in: *The Functional and Evolutionary Biology of Primates* (R. Tuttle, ed.), Aldine–Atherton, Chicago, pp. 175–186.

Radinsky, L., 1973a, *Aegyptopithecus* endocasts: Oldest record of a pongid brain, *Am. J. Phys. Anthropol.* **39:**239–248.

Radinsky, L., 1973b, Are stink badgers skunks? Implications of neuroanatomy for mustelid phylogeny, *J. Mammol.* **54:**585–593.

Radinsky, L., 1973c, Evolution of the canid brain, *Brain Behav. Evol.* **7:**169–202.

Radinsky, L., 1974, Prosimian brain morphology: Functional and phylogenetic implications, in: *Prosimian Biology* (R. D. Martin, G. A. Doyle, and A. C. Walker, eds.), Duckworth, London, pp. 781–798.

Radinsky, L., 1975a, Evolution of the felid brain, *Brain Behav. Evol.* **11:**214–254.

Radinsky, L., 1975b, Primate brain evolution, *Am. Sci.* **63:**656–663.

Radinsky, L., 1975c, Viverrid neuroanatomy: Phylogenetic and behavioral implications, *J. Mammol.* **56:**130–150.

Radinsky, L., 1976a, The brain of *Mesonyx*, a middle Eocene mesonychid condylarth, *Fieldiana Geol.* **33:**323–337.

Radinsky, L., 1976b, Cerebral clues, *Nat. Hist.* **85:**54–59.

Radinsky, L., 1976c, New evidence of ungulate brain evolution, *Am. Zool.* **16:**207.

Radinsky, L., 1976d, Oldest horse brains: More advanced than previously realized, *Science* **194:**626–627.

Radinsky, L., 1977a, Brains of early carnivores, *Paleobiology* **3:**333–349.

Radinsky, L., 1977b, Early primate brains: Facts and fiction, *J. Hum. Evol.* **6:**79–86.

Radinsky, L., 1978, Evolution of brain size in carnivores and ungulates, *Am. Nat.* **112:**815–831.

Radinsky, L., 1979, *The Fossil Record of Primate Brain Evolution*, American Museum of Natural History, New York, pp. 1–27.

Radinsky, L., 1980, Endocasts of amphicyonid carnivorans, *Am. Mus. Novit.* **2694:**1–11.

Radinsky, L., 1981, Brain evolution in extinct South American ungulates, *Brain Behav. Evol.* **18:**169–187.

Radinsky, L., 1982, Some cautionary notes on making inferences about relative brain size, in: *Primate Brain Evolution: Methods and Concepts* (E. Armstrong and D. Falk, eds.), Plenum Press, New York, pp. 29–37.

Rakic, P., 1974, Neurons in rhesus monkey visual cortex: Systematic relation between time of origin and eventual disposition, *Science* **183:**425–427.

Rakic, P., 1975a, Local circuit neurons, *Neurosci. Res. Progr. Bull.* **13:**290–446.

Rakic, P., 1975b, Timing of major ontogenetic events in the visual cortex of the rhesus monkey, in: *Brain Mechanisms in Mental Retardation* (N. A. Buchwald and M. A. B. Brazier, eds.), Academic Press, New York, pp. 3–40.

Rakic, P., 1976, Differences in the time of origin and in eventual distribution in areas 17 and 18 of visual cortex in rhesus monkey, in: *Afferent and Intrinsic Organization of Laminated Structures in the Brain* (O. Creutzfeldt, ed.), Springer-Verlag, Berlin, pp. 244–248.

Rakic, P., 1978, Neuronal migration and contact guidance in the primate telencephalon, *Postgrad. Med. J.* **54:**25–40.

Rakic, P., 1979, Genetic and epigenetic determinants of local neuronal circuits in the mammalian central nervous system, in: *The Neurosciences: Fourth Study Program* (F. O. Schmitt and F. G. Worden, eds.), MIT Press, Cambridge, Mass., pp. 109–127.

Rakic, P., 1981, Developmental events leading to laminar and areal organization of the neocortex, in: *The Organization of the Cerebral Cortex: Proceedings of a Neurosciences Research Program Colloquium* (F. O. Schmitt, F. G. Worden, G. Adelman, and S. G. Dennis, eds.), MIT Press, Cambridge, Mass., pp. 7–28.

Rakic, P., 1985, Contact regulation of neuronal migration, in: *The Cell in Contact: Adhesion and Junctions as Morphogenetic Determinants* (G. M. Edelman and J.-P. Thiery, eds.), Wiley, New York, pp. 67–91.

Rakic, P., 1988, Specification of cerebral cortical areas, *Science* **241:**170–176.

Rakic, P., and Goldman-Rakic, P. S. 1982, Development and modifiability of the cerebral cortex, *Neurosci. Res. Progr. Bull.* **20:**427–611.

Rakic, P., and Yakovlev, P. I., 1968, Development of the corpus callosum and cavum septi in man, *J. Comp. Neurol.* **132:**45–72.

Rakic, P., Bourgeois, J.-P., Eckenhoff, M. F., Zecevic, N., and Goldman-Rakic, P. S., 1986, Concurrent overproduction of synapses in diverse regions of the primate cerebral cortex, *Science* **232:**232–235.

Ranke, O., 1910, Beiträge zur Kenntnis der normalen und pathologischen Hirnrindenbildung, *Beitr. Pathol. Anat.* **47:**51–125.

Rasmussen, A. T., 1947, *Some Trends in Neuroanatomy,* Brown, Dubuque, Iowa.

Ray, R. H., and Craner, S. L., 1988, The development of the topographic organization of the sensory cortices of the neonatal pig, *Soc. Neurosci. Abstr.* **14:**224.

Reep, R. L., and Goodwin, G. S., 1988, Layer VII of rodent cerebral cortex, *Neurosci. Lett.* **90:**15–20.

Reinoso-Suárez, F., 1984, Connectional patterns in parietotemporooccipital association cortex of the feline cerebral cortex, in: *Cortical Integration* (F. Reinoso-Suárez and C. Ajmone-Marsan, eds.), Raven Press, New York, pp. 255–278.

Reinoso-Suárez, F., and Ajmone-Marsan, C. (eds.), 1984, *Cortical Integration. Basic, archicortical, and Cortical Association Levels of Neural Integration,* Raven Press, New York.

Rensch, B., 1948, Histological changes correlated with evolutionary changes of body size, *Evolution* **2:**218–230.

Retzius, A., 1891, Ueber den Bau der Oberflachenschicht der Grosshirnrinde beim Menschen und bei den Säugethieren, *Verh. Biol. Ver.* **3:**90–103.

Richman, D. P., Stewart, R. M., and Caviness, V. S., Jr., 1973, Microgyria, lissencephaly, and neuron migration to the cerebral cortex: An architectonic approach, *Proc. Am. Acad. Neurol.* **23:**413.

Richman, D. P., Stewart, R. M., and Caviness, V. S., Jr., 1974, Cerebral microgyria in a 27-week fetus: An architectonic and topographic analysis, *J. Neuropathol. Exp. Neurol.* **33:**374–399.

Richman, D. P., Stewart, R. M., Hutchinson, J. W., and Caviness, V. S., Jr., 1975, Mechanical model of brain convolutional development. Pathologic and experimental data suggest a model based on differential growth within the cerebral cortex, *Science* **189:**18–21.

Rickmann, M., Chronwall, B. M., and Wolff, J. R., 1977, On the development of non-pyramidal neurons and axons outside the cortical plate: The early marginal zone as a pallial anlage, *Anat. Embryol.* **151:**285–307.

Ridgway, S. H., 1986, Physiological observations on dolphin brains, in: *Dolphin Cognition and Behavior: A Comparative Approach* (R. J. Schusterman, J. A. Thomas, and F. G. Wood, eds.), Erlbaum, Hillsdale, N.J., pp. 31–59.

Riley, F., and Riley, H. A., 1921, *The Form and Functions of the Central Nervous System: An Introduction to the Study of Nervous Diseases,* Hoeber, New York.

Roberts, M. P., Hanaway, J., and Morest, D. K., 1987, *Atlas of the Human Brain in Section,* 2nd ed., Lea & Febiger, Philadelphia.

Roberts, T. S., and Akert, K., 1963, Insular and opercular cortex and its thalamic projection in Macaca mulatta, *Schweiz. Arch. Neurol. Neurochir. Psychiatr.* **92:**1–43.

Rockel, A. J., Hiorns, R. W., and Powell, T. P. S., 1980, The basic uniformity in the structure of the neocortex, *Brain* **103:**221–244.

Romer, A. S., and Edinger, T., 1942, Endocranial casts and brains of living and fossil amphibia, *J. Comp. Neurol.* **77:**355–389.

Rose, J. E., 1949, The cellular structure of the auditory region of the cat, *J. Comp. Neurol.* **91:**409–440.

Rose, J. E., and Woolsey, C. N., 1949, The relations of thalamic connections, cellular structure and evocable electrical activity in the auditory region of the cat, *J. Comp. Neurol.* **91:**441–466.

Rose, M., 1928, Die Inselrinde des Menschen und der Tiere, *J. Psychol. Neurol.* **37:**467–624.

Rosenquist, A. C., 1985, Connections of visual cortical areas in the cat, in: *Cerebral Cortex,* Volume 3 (A. Peters and E. G. Jones, eds.), Plenum Press, New York, pp. 81–117.

Rubel, W. W., 1971, A comparison of somatotopic organization in sensory neocortex of newborn kittens and adult cats, *J. Comp. Neurol.* **143:**447–480.

Rubens, A. B., 1977, Anatomical asymmetries of human cerebral cortex, in: *Lateralization in the Nervous System* (S. Harnad, R. W. Doty, L. Goldstein, J. Jaynes, and G. Krauthamer, eds.), Academic Press, New York, pp. 503–516.

Rubinstein, H. S., 1934, The relation of brain weight to body size. The mathematical basis for the Dubois formula, *Bull. School Med (Univ. Maryland)* **19:**1–4.

Sacher, G. A., 1970, Allometric and factorial analysis of brain structure in insectivores and primates, in: *The Primate Brain* (C. R. Noback and W. Montagna, eds.), Appleton–Century–Crofts, New York, pp. 245–287.

Sacher, G. A., 1982, The role of brain maturation in the evolution of the primates, in: *Primate Brain Evolution: Methods and Concepts* (E. Armstrong and D. Falk, eds.), Plenum Press, New York, pp. 97–112.

Sakai, S. T., 1982, The thalamic connectivity of the primary motor cortex (MI) in the raccoon, *J. Comp. Neurol.* **204:**238–252.

Sanides, F., 1962, Die Architektonik des Menschlichen Stirnhirns. Zugleich eine Darstellung der Prinzipien seiner Gestaltung al Spiegel der Stammesgeschichtlichen Differenzierung der Grosshirnrinde, *Gesamtgebiete Neurol. Psychiatr. (Monogr.)* **98.**

Sanides, F., 1964, The cyto-myeloarchitecture of the human frontal lobe and its relation to phylogenetic differentiation of the cerebral cortex, *J. Hirnforsch.* **6:**269–282.

Sanides, F., 1969a, Comparative architectonics of the neocortex of mammals and their evolutionary interpretation, *Ann. N.Y. Acad. Sci.* **167:**404–423.

Sanides, F., 1969b, Cyto- and myeloarchitecture of the visual cortex of the cat and of the surrounding integration cortices, *J. Hirnforsch.* **11:**79–104.

Sanides, F., 1970a, Functional architecture of motor and sensory cortices in primates in the light of a new concept of neocortex evolution, in: *The Primate Brain* (C. R. Noback and W. Montagna, eds.), Appleton–Century–Crofts, New York, pp. 137–208.

Sanides, F., 1970b, Evolutionary aspect of the primate neocortex, *Proc. 3rd Int. Congr. Primat. (Zurich)* **1:**92–98.

Sanides, F., 1975, Comparative neurology of the temporal lobe in primates including man with reference to speech, *Brain Lang.* **2:**396–419.

Sanides, F., and Krishnamurti, A., 1967, Cytoarchitectonic subdivisions of sensorimotor and prefrontal regions and of bordering insular and limbic fields in slow loris (*Nycticebus coucang coucang*), J. Hirnforsch. **9:**225–252.

Santee, H. E., 1914, The brain of a black monkey, Macacus maurus: The relative prominence of different gyri, *Anat. Rec.* **8:**257–266.

Saraiva, P. E. S., and Magalhães-Castro, B., 1975, Sensory and motor representation in the cerebral cortex of the three-toed sloth (*Bradypus tridactylus*), Brain Res. **90:**181–193.

Sarkissov, S. A., Filimonoff, I. N., Kononowa, W. P., Preobraschenskaja, I. S., and Kukuew, L. A., 1955, *Atlas of the Cytoarchitectonics of the Human Cerebral Cortex*, Medgiz., Moscow.

Sawaguchi, T., 1988, Correlations of cerebral indices for 'extra' cortical parts and ecological variables in primates, *Brain Behav. Evol.* **32:**129–140.

Schaffer, K., 1918a, Über normale und pathologische Hirnfurchung, *Z. Gesamte Neurol. Psychiatr.* **38:**1–78.

Schaffer, K., 1918b, Zum Mechanismus der Furchenbildung, *Z. Gesamte Neurol. Psychiatr.* **38:**79–84.

Schaffer, K., 1923, Histogenese der Hirnfurchung, *Z. Anat. Entwicklungsgesch.* **69:**467–482.

Schaltenbrand, G., and Woolsey, C. N., (eds.), 1964, *Cerebral Localization and Organization*, University of Wisconsin Press, Madison.

Schiller, F., 1965, The rise of the "enteroid processes" in the 19th century: Some landmarks in cerebral nomenclature, *Bull. Hist. Med.* **39:**326–338.

Schmidt, F., 1862, Beiträge zur Entwicklungsgeschichte des Gehirns, *Z. Wiss. Zool.* **11:**43–61.

Schmidt-Nielsen, K., 1984, *Scaling: Why Is Animal Size so Important?* Cambridge University Press, London.

Schmitt, F. O., Worden, F. G., Adelman, G., and Dennis, S. G. (eds.), 1981, *The Organization of the Cerebral Cortex: Proceedings of a Neuroscience Research Program Colloquium*, MIT Press, Cambridge, Mass.

Scollo-Lavizzari, G., and Akert, K., 1963, Cortical area 8 and its thalamic projection in *Macaca mulatta*, *J. Comp. Neurol.* **121:**259–269.

Seitz, J., 1887, Ueber die Bedeutung der Gehirnfurchung, *Jahrb. Psychiatr. Neurol.* **7:**225–288.

Seltzer, B., and Pandya, D. N., 1978, Afferent cortical connections and architectonics of the superior temporal sulcus and surrounding cortex in rhesus monkey, *Brain Res.* **149:**1–24.

Sessle, B. J., and Wiesendanger, M., 1982, Structural and functional definition of the motor cortex in the monkey (*Macaca fascicularis*), *J. Physiol. (London)* **323:**245–265.

Shanks, M. F., Rockel, A. J., and Powell, T. P. S., 1975, The commissural fibre connections of the primary somatic sensory cortex, *Brain Res.* **98:**166–171.

Shariff, G. A., 1953, Cell counts in the primate cerebral cortex, *J. Comp. Neurol.* **98:**381–400.

Shellshear, J. L., 1927, The evolution of the parallel sulcus, *J. Anat.* **61:**268–279.

Sherk, H., 1986, The claustrum and the cerebral cortex, in: *Cerebral Cortex*, Volume 5 (E. G. Jones and A. Peters, eds.), Plenum Press, New York, pp. 467–499.

Sholl, D. A., 1948, The quantitative investigation of the vertebrate brain and the applicability of allometric formulae to its study, *Proc. R. Soc. London (Biol.)* **135:**243–258.

Sholl, D. A., 1956, *The Organization of the Cerebral Cortex*, Wiley, New York.

Sholl, D. A., 1960, Anatomical heterogeneity in the cerebral cortex, in: *Structure and Function of the Cerebral Cortex* (D. B. Tower and J. P. Schadé, eds.), Elsevier, Amsterdam, pp. 21–27.

Sidman, R. L., and Rakic, P., 1973, Neuronal migration, with special reference to developing human brain: A review, *Brain Res.* **62:**1–35.

Sidman, R. L., and Rakic, P., 1982, Development of the human nervous system in: *Histology and Histopathology of the Nervous System* (W. Haymaker and R. D. Adams, eds.), Thomas, Springfield, Ill., pp. 3–145.

Sievers, J., and Raedler, A., 1981, Light and electron microscopical studies on the development of horizontal cells of Cajal–Retzius, *Bibl. Anat.* **19:**161–166.

Simpson, G. G., 1961, *Principles of Animal Taxonomy*, Columbia University Press, New York.

Siuta, J., 1967, Preliminary allometric studies on the fissural cortex, *Acta Biol. Cracov. Ser. Zool.* **10:**227–231.

Smart, I. H. M., and McSherry, G. M., 1986a, Gyrus formation in the cerebral cortex of the ferret. I. Description of the external changes, *J. Anat.* **146:**141–152.

Smart, I. H. M., and McSherry, G. M., 1986b, Gyrus formation in the cerebral cortex of the ferret. II. Description of the internal histological changes, *J. Anat.* **147:**27–43.

Smith, G. E., 1902a, Descriptive and illustrated catalogue of the physiological series of comparative anatomy contained in the Museum of the Royal College of Surgeons of England, 2nd ed., Taylor & Francis, London.

Smith, G. E., 1902b, On the homologies of the cerebral sulci, *J. Anat. Physiol.* **36:**309–319.

Smith, G. E., 1902c, X. On the morphology of the brain in the Mammalia, with special reference to that of the lemurs, recent and extinct, *Trans. Linn. Soc. (Biol.)* **8:**319–432.

Smith, G. E., 1907a, New studies on the folding of the visual cortex and the significance of the occipital sulci in the human brain, *J. Anat.* **41:**198–207.

Smith, G. E., 1907b, A new topographical survey of the human cerebral cortex, being an account of the distribution of the anatomically distinct cortical areas and their relationship to the cerebral sulci, *J. Anat. Physiol.* **61:**237–254.

Smith, G. E., 1929, The variations in the folding of the visual cortex in man, in: *Contributions to Psychiatry, Neurology and Sociology (Dedicated to the Late Sir Frederick Mott)*, Lewis, London, pp. 57–66.

Smith, G. E., 1931, The central nervous system, in: *Cunningham's Textbook of Anatomy* (A. Robinson, ed.), Oxford University Press, London, pp. 505–679.

Smith, R. J., 1985, The present as a key to the past: Body weight of Miocene hominids as a test of allomeric methods for paleontological inference, in: *Size and Scaling in Primate Biology* (W. L. Jungers, ed.), Plenum Press, New York, pp. 437–448.

Snell, O., 1891, Abhängigkeit des Hirngewichtes von dem Korpergewicht und den geistigen Fahigkeiten, *Arch. Psychiatr. Nervenkr.* **23:**436–446.

Starck, D., 1963, Morphologische Untersuchungen am Kopf der Säugetiere, besonders der *Prosimier*, ein Beitrag zum Problem des Formwandels des Säugerschädels, *Z. Wiss. Zool.* **157:**169–219.

Stephan, H., 1954, Vergleichend-anatomische Untersuchungen an Hirnen von Wild- und Haustieren. II. Die oberfläschen des Allocortex bei Wild-und Hausform von *Epimys norvegicus* Erxl, *G. Morphol. Jahrb.* **93s:**125–471.

Stephan, H., 1960, Methodische Studien über den quantitativen Vergleich architektonischer Struktureinheiten des Gehirns, *Z. Wiss. Zool.* **164:**143–172.

Stephan H., Bauchot, R., and Andy, O. J., 1970, Data on size of the brain and of various brain parts in insectivores and primates, in: *The Primate Brain* (C. R. Noback and W. Montagna, eds.), Appleton–Century–Crofts, New York, pp. 289–297.

Stephan, H., Frahm, H. D., and Stephan, M., 1982, Comparison of brain structure volumes in Insectivora and Primates, *J. Hirnforsch.* **23:**375–389.

Stephan H., Baron, G., Frahm, H. D., and Stephan, M., 1986, Grossenvergleiche an Gehirnen und Hirnstrukturen von Säugern, *Z. Mikrosk. Anat. Forsch.* **100:**189–212.

Steudel, K., 1985, Allometric perspectives on fossil catarrhine morphology, in: *Size and Scaling in Primate Biology* (W. L. Jungers, ed.), Plenum Press, New York, pp. 449–475.

Stewart, R. M., Richman, D. P., and Caviness, V. S., Jr., 1975, Lissencephaly and pachygyria. An architectonic and topographical analysis, *Acta Neuropathol.* **31:**1–12.

Strasburger, E. H., 1937, Die myeloarchitektonische Gliederung des Stirnhirns beim Menschen und Schimpansen. Teil I. Myeloarchitectonische Gliederung des Menschlishen Stirnhirn, *J. Psychol. Neurol.* **47:**461–491.

Strick, P. L., and Sterling, P., 1974, Synaptic termination of afferents from the ventrolateral nucleus of the thalamus in the cat motor cortex. A light and electron microscope study, *J. Comp. Neurol.* **153**:77–106.

Symington, J., 1915, On the relations of the inner surface of the cranium to the cranial aspect of the brain, *Edinburgh Med. J.* **14**:85–100.

Symington, J., 1916, Endocranial casts and brain form: A criticism of some recent speculations, *J. Anat. Physiol.* **50**:111–130.

Symonds, L. L., and Rosenquist, A. C., 1984a, Corticocortical connections among visual areas in the cat, *J. Comp. Neurol.* **229**:1–38.

Symonds, L. L., and Rosenquist, A. C., 1984b, Laminar origins of visual corticocortical connections in the cat, *J. Comp. Neurol.* **229**:39–47.

Szentágothai, J., 1969, Architecture of the cerebral cortex, in: *Basic Mechanisms of the Epilepsies* (H. H. Jasper, A. A. Ward, and A. Pope, eds.), Little, Brown, Boston, pp. 13–28.

Tan, U., and Çalişkan, S. 1987, Asymmetries in the cerebral dimensions and fissures of the dog, *Int. J. Neurosci.* **32**:943–952.

Temkin, O., 1947, Gall and the phrenological movement, *Bull. Hist. Med.* **21**:275–321.

Thatcher, R. W., Walker, R. A., and Guidice, S., 1987, Human cerebral hemispheres develop at different rates and ages, *Science* **236**:1110–1113.

Thompson, D. W., 1942 (new ed.), *On Growth and Form*, Macmillan & Co., London.

Thompson, R. A., and Green, J. R. (eds.), 1982, *New Perspectives in Cerebral Localization*, Raven Press, New York.

Thompson, R. A., and Green, R. (eds.), 1985, *Prenatal Neurology and Neurosurgery*, Spectrum, New York.

Tizard, B., 1969, Theories of brain localization from Flourens to Lashley, *Med. Hist.* **3**:132–142.

Tobias, P. V., 1968, Cranial capacity in anthropoid apes, Australopithecus and Homo habilis, with comments on skewed samples, *S. Afr. J. Sci.* **64**:81–91.

Tobias, P. V., 1971, *The Brain in Hominid Evolution*, Columbia University Press, New York.

Todd, P. H., 1982, A geometric model for the cortical folding pattern of simple folded brains, *J. Theor. Biol.* **97**:529–538.

Tömböl, T., 1984, Layer VI cells, in: *Cerebral Cortex*, Volume 1 (A. Peters and E. G. Jones, eds.), Plenum Press, New York, pp. 479–519.

Tower, D. B., 1954, Structural and functional organization of mammalian cerebral cortex: The correlation of neuron density with brain size, *J. Comp. Neurol.* **101**:19–51.

Tower, D. B., and Schadé, J. P. (eds.), 1960, *Structure and Function of the Cerebral Cortex, Proceedings of the Second International Meeting of Neurobiologists, Amsterdam, 1959*, Elsevier, Amsterdam.

Turner, W., 1890, The convolutions of the brain: A study in comparative anatomy, *J. Anat. Physiol.* **25**:105–153.

Tusa, R. J., Palmer, L. A., and Rosenquist, A. C., 1982, Multiple cortical visual areas. Visual field topography in the cat, in: *Cortical Sensory Organization*, Volume 2 (C. N. Woolsey, ed.), Humana Press, Clifton, N.J., pp. 1–31.

Uylings, H. B. M., Verwer, R. W. H., and Van Pelt, J., 1986, Morphometry and stereology in neurosciences, *J. Neurosci. Methods* **18**.

Valverde, F., 1985, The organizing principles of the primary visual cortex in the monkey, in: *Cerebral Cortex*, Volume 3 (A. Peters and E. G. Jones, eds.), Plenum Press, New York, pp. 207–257.

Valverde, F., 1986, Intrinsic neocortical organization: Some comparative aspects, *Neuroscience* **18**:1–23.

Van der Loos, H., 1979, The development of topological equivalences in the brain, in: *Neural Growth and Differentiation* (E. Meisami and M. A. B. Brazier, eds.), Raven Press, New York, pp. 331–336.

Van Essen, D. C., 1985, Functional organization of primate visual cortex, in: *Cerebral Cortex*, Volume 3 (A. Peters and E. G. Jones, eds.), Plenum Press, New York, pp. 259–329.

Van Essen, D. C., and Maunsell, J. H. R., 1980, Two-dimensional maps of the cerebral cortex, *J. Comp. Neurol.* **191**:255–281.

Van Essen, D. C., Maunsell, J. H. R., and Bixby, J. L., 1981, The middle temporal visual area in the macaque: Myeloarchitecture, connections, functional properties and topographic organization, *J. Comp. Neurol.* **199**:293–326.

Vicario, D. S., Martin, J. H., and Ghez, C., 1983, Specialized subregions in the cat motor cortex: A single unit analysis in the behaving animal, *Exp. Brain Res.* **51**:351–367.

Vinken, P. J., Bruyn, G. W., and Myrianthopoulos, N., 1977, Congenital malformations of the brain and skull, in: *Handbook of Clinical Neurology* (P. J. Vinken and G. W. Bruyn, eds.), North-Holland, Amsterdam (selected pages).

Vogt, B. A., 1985, Cingulate cortex, in: *Cerebral Cortex,* Volume 4 (A. Peters and E. G. Jones, eds.), Plenum Press, New York, pp. 89–149.

Vogt, O., 1910, Die myeloarchitektonische Felderung des menschlichen Stirnhirns, *J. Psychol. Neurol.* **15:**221.

Vogt, O., 1923, Furchenbildung und architektonische Rindenfelderung, *J. Psychol. Neurol.* **29:**438.

Vogt, O., 1943, Der heutige Stand der cerebralen Organologie und die zukünftige Hirnforschung, *Anat. Anz.* **94:**49–73.

Volpe, J. J., 1987, *Neurology of the Newborn,* Saunders, Philadelphia, pp. 33–68.

Wall, J. T., 1988, Development and maintenance of somatotopic maps of the skin: A mosaic hypothesis based on peripheral and central contiguities, *Brain Behav. Evol.* **31:**252–268.

Warren, S., and Pubols, B. H., Jr., 1984, Somatosensory thalamocortical connections in the raccoon: An HRP study, *J. Comp. Neurol.* **227:**597–606.

Washburn, S. L., 1947, The relation of the temporal muscle to the form of the skull, *Anat. Rec.* **99:**239–248.

Webster, D. B., 1976, On the comparative method of investigation, in: *Evolution, Brain, and Behavior: Persistent Problems* (R. B. Masterton, W. Hodos, and H. Jerison, eds.), Erlbaum, Hillsdale, N.J., pp. 1–11.

Webster, W. G., 1977, Hemispheric asymmetry in cats, in: *Lateralization in the Nervous System* (S. Harnad, R. W. Doty, L. Goldstein, J. Jaynes, and G. Krauthamer, eds.), Academic Press, New York, pp. 471–480.

Weibel, E. R. 1979, *Stereological Methods. Practical Methods for Biological Morphometry,* Academic Press, New York.

Weidenreich, F., 1940, The brain and its role in the phylogenetic transformation of the human skull, *Trans. Am. Philos. Soc.* **31:**321–442.

Weinberg, R., 1902, Die Interzentralbrücke der Carnivoren und der sulcus Rolandi, *Anat. Anz.* **22:**268–280.

Weiss, P., 1955, Nervous system (neurogenesis), Section VII (special vertebrate organogenesis, in: *Analysis of Development* (B. H. Willier, P. A., Weiss, and V. Hamburger, eds), Saunders, Philadelphia, pp. 346–401.

Weiss, P., 1967, 1 + 1 = 2 (one plus one does not equal two), in: *The Neurosciences* (G. C. Quarton, T. Melnechuk, and F. O. Schmitt, eds.), Rockefeller University Press, New York, pp. 801–821.

Weiss, P. A., 1970, Neural development in biological perspective, in: *The Neurosciences: Second Study Program* (F. O. Schmitt, ed.), Rockefeller University Press, New York, pp. 53–61.

Welker, W. I., 1976, Mapping the brain. Historical trends in functional localization, *Brain Behav. Evol.* **13:**327–343.

Welker, W., 1990, The significance of foliation and fissuration of cerebellar cortex. The cerebellar folium as a fundamental unit of sensorimotor integration, *Arch. Ital. Biol.,* **128:**87–109.

Welker, W. I., and Campos, G. B., 1963, Physiological significance of sulci in somatic sensory cortex of mammals of the family Procyonidae, *J. Comp. Neurol.* **120:**19–36.

Welker, W. I., and Carlson, M., 1976, Somatic sensory cortex of hyrax (*Procavia*), Brain Behav. Evol. **13:**294–301.

Welker, W. I., and Johnson, J. I., Jr., 1965, Correlation between nuclear morphology and somatotopic organization in ventro-basal complex of the raccoon's thalamus, *J. Anat.* **99:**761–790.

Welker, W., and Lende, R. A., 1980, Thalamocortical relationships in echidna (*Tachyglossus aculeatus*), in: *Comparative Neurobiology of the Telencephalon* (S. O. E. Ebbesson, ed.), Plenum Press, New York, pp. 449–481.

Welker, W. I., and Seidenstein, S., 1959, Somatic sensory representation in the cerebral cortex of the raccoon (*Procyon lotor*), J. Comp. Neurol. **111:**469–501.

Welker, W. I., Johnson, J. I., Jr., and Pubols, B. H., Jr., 1964, Some morphological and physiological characteristics of the somatic sensory system in raccoons, *Am. Zool.* **4:**75–96.

Welker, W. I., Adrian, H. O., Lifschitz, W., Kaulen, R., Caviedes, E., and Gutman, W., 1976, Somatic sensory cortex of llama (*Lama glama*), Brain Behav. Evol. **13:**284–293.

Weller, R. E., and Kaas, J. H., 1983, Retinotopic patterns of connections of areas 17 with visual areas V–II and MT in macaque monkeys, *J. Comp. Neurol.* **220:**253–279.

Weller, R. E., and Kaas, J. H., 1985, Cortical projections of the dorsolateral visual area in owl monkeys: The prestriate relay to inferior temporal cortex, *J. Comp. Neurol.* **234:**35–59.

Whitaker, H. A., and Selnes, O. A., 1976, Anatomic variations in the cortex: Individual differences and the problem of the localization of language functions, in: *Origins and Evolution of Language and Speech* (S. R. Harnad, H. D. Steklis, and J. Lancaster, eds.), New York Academy of Sciences, New York, pp. 844–854.

Whitney, G., 1976, Genetic considerations in studies of the evolution of the nervous system and behavior, in: *Evolution, Brain, and Behavior: Persistent Problems*, (R. B. Masterton, W. Hodos, and H. Jerison, eds.), Erlbaum, Hillsdale, N.J., pp. 79–106.

Wiener, S. I., Johnson, J. I., and Ostapoff, E. M., 1987a, Mechanosensory projection zones in the ventrobasal thalamus of raccoons: Distributions of cytochrome oxidase activity, myelin, acetylcholinesterase activity and Nissl substance in electrophysiologically mapped tissues, *J. Comp. Neurol.* **258**:509–526.

Wiener, S. I., Johnson, J. I., and Ostapoff, E. M., 1987b, Organization of postcranial kinesthetic projections to the ventrobasal thalamus in raccoons, *J. Comp. Neurol.* **258**:496–508.

Wiesendanger, M., 1981, Organization of secondary motor areas of cerebral cortex, in: *Handbook of Physiology*, Section 1, Volume II, Part 1 (M. Wiesendanger, ed.), American Physiological Society, Bethesda, pp. 1121–1147.

Wilder, B. G., 1895, The cerebral fissures of two philosophers, Chauncy Wright and James Edward Oliver, *J. Comp. Neurol.* **5**:124–125.

Williams, R. S., Ferrante, R. J., and Caviness, V. S., Jr., 1976, The cellular pathology of microgyria. A Golgi analysis, *Acta Neuropathol.* **36**:269–283.

Williams, R. W., and Herrup, K., 1988, The control of neuron number, *Annu. Rev. Neurosci.* **11**:423–453.

Williams, R. W., Ryder, K., and Rakic, P., 1987, Emergence of cytoarchitectonic differences between areas 17 and 18 in the developing rhesus monkey, *Soc. Neurosci. Abstr.* **14**:1044.

Willier, B. H., Weiss, P. A., and Hamburger, V., 1955, *Analysis of Development*, Saunders, Philadelphia.

Wirz, K., 1950, Studien uber die Cerebralisation: Zur quantitativen Bestimmung der Rangordnung bei Säugetieren, *Acta Anat.* **9**:134–196.

Wise, S. P., 1985, The primate premotor cortex: Past, present, and preparatory, *Annu. Rev. Neurosci.* **8**:1–19.

Wolff, J. R., 1978, Ontogenetic aspects of cortical architecture: Lamination, in: *Architectonics of the Cerebral Cortex* (M. A. B. Brazier and H. Petsche, eds.), Raven Press, New York, pp. 159–173.

Wong, W. C., 1967, The tangential organization of dendrites and axons in three auditory areas of the cat's cerebral cortex, *J. Anat.* **101**:419–433.

Woolsey, C. N., 1960a, Organization of cortical auditory system: A review and a synthesis, in: *Neural Mechanisms of the Auditory and Vestibular Systems* (G. L. Rasmussen and W. F. Windle, eds.), Thomas, Springfield, Ill., pp. 165–180.

Woolsey, C. N., 1960b, Some observations on brain fissuration in relation to cortical localization of function, in: *Structure and Function of the Cerebral Cortex* (D. B. Tower and J. P. Schadé, eds.), Elsevier, Amsterdam, pp. 64–68.

Woolsey, C. N., 1963, Comparative studies on localization in precentral and supplementary motor areas, *Int. J. Neurol.* **4**:13–20.

Woolsey, C. N., 1964, Cortical localization as defined by evoked potential and electrical stimulation studies, in: *Cerebral Localization and Organization* (G. Schaltenbrand and G. N. Woolsey, eds.), University of Wisconsin Press, Madison, pp. 17–26.

Woolsey, C. N., (ed.), 1981a, *Cortical Sensory Organization*, Volume 1, *Multiple Somtic Areas*, Humana Press, Clifton, N.J.

Woolsey, C. N., (ed.), 1981b, *Cortical Sensory Organization*, Volume 2, *Multiple Somtic Areas*, Humana Press, Clifton, N.J.

Woolsey, C. N., (ed.), 1981c, *Cortical Sensory Organization*, Volume 3, *Multiple Somtic Areas*, Humana Press, Clifton, N.J.

Woolsey, C. N., 1984, Comparative evoked potential studies on somatosensory cortex of animals, in: *Somatosensory Mechanisms* (C. von Euler, O. Franzen, U. Lindblom, and D. Ottoson, eds.), Macmillan & Co., London, pp. 19–49.

Woolsey, C. N., and Fairman, D., 1946, Contralateral, ipsilateral and bilateral representation of cutaneous receptors in somatic areas I and II of the cerebral cortex of pig, sheep and other mammals, *Surgery* **19**:684–702.

Wree, A., Zilles, K., and Schleicher, A., 1981, A quantitative approach to cytoarchitectonics. VII. The areal pattern of the cortex of the guinea pig, *Anat. Embryol.* **162**:81–103.

Wree, A., Zilles, K., and Schleicher, A., 1983, A quantitative approach to cytoarchitectonics. VIII. The areal pattern of the cortex of the albino mouse, *Anat. Embryol.* **166**:333–353.

Wright, R. D., 1934, Some mechanical factors in the evolution of the central nervous system, *J. Anat.* **69**:86–88.

Yakovlev, P. I., 1959, Pathoarchitectonic studies of cerebral malformations. III. Arrhinencephalies (holotelencephalies), *J. Neuropathol. Exp. Neurol.* **18**:22–55.

Yakovlev, P. I., 1968, Telencephalon "impar," "semipar" and "totopar," *Int. J. Neurol.* **6:**245–265.

Yakovlev, P. I., and Lecours, A.-R., 1967, The myelogenetic cycles of regional maturation of the brain, in: *Regional Development of the Brain in Early Life* (A. Minkowski, ed.), Blackwell, Oxford, pp. 3–70.

Yakovlev, P. I., and Wadsworth, R. C., 1946a, Schizencephalies. A study of the congenital clefts in the cerebral mantle. I. Clefts with fused lips. *J. Neuropathol. Exp. Neurol.* **5:**116–130.

Yakovlev, P. I., and Wadsworth, R. C., 1946b, Schizencephalies. A study of the congenital clefts in the cerebral mantle. II. Clefts with hydrocephalus and lips separated, *J. Neuropathol. Exp. Neurol.* **5:**169–206.

Yeni-Komshian, G. H., and Benson, D. A., 1976, Anatomical study of cerebral asymmetry in the temporal lobe of humans, chimpanzees, and rhesus monkeys, *Science* **192:**387–389.

Young, R. M., 1970, *Mind, Brain and Adaptation in the Nineteenth Century: Cerebral Localization and Its Biological Context from Gall to Ferrier,* Oxford University Press (Clarendon), London.

Zecevic, N., and Rakic, P., 1985, Changes in the organization and density of synaptic contacts in motor cortex during pre- and postnatal life of rhesus monkeys, *Soc. Neurosci. Abstr.* **11:**1288.

Ziehen, T., 1896, Ueber die Grosshirnfurchung der Halbaffen und die Deutung einiger Furchen des menschlichen Gehirns, *Arch. Psychiatr. Nervenkr.* **28:**898–930.

Zilles, K., Stephan H., and Schleicher, A., 1982, Quantitative cytoarchitectonics of the cerebral cortices of several prosimian species, in: *Primate Brain Evolution: Methods and Concepts* (E. Armstrong and D. Falk, eds.), Plenum Press, New York, pp. 177–201.

Zilles, K., Werners, R., Büsching, U., and Schleicher, A., 1986, Ontogenesis of the laminar structure in areas 17 and 18 of the human visual cortex, *Anat. Embryol.* **174:**339–353.

Zilles, K., Armstrong, E., and Schleicher, A., 1988, The human pattern of gyrification in the cerebral cortex, *Anat. Embryol.* **179:**173–179.

Zilles, K., Armstrong, E., Moser, K. H., and Stephan, H., 1989, Gyrification in the cerebral cortex of primates, *Brain Beh. Evol.* **34:**143–150.

Zulch, K. J., Creutzfeldt, O., and Galbraith, G. C., 1975, *Cerebral Localization: An Otfrid Foerster Symposium,* Springer, Berlin.

Zurabashvili, A. D., 1964, On some vital problems of synaptoarchitectonics, *J. Hirnforsch.* **7:**385–391.

11

Comparative Aspects of Olfactory Cortex

LEWIS B. HABERLY

1. Introduction

Three different types of cerebral cortex have traditionally been distinguished on the basis of structural, phylogenetic, and ontogenetic considerations (Ariëns Kappers *et al.*, 1936): neocortex, hippocampal archicortex, and olfactory paleocortex. An often-stated speculation with little experimental or theoretical support is that the neocortex evolved through "elaboration" of the olfactory cortex and/or hippocampal cortex. Errors by early anatomists concerning the spatial extent of olfactory projections in sharks and amphibians also led to the now questionable view that the cerebral cortex and other telencephalic structures were largely an outgrowth of the olfactory system (see Northcutt, 1981). However, in spite of the apparently less than pivotal role of the olfactory sense in evolution of the telencephalon beyond jawless fishes (Northcutt and Puzdrowski, 1988), recent studies have revealed close parallels in the morphology, physiology, and pharmacology of the neuronal circuitry in mammalian olfactory cortex with that in both neocortex and hippocampal cortex. This chapter was undertaken to explore the nature, roots, and implications of these parallels by comparative analysis of the olfactory cortex in sharks, amphibians, reptiles, and mammals.

LEWIS B. HABERLY • Department of Anatomy, University of Wisconsin Medical Sciences Center, Madison, Wisconsin 53706.

2. Definition of Olfactory Cortex

While olfactory cortex has been defined in a number of different ways, in the present chapter it will be considered to be those paleocortical derivatives that receive direct afferents from the olfactory bulb (Fig. 1). In mammals this definition includes the piriform cortex, olfactory tubercle, anterior and lateral portions of the cortical amygdala, and cortical areas within the anterior olfactory "nucleus" (Heimer, 1968; Price, 1973; Broadwell, 1975; Skeen and Hall, 1977; Davis *et al.*, 1978; Turner *et al.*, 1978; Shammah-Lagnado and Negrao, 1981; Shipley and Adamek, 1984; see reviews by Scott, 1986; Switzer *et al.*, 1986). Posterior and medial portions of the cortical amygdala also receive projections from the accessory olfactory bulb (Scalia and Winans, 1975; Skeen and Hall, 1977), which receives its input from the vomeronasal (Jacobson) organ. Recent evidence indicates that this so-called accessory olfactory system plays a major role in mediation of pheromone-dependent behavior (Meredith, 1983; Halpern and Kubie, 1984). Other areas of mammalian cortex that receive direct olfactory bulb afferents, and therefore have been considered to be olfactory cortex in certain accounts, are the taenia tecta (Price, 1973), indusium griseum (Wyss and Sripanidkulchai, 1983; Adamek *et al.*, 1984), lateral entorhinal cortex (Heimer, 1968; Price, 1973; Scalia and Winans, 1975; Kosel *et al.*, 1981), and insular cortex bordering on the rhinal sulcus (Meyer, 1981; Shammah-Lagnado and Negrao, 1981; Shipley and Geinisman, 1984). While the taenia tecta (anterior hippocampal rudiment) is spatially contiguous with the anterior olfactory nucleus, both it and the indusium griseum (dorsal hippocampal rudiment) are archicortex deriv-

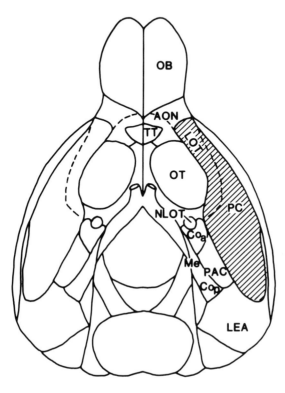

Figure 1. Cortical areas receiving monosynaptic olfactory bulb (OB) input in the rat; ventral view. Olfactory cortical areas as defined in the text are the piriform cortex (PC) (shaded area), olfactory tubercle (OT), anterior olfactory nucleus (AON), and amygdaloid areas: nucleus of the lateral olfactory tract (NLOT), anterior cortical nucleus of the amygdala (Coa), and periamygdaloid cortex (PAC). Other areas receiving input from the olfactory bulb are the lateral entorhinal area (LEA), taenia tecta (TT) (anterior hippocampal rudiment), indusium griseum (dorsal hippocampal rudiment) (not illustrated), and agranular insula (not illustrated). Areas receiving input from the accessory olfactory bulb are the posterior cortical nucleus of the amygdala (Cop) and medial nucleus of the amygdaloid (Me). LOT, lateral olfactory tract. Modified, with permission, from Luskin and Price (1983a).

atives. The lateral entorhinal cortex has a unique multilaminar cytoarchitecture that cannot be readily classed with any of the traditional types of cerebral cortex and receives inputs from other sensory modalities in addition to olfaction; therefore, it is not usually classified as olfactory cortex. The insular cortex is clearly neocortical in structure and receives gustatory as well as olfactory input (Shipley and Geinisman, 1984).

Given the paucity of experimental data on most olfactory cortical areas, this chapter will, of necessity, focus on the largest subdivision, termed piriform cortex in mammals*. Wherever possible, however, data on other olfactory areas will also be presented.

3. Comparative Anatomy and Physiology

3.1. Mammals

3.1.1. Cytoarchitecture

The cytoarchitecture of most olfactory cortical areas is similar in monotreme, marsupial, and placental mammals including primates, but the proportion of the cerebral cortex that is concerned with olfaction varies over a wide range (lower two panels in Fig. 2). Three layers are usually distinguished: layer I is a superficial plexiform layer, layer II, a compact cell body layer, and layer III, a deep, sparsely packed cell body layer. In the piriform cortex, studies using axon tracing techniques, Golgi methods, immunocytochemistry, and current source density analysis have revealed clearly defined sublayers (Fig. 3). The plexiform layer can be subdivided into layer Ia, a superficial sublamina dominated by afferent fibers from the olfactory bulb, and layer Ib, a deep sublamina dominated by association fibers of intrinsic origin (Heimer, 1968; Haberly and Shepherd, 1973; Price, 1973). Both sublaminae also contain small numbers of morphologically diverse GABAergic neuron somata (Section 3.1.3). Layer II can be subdivided into a superficial sublamina termed layer IIa by Haberly and Price (1978a) that contains predominantly pyramidal-type cells lacking basal dendrites (Section 3.1.2) and a deep sublamina termed layer IIb that is dominated by pyramidal cells, but also contains a low percentage of small GABAergic and peptidergic nonpyramidal cells. In the opossum this subdivision can only be visualized in Golgi-stained material (Haberly, 1983), but in the rat, layers IIa and IIb are readily apparent in Nissl-stained sections over portions of the piriform cortex (Fig. 3). Finally, layer III can be subdivided into a superficial part that is dominated by pyramidal cells and a deep part that is dominated by polymorphic cells (Ramón y Cajal, 1911; O'Leary, 1937; Valverde, 1965; Haberly, 1983; Tseng and Haberly, 1989a), many of which are GABAergic and peptidergic (Section 3.1.3). This sublamination within layer III cannot be readily distinguished in normal Nissl-stained material. Deep to layer III is a concentration of cells now commonly termed the endopiriform nucleus. Recent studies have revealed interconnections between the endopiriform nucleus and overlying cortex (Krettek

*Alternative terms include prepiriform, prepyriform, and primary olfactory cortex, although in recent years the majority of reports have used the terms piriform or pyriform.

and Price, 1977; Haberly and Price, 1978a; Haberly and Presto, 1986) and close similarities in the morphology and physiology of its cells with those in the deep part of layer III (Tseng and Haberly, 1989a,b).

Other olfactory cortical areas also display a condensed layer II and relatively cell-sparse layer III with the exception of the anterior olfactory nucleus, in which a single cell body layer is usually distinguished. However, the cell layer over most

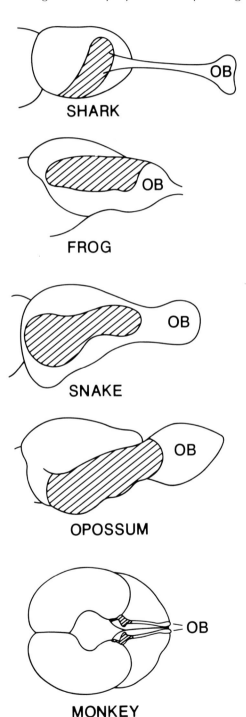

Figure 2. Comparison of telencephalic projection zones of the olfactory bulb (OB) in the nurse shark (Heimer, 1969), bullfrog (Northcutt and Royce, 1975; Scalia, 1976), sand boa (Ulinski, 1974), opossum, and rhesus monkey (Turner *et al.*, 1978). All views are from the lateral aspect with the exception of the rhesus monkey, which is a ventral view.

of the anterior olfactory nucleus can be subdivided into a superficial portion dominated by pyramidal-type cells (Haberly and Price, 1978b) that is comparable to layers II and superficial III in the piriform cortex, and a deep portion that contains a high percentage of polymorphic GABAergic cells that is comparable to deep layer III in the piriform cortex (Haberly et al., 1987).

In the rhesus monkey, portions of the anterior olfactory nucleus and olfactory tubercle have poorly defined laminae (Turner et al., 1978). Nevertheless, other olfactory cortical areas are similar to their counterparts in nonprimate mammals. In man, only a small part of the olfactory tubercle has a recognizable trilaminar structure (Crosby and Humphrey, 1941) and portions of layer II in the piriform cortex have an irregular patchy appearance (Bailey and von Bonin, 1951).

3.1.2. Pyramidal Neurons

As in other types of cerebral cortex, pyramidal cells are the dominant cell type in the piriform cortex and other parts of the olfactory cortex. Pyramidal cells in deep layer II and layer III of the piriform cortex have the classical form with a highly branched, profusely spiny apical dendritic tree that originates as a single trunk, finer-caliber basal dendrites that are also covered with a high density of spines, and a myelinated axon that is directed toward the deep pole of the cortex (Fig. 4A). The bulk of pyramidal cell spines are single knobs with thin necks as in other parts of the cerebral cortex, although in the opossum occasional long beaded spines are observed (Haberly, 1983). Synaptic distribution patterns in piriform cortex (Figs. 5 and 6) (Westrum, 1966; Haberly and Feig, 1983; Haberly and Presto, 1986) are also typical for pyramidal cells in other parts of the cerebral cortex (e.g., Peters et al., 1968; Jones and Powell, 1969; Gottlieb and Cowan, 1972; LeVay, 1973; Parnuvelas et al., 1977; Sloper and Powell, 1979;

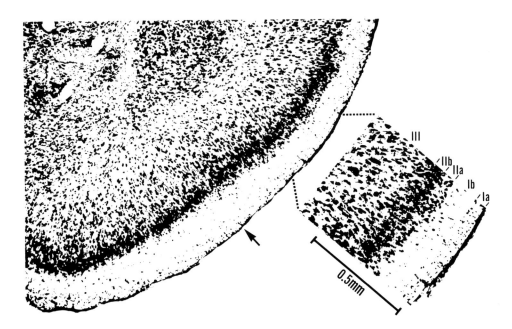

Figure 3. Photomicrograph of the posterior part of the rat piriform cortex; Nissl stain. Reprinted, with permission, from Haberly and Price (1978a).

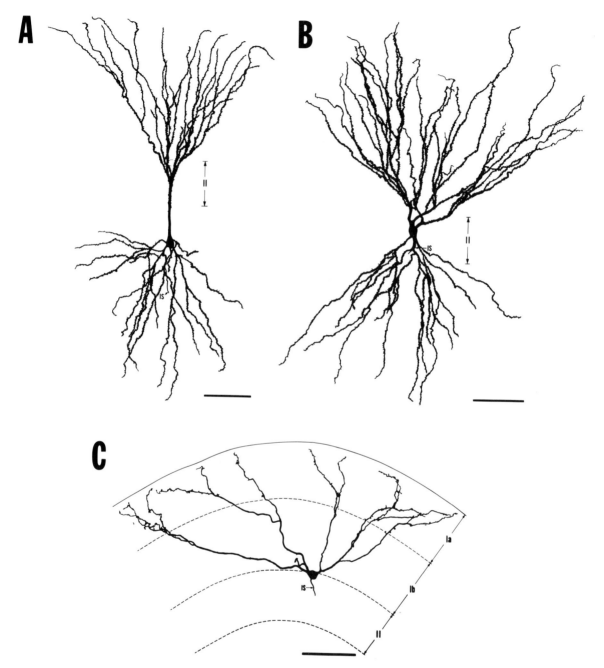

Figure 4. Pyramidal-type cells in the piriform cortex of the opossum; Golgi stain. (A) Pyramidal cell with classical form in layer III. (B) Layer II "pyramidal" cell with secondary apical dendrites emanating directly from the cell body. (C) Semilunar cell from superficial layer II. IS, axon initial segment; Roman numerals denote cortical layers. Bars = 100 μm. Reprinted, with permission, from Haberly (1983).

Kosaka, 1980; Hersch and White, 1981; Peters, 1985; Lacaille *et al.*, 1987): asymmetrical synapses with associated round vesicles are concentrated on dendritic spines and completely excluded from somata; symmetrical synapses with associated pleomorphic vesicles are found at very high density on axon initial segments and at a moderate density over all other parts including somata and both apical and basal dendrites. Axons of pyramidal cells in the piriform cortex (Haberly and Presto, 1986), like those in the neocortex (Winfield *et al.*, 1981; McGuire *et al.*, 1984), give rise to both terminal and en passant boutons that

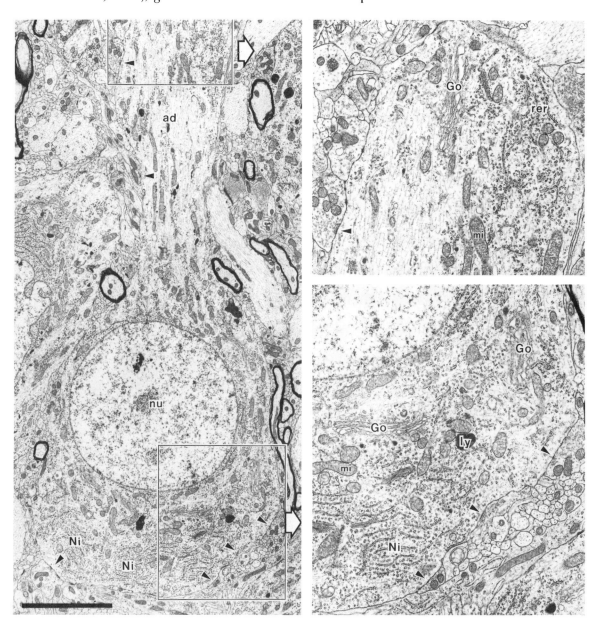

Figure 5. Electron micrograph of typical layer III pyramidal cell from the opossum. ad, apical dendrite; Go, Golgi apparatus; ly, lysozome; Ni, Nissl bodies; nu, nucleus; arrowheads denote symmetrical synapses on the soma and proximal dendrites. Bar = 5 μm. Reprinted, with permission, from Haberly and Feig (1983).

make asymmetrical synapses onto pyramidal as well as nonpyramidal cells. The ultrastructure of pyramidal cells in the piriform cortex (Figs. 5 and 6) (Haberly and Feig, 1983) also resembles that of small to medium pyramids in other parts of the cerebral cortex (e.g., Jones and Powell, 1970; Peters and Kaiserman-Abramof, 1970; Peters and Kara, 1985). Apical dendrites of pyramidal cells in the piriform cortex branch into secondary trunks at approximately the layer I–II border. As a consequence, the length of apical trunks is determined by the depth of somata. Pyramidal cells with somata in the deep part of layer III have long apical trunks (Fig. 4A), while many of those in the superficial part of layer II lack apical trunks so that secondary apical dendrites originate directly from somata (Fig. 4B). Similar pyramidal cells that lack apical trunks are found in layer II of the neocortex (Sanides and Sanides, 1972; Peters and Kara, 1985; Valverde and Facal-Valverde, 1986).

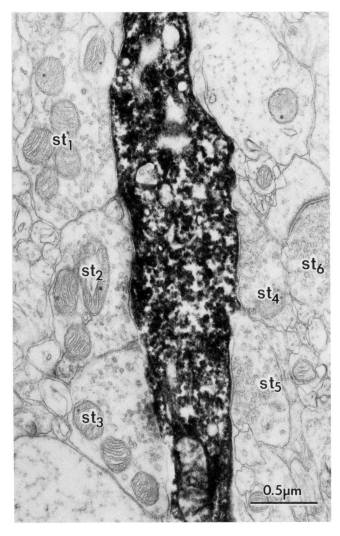

Figure 6. Axon initial segment of a layer II pyramidal cell from opossum piriform cortex labeled by intracellular injection of horseradish peroxidase. St_1 to St_5 are synaptic terminals with pleomorphic vesicles. Reprinted, with permission, from Haberly and Presto (1986).

Layer IIa cells resemble pyramidal cells by virtue of apical dendritic trees, deep-directed axons, and similar somatic ultrastructure, but lack basal dendrites (Fig. 4C) (Calleja, 1893; Ramón y Cajal, 1911; Haberly, 1983; Haberly and Feig, 1983). These cells have been termed semilunar cells by Valverde (1965) as a consequence of the shape of their somata. Apical dendrites of semilunar cells give rise to spines that, like pyramidal cells, receive asymmetrical synaptic contacts from afferent fibers (Haberly and Behan, 1983); however, the morphology and distribution of these spines, in the opposum at least (Haberly, 1983), are not typical of pyramidal cells. Spines on distal dendritic segments in layer Ia are large and flattened while those on proximal segments in layer Ib are small and sparse. An intriguing feature of these cells is that they undergo a rapid transsynaptic degeneration after removal of the olfactory bulb (Heimer and Kalil, 1978; Friedman and Price, 1986), perhaps in part as a consequence of the dominance of afferent synaptic inputs in layer Ia.

3.1.3. Nonpyramidal Neurons

Golgi studies of the piriform cortex in rodent species (Ramón y Cajal, 1911; O'Leary, 1937; Valverde, 1965), the opossum (Haberly, 1983), and the cat (Stevens, 1969), and an intracellular dye injection study in the rat (Tseng and Haberly, 1989a) have revealed a great diversity in types of nonpyramidal cells (Fig. 7). These include multipolar cells with both smooth and profusely spiny dendrites that are concentrated in the deep part of layer III, small globular soma cells with smooth dendrites concentrated in layers I and II, and large horizontal cells confined to layer Ia with a striking resemblance to Cajal–Retzius cells in neocortex.

A study of opossum piriform cortex with antisera to glutamic acid decarboxylase (GAD) and GABA has revealed several populations of presumed GABAergic cells that are distinctive by virtue of laminar distribution and somatic morphology (Haberly et al., 1987). These include large horizontal cells that clearly correspond to the Cajal–Retzius-like cells in layer Ia, small globular soma cells in layers I and II that appear to correspond at least in part to the small, smooth dendrite cells observed in Golgi studies, and large numbers of multipolar cells in the deep part of layer III and the subjacent endopiriform nucleus with uncertain correspondence to morphologically defined cell types. Reports describing the laminar distribution of GABAergic cells (Mugnaini and Oertel, 1985; Westenbroek et al., 1987) and a study of cell morphology (Haberly and Feig, unpublished) indicate that similar populations of probable GABAergic cells are present in the rat.

Nonpyramidal cells displaying immunoreactivity to many neuropeptides have been described in layers II and III of the piriform cortex and in the endopiriform nucleus. These include somatostatin, neuropeptide Y, cholecystokinin (CCK), vasoactive intestinal peptide (VIP), neurotensin, corticotropin-releasing factor, substance P, and several opioids (reviewed by Haberly, 1990).

3.1.4. Afferent Fiber Systems

The projection from the olfactory bulb terminates exclusively in the superficial part of the plexiform layer (layer Ia) (Figs. 3, 8, and 9) in all olfactory areas in all species that have been examined including the rat (Price, 1973), hamster (Davis *et al.,* 1978), mouse (Shipley and Adamek, 1984), rabbit (Broadwell, 1975), opossum (Shammah-Lagnado and Negrao, 1981), tree shrew (Skeen and Hall, 1977), and rhesus monkey (Turner *et al.,* 1978). Physiological studies have shown that afferent fibers mediate a monosynaptic EPSP in distal apical dendritic segments of superficial and deep pyramidal cells in piriform cortex as well as monosynaptically exciting certain nonpyramidal cells (semilunar and GABAergic cells) (Biedenbach and Stevens, 1969; Satou *et al.,* 1982; Haberly and Bower,

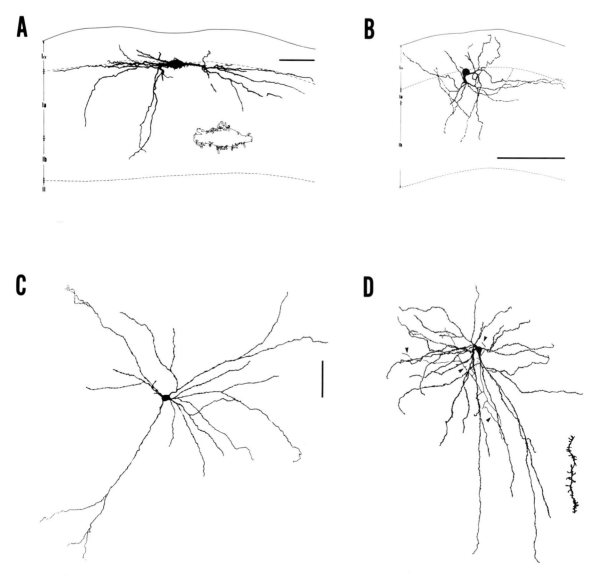

Figure 7. Nonpyramidal cells in the piriform cortex. (A) Large superficial horizontal cell resembling neocortical Cajal–Retzius cells. (B) Small layer I globular soma neuron with smooth dendrites. (C) Layer III multipolar neuron with aspiny dendrites. (D) Layer III multipolar neuron with spiny dendrites; arrowheads denote axon collaterals. Neurons in A to C were stained with the Golgi method in the opossum; reprinted from Haberly (1983) with permission. The neuron in D was stained by intracellular injection in the rat; reprinted from Tseng and Haberly (1989a) with permission. Bars = 100 μm; bar in C also applies to D.

1984; Tseng and Haberly, 1988, 1989a). Two striking features of the afferent system that distinguish it from the sensory afferent projections to the neocortex are a tangential pattern of spread across the surface that provides sequential rather than synchronous activation (Freeman, 1959, Haberly, 1973b) and a relative lack of topographical organization (Haberly and Price, 1977; Skeen and Hall, 1977; Scott *et al.*, 1980). While there is a topographical organization in the reciprocal connections between pars externa of the anterior olfactory nucleus and the olfactory bulb (Schoenfeld and Macrides, 1984; Scott *et al.*, 1985), the afferent input to all other projection areas is highly distributed in nature.

In addition to the principal afferent system from the olfactory bulb, olfactory cortical areas also receive inputs from nonadrenergic cells in the locus co-

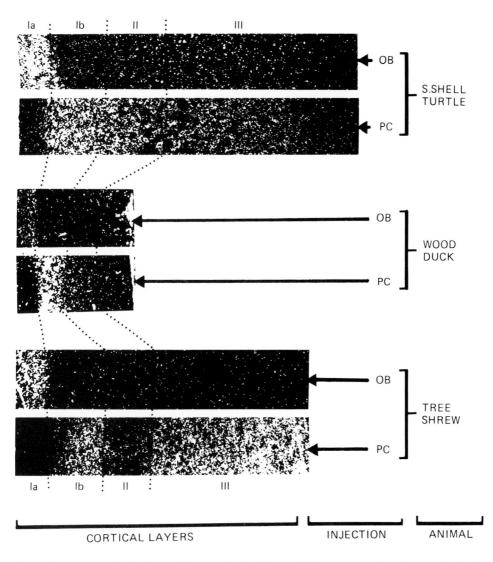

Figure 8. Laminar distribution of olfactory bulb afferents (OB) and association fibers of intrinsic origin (PC) in the piriform cortex of the soft-shelled turtle, wood duck, and tree shrew. Note the complementary lamination of these two fiber systems in layer I. Reprinted, with permission, from Skeen *et al.* (1984).

eruleus, serotonergic cells in raphé nuclei, dopaminergic cells in the ventral tegmental area, cholinergic cells in the basal forebrain, histaminergic cells in the hypothalamus, and a small number of widely distributed cells in the thalamus (reviewed by Haberly, 1990).

3.1.5. Association Fiber Systems

With the exception of the olfactory tubercle, all olfactory cortical areas as well as the lateral entorhinal cortex and taenia tecta give rise to corticocortical "associational" projections to other areas that receive olfactory bulb inputs (Heimer, 1968; Price, 1973; Krettek and Price, 1977; Haberly and Price, 1978a; Luskin and Price, 1983a,b). The olfactory tubercle receives, but does not give rise to, such connections. Commissural connections between different cortical areas that receive olfactory bulb inputs are also present. An intriguing spatial offset is present in the commissural projection to the piriform cortex: the anterior part receives input from the opposite anterior olfactory nucleus, while the posterior part and adjacent areas receive input from the opposite anterior piriform cortex (Haberly and Price, 1978a; Luskin and Price, 1983a). Like the afferent projections from the olfactory bulb, both asociational and commissural inputs spread tangentially across target areas and are highly distributed in the horizontal dimension (Haberly and Price, 1978a; Luskin and Price, 1983a). The broad topographical order in these systems clearly does not allow transfer of a surface "map" between areas but rather may be involved in ordering the relative times of arrival of mono- and disynaptic inputs to pyramidal cells (Haberly and Price, 1978a).

Within the piriform cortex an intriguing multicomponent system of intrinsic association fibers has been demonstrated in the opossum and rat (Fig. 9). Like the primary afferent system and association fibers of extrinsic origin, the intrinsic association fibers are distributed in a precisely ordered way in the laminar

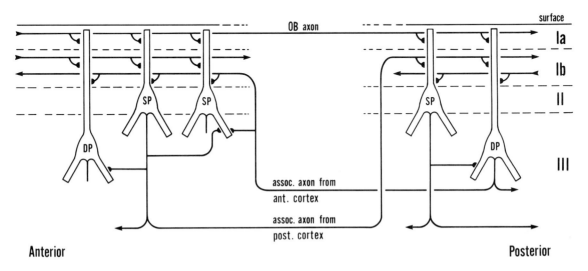

Figure 9. Schematic diagram of excitatory inputs to pyramidal cells in piriform cortex. DP, deep pyramidal cells; OB, olfactory bulb; SP, superficial pyramidal cells. Modified, with permission, from Haberly (1985).

dimension, but are highly distributed in the horizontal dimension (parallel to the surface) (Heimer, 1968; Price, 1973; Haberly and Price, 1978a; Luskin and Price, 1983a,b). These fibers have been shown to originate from, and terminate on pyramidal cells (Haberly and Price, 1978a; Haberly and Behan, 1983; Haberly and Bower, 1984). Over short distances, associational axons terminate in layer III on basal dendrites of pyramidal cells and deep nonpyramidal cells (Haberly and Presto, 1986); over long distances they terminate on apical dendrites of pyramidal cells in layer Ib (Haberly and Behan, 1984). Long projections from different parts of piriform cortex are concentrated at different depths within layer Ib as illustrated in Fig. 9. Evidence from intracellular recording (Haberly and Bower, 1984; Tseng and Haberly, 1989a) and current source-density analysis (Haberly and Shepherd, 1973; Rodriguez and Haberly, 1989) indicates that following activation of afferent fibers, both superficial and deep pyramidal cells in the piriform cortex receive a series of EPSPs in different dendritic segments: a monosynaptic EPSP in distal-most apical segments from afferent fibers and several successive disynaptic EPSPs in different dendritic segments via short and long associational fiber system components. As discussed in recent reviews (Haberly, 1985; Haberly and Bower, 1989; Haberly, 1990), such a convergence onto the same neuronal elements of the monosynaptic excitation provided by the distributed afferent fiber system and the distributed positive feedback provided by the intrinsic association fiber systems could be the substrate for a so-called content addressable memory for analysis of the spatially distributed olfactory code.

3.1.6. Inhibitory Systems

There is little direct evidence concerning inhibitory circuitry in the piriform cortex, but inferences have been made on the basis of evidence from studies with physiological, Golgi, and immunocytochemical methods. Physiological studies have revealed that pyramidal cells receive inhibition by way of feedforward interneurons that are directly activated by afferent fibers (Haberly and Bower, 1984; Tseng and Haberly, 1988) and feedback interneurons that are excited via pyramidal cell axons (Biedenbach and Stevens, 1969; Haberly, 1973a; Satou *et al.*, 1983; Haberly and Bower, 1984; Tseng and Haberly, 1988). Both feedforward and feedback processes consist of a fast chloride-dependent component that is mediated by $GABA_A$ receptors and a slow potassium-dependent component mediated by $GABA_B$ receptors (Tseng and Haberly, 1988; Hoffman and Haberly, 1989). Candidates for interneurons mediating feedforward processes include the large Cajal–Retzius-like cells and the superficial globular soma cells. Candidate interneurons for feedback inhibition include multipolar cells in layer III and the endopiriform nucleus, and small globular soma cells in layer II (Haberly *et al.*, 1987). Electron microscopic studies have revealed that possible inhibitory synapses with symmetrical contacts and associated pleomorphic vesicles are found on all parts of pyramidal cells including distal dendrites. The density of symmetrical synapses is highest on axon initial segments (Fig. 6), but total numbers are highest on dendrites (Haberly and Feig, 1983; Haberly and Presto, 1986). Physiological studies have also provided evidence for both dendritic and somatic inhibition—the fast chloride-mediated process appears to be concentrated in the vicinity of cell bodies and the slow potassium-mediated process on dendrites (Tseng and Haberly, 1988).

3.1.7. Output Fiber Systems

Outputs from cortical areas that receive direct olfactory input are direct to many different brain systems. There are outputs to the medial dorsal nucleus of the thalamus and lateral hypothalamus from the piriform cortex and other olfactory cortical areas, outputs to the corpus striatum via the olfactory tubercle, direct and relayed outputs to the neocortex from the piriform cortex, outputs to limbic and other areas of the forebrain from the amygdala, and outputs to the hippocampal formation via the lateral entorhinal cortex (reviewed by Price, 1985; Takagi, 1986). Piriform cortex and other olfactory cortical areas also project back to the olfactory bulb (Luskin and Price, 1983a,b).

3.2. Reptiles

The projection of the olfactory bulb to cortical areas has been examined with experimental methods in lizards (Gambel, 1952; Heimer, 1969; Ulinski and Peterson, 1981; Martinez-Garcia *et al.*, 1986; Lohman *et al,* 1988), snakes (Fig. 2) (Halpern, 1976b; Ulinski and Rainey, 1980), turtles (Rolon and Skeen, 1980; Skeen et al., 1984; Reiner and Karten, 1985), and crocodilians (Scalia *et al.*, 1969). In all species examined, representing three of the four orders of reptiles, the olfactory bulb projects to four different cortical areas: the lateral cortex, which closely resembles the piriform cortex of mammals, the olfactory tubercle, the anterior olfactory nucleus, and a rostral subdivision of the medial cortex that may be homologous to the taenia tecta of mammals. In at least certain crocodilians (Scalia *et al.*, 1969), turtles (Reiner and Karten, 1985), and lizards (Lohman *et al.*, 1988), but not the snakes that have been studied, there is also a projection to cortical parts of the amygdala. Projections from the olfactory bulb have been inconsistently described to the rostral part of the septal area (see discussion by Ulinski and Peterson, 1981). Olfactory projections in the duck (Skeen *et al.*, 1984) and pigeon (Reiner and Karten, 1985) are similar to those in reptiles.

In lizards and snakes the accessory olfactory bulb can be as large as the olfactory bulb (Northcutt, 1978); in crocodilians and many turtles it is absent (Northcutt, 1981). The accessory olfactory bulb in lizards and snakes projects predominantly to the nucleus sphericus (Heimer, 1969; Ulinski and Kanarek, 1973; Halpern, 1976b) (see also Fig. 3 in Ulinski, 1974). The primary projection target of this nucleus is the medial hypothalamus (Halpern and Silfen, 1974), which is also the primary target of the portion of the amygdala that receives accessory olfactory bulb input in mammals (Leonard and Scott, 1971; de Olmos and Ingram, 1972).

Studies of cell morphology in the olfactory part of the lateral cortex of snakes (Ulinski, 1974; Ulinski and Rainey, 1980) and lizards (Ebbesson and Voneida, 1969; Ulinski and Peterson, 1981) have revealed close parallels with the piriform cortex of mammals: Layer I is a plexiform layer with a small number of predominantly stellate cells. Layer II is a condensed cell body layer that contains "bowl" cells resembling semilunar cells in mammals (Fig. 10), and stellate cells. Layer III, as in mammals, contains pyramidal cells with single apical trunks in its superficial part and a variety of stellate and fusiform cells concentrated in its deep part, some of which have sparsely spiny dendrites. Dendrites from bowl cells and pyramidal-type cells in layers II and III extend into layer I.

Afferent fibers from the olfactory bulb to the lateral cortex in all reptilian species that have been examined are tangentially distributed and terminate exclusively in a superficial sublamina (Ia) of the plexiform layer as in mammals (Fig. 8). Analysis of transport patterns from small amino acid injections in the turtle (Skeen *et al.*, 1984) has revealed a lack of topographical order as in mammals. Limited physiological (Orrego and Lissenby, 1962) and electron microscopic (Ulinski and Rainey, 1980) evidence is consistent with the finding for mammals that olfactory bulb afferents monosynaptically excite pyramidal-type cells via spines on distal dendritic segments. Counterparts to most of the other afferent systems to the olfactory cortex in mammals have also been reported in reptiles. These include serotonergic, noradrenergic, and dopaminergic cells in brain-stem nuclei (reviewed by Hoogland and Vermeulen-Van der Zee, 1988) and possible cholinergic cells in the basal forebrain (Bruce and Butler, 1984a; Martinez-Garcia *et al.*, 1986). Light projections to the turtle olfactory cortex have been described from the thalamus and hypothalamus (Bruce and Butler, 1984a) as in mammals (Section 3.1.4), although Martinez-Garcia *et al.* (1986) have questioned the presence of these pathways based on their findings in the lizard.

As in the mammalian piriform cortex, an extensive, highly distributed intrinsic associational fiber system has been demonstrated in the lateral cortex in the soft-shelled turtle. This system terminates in a deep sublamina (Ib) of the plexiform layer that is complementary to the afferent fiber projection, as well as in deeper layers (Fig. 8) (Skeen *et al.*, 1984). Limited observations with degenera-

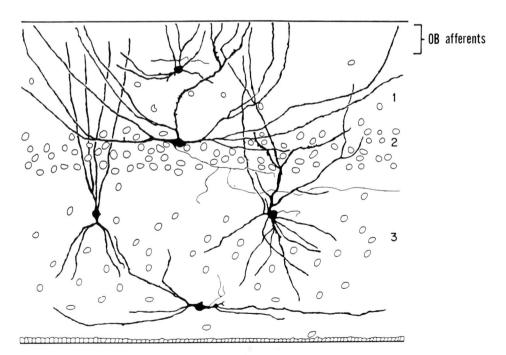

Figure 10. Semidiagrammatic view of cytoarchitecture and cell types in the snake lateral (piriform) cortex. Reprinted, with permission, from Ulinski and Rainey (1980).

tion methods (Halpern, 1976b) suggest that a similar system is present in snakes. As in mammals (Friedman and Price, 1984), only the deep sublamina of layer I stains with Timm's method in the lizard (Pérez-Clausell and Fredens, 1988), suggesting that zinc is confined to association fiber terminals. The presence of a diphasic surface negative response to surface olfactory bulb or olfactory tract stimulation (Orrego and Lissenby, 1962) that closely resembles the mammalian response, provides preliminary evidence that the association fiber system mediates a disynaptic reactivation that follows the monosynaptic afferent activation as in mammals (Section 3.1.5).

The only outputs from the lateral cortex that have been described in reptiles are a projection to the ipsilateral olfactory bulb (Halpern, 1976a) as in mammals (de Olmos et al., 1978; Davis and Macrides, 1981; Luskin and Price, 1983a; Shipley and Adamek, 1984) and a heavy projection to the plexiform layer of the medial (hippocampal) cortex from the dorsal part of the lateral cortex (Ulinski, 1976; Bruce and Butler, 1984a; Martinez-Garcia et al., 1986; Desan, 1988). On the basis of this latter projection, Martinez-Garcia et al. (1986) have postulated that the dorsal portion of the lateral cortex is homologous to the entorhinal cortex of mammals, which also receives a direct olfactory bulb input and projects to the hippocampal formation (Section 2 and 3.1.7).

While there are many parallels in the organization of the olfactory cortex in reptiles and mammals, there is one striking difference. In contrast to mammals where commissural connections originate from secondary olfactory areas, in all reptile species examined a projection has been observed that originates from the olfactory bulb, crosses in the habenular rather than anterior commissure, and is distributed to layer Ia rather than layer Ib of the olfactory cortex (Heimer, 1969; Scalia et al., 1969; Halpern, 1976b; Ulinski and Peterson, 1981; Skeen et al., 1984; Reiner and Karten, 1985). Recent studies of the lateral cortex of three lizard species using axon transport methods (Bruce and Butler, 1984a; Martinez-Garcia et al., 1986) have revealed that a homotopic interhemispheric connection is also present.

3.3. Amphibians

Many early reports described olfactory bulb projections to widespread telencephalic areas. However, more recent studies using degeneration methods in frogs and the tiger salamander (Scalia et al., 1968; Northcutt and Royce, 1975; Northcutt and Kicliter, 1980) have revealed a restricted termination zone in the lateral pallium (Fig. 2), confirming in large part the Golgi observations of Herrick (1921, 1948). While the relatively poor cytoarchitectonic definition of the lateral and dorsal pallia in amphibians has led to confusion in terminology, the homology of at least a portion of the olfactory projection area to the mammalian piriform cortex is generally accepted (Northcutt, 1974; Kicliter and Ebbesson, 1976). Projections have also been described to the plexiform layer overlying an area that has been considered to be a homologue of the corpus striatum based on histochemical observations (Northcutt, 1974) and to a ventural extension of the lateral pallium that has been termed pars lateralis of the amygdala by Northcutt and Royce (1975) (see also Northcutt, 1974). However, the Golgi observations of Scalia (1976) and Kicliter and Ebbesson (1976) suggest that synaptic terminals in these regions are on obliquely oriented dendrites from the adjoining lateral pallium. Medial projections from the olfactory bulb have been described to a possible homologue of the olfactory tubercle (Northcutt and Kicliter, 1980) and to rostral portions of the medial pallium and septal area as in reptiles (Scalia *et al.*, 1968; Northcutt and Royce, 1975). There appears to be no homologue of the anterior olfactory nucleus in frogs and salamanders (Scalia, 1976; Northcutt and Kicliter, 1980). Commissural projections are similar to those in reptiles with a direct olfactory bulb projection to the superficial part of the plexiform layer in olfactory cortical areas by way of the habenular commissure (Northcutt and Royce, 1975). The accessory olfactory bulb of frogs and salamanders projects heavily to the plexiform layer overlying the entire rostral to caudal extent of pars lateralis of the amygdala (Scalia, 1972; Northcutt and Kicliter, 1980).

In contrast to the three-layered plan of reptiles and mammals, the amphibian paleopallium consists of two layers (Fig. 11): a superficial plexiform layer and a single deep cell layer that directly adjoins the lateral ventricle and is poorly demarcated from the plexiform layer. The principal cell type is an "extraverted" neuron with an exclusively apical dendritic tree that extends into the plexiform

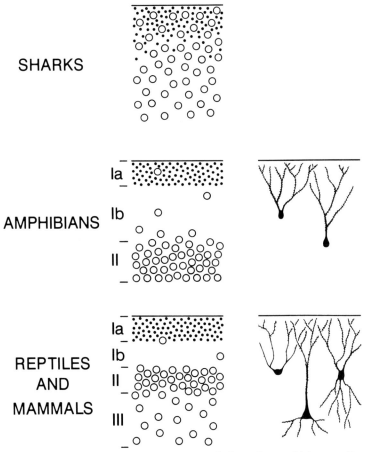

Figure 11. Schematic view of the cytoarchitecture, morphology of pyramidal-type cells, and laminar distribution of afferents from the olfactory bulb (stippling) in the lateral (piriform) cortex of sharks, amphibians, reptiles, and mammals. *Circles* denote cell bodies. There are no published data on cell morphology in sharks.

layer and a deep-directed axon (Fig. 11) (Herrick, 1948; Kicliter and Ebbesson, 1976). Since pyramidal cells display a similar appearance in embryonic mammalian cerebral cortex, it has been argued that these neurons represent phylogenetically primitive pyramidal cells (Ramón y Cajal, 1911; Sanides and Sanides, 1972). As described above (Sections 3.1.2 and 3.2), cells with this dendritic form are found in the superficial part of layer II of adult piriform (lateral) cortex in mammals and reptiles.

As in mammals and reptiles, the olfactory bulb projection in frogs and salamanders is confined to the superficial part of the molecular layer (Northcutt and Royce, 1975; Northcutt and Kicliter, 1980). Widespread associational connections reciprocally linking the lateral pallium with both the medial and dorsal pallia have been reported with Golgi methods, although only a projection from the lateral pallium to the medial pallium that passes through the deep part of the plexiform layer of the dorsal pallium has thus far been verified with modern experimental methods (Scalia, 1976). No studies of possible intrinsic connections of the lateral pallium have been carried out and no output pathways other than the projection to the medial pallium have been experimentally demonstrated.

3.4. Sharks

For comparative study of the cerebral cortex, sharks and other cartilaginous fishes offer an advantage over most bony fishes for comparative study: the presence of an "evaginated" telencephalon with a centrally located lateral ventricle like that of higher vertebrates. By contrast, in teleosts and other ray-finned fishes cortical layers are inverted relative to other vertebrates as a result of an "everted" development of the telencephalon (Northcutt, 1981).

As in amphibians and reptiles, the shark pallium is commonly divided into lateral, dorsal, and medial parts, although in certain species including the commonly studied nurse shark, an extreme thickening of the dorsal pallium tends to obscure these subdivisions (see Fig. 5 in Northcutt, 1981). Early workers employing simple axon staining methods came to the erronous conclusion that the olfactory bulb projects over virtually the entire extent of the shark telencephalon (reviewed by Smeets et al., 1983). Studies with degeneration techniques have revealed that the secondary projection is spatially restricted, although variable in different species.* In the three shark species in which experimental studies have been carried out (Ebbesson and Heimer, 1970; Bodznick and Northcutt, 1979; Smeets, 1983), as well as the horned ray (Smeets, 1983), the olfactory bulb projects to a restricted portion of the lateral pallium (Fig. 2) termed the lateral olfactory area by Ebbesson and Heimer (1970). In the nurse shark (Heimer, 1969; Ebbesson and Heimer, 1970; Ebbesson, 1972) and spotted dogfish (Smeets, 1983), but not the horn shark (Bodznick and Northcutt, 1979; Northcutt, 1981), there is also a projection to the lateral part of the area superficialis of Johnston (1911) at the base of the telencephalon (termed the olfactory tubercle by Dart, 1920). In the spotted dogfish (Smeets, 1983), but not the nurse or horn shark, olfactory bulb projections have been described to restricted portions of the dorsal pallium on both ipsilateral

---

*It should be noted, however, that early studies with degeneration methods on mammalian olfactory pathways yielded inconsistencies as a consequence of transneuronal degeneration. These inconsistencies were only resolved after application of axon transport methods.

and contralateral sides and to the opposite olfactory bulb via a unique superficial tract termed the superior olfactory commissure. A projection to possible homologues of septal nuclei has also been described in the horn shark (Northcutt, 1981).

The lateral olfactory area of Ebbesson and Heimer lacks a superficial plexiform layer like that in higher vertebrates, although a subtle cellular sublamination in a portion of this area has been described in the horn shark by Bodznick and Northcutt (1979). By contrast, the area superficialis basalis has a distinctly cortical appearance by virtue of a superficial plexiform layer and compact cell body layer.

In marked contrast to higher vertebrates in which the olfactory bulb projection is to a sharply delimited superficial sublamina, the projection to the lateral olfactory area in sharks, while concentrated superficially, is intermingled with cell bodies and gradually decreases in intensity over depth (Ebbesson and Heimer, 1970) (Fig. 11). The projection to the lateral part of the area superficialis basalis is restricted to the plexiform layer, but in contrast to higher vertebrates is distributed throughout the depth of this layer (Fig. 2 in Smeets, 1983).

Extensive connections between the different pallial subdivisions in the horn shark have been described with anterograde and retrograde axon transport methods. As in mammals, these connections are crossed as well as uncrossed. The lateral pallium projects to the ipsilateral and contralateral area superficialis basalis and contralateral lateral and dorsal pallia as well as to both ipsilateral and contralateral olfactory bulbs (Ebbesson, 1972; Bodznick and Northcutt, 1979). The lateral pallium receives projections from the ipsilateral and contralateral medial and dorsal pallia in addition to the opposite lateral pallium (Bodznick and Northcutt, 1979). Unfortunately, there are no descriptions of the laminar distributions of these projections.

4. Comparison of Olfactory Cortex to Other Types of Cerebral Cortex

4.1. Comparison to Hippocampal Cortex

The olfactory cortex and hippocampal formation have much in common in amphibians through mammals. Both types of cortex appear to have attained a three-layered structure in stem reptiles that was retained through mammals (Fig. 12) (Sections 3.1.1 and 3.2; Ulinski, 1977). Both have a predominantly horizontal organization of afferent and association fiber systems in amphibians through mammals and a precise complementarity in the arrangement of fiber systems over depth in reptiles and mammals (Sections 3.1.5, 3.2, and 3.3; Herrick, 1948; Lohman and Mentink, 1972; Scalia, 1976; Ulinski, 1976; Shepherd, 1979). Pyramidal-type cells are similar morphologically in amphibians through mammals (Sections 3.1.2, 3.2, and 3.3; Northcutt, 1967; Kicliter and Ebbesson, 1976; Ulinski, 1977; Shen and Kriegstein, 1986), and in mammals the differential distribution of symmetrical and asymmetrical synapses across their surfaces is strikingly similar (Section 3.1.2; Schwartzkroin et al., 1982; Somogyi et al., 1983; Lacaille et al., 1987).

Physiologically, there are similarities in both excitatory and inhibitory synaptic potentials and in properties imparted by voltage-dependent channels (see reviews by Haberly, 1990; Brown and Zador, 1990). In both types of cortex there are feedback and feedforward inhibitory processes which are mediated by GABA (Section 3.1.6; Knowles and Schwartzkroin, 1981; Alger and Nicoll, 1982; Lacaille and Schwartzkroin, 1988) and the same peptides are found in nonpyramidal cells (Section 3.1.3; Brown and Zador, 1990).

While there are many similarities between the olfactory cortex and hippocampus, there are important differences as well. The mammalian olfactory cortex has pyramidal cells in layers II and III, whereas pyramidal cells in the mammalian hippocampus (Ammon's horn) are restricted to the middle cell layer (stratum pyramidale, Fig. 12). A second difference is that pyramidal-type cells that lack basal dendrites are confined in a cytoarchitectonically distinct subregion of the hippocampal formation, the dentate gyrus, but segregated over depth in layer IIa of piriform cortex. Finally, there is no counterpart in olfactory cortex to the mossy fiber system of the hippocampal formation.

4.2. Comparison to Neocortex

Given the marked differences in cytoarchitecture between the olfactory cortex and neocortex in mammals, a rather surprising observation is the close similarity of the mammalian olfactory cortex to the reptilian dorsal cortex—the traditional homologue of neocortex (Ariëns Kappers *et al.*, 1936) (Fig. 13). Features that the reptilian dorsal cortex has in common with the mammalian olfactory cortex include a three-layered architecture (Section 3.1.1; Ulinski, 1974; Connors and Kriegstein, 1986), segregation of the principal afferent input to a precisely defined superficial sublamina of the plexiform layer (Section 3.1.4;

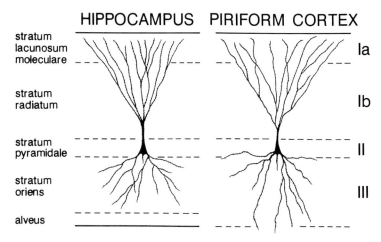

Figure 12. Comparison of terminology for hippocampus (Ammon's horn) and piriform cortex. Layer Ia of piriform cortex and stratum lacunosum-moleculare of hippocampus receive afferents of extrinsic origin; layer Ib and stratum radiatum receive intrinsic associational and commissural fibers; layer II and stratum pyramidale are densely packed laminae of pyramidal-type cell somata; layer III and stratum oriens both contain basal dendrites from overlying pyramidal cells and GABAergic and peptidergic nonpyramidal cells, but layer III of piriform cortex contains pyramidal cells in its superficial part while stratum oriens of hippocampus does not.

Hall and Ebner, 1970; Butler and Ebner, 1972), extensive associational connections that terminate in the deep part of the plexiform layer (Section 3.1.5; Lohman and Mentink, 1972; Ulinski, 1976, 1988), a tangential spread of both afferent and association fiber systems within the plexiform layer (Sections 3.1.4 and 3.1.5; Lohman and Mentink, 1972; Ulinski, 1976), similarities in the morphology of both pyramidal and nonpyramidal neurons (Sections 3.1.2 and 3.1.3; Ulinski, 1974; Connors and Kriegstein, 1986), and a tendency for segregation of nonpyramidal cells into superficial and deep layers (Section 3.1.3; Connors and Kriegstein, 1986). It must be pointed out, however, that while recent studies have demonstrated similarities in connections and physiology between the dorsal cortex and mammalian striate visual cortex (Orrego and Lissenby, 1962; Hall and Ebner, 1970; Northcutt, 1974; Smith *et al.,* 1980; Ouimet and Ebner, 1981; Connors and Kriegstein, 1986), parallels with the hippocampus have also been pointed out (Martinez-Garcia and Olucha, 1988), and there is increasing evidence that the dorsal ventricular ridge of reptiles is the functional equivalent for much of the mammalian neocortex. In spite of its subcortical location and noncortical appearance, the dorsal ventricular ridge has striking similarities in connections with mammalian neocortex including inputs from visual, auditory, and somatic sensory thalamic relay nuclei (reviewed by Ulinski, 1983; see also Bruce and Butler, 1984b). On the basis of embryological and histochemical observations, it has been postulated that the neocortex of mammals evolved, at least in part, from the dorsal ventricular ridge of an ancestral reptile (Kallen, 1951; Karten, 1969; Nauta and Karten, 1970; Bruce and Butler, 1984b) or, alternatively, that both the neocortex of mammals and the dorsal ventricular ridge of present-day reptiles developed from the same lateral pallial region in a common ancestor by outward and inward cell migrations, respectively (Northcutt, 1969). Northcutt (1969) has further postulated that the piriform cortex evolved from the ventral part of the lateral pallial region that gave rise to the neocortex and dorsal ventricular ridge. There is little evidence to support the view of Abbie

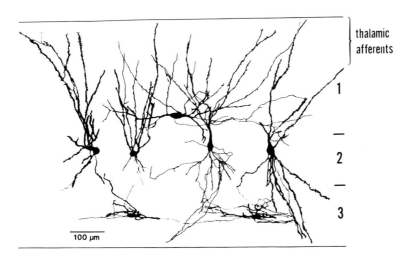

thalamic
afferents

1

2

3

100 µm

Figure 13. Laminar distribution of pyramidal-type and nonpyramidal cells in the turtle dorsal cortex. As described in the text, the dorsal cortex of reptiles resembles the lateral (piriform) cortex of reptiles and mammals in many important respects. Modified from Connors and Kriegstein (1986) with permission from the Society for Neuroscience.

(1942) (see also Sanides, 1969) that the neocortex had a dual origin via "circumferential differentiation" from the paleocortex laterally and archicortex medially.

In spite of the differences in cytoarchitecture between the olfactory cortex and neocortex in mammals, there are important similarities at the level of neuronal circuitry in keeping with the postulated evolutionary relationship. These similarities are especially striking for pyramidal cells. As described above (Section 3.1.2) there are close similarities in morphology, synaptic distribution patterns, and ultrastructural features of olfactory cortical and neocortical pyramidal cells. Furthermore, while pyramidal cells in olfactory cortex resemble those in hippocampal cortex in physiological properties (Section 4.1), the parallels are even closer with neocortex (see reviews by Douglas and Martin, 1990; Haberly, 1990): First, as a consequence of more depolarized resting membrane potentials, at least *in vitro*, synaptically mediated chloride-dependent IPSPs in slices of hippocampal cortex are consistently hyperpolarizing while those in both olfactory cortex and neocortex have little associated potential change or are depolarizing in sign so that the inhibitory action is via current shunting (Scholfield, 1978; Tseng and Haberly, 1988; Connors *et al.*, 1988). Second, pyramidal cells with differing properties imparted by voltage-dependent channels tend to be segregated over depth in both piriform cortex and neocortex (McCormick *et al.*, 1985; Tseng and Haberly, 1989a,b), but spatially segregated in the hippocampal formation (e.g., dentate gyrus, CA1, CA3). While data are insufficient for detailed comparison, there are also at least superficial similarities in the morphology of nonpyramidal cells. Many GABAergic cells in both the olfactory cortex and neocortex have smooth dendrites and receive both symmetrical and asymmetrical synapses on their somata. "Chandelier" cells that synapse selectively on axon initial segments are present in both types of cortex, the large layer Ia horizontal cells in the piriform cortex are strikingly similar to Cajal–Retzius cells in the neocortex, and the same types of neuropeptides are present in nonpyramidal cells (Section 3.1.3; Somogyi *et al.*, 1982; Haberly, 1983; Emson and Hunt, 1984; Fairén *et al.*, 1984; Haberly *et al.*, 1987; Haberly, 1990; Douglas and Martin, 1990). While afferent and corticocortical inputs to the neocortex enter from the deep pole and spread predominantly in the radial (vertical) dimension, it has become increasingly clear that intrinsic horizontal connections are also present as in the olfactory cortex (Gilbert, 1985). Intrinsic horizontal connections may be especially well developed in "association" areas. For example, in the cat suprasylvian gyrus, a region that receives multimodality inputs, there are dense horizontal connections of intrinsic origin that extend for up to 10 mm—a distance comparable to the lengths of associational connections in the olfactory cortex (Callahan and Haberly, 1987). In contrast to the olfactory cortex, however, these connections have an irregular patchy rather than continuous distribution.

An intriguing question is why the mammalian olfactory cortex has retained the organizational plan of the reptilian pallium while the neocortex underwent dramatic changes during the evolution of mammals. One obvious consequence of the shift to a predominantly radial afferent fiber distribution pattern in the mammalian neocortex from the primitive tangential pattern is that it allows a synchronous rather than sequential activation of cortical areas. For the olfactory cortex, which has only a broad overlapping topographical order and operates on a slow time scale, a tangential organization is clearly adequate, but for nonchemical senses the switch to a synchronous activation pattern presumably enhanced discrimination capabilities. Furthermore, the addition of multiple layers with radial connections greatly increased the information processing capabilities of neocortex. The presence of a substantial vertical dimension in the neocortex allows processing of different aspects of sensory input patterns in spatially segregated "columns" within single topographically organized cortical areas. For discrimination of olfactory stimuli a direct transfer of the output from the olfactory bulb to a distributed cortical processor (Section 3.1.5) is clearly adequate, but for other sensory modalities it appears that preliminary stages of topographically organized processing are essential to enhance the feature detection capabilities of individual cells before the final stages of distributed pattern analysis.

Another important question concerns the extent to which the basic principles of information processing differ in three-layered pallia and the neocortex. Given the great complexity of the neocortex and the poor segregation of neuronal elements over depth, analysis of its neuronal circuitry with present methods is very difficult. By contrast, the three-layered types of cerebral cortex are comparatively easy to analyze physiologically and anatomically, and it is therefore important to ask to what extent they can serve as model systems for analysis of neuronal processes in neocortex. Recent studies on the turtle dorsal cortex have revealed that this system has much in common with the mammalian neocortex (Connors and Kriegstein, 1986; Kriegstein and Connors, 1986), although there are certain differences in the physiological properties of its pyramidal cells. Similarly, the olfactory cortex and, to a lesser extent, the hippocampus display parallels to the neocortex at the local circuit level. The major difference between the neocortex and these three simple cortices is obviously the vertical-columnar versus tangential-continuous organization of fiber systems. However, as described above, there are strong horizontal connections in "association" areas of the neocortex that may have a distributed rather than topographically ordered organization. This raises the possibility that the olfactory cortex could serve as a model for analysis of neuronal mechanisms underlying the processing of spatially distributed activity patterns (see comments on content addressable memory, Section 3.1.5) in addition to membrane, cellular, and local circuit level processes.

5. Summary and Conclusions

In sharks, amphibians, reptiles, and mammals, the cortical areas that receive olfactory input comprise a spatially restricted part of the cerebral hemisphere. In the poorly differentiated pallia of sharks and amphibians, homologies for most cortical areas are difficult to establish, but a specialization of olfactory recipient zones is apparent. In reptiles, most of the olfactory cortical areas of mammals are clearly recognizable. Distinct cortical laminae are absent over much of the olfactory projection zone in sharks, a single cellular lamina with an overlying plexiform layer is present in amphibians, and two cellular layers are present in reptiles as in mammals. Afferent fibers are poorly segregated over depth in sharks, but in amphibians, reptiles, and mammals they are restricted to a precisely defined superficial sublamina. In reptiles and mammals, and possibly amphibians, association fibers are confined to a deep sublamina of the plexiform layer that is complementary to the afferent fiber projection zone. In amphibians, pyramidal-type cells are present, but in the lateral pallium they lack basal dendrites. In reptiles, the major variants of pyramidal-type and nonpyramidal cells that have been recognized in mammals appear to be present. Association fiber systems in the olfactory cortex are well developed in sharks through mammals. Commissural fibers are present in sharks through mammals, although the origins, routes, and sites of termination of these pathways are virtually unique in each vertebrate group.

An intriguing finding from comparative studies is the close similarity in morphology and connections of the olfactory cortex in three orders of reptiles and mammals. This suggests that in contrast to the visual, auditory, and somatic sensory systems which underwent dramatic changes during the evolution of mammals, a nearly optimal solution to the processing of olfactory information at the level of the primary cortex was achieved at least 200 million years ago in an ancestor common to reptiles and mammals. Certain features of olfactory cortex organization also appear to have been conserved from Devonian times (approximately 300 million years ago) including the spatial restriction of the olfactory bulb input to the telencephalon, the differentiation of the olfactory cortex into multiple, apparently specialized regions, the high degree of associational interconnection, and the tangential pattern of spread of afferent and association fibers.

The lateral, medial, and dorsal pallia display parallel increases in organizational complexity in extant sharks through reptiles: the differentiation of a discrete plexiform layer, development of a complementary lamination of tangentially distributed afferent and association fiber systems, differentiation of a cell-sparse deep layer, and the appearance of basal dendrites on pyramidal-type cells. While the olfactory and hippocampal cortices are similar in reptiles and mammals, the neocortex of mammals has a predominantly vertical rather than tangential pattern of fiber inputs and multiple cellular layers. Nevertheless, the strong horizontal organization appears to have been retained, especially in higher-order " association" areas, and there are many similarities in neurons, synaptic relationships, neurotransmitters, local circuitry, and physiological properties, particularly in the olfactory cortex. While the evolutionary origins of these parallels remain obscure, their presence makes the olfactory cortex a potentially useful model for study of certain general principles of operation of the neocortex.

Note Added in Proof

For additional discussion of parallels between olfactory cortex and other types of cerebral cortex, see Shepherd, G. M., 1988, A basic circuit of cortical organization, in: *Perspectives in Memory Research* (M. S. Gazzaniga, ed.), MIT Press, Cambridge, Massachusetts, pp. 93–134.

ACKNOWLEDGMENTS. I thank Dr. Philip Ulinski for critically reading the manuscript, and the Department of Neurophysiology at the University of Wisconsin for use of their extensive collection of vertebrate brain sections.

6. References

Abbie, A. A., 1942, Cortical lamination in a poliprodont marsupial, *Perameles natusa, J. Comp. Neurol.* **76**:509–536.

Adamek, G. D., Shipley, M. T., and Sanders, M. S., 1984, The indusium griseum in the mouse: Architecture, Timm's histochemistry and some afferent connections, *Brain Res. Bull.* **12**:657–668.

Alger, B. E., and Nicoll, R. A., 1982, Feedforward dendritic inhibition in rat hippocampal pyramidal cells studied *in vitro, J. Physiol. (London)* **328**:105–123.

Ariens Kappers, C. U., Huber, G. C., and Crosby, E. C., 1936, *The Comparative Anatomy of the Nervous System of Vertebrates Including Man,* Macmillan Co., New York.

Bailey, P., and von Bonin, G., 1951, *The Isocortex of Man,* University of Illinois Press, Urbana.

Biedenbach, M. A., and Stevens, C. F., 1969, Synaptic organization of the cat olfactory cortex as revealed by intracellular recording, *J. Neurophysiol.* **32**:204–214.

Bodznick, D., and Northcutt, R. G., 1979, Some connections of the lateral olfactory area of the horn shark, *Soc. Neurosci. Abstr.* **5**:139.

Broadwell, R. D., 1975, Olfactory relationships of the telencephalon and diencephalon in the rabbit. I. An autoradiographic study of the efferent connections of the main and accessory olfactory bulb, *J. Comp. Neurol.* **163**:329–345.

Brown, T. H., and Zador, A. M., 1990, Hippocampus, in: *The Synaptic Organization of the Brain* (G. M. Shepherd, ed.), Oxford University Press, London, pp. 346–388.

Bruce, L. L., and Butler, A. B., 1984a, Telencephalic connections in lizards. I. Projection to cortical areas, *J. Comp. Neurol.* **229**:585–601.

Bruce, L. L., and Butler, A. B., 1984b, Telencephalic connections in lizards. II. Projections to anterior dorsal ventricular ridge, *J. Comp. Neurol.* **229**:602–615.

Butler, A. B., and Ebner, F. F., 1972, Thalamotelencephalic projections in the lizard *Iguana iguana, Anat. Rec.* **172**:282.

Callahan, E. C., and Haberly, L. B., 1987, An extensive intrinsic association fiber system within cat area 7 revealed by anterograde and retrograde axon tracing methods, *J. Comp. Neurol.* **258**:125–137.

Calleja, C., 1893, *La Region Olfactoria del Cerebro,* Moya, Madrid, pp. 4–40.

Connors, B. W., and Kriegstein, A. R., 1986, Cellular physiology of the turtle visual cortex: Distinctive properties of pyramidal and stellate neurons, *J. Neurosci.* **6**:164–177.

Connors, B. W., Malenka, R. C., and Silva, L. R., 1988, Inhibition of neocortical pyramidal neurones in rat and cat: two types of postsynaptic potentials, and GABA A and GABA B receptor mediated responses, *J. Neurophysiol.* **406**:443–468.

Crosby, E. C., and Humphrey, T., 1941, Studies of the vertebrate telencephalon. II. The nuclear pattern of the anterior olfactory nucleus, tuberculum olfactorium, and the amygdaloid complex in adult man, *J. Comp. Neurol.* **74**:309–352.

Dart, R. A., 1920, A contribution to the morphology of the corpus striatum, *J. Anat.* **55**:1–26.

Davis, B. J., and Macrides, F., 1981, The organization of centrifugal projections from the anterior olfactory nucleus, ventral hippocampal rudiment, and piriform cortex to the main olfactory bulb in the hamster: An autoradiographic study, *J. Comp. Neurol.* **203**:475–493.

Davis, B. J., Macrides, F., Youngs, W. M., Schneider, S. P., and Rosene, D. L., 1978, Efferents and centrifugal afferents of the main and accessory olfactory bulbs in the hamster, *Brain Res. Bull.* **3**:59–72.

de Olmos, J. S., and Ingram, W. R., 1972, The projection field of the stria terminalis in the rat brain. An experimental study, *J. Comp. Neurol.* **146**:303–334.

de Olmos, J., Hardy, H., and Heimer, L., 1978, The afferent connections of the main and accessory olfactory formations in the rat: An experimental HRP-study, *J. Comp. Neurol.* **181**:213–244.

Desan, P. H., 1988, Organization of the cerebral cortex in turtle, in: *The Forebrain of Reptiles* (W. K. Schwerdtfeger and W. J. A. J. Smeets, eds.), Karger, Basel, pp. 1–11.

Douglas, R. J., and Martin, K. A. C., 1990, Neocortex, in: *The Synaptic Organization of the Brain* (G. M. Shepherd, ed.), Oxford University Press, London, pp. 389–438.

Ebbesson, S. O. E., 1972, New insights into the organization of the shark brain, *Comp. Biochem. Physiol.* **42A**:121–129.

Ebbesson, S. O. E., and Heimer, L., 1970, Projections of the olfactory tract fibers in the nurse shark *Ginglymostoma cirratum), Brain Res.* **17**:47–55.

Ebbesson, S. O. E., and Voneida, T. J., 1969, The cytoarchitecture of the pallium in the tegu lizard *Tupinambis nigropunctatus, Brain Behav. Evol.* **2**:431–466.

Emson, P. C., and Hunt, S. P., 1984, Peptide-containing neurons of the cerebral cortex, in: *Cerebral Cortex,* Volume 2 (E. G. Jones and A. Peters, eds.), Plenum Press, New York, pp. 145–169.

Fairén, A., Defilipe, J., and Regidor, J., 1984, Nonpyramidal neurons, general account, in: *Cerebral Cortex,* Volume 1 (A. Peters and E. G. Jones, eds.), Plenum Press, New York, pp. 201–253.

Freeman, W. J., 1959, Distribution in time and space of prepyriform electrical activity, *J. Neurophysiol.* **22**:644–665.

Friedman, B., and Price, J. L., 1984, Fiber systems in the olfactory bulb and cortex: A study in adult and developing rats, using the Timm method with the light and electron microscope, *J. Comp. Neurol.* **223**:88–109.

Friedman, B., and Price, J. L., 1986, Age-dependent cell death in the olfactory cortex: Lack of transneuronal degeneration in neonates, *J. Comp. Neurol.* **246**:20–31.

Gamble, H. J., 1952, An experimental study of the secondary olfactory connexions in *Lacerta oridis, J. Anat.* **86**:180–196.

Gilbert, C. D., 1985, Horizontal integration in the neocortex, *Trends Neurosci.* **8**:160–165.

Gottlieb, D. I., and Cowan, W. M., 1972, On the distribution of axonal terminals containing spheroidal and flattened synaptic vesicles in the hippocampus and dentate gyrus of the rat and cat, *Z. Zellforsch.* **129**:413–429.

Haberly, L. B., 1973a, Unitary analysis of opossum prepyriform cortex, *J. Neurophysiol.* **36**:762–774.

Haberly, L. B., 1973b, Summed potentials evoked in opossum prepyriform cortex, *J. Neurophysiol.* **36**:775–778.

Haberly, L. B., 1983, Structure of the piriform cortex of the opossum. I. Description of neuron types with Golgi methods, *J. Comp. Neurol.* **213**:163–187.

Haberly, L. B., 1985, Neuronal circuitry in olfactory cortex: Anatomy and functional implications, *Chem. Senses* **10**:219–238.

Haberly, L. B., 1990, Olfactory cortex, in: *Synaptic Organization of the Brain* (G. M. Shepherd, ed.), Oxford University Press, London, pp. 317–345.

Haberly, L. B., and Behan, M., 1983, Structure of the piriform cortex of the opossum. III. Ultrastructural characterization of synaptic terminals of association and olfactory bulb afferent fibers, *J. Comp. Neurol.* **219**:448–460.

Haberly, L. B., and Bower, J. M., 1984, Analysis of association fiber system in piriform cortex with intracellular recording and staining techniques, *J. Neurophysiol.* **51**:90–112.

Haberly, L. B., and Bower, J. M., 1989, Olfactory cortex: Model circuit for study of associative memory? *Trends Neurosci.* **12**:258–264.

Haberly, L. B., and Feig, S., 1983, Structure of the piriform cortex of the opossum. II. Fine structure of cell bodies and neuropil, *J. Comp. Neurol.* **216**:69–88.

Haberly, L. B., and Presto, S., 1986, Ultrastructural analysis of synaptic relationships of intracellularly stained pyramidal cell axons in piriform cortex, *J. Comp. Neurol.* **284**:464–474.

Haberly, L. B., and Price, J. L., 1977, The axonal projection patterns of the mitral and tufted cells of the olfactory bulb in the rat, *Brain Res.* **129**:152–157.

Haberly, L. B., and Price, J. L., 1978a, Association and commissural fiber systems of the olfactory cortex of the rat. I. Systems originating in the piriform cortex and adjacent areas, *J. Comp. Neurol.* **178**:711–740.

Haberly, L. B., and Price, J. L., 1978b, Association and commissural fiber systems of the olfactory cortex of the rat. II. Systems originating in the olfactory peduncle, *J. Comp. Neurol.* **181**:781–808.

Haberly, L. B., and Shepherd, G. M., 1973, Current density analysis of opossum prepyriform cortex, *J. Neurophysiol.* **36**:789–802.

Haberly, L. B., Hansen, D. J., Feig, S. L., and Presto, S., 1987, Distribution and ultrastructure of neurons in opossum piriform cortex displaying immunoreactivity to GABA and GAD and high affinity tritiated GABA uptake, *J. Comp. Neurol.* **266**:269–290.

Hall, W. C., and Ebner, F. F., 1970, Thalamotelencephalic projections in the turtle (Pseudemys scripta), *J. Comp. Neurol.* **140**:101–122.

Halpern, M., 1976a, Efferent connections of the lateral and dorsal cortices of snakes of the genus *Thamnophis, Anat. Rec.* **184**:421.

Halpern, M., 1976b, The efferent connections of the olfactory bulb and accessory olfactory bulb in the snakes, *Thamnophis sirtalis* and *Thamnophis radix, J. Morphol.* **150**:553–578.

Halpern, M., and Kubie, J. L., 1984, The role of the ophidian vomeronasal system in species-typical behavior, *Trends Neurosci.* **7**:472–477.

Halpern, M., and Silfen, R., 1974, The efferent connections of the nucleus sphericus in the garter snake, *Thamnophis sirtalis, Anat. Rec.* **178**:368.

Heimer, L., 1968, Synaptic distribution of centripetal and centrifugal nerve fibers in the olfactory system of the rat. An experimental anatomical study, *J. Anat.* **103**:413–432.

Heimer, L., 1969, The secondary olfactory connections in mammals, reptiles and sharks, *Ann. N.Y. Acad. Sci.* **167**:129–146.

Heimer, L., and Kalil, R., 1978, Rapid transneuronal degeneration and death of cortical neurons following removal of the olfactory bulb in adult rats, *J. Comp. Neurol.* **178**:559–609.

Herrick, C. J., 1921, The connections of the vomeronasal nerve, accessory olfactory bulb and amygdala in amphibia, *J. Comp. Neurol.* **33**:213–280.

Herrick, C. J., 1948, *The Brain of the Tiger Salamander,* University of Chicago Press, Chicago.

Hersch, S. M., and White, E. L., 1981, Quantification of synapses formed with apical dendrites of Golgi-impregnated pyramidal cells: Variability in thalamocortical inputs, but consistency in the ratios of asymmetrical to symmetrical synapses, *Neuroscience* **6**:1043–1051.

Hoffman, W. H., and Haberly, L. B., 1989, Do changes in synaptic excitation or inhibition underlie generation of long-lasting bursting-induced late EPSPs in piriform cortex? *Soc. Neurosci. Abstr.* **15**:700.

Hoogland, P. V., and Vermeulen-Van der Zee, E., 1988, Intrinsic and extrinsic connections of the cerebral cortex of lizards, in: *The Forebrain of Reptiles* (W. K. Schwerdtfeger and W. J. A. J. Smeets, eds.), Karger, Basel, pp. 20–29.

Johnston, J. B., 1911, The telencephalon of selachians, *J. Comp. Neurol.* **21**:1–113.

Jones, E. G., and Powell, T. P. S., 1969, Synapses on the axon hillocks and initial segments of pyramidal cell axons in the cerebral cortex, *J. Cell Sci.* **5**:495–507.

Jones, E. G., and Powell, T. P. S., 1970, Electron microscopy of the somatic sensory cortex of the cat. I. Cell types and synaptic organization, *Philos. Trans. R. Soc. London Ser. B* **257**:1–11.

Kallen, B., 1951, On the ontogeny of the reptilian forebrain. Nuclear structures and ventricular sulci, *J. Comp. Neurol.* **95**:307–347.

Karten, H. J., 1969, The organization of the avian telencephalon and some speculations on the phylogeny of the amniote telencephalon, *Ann. N.Y. Acad. Sci.* **167**:164–179.

Kicliter, E., and Ebbesson, S. O. E., 1976, Organization of the "nonolfactory" telencephalon, in: *Frog Neurobiology* (R. Llinas and W. Precht, eds.), Springer-Verlag, Berlin, pp. 946–972.

Knowles, W. D., and Schwartzkroin, P. A., 1981, Local circuit interactions in hippocampal brain slices, *J. Neurosci.* **1**:318–322.

Kosaka, T., 1980, The axon initial segment as a synaptic site—Ultrastructure and synaptology of the initial segment of the pyramidal cell in the rat hippocampus (CA3 region), *J. Neurocytol.* **9**:861–882.

Kosel, K. C., Van Hoesen, G., and West, J. R., 1981, Olfactory bulb projection to the parahippocampal area of the rat, *J. Comp. Neurol.* **198**:467–482.

Krettek, J. E., and Price, J. L., 1977, Projections from the amygdaloid complex and adjacent olfactory structures to the entorhinal cortex and to the subiculum in the rat and cat, *J. Comp. Neurol.* **172**:723–752.

Kriegstein, A. R., and Connors, B. W., 1986, Cellular physiology of the turtle visual cortex: Synaptic properties and intrinsic circuitry, *J. Neurosci.* **6**:178–191.

Lacaille, J.-C., and Schwartzkroin, P. A., 1988, Stratum lacunosum-moleculare interneurons of hippocampal CA1 region. II. Intrasomatic and intradendritic recordings of local circuit synaptic interactions, *J. Neurosci.* **8**:1411–1424.

Lacaille, J.-C., Kunkel, D. D., and Schwartzkroin, P. A., 1987, Local circuit interactions between oriens/alveus interneurons and CA1 cells in hippocampal slices: Electrophysiology and morphology, *J. Neurosci.* **7**:1979–1993.

Leonard, C. M., and Scott, J. W., 1971, Origin and distribution of the amygdalofugal pathways in the rat: An experimental neuroanatomical study, *J. Comp. Neurol.* **141**:313–330.

LeVay, 1973, Synaptic patterns in the visual cortex of the cat and monkey. Electron microscopy of Golgi preparations, *J. Comp. Neurol.* **150**:53–86.

Lohman, A. H. M., and Mentink, G. M., 1972, Some cortical connections of the tegu lizard *(Tupinambis tequizin), Brain Res.* **45**:325–344.

Lohman, A. H. M., Hoogland, P. V., and Witjes, R. J. G. M., 1988, Projections from the main and accessory olfactory bulbs to the amygdaloid complex in the lizard *Gekko gecko,* in: *The Forebrain of Reptiles* (W. K. Schwerdtfeger and W. J. A. J. Smeets, eds.), Karger, Basel, pp. 41–49.

Luskin, M. B., and Price, J. L., 1983a, The topographic organization of associational fibers of the olfactory system in the rat, including centrifugal fibers to the olfactory bulb, *J. Comp. Neurol.* **216:**264–291.

Luskin, M. B., and Price, J. L., 1983b, The laminar distribution of intracortical fibers originating in the olfactory cortex of the rat, *J. Comp. Neurol.* **216:**292–302.

McCormick, D. A., Connors, B. W., Lighthall, J. W., and Prince, D. A., 1985, Comparative electrophysiology of pyramidal and sparsely spiny stellate neurons of the neocortex, *J. Neurophysiol.* **54:**782–806.

McGuire, B. A., Hornung, J.-P., and Gilbert, C. D., 1984, Patterns of synaptic input to layer 4 of cat striate cortex, *J. Neurosci.* **4:**3021–3033.

Martinez-Garcia, F., and Olucha, F. E., 1988, Afferent projections to the Timm-positive cortical areas of the telencephalon of lizards, in: *The Forebrain of Reptiles* (W. K. Schwerdtfeger and W. J. A. J. Smeets, eds.), Karger, Basel, pp. 30–40.

Martinez-Garcia, F., Amiguet, M., Olucha, F., and Lopez-Garcia, C., 1986, Connections of the lateral cortex in the lizard, *Podarcis hispanica, Neurosci. Lett.* **63:**39–44.

Meredith, M., 1983, Sensory physiology of pheromone communication, in: *Pheromones and Reproduction in Mammals* (J. G. Vandebergh, ed.), Academic Press, New York, pp. 199–252.

Meyer, R. P., 1981, Central connections of the olfactory bulb in the American opossum (*Didelphys virginiana*): A light microscopic degeneration study, *Anat. Rec.* **201:**141–156.

Mugnaini, E., and Oertel, W. H., 1985, An atlas of the distribution of GABAergic neurons and terminals in the rat CNS as revealed by GAD immunohistochemistry, in: *Handbook of Chemical Neuroanatomy*, Volume 4, Part I (A. Björklund and T. Hökfelt, eds.), Elsevier, Amsterdam, pp. 436–622.

Nauta, W. J. H., and Karten, H. J., 1970, A general profile of the vertebrate brain with sidelights on the ancestry of cerebral cortex, in: *The Neurosciences: Second Study Program* (F. O. Schmidt, ed.), Rockefeller University Press, New York, pp. 7–26.

Northcutt, R. G., 1967, Architectonic studies of the telencephalon of *Iguana iguana, J. Comp. Neurol.* **130:**109–148.

Northcutt, R. G., 1969, Discussion of the preceding paper, *Ann. N.Y. Acad. Sci.* **167:**180–185.

Northcutt, R. G., 1974, Some histochemical observations of the telencephalon of the bullfrog, *Rana catesbeiana shaw, J. Comp. Neurol.* **157:**379–390.

Northcutt, R. G., 1978, Forebrain and midbrain organization in lizards and its phylogenetic significance, in: *Behavior and Neurology of Lizards* (N. Greenberg and P. D. Mac Lean, eds.), NIMH, Washington, D.C., pp. 11–64.

Northcutt, R. G., 1981, Evolution of the telencephalon in nonmammals, *Annu. Rev. Neurosci.* **4:**301–350.

Northcutt, R. G., and Kicliter, E., 1980, Organization of the amphibian telencephalon, in: *Comparative Neurology of the Telencephalon* (S. O. E. Ebbesson, ed.), Plenum Press, New York, pp. 203–255.

Northcutt, R. G., and Puzdrowski, R. L., 1988, Projections of the olfactory bulb and nervus terminalis in the silver lamprey, *Brain Behav. Evol.* **32:**96–107.

Northcutt, R. G., and Royce, G. J., 1975, Olfactory bulb projections in the bullfrog *Rana catesbeiana, J. Morphol.* **145:**251–268.

O'Leary, J. L., 1937, Structure of the primary olfactory cortex of the mouse, *J. Comp. Neurol.* **150:**217–238.

Orrego, F., and Lissenby, D., 1962, The reptilian forebrain. IV. Electrical activity of the turtle cortex, *Arch. Ital. Biol.* **100:**17–30.

Ouimet, C. C., and Ebner, F. F., 1981, Extrathalamic inputs to the cerebral cortex of the turtle, *Pseudemys scripta, Anat. Rec.* **199:**189A.

Parnavelas, J. G., Sullivan, K., Lieberman, A. R., and Webster, K. E., 1977, Neurons and their synaptic organization in the visual cortex of the rat, *Cell Tissue Res.* **183:**499–517.

Pérez-Clausell, J., and Fredens, K., 1988, Chemoarchitectonics in the telencephalon of the lizard *Podarcis hispanica*, in: *The Forebrain of Reptiles* (W. K. Schwerdtfeger and W. J. A. J. Smeets, eds.), Karger, Basel, pp. 85–96.

Peters, A., 1985, The visual cortex of the rat, in: *Cerebral Cortex*, Volume 3 (A. Peters and E. G. Jones, eds.), Plenum Press, New York, pp. 19–80.

Peters, A., and Kaiserman-Abramof, I. R., 1970, The small pyramidal neuron of the rat cerebral cortex. The perikaryon, dendrites and spines, *Am. J. Anat.* **127:**321–356.

Peters, A., and Kara, D. A., 1985, The neuronal composition of area 17 of rat visual cortex. I. The pyramidal cells, *J. Comp. Neurol.* **234:**218–241.

Peters, A., Proskauer, C. C., and Kaiserman-Abramof, I. R., 1968, The small pyramidal neuron of the rat cerebral cortex. The axon hillock and initial segment, *J. Cell Biol.* **39**:604–619.

Price, J. L., 1973, An autoradiographic study of complementary laminar patterns of termination of afferent fibers to the olfactory cortex, *J. Comp. Neurol.* **150**:87–108.

Price, J. L., 1985, Beyond the primary olfactory cortex: Olfactory-related areas in the neocortex, thalamus and hypothalamus, *Chem. Senses* **10**:239–258.

Ramón y Cajal, S., 1911, *Histologie due Système Nerveux de l'Homme et des Vertébrés,* Maloine, Paris.

Reiner, A., and Karten, H. J., 1985, Comparison of olfactory bulb projections in pigeons and turtles, *Brain Behav. Evol.* **27**:11–27.

Rodriguez, R., and Haberly, L. B., 1989, Analysis of synaptic events in the opossum piriform cortex with improved current source density techniques, *J. Neurophysiol.* **61**:702–718.

Rolon, R. R., and Skeen, L. C., 1980, Afferent and efferent connections of the olfactory bulb in the soft-shelled turtle (*Trionyx spinifer spinifer*), *Soc. Neurosci. Abstr.* **6**:305.

Sanides, F., 1969, Comparative architectonics of the neocortex of mammals and their evolutionary interpretation, *Ann. N.Y. Acad. Sci.* **167**:405–423.

Sanides, F., and Sanides, D., 1972, The "extraverted neurons" of the mammalian cerebral cortex, *Z. Anat. Entwicklungsgesch.* **136**:272–293.

Satou, M., Mori, K., Tazawa, Y., and Takagi, S. F., 1982, Two types of postsynaptic inhibition in pyriform cortex of the rabbit: Fast and slow inhibitory postsynaptic potentials, *J. Neurophysiol.* **48**:1142–1156.

Satou, M., Mori, K., Tazawa, Y., and Takagi, S. F., 1983, Interneurons mediating fast postsynaptic inhibition in pyriform cortex of the rabbit, *J. Neurophysiol.* **50**:89–101.

Scalia, F., 1972, The projection of the accessory olfactory bulb in the frog, *Brain Res.* **36**:409–411.

Scalia, F., 1976, Structure of the olfactory and accessory olfactory systems, in: *Frog Neurobiology* (R. Llinas and W. Precht, eds.), Springer-Verlag, Berlin, pp. 213–233.

Scalia, F., and Winans, S. S., 1975, The differential projections of the olfactory bulb and accessory olfactory bulb in mammals, *J. Comp. Neurol.* **161**:31–56.

Scalia, F., Halpern, M., Knapp, H., and Riss, W., 1968, The efferent connexions of the olfactory bulb in the frog: A study of degenerating unmyelinated fibers, *J. Anat.* **103**:245–262.

Scalia, F., Halpern, M., and Riss, W., 1969, Olfactory bulb projections in the South American caiman, *Brain Behav. Evol.* **2**:238–262.

Schoenfeld, T. A., and Macrides, F., 1984, Topographical organization of connections between the main olfactory bulb and pars externa of the anterior olfactory nucleus in the hamster, *J. Comp. Neurol.* **227**:121–135.

Scholfield, C. N., 1978, A depolarizing inhibitory potential in neurones of the olfactory cortex *in vitro, J. Physiol. (London)* **279**:547–557.

Schwartzkroin, P. A., Kunkel, D. D., and Mathers, L. H., 1982, Development of rabbit hippocampus: Anatomy, *Dev. Brain Res.* **2**:453–468.

Scott, J. W., 1986, The olfactory bulb and central pathways, *Experientia* **42**:223–232.

Scott, J. W., McBride, R. L., and Schneider, S. P., 1980, The organization of projections from the olfactory bulb to the piriform cortex and olfactory tubercle in the rat, *J. Comp. Neurol.* **194**:519–534.

Scott, J. W., Rainer, E. C., Pemberton, J. L., Orona, E., and Mouradian, L. E., 1985, Pattern of rat olfactory bulb mitral and tufted cell connections to the anterior olfactory nucleus pars externa, *J. Comp. Neurol.* **242**:415–424.

Shammah-Lagnado, S. J., and Negrao, N., 1981, Efferent connections of the olfactory bulb in the opossum (*Didelphis marsupialis aurita*): A Fink–Heimer study, *J. Comp. Neurol.* **201**:51–63.

Shen, J. M., and Kriegstein, A. R., 1986, Turtle hippocampal cortex contains distinct cell types, burst-firing neurons, and an epileptogenic subfield, *J. Neurophysiol.* **56**:1626–1649.

Shepherd, G. M., 1979, *The Synaptic Organization of the Brain,* Oxford University Press, London.

Shipley, M. T., and Adamek, G. D., 1984, The connections of the mouse olfactory bulb: A study using orthograde and retrograde transport of wheat germ agglutinin conjugated to horseradish peroxidase, *Brain Res. Bull.* **12**:669–688.

Shipley, M. T., and Geinisman, Y., 1984, Anatomical evidence for convergence of olfactory, gustatory, and visceral afferent pathways in mouse cerebral cortex, *Brain Res. Bull.* **12**:221–226.

Skeen, L. C., and Hall, W. C., 1977, Efferent projections of the main and accessory olfactory bulb in the tree shrew (*Tupaia glis*), *J. Comp. Neurol.* **172**:1–36.

Skeen, L. C., Pindzola, R. R., and Schofield, B. R., 1984, Tangential organization of olfactory, association, and commissural projections to olfactory cortex in a species of reptile (*Trionyx spiniferns*), bird (*Aix sponsa*), and mammal (*Tupaia glis*), *Brain Behav. Evol.* **25**:206–216.

Sloper, J. J., and Powell, T. P. S., 1979, A study of the axon initial segment and proximal axon of neurons in the primate motor and somatic sensory cortices, *Philos. Trans. R. Soc. London Ser. B* **285**:173–197.

Smeets, W. J. A. J., 1983, The secondary olfactory connections in two chondrichthians, the shark *Scyliorhinus canicula* and the ray *Raja clavata, J. Comp. Neurol.* **218**:334–344.

Smeets, W. J. A. J., Nieuwenhuys, R., and Roberts, B. L., 1983, *The Central Nervous System of Cartilaginous Fishes*, Springer-Verlag, Berlin.

Smith, L. M., Ebner, F. F., and Colonnier, M., 1980, The thalamocortical projection in *Pseudemys* turtles: A quantitative electron microscopic study, *J. Comp. Neurol.* **190**:445–461.

Somogyi, P., Freund, T. F., and Lowey, A., 1982, The axo-axonic interneuron in the cerebral cortex of the rat, cat, and monkey, *Neuroscience* **7**:2577–2607.

Somogyi, P., Smith, A. D., Nungi, M. G., Gorio, A., Takagi, H., and Wu, J. Y., 1983, Glutamate decarboxylase immunoreactivity in the hippocampus of the cat: Distribution of immunoreactive synaptic terminals with special reference to the axon initial segment of pyramidal neurons, *J. Neurosci.* **3**:1450–1468.

Stevens, C. F., 1969, Structure of cat frontal olfactory cortex, *J. Neurophysiol.* **32**:184–192.

Switzer, R. C., de Olmos, J., and Heimer, L., 1986, The olfactory system, in: *The Rat Nervous System: Forebrain and Midbrain*, Volume 1 (G. Paxinos, ed.), Academic Press, New York.

Takagi, S. F., 1986, Studies on the olfactory nervous system of the old world monkey, *Prog. Neurobiol.* **27**:195–250.

Tseng, G.-F., and Haberly, L. B., 1988, Characterization of synaptically mediated fast and slow inhibitory processes in piriform cortex in an in vitro slice preparation, *J. Neurophysiol.* **59**:1352–1376.

Tseng, G.-F., and Haberly, L. B., 1989a, Deep neurons in piriform cortex. I. Morphology and synaptically evoked responses including a unique high amplitude paired shock facilitation, *J. Neurophysiol.* **62**:369–385.

Tseng, G.-F., and Haberly, L. B., 1989b, Deep neurons in piriform cortex. II. Membrane properties that underlie unusual synaptic responses, *J. Neurophysiol.* **62**:386–400.

Turner, B. H., Gupta, K. C., and Mishkin, M., 1978, The locus and cytoarchitecture of the projection areas of the olfactory bulb in *Macaca mulatta, J. Comp. Neurol.* **177**:381–396.

Ulinski, P. S., 1974, Cytoarchitecture of cerebral cortex in snakes, *J. Comp. Neurol.* **158**:243–266.

Ulinski, P. S., 1976, Intracortical connections in the snakes *Natrix sipedon* and *Thamnophis sirtalis, J. Morphol.* **150**:463–484.

Ulinski, P. S., 1977, Intrinsic organization of snake medial cortex: An electron microscopic and Golgi study, *J. Morphol.* **152**:247–280.

Ulinski, P. S., 1983, *Dorsal Ventricular Ridge: A Treatise on Forebrain Organization in Reptiles and Birds*, Wiley, New York.

Ulinski, P. S., 1988, Functional architecture of turtle visual cortex, in: *The Forebrain of Reptiles* (W. K. Schwerdtfeger and W. J. A. J. Smeets, eds.), Karger, Basel, pp. 151–161.

Ulinski, P. S., and Kanarek, D. A., 1973, Cytoarchitecture of nucleus sphericus in the common boa, *Constrictor constrictor, J. Comp. Neurol.* **151**:149–174.

Ulinski, P. S., and Peterson, E. H., 1981, Patterns of olfactory projections in the desert iguana *Dipsosaurus dorsalis, J. Morphol.* **168**:189–227.

Ulinski, P. S., and Rainey, W. T., 1980, Intrinsic organization of snake lateral cortex, *J. Morphol.* **165**:85–116.

Valverde, F., 1965, *Studies on the Piriform Lobe*, Harvard University Press, Cambridge, Mass.

Valverde, F., and Facal-Valverde, M. V., 1986, Neocortical layers I and II of the hedgehog *Erinaceus europaeus*. I. Intrinsic organization, *Anat. Embryol.* **173**:413–430.

Westenbroek, R. E., Westrum, L. E., Hendrickson, A. E., and Wu, J.-Y., 1987, Immunocytochemical localization of cholecystokinin and glutamic acid decarboxylase during normal development in the prepyriform cortex of rats, *Dev. Brain Res.* **34**:191–206.

Westrum, L. E., 1966, Synaptic contacts on axons in the cerebral cortex, *Nature* **210**:1289–1290.

Winfield, D. A., Brooke, R. N. L., Sloper, J. J., and Powell, T. P. S., 1981, A combined Golgi–electron microscopic study of the synapses made by the proximal axon and recurrent collaterals of a pyramidal cell in the somatic sensory cortex of the monkey, *Neuroscience* **6**:1217–1230.

Wyss, J. M., and Sripanidkulchai, K., 1983, The indusium griseum and anterior hippocampal continuation in the rat, *J. Comp. Neurol.* **219**:251–272.

12

Comparative Anatomy of the Hippocampus

With Special Reference to Differences in the Distributions of Neuroactive Peptides

CHRISTINE GALL

1. Introduction

Experimental work beginning in the last century and carried on with increasing intensity in recent times has provided ever more precise accounts of the anatomical, physiological, and biochemical properties of the various subfields and interconnections of the hippocampal formation. Indeed, hippocampus is now one of the most thoroughly described regions in mammalian brain. Despite this, it has not been possible to link the specific neurobiological features of the structure to its contributions to behavior; this is quite possibly one of the reasons that the role of hippocampus in processes such as learning and memory remains a subject of continuing controversy.

Comparative studies have historically been of value in identifying possible functional linkages between particular elements in multiple component biological systems as well as in developing hypotheses regarding the associations between those elements and behavior. Examination of a variety of species allows one to detect features that covary as well as those that do not, data that are useful in formulating ideas about functional interrelationships. Moreover, the com-

CHRISTINE GALL • Department of Anatomy and Neurobiology, University of California–Irvine, California 92717.

parative approach often points to correlations between behavioral specializations of particular animals and distinctive features of the biological system of interest.

While there is a long history of comparative research on the relationship between brain and body size (see Jerison, 1973, for a review), much less attention has been given to cross-species differences in the size and organization of particular brain regions. Nonetheless, pertinent observations have slowly accumulated and there is now sufficient material to begin constructing a comparative picture of hippocampus and certain other brain areas. As will be discussed, the collected results of many different studies do suggest certain phylogenetic trends, but perhaps equally important they indicate areas in which additional work is badly needed if a systematic description is to be obtained.

As will be reviewed in the pages which follow, select aspects of hippocampal anatomy and neurochemistry have been evaluated in a number of species. Much of this information suggests that, in contrast to many other areas of telencephalon, the major features of hippocampal anatomy are remarkably consistent across the mammalian radiations. While the neocortex has evolved from a small, rather diffusely organized dorsal pallium, as seen in primitive mammals, to become a highly laminated and complex structure which occupies approximately 95% of the human forebrain (Stephan, 1983), the hippocampus has remained recognizable with the same principal cell types, cytoarchitectonic laminae, and innervation patterns across several orders of mammals. However, as one examines hippocampal anatomy more closely, and more selectively, phylogenetic changes are evident. Most particularly, the use of axonal tracing and immunohistochemical techniques has demonstrated clear interspecies differences both in the innervation topographies of major hippocampal afferents and in the distribution of neuroactive substances within hippocampal circuitry.

The present chapter will focus on three basic features of hippocampal organization in a number of mammalian species which reflect both the extreme phylogenetic stability of some anatomical characters and the apparent inconsistency of others. After a brief summary of hippocampal organization and nomenclature, the issue of how the size of various hippocampal subfields change as a function of the size of hippocampus (i.e., the allometry of hippocampus and hippocampal subfields) will be considered. This material is followed by a discussion of the comparative differences in the distributions of the major systems of intrinsic and extrinsic hippocampal afferents. Finally, recently observed comparative differences in the immunocytochemical properties of hippocampal systems will be discussed. The material reviewed leads to the conclusion that the stability of some of the more conspicuous features of hippocampal organization should not be interpreted to indicate consistent functional properties. Simple differences in the size of hippocampus between animals predict basic differences in the proportions of various subfields and changes in neuronal density which might influence the fundamental computational properties of the structure. Differences in the distribution of the principle afferent systems between animals, most particularly changes in the hippocampal commissural projections, suggest the tendency toward hemispheric isolation of hippocampus in primates. Finally, striking comparative differences in the distribution of neuroactive peptides within aspects of hippocampal circuitry indicate there may be major differences in the synaptic physiology of phylogenetically conserved axonal systems between animals.

Detailed descriptions of comparative differences in hippocampal cytoarchitectonics and the distributions of the numerically more minor hippocampal afferents are beyond the scope of the present chapter. For further information on these topics the reader is referred to the review of Rosene and Van Hoesen (1987).

169

COMPARATIVE
ANATOMY OF THE
HIPPOCAMPUS

2. Cytoarchitectonics

The hippocampus is a long arcing structure which, in rat, lies with its rostral, or septal, pole in continuity with the fornix immediately caudal to the septal region, and its temporal pole lying ventrolateral to the diencephalon near the amygdala. In mammals with bigger brains, the entire structure appears to have shifted ventrally and laterally into the temporal lobe such that in monkey and man the temporal pole of hippocampus is found within the rostral temporal lobe, immediately caudal to the amygdala, and the region homologous to the "septal pole" in rodent lies within the more caudal temporal lobe. The simple stereotypic organization of hippocampal cytoarchitectonics is best appreciated in sections cut perpendicular to the long axis of the structure. In virtually all such cross sections through "septal" or "temporal" regions, hippocampal cytoarchitectonics can be characterized as two interlocking "C's" formed by the compact layer of granule cells (stratum granulosum) of the fascia dentata and the broader curving layer of pyramidal cells (stratum pyramidale) of the hippocampus proper (Fig. 1). The dendrites of these two principal cell types are aligned to form relatively cell-free molecular layers within which the major hippocampal afferents terminate (Fig. 1B). The granule cell dendrites radiate to the outside of the curving granule cell layer to form the molecular layer of the fascia dentata. The hilar region, which lies to the inside of the curve of granule cells, and fascia dentata together constitute the dentate gyrus (Geneser, 1987). The pyramidal cells are oriented with apical dendrites toward the inside of the curving cell layer and basal dendrites toward the hippocampal surface. In addition to the principal cell types, morphologically heterogeneous interneurons and some efferent neurons are scattered through all laminae of the structure (Lorente de Nó, 1934; Schwerdtfeger and Buhl, 1986).

The granule cells of the dentate gyrus are relatively homogeneous and do not segregate themselves into subfields. Although the dendritic arborizations of the granule cells vary depending on the depth of the cell body within stratum granulosum, these differences do not warrant attempts to divide the cell body layer into sublaminae. The hilus of the dentate gyrus contains a bewildering array of cell types and extrinsic afferents and, largely due to species differences in cytoarchitectonics, the limits of this field have been the subject of some controversy (see Geneser, 1987, for discussion). The area immediately subjacent to the granule cells contains basket cell interneurons of the type found throughout hippocampus and the rest of the telencephalon (Ribak and Seress, 1983). In rat, the more central hilus contains a variety of interneurons as well as polymorph neurons that generate the dentate gyrus commissural and associational projections (see Section 4.1.2). At least some of these hilar cell types are innervated by the much more numerous granule cells via the mossy fiber system (Amaral, 1978). The core of the hilus abuts the free end of the hippocampal pyramidal cell layer.

The most conspicuous comparative differences in the organization of the dentate gyrus are to be found in the relative degree of stratification within the

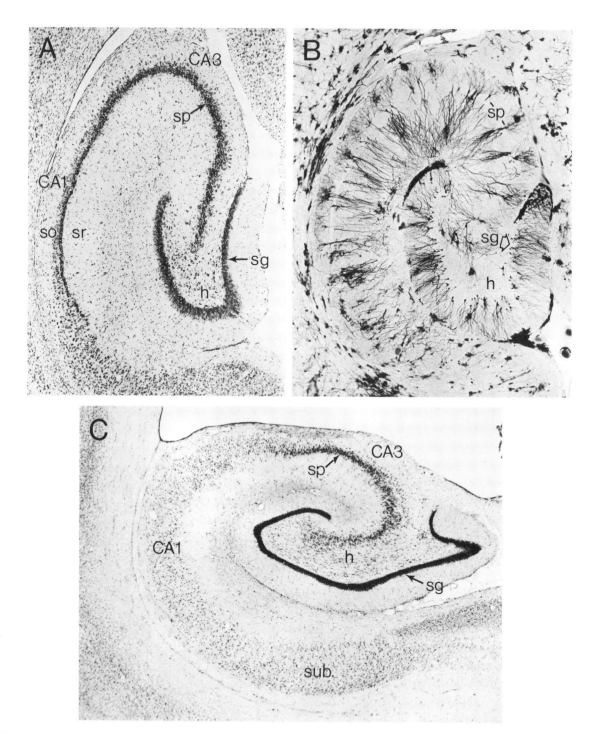

Figure 1. Low-magnification photomicrographs of Nissl-stained (A, C) and Golgi-impregnated (B) sections through rat (A, B) and Old World monkey (C) hippocampus which illustrate the cytoarchitectonic organization and stereotypic dendritic arborization patterns described in the text. Note that in a comparison of the Nissl-stained sections shown in panels A and C, the most conspicuous difference in the cytoarchitectonic organization of rat and monkey hippocampus is in the density of cell packing within stratum pyramidale of region CA1 and the associated absence of a cell-free stratum oriens in this region of monkey.

hilus. In the hilar region of both the rat and mouse, no clear lamination is evident in either the cytoarchitectonics or the distribution of axonal systems. In contrast, in the guinea pig, rabbit, monkey, and man, hilar neurons conform to reasonably well-defined strata, and histochemically distinct axonal systems, which are diffusely distributed across the full hilus of the rat, appear targeted to particular cytoarchitectonic laminae (Geneser, 1987; Rosene and Van Hoesen, 1987). There has been much less discussion of comparative differences in the organization of the granule cells and their dendritic fields, and one gains the impression that this neuronal population is relatively invariant across species. However, it has recently been reported that one very striking and characteristic feature of the granule cell in rodents, the lack of basal dendrites, does not hold in the primate (Seress and Mrzljak, 1987). In addition, recent immunocytochemical work has identified major between-species differences in the neuropeptide chemistry of the granule cells, a subject that will be discussed at length in a later section.

The pyramidal cells of hippocampus, in contrast to the granule cells, do exhibit sufficient regional differences to suggest natural subdivisions around the arc of the curving cell layer and these differences in neuronal morphology are correlated with marked variations in the organization of afferent and efferent projections. Ramón y Cajal (1911, 1968) recognized two subdivisions based on the size and dendritic arborization patterns of the pyramidal cells, i.e., a field of small pyramidal cells, the regio superior, and a large cell field, the regio inferior. Lorente de Nó (1934) made a finer classification scheme consisting of CA1a, b, and c (CA: Cornu Ammonis); CA2; CA3a, b, and c; and CA4. The existence of CA2 and CA4 has long been a subject of controversy and need not occupy us here except to note that Lorente de Nó considered that the area he defined as region CA4, comprised of the "reflected blades" of stratum pyramidale within the curve of the dentate gyrus, changed drastically from small- to large-brained animals. Region CA4 of Lorente de Nó generally corresponds to what is now considered the hilar region of the dentate gyrus by most modern investigators (Amaral, 1978; Geneser, 1987). The remainder of the system of nomenclature has proven its utility and is widely employed today.

In the hippocampus proper, the greatest cytoarchitectonic difference seen between species is in the depth, or what might be seen as the density of cell packing, in stratum pyramidale (Stephan, 1983; Rosene and Van Hoesen, 1987; Stephan and Manolescu, 1980). In less encephalized mammals such as the rat, the small pyramidal neurons of region CA1 are collected into a compact lamina and are separated from the alveus, at the surface of hippocampus, by a well-defined, cell-poor stratum oriens (Fig. 1A). In larger-brained mammals, the CA1 pyramidal cell layer becomes dispersed into stratum oriens such that, with the great enlargement of the region seen in man, stratum oriens is virtually obliterated and the transition from region CA1 to the subiculum is difficult to identify in Nissl preparations (Fig. 1C).

3. Allometric Relationships

Before taking up the question of comparative differences in the sizes of the components of hippocampus, a brief comment on the size of the structure as a whole is appropriate. As has been known since the end of the 19th century, brain size in mammals scales to body size with an exponent of ⅔ to ¾ (Armstrong, 1982). Most of the increase is due to expansion of neocortex and as a result the hippocampus, though growing absolutely larger with increasing body size, accounts for an ever-decreasing percentage of total brain as brain increases. This point is evident in Fig. 2 which shows log–log plots of hippocampal versus total brain size for two orders of mammals (insectivores and two suborders of primates). The steeper slope for hippocampal size increase in insectivores and prosimians results from the fact that brain and neocortex do not increase with body size to the same degree in these groups as they do in the simian primates; in essence the difference between the curves does not reflect a failure of hippocampus to keep pace with body size in the simians but rather its failure to keep pace with neocortical expansion. In fact, as shown by Stephan and colleagues (Ste-

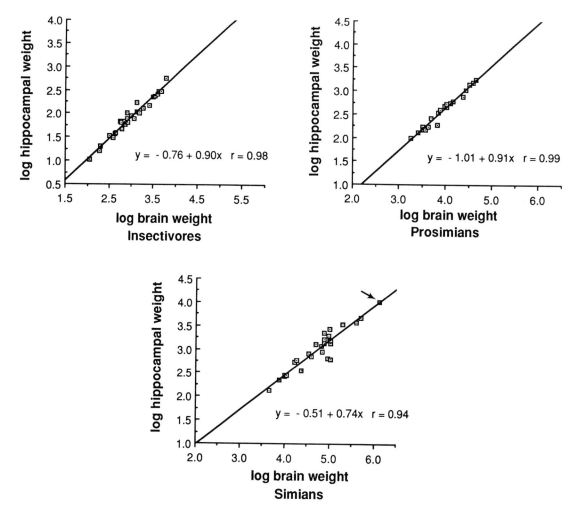

Figure 2. Log hippocampal weight is plotted against log brain weight for a sample of 28 insectivores, 21 prosimians, and 27 simians including man (arrow) (from data of Stephan *et al.*, 1981). Equations describe the line which best fits the data for each group (*y* is log hippocampal weight, *x* is log brain weight, the value preceding *x* is the slope of the line, and *r* is the correlation coefficient).

phan, 1983; Stephan and Manolescu, 1980; Stephan *et al.*, 1981), the hippocampus of humans is four times larger than it would be in a hypothetical insectivore of equivalent body size, and for this reason can be considered as a "progressive" structure.

One interesting point made by Fig. 2 is that human hippocampus is about the size that would be expected for a generalized simian brain of the volume of human brain. In other words, the allometric equation relating hippocampus to brain size for the simian primate suborder accurately predicts the size of human hippocampus; this observation points to the conclusion that evolutionary pressures have not had a powerful effect on the absolute volume of this structure in humans.

Figure 3, which is based on data published by Stephan and Manolescu (1980), illustrates the relationship in primates between the size of three hippocampal subfields to an estimate of the size of hippocampus. The correlation coefficients between the size of the part and the size of the whole are extremely high, a point that is all the more surprising since the sample includes values for prosimians and simians, including human. It would appear then that a basic hippocampal form exists for primates and that none of the representatives included in Fig. 3 deviate significantly from this plan.

It will be noted that in primates the slope for the size increase of field CA1 is slightly steeper than that for CA3 or dentate gyrus. This changes the ratio of CA1 to the other subfields as a function of primate brain and hippocampal size [e.g., CA1/CA3 in humans is 273% while in *Callithrix jacchus* (New World monkey) it is 128%]. With the caveat that the sample size used to generate the curves is small and includes only one large primate (human), these observations illustrate the point that allometric relationships can generate substantial differences between species in the absence of selective evolutionary pressures on those species other than for absolute size. They also indicate that differences within a brain area between two species cannot be taken as evidence of evolutionary specializations in the absence of considerations of size differences and allometric relationships.

Allometrically derived alterations of this type are known to have profound effects in many areas of biology; the ratio of surface area to body size, for example, decreases with increasing body size and has a major impact on heat retention and loss, factors that in turn surely affect behavior. The possible func-

Figure 3. The logs of the areas (mm²) of hippocampal subfields CA1, CA3, and dentate gyrus are plotted against the log of total hippocampal area for eight primates including four prosimians, three nonhuman simians, and man (arrow) (from data of Stephan and Manolescu, 1980). Note that in man the size of each subfield is consistent with the trend in this relatively small group of primates and that the slope describing the increase in the size of hippocampal region CA1 (1.15) is greater than the slope for CA3 or the dentate gyrus.

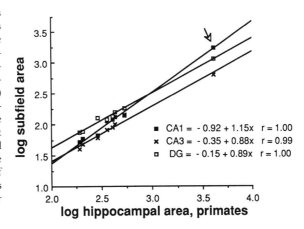

$$CA1 = -0.92 + 1.15x \quad r = 1.00$$
$$CA3 = -0.35 + 0.88x \quad r = 0.99$$
$$DG = -0.15 + 0.89x \quad r = 1.00$$

tional consequences of the changes in the balance of hippocampal subdivisions occurring with increasing hippocampal size should be borne in mind when considering possible differences in the contributions of hippocampus to behavior of humans versus smaller-brained animals.

Figure 4 summarizes the relationships between the sizes of field CA1, field CA3, and the dentate gyrus with absolute hippocampal size in the insectivores. It is again evident that an excellent correlation exists among these variables, strongly suggesting that the various species have retained with little modification a basic plan for the order. With the proviso that the sample size is small, it appears that this plan deviates from that of the primates in that the slope of the curve relating field CA3 to hippocampal size is steeper than that for field CA1, the reverse of the situation for primates. If confirmed with further work, this observation would point to the conclusion that evolutionary pressures early in phylogeny did operate upon the hippocampus in one or both of these orders. This would then raise the question of how insectivores as an order differ in their behavior or adaptations to their ecology from primates as an order. Is a feature such as dependence on vision versus olfaction responsible for what may be a shift in the relative balance of CA1 versus CA3? Issues such as this would be greatly clarified by construction of allometric curves for other orders and increased sampling, particularly of the primates.

It should be noted that allometric relationships are known to exist between the size of a region and the cellular features of that region. For example, the length of dendrites in neocortex is reported to scale to the 0.3 power of cortical volume while the density of cells decreases with increasing cortical size (see Jerison, 1973, for discussion of these and other such features). It appears likely that similar relationships also hold for hippocampus. In a comparison of rats and mice, West and Andersen (1980) found that both the number of granule cells per unit volume and the length of granule cell dendrites are correlated with the size of the fascia dentata, such that granule cell density decreases with the enlargement of the area. This has important implications for the interpretation of the between-species cytoarchitectonic differences noted earlier since it is possible that these are to some extent simple reflections of size rather than evolutionary specializations.

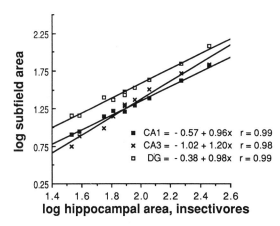

Figure 4. The logs of the areas (mm²) of hippocampal subfields CA1, CA3, and dentate gyrus (calculated from linear measurements through the cell layers) are plotted against the log of the total hippocampal area for a group of ten insectivores (from data of Stephan and Manolescu, 1980). Equations describe the "best-fit" lines for each subfield as in Fig. 2. Note that the slope describing the increase in the size of region CA3 with increased hippocampal size (1.20) is greater than that for either region CA1 or the dentate gyrus.

To summarize, analysis of the comparative data collected by Stephan and colleagues suggests the following:

1. The hippocampus appears to be a relatively "conservative" structure in that individual species of primates do not deviate greatly from a general pattern that operates across the order.
2. Relatively slight differences in the allometric relationships between CA1, CA3, and dentate gyrus with the size of hippocampus appear to be present in primates and result in changes in the relative proportions of these areas across hippocampi of different sizes. It might then be expected that significant differences in the internal organization of the hippocampus could exist in primates of different brain sizes purely as a consequence of allometry.
3. The general plan for primates may differ from that for insectivores, suggesting that evolutionary changes occurred early in the history of these orders and were retained across the subsequent course of phylogeny.
4. Further comparative work may point to hypotheses about the functional consequences of the order-level differences as well as identifying within-order differences in hippocampal anatomy that are not predicted by allometry.

4. Comparative Differences in Afferent Topographies

4.1. Major Intrinsic Afferent Systems

As with the cytoarchitectonics, a simple, stereotypic plan of hippocampal organization is evident in the pattern of afferent termination as well. This stratified organization is well illustrated in sections through rat hippocampus processed by Timm's stain for heavy metals (Fig. 5) in which bands of differential staining intensity correspond quite precisely with the laminar termination of the major afferent systems within the principal dendritic fields (Haug, 1974; Zimmer, 1973). Both the hippocampus proper and the fascia dentata receive the vast majority of their innervation from the entorhinal cortex and from within the hippocampus itself. As observed in the rat, the three major afferent systems which arise from within the hippocampus include: (1) the collateral commissural and ipsilateral associational projections from polymorph hilar neurons that innervate the proximal molecular layer of the dentate gyrus (Blackstad, 1956; Zimmer, 1971; Gottlieb and Cowan, 1973; Hjorth-Simonsen and Laurberg, 1977; Laurberg and Sørensen, 1981; Swanson *et al.*, 1981), (2) the commissural and ipsilateral Schaffer collateral projections from the pyramidal cells of region CA3 that innervate strata radiatum and oriens of the hippocampus proper (regions CA3, CA2, CA1) (Blackstad, 1956; Hjorth-Simonsen, 1972a, 1977; Swanson *et al.*, 1978), and (3) the strictly ipsilateral mossy fiber projections of the dentate gyrus granule cells which terminate within the hilus and stratum lucidum of field CA3 (see Figs. 1 and 5 for nomenclature; Fig. 7). In the latter area, the mossy fibers innervate the proximal dendrites and thorny spines of the regio inferior pyramidal cells (Gaarskjaer, 1978; Blackstad and Kjaerheim, 1961; Laatsch and Cowan, 1965; Blackstad *et al.*, 1970; Haug *et al.*, 1971). In the rat, intrinsic afferent fields abut, but do not overlap, the zones in which afferent axons from the entorhinal cortex terminate; in both the dentate gyrus and hippocampus proper the hippocampal afferents occupy the more proximal dendritic fields whereas the entorhinal afferents terminate more distally (Fig. 6).

On the basis of physiological analyses in rabbit, Andersen *et al.* (1971) proposed that the major axonal systems within hippocampus (mossy fibers, hippocampal commissural and Schaffer collateral projections, and entorhinal "perforant path" afferents) were oriented approximately perpendicular to the long axis of the structure giving rise to nonoverlapping "lamellae," or what might be seen as thin slices through hippocampus, each of which contained an equivalent trisynaptic circuit consisting of perforant path projections to dentate gyrus granule cells to CA3 pyramidal cells (via mossy fibers) to CA1 pyramidal cells (via Schaffer collaterals) (Fig. 7) (Rawlins and Green, 1977). We now know there is much greater septotemporal spread in these projections than originally appreciated.

4.1.1. The Mossy Fibers

The distribution of the mossy fiber projections most closely approximates the transverse lamellae proposed by Andersen *et al.* (1971). In the rat, the mossy fiber axons of the dentate gyrus granule cells fill the hilus, course within stratum

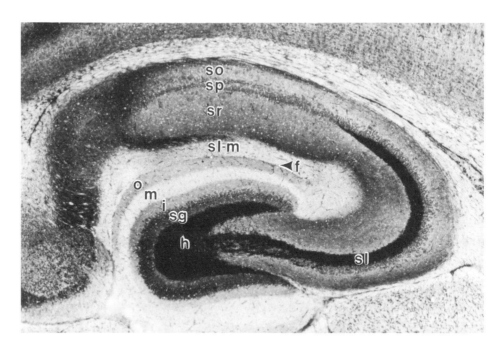

Figure 5. Horizontal section through rat hippocampus processed by Timm's stain for the localization of heavy metals which illustrates the principal hippocampal laminae discussed in the text. The dense reaction product in the hilus and stratum lucidum is associated with mossy fiber terminal boutons. In the rat, the laminae of differing staining intensity in other fields correspond with the laminated termination of the major afferent systems of entorhinal and hippocampal origin. For abbreviations see Section 7.

lucidum in the proximal apical dendritic field of regio inferior, and innervate the dendritic shafts and thorny excrescences of the large CA3 pyramidal cells across the full septotemporal extent of hippocampus (Gaarskjaer, 1978; Laatsch and Cowan, 1965; Blackstad *et al.*, 1970; West *et al.*, 1982). The unusually large, mossy fiber terminal boutons formed by these axons contain relatively high concentrations of zinc. As such, it has been possible to exploit Timm's silver sulfide technique for the localization of heavy metals to analyze the distribution of the mossy fibers in the rat, mouse, European hedgehog, hamster, rabbit, guinea pig, cat, tree shrew, marmoset, and monkey (Gaarskjaer, 1978; Haug, 1974; Rosene and Van Hoesen, 1987; West and Schwerdtfeger, 1985; Geneser-Jensen *et al.*, 1974; Haug *et al.*, 1971; Gall, unpublished observations). With two rather minor exceptions to be mentioned below, the mossy fibers in each of these animals exhibit essentially the same distribution as found in the rat. In this rodent, the major portion of the mossy fiber system is sharply topographic with axons coursing roughly perpendicular to the long axis of hippocampus to innervate CA3 pyramidal cells within, and somewhat rostral to, their septotemporal plane of origin (Gaarskjaer, 1978; Blackstad *et al.*, 1970; Haug *et al.*, 1971; West *et al.*, 1982). Only a small component of the system deviates from this plane: within mid-septotemporal hippocampus, some mossy fibers in the CA3a/CA2 region arc to course temporally for several hundred micrometers, thereby creating a small "longitudinal" portion of the system (West, 1983; Swanson *et al.*, 1978).

The differences in the distribution of the mossy fibers between animals involve the spread of the system within the hilus and the extension of mossy fiber axons, in two cases, into regio superior. In animals with diffusely organized hilar regions such as the rat, mouse, and hamster, the mossy fibers occupy the full hilus and form fairly sharp boundaries directly against both stratum granulosum

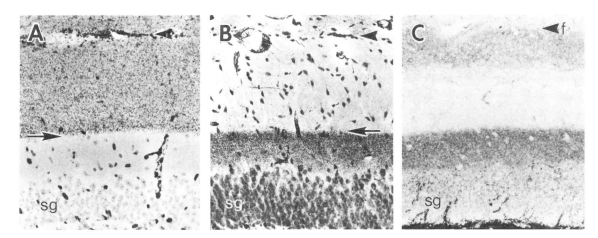

Figure 6. Photomicrographs of equivalent fields through rat dentate gyrus molecular layer showing the laminated distribution of (A) entorhinal and (B) commissural innervation as seen by silver impregnation of terminal degeneration following (A) ablation of the ipsilateral entorhinal cortex and (B) removal of the contralateral hippocampus (Fink–Heimer technique). Panel C shows the distribution of heavy metals in this field in tissue processed by Timm's technique. The hippocampal fissure is indicated by an arrowhead at the top of each micrograph. Arrows in A and B indicate the proximal limit of the entorhinal terminal field and the distal limit of the commissural terminal field, respectively. Note the exclusive lamination of (A) entorhinal and (B) commissural afferent innervation and the correspondence between inner molecular layer fields of commissural afferent termination and heavy metal staining.

and strata radiatum and oriens of regio inferior (Fig. 5). In contrast, in animals in which the hilar region is cytoarchitectonically stratified, such as the guinea pig and rabbit, the mossy fibers are offset from stratum granulosum and lie central to the intervening "plexiform zone" of Ramón y Cajal (Geneser-Jensen *et al.*, 1974; see also Fig. 15B).

As in the rat, termination of the mossy fiber system within hippocampus proper of the rabbit, guinea pig, and monkey is restricted to regio inferior. However, in the European hedgehog the mossy fibers extend beyond regio inferior to innervate, in a continuous fashion, the smaller pyramidal cells of region CA1 (Gaarskjaer *et al.*, 1982). In the cat, the mossy fibers of the more septal hippocampus also continue past the regio inferior border and course within temporally directed fascicles in proximal stratum radiatum of region CA1. Mossy fiber axons are not observed within region CA1 of the more temporal cat hippocampus (Laurberg and Zimmer, 1980).

4.1.2. The Commissural and Associational Systems

In the rat, the commissural and associational projections of the CA3 pyramidal cells and hilar polymorph neurons both arise from and innervate the full length of hippocampus and, as mentioned above, predominate in the innervation of broad fields of hippocampus (strata oriens and radiatum), and the dentate gyrus inner molecular layer, respectively. Autoradiographic analyses have demonstrated that, in contrast to the mossy fibers, there is a great deal of septotemporal spread in these projections (Fricke and Cowan, 1978; Van Groen and Wyss, 1988). For example, in the study of Van Groen and Wyss, injections of

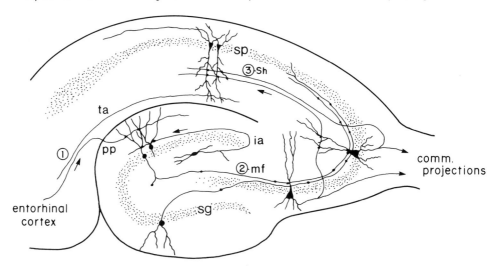

Figure 7. Schematic illustration of the major hippocampal afferent systems discussed in the text. Numbers indicate the relays in the excitatory trisynaptic circuit which were considered by Andersen *et al.* (1971) to define the hippocampal lamellae: (1) the afferents from entorhinal cortex which form the perforant path innervation of the dentate gyrus granule cells, (2) the mossy fiber axons of the dentate gyrus granule cells which innervate the pyramidal cells of region CA3, and (3) the Schaffer collaterals of the CA3 pyramidal cells which innervate the pyramidal cells of region CA1. Also illustrated are the temperoammonic innervation of the hippocampus proper and the dentate gyrus ipsilateral associational system which arises from polymorph cells of the hilus and innervates the inner dentate gyrus molecular layer.

tritiated amino acids which spanned 15 to 20% of the longitudinal extent of either the dentate gyrus or region CA3 gave rise to labeling of commissural and ipsilateral projections across 70 to 80% of the longitudinal extent of the dentate gyrus molecular layer or hippocampus proper (CA3 to CA1), respectively. The spread of these commissural projections was found to be similar following injections into either the septal or temporal third of hippocampus.

The hippocampal commissural projections in the mouse (Stanfield *et al.*, 1979; West *et al.*, 1979), rabbit (Hjorth-Simonsen, 1977; Van Groen and Wyss, 1988), cat, and guinea pig (Van Groen and Wyss, 1988) have been found to follow the same general scheme (origin, termination, topography) observed in the rat although there are some differences in the density of termination to different laminae (i.e., stratum oriens as compared to stratum radiatum; Van Groen and Wyss, 1988). However a very different pattern of commissural innervation is observed in primates. Amaral *et al.* (1984) have found that in Old World monkeys (*Macaca fascicularis*), hippocampal commissural projections only arise from, and project to, the "uncal" (or, most rostral) extremity of hippocampus— that portion of hippocampus homologous to the temporal extreme of hippocampus in the rat. Surprisingly, the greater portion of hippocampus and dentate gyrus was not found to receive any commissural innervation. The limited commissural projections present in the monkey do retain some aspects of the topography observed in the rat: the dentate gyrus molecular layer receives input from contralateral hilar neurons whereas hippocampal stratum radiatum is innervated by contralateral hippocampal region CA3. As in the rat, no commissural projections arise from the pyramidal cells of regio superior.

In contrast to the limited distribution of commissural connections, Amaral *et al.* (1984) found robust associational (i.e., ipsilateral) projections to both hippocampus and dentate gyrus throughout monkey hippocampus. As such, dendritic zones of "hippocampal afferent" termination are retained throughout both the dentate gyrus molecular layer and strata radiatum and oriens of hippocampus proper; in the uncal hippocampus these fields contain both commissural and ipsilateral associational innervation whereas throughout the body of the structure "hippocampal" innervation is purely associational. Rosene and Van Hoesen (1987) have found that, as in the rat, there is considerable longitudinal spread in the distribution of the dentate gyrus associational afferents in the monkey; following injections of tritiated amino acids into the uncal extreme of the dentate gyrus, associational afferents to the dentate inner molecular layer were labeled across the full longitudinal extent of the structure.

4.2. Afferents from Entorhinal Cortex

Entorhinal cortex is the major source of extrinsic afferents to the hippocampal formation. The majority of these projections are ipsilateral although there is a small contralateral component as will be described below. In the rat, the ipsilateral temporoammonic and perforant path afferents distribute across hippocampal stratum lacunosum-moleculare and densely innervate the distal 75% of the dentate gyrus molecular layer, respectively (Hjorth-Simonsen and Jeune, 1972). In both the dentate gyrus and regio inferior, entorhinal afferents terminate in an orderly laminated fashion: afferents from the medial entorhinal cortex lie adjacent and distal to the fields of commissural/associational innervation whereas afferents from the lateral entorhinal cortex terminate in the more distal field and extend to the hippocampal fissure (Hjorth-Simonsen, 1972b; Steward, 1976). Although there are indications of gradients within this topography (i.e., intermediate entorhinal cortex projecting to a zone lying between the fields of more medial and more lateral entorhinal innervation), the dentate gyrus molecular layer is generally considered to include three distinct laminae that are defined by the laminated termination of the principal afferent systems: that is, the inner, middle, and outer molecular layers which are innervated by the hippocampal commissural/associational, medial entorhinal, and lateral entorhinal afferents, respectively. In regio superior, the gradient from medial to lateral entorhinal innervation extends from CA2 to the subicular limit of region CA1 stratum lacunosum-moleculare; as such the afferents from medial and lateral entorhinal cortex are not proximodistally laminated in this region (Steward, 1976; Wyss, 1981).

As mentioned above, the entorhinal cortex also gives rise to much more modest projections to the contralateral hippocampal formation. In the rat, these crossed projections arise from all but the most ventral entorhinal cortex (Wyss, 1981) and are most densely distributed within contralateral region CA1. Contralateral projections to regio inferior and the dentate gyrus are very sparse and are restricted to the dorsal (more septal) hippocampus (Steward, 1976; Goldowitz et al., 1975) but within these regions exhibit basically the same topography as the projections to ipsilateral hippocampus. That is, crossed afferents from medial and lateral entorhinal cortex are proximodistally distributed within the dentate gyrus molecular layer and distributed across the CA2 to subicular regions of stratum lacunosum-moleculare of hippocampal region CA1.

Early reports of the distribution of the major afferents to hippocampus of the rabbit, mouse, and monkey encouraged the assumption that the pattern of innervation observed in the rat was followed quite faithfully in other mammals as well. This assumption still appears valid in regard to the laminated termination of afferents from the entorhinal cortex to the dentate gyrus. In the mouse (Stanfield et al., 1979), hamster (see Section 4.3), cat (Habets et al., 1980), and monkey (Van Hoesen and Pandya, 1975), the entorhinal cortical afferents terminate within a sharply defined field occupying the distal two thirds to three quarters of the dentate gyrus molecular layer. In each of these animals, as in the rat, the more medial entorhinal cortex innervates the middle molecular layer whereas the lateral entorhinal and perirhinal cortices innervate the contiguous distal molecular layer. However, species differences have been observed in the magnitude of the entorhinal projection to the contralateral hippocampus and dentate gyrus.

Crossed projections from entorhinal cortex to hippocampus in the Old World monkey and rabbit are distributed differently than in the rat. It will be remembered that in the rat, modest contralateral projections from both medial and lateral entorhinal cortex most densely innervate stratum lacunosum-moleculare of region CA1, and are only very sparsely distributed within the dentate gyrus molecular layer of septal hippocampus. In the rabbit, the dentate gyrus molecular layers fuse across the midline at the septal pole of hippocampus and, seemingly through this region of continuity, perforant path axons course into the dentate gyrus molecular layer contralateral to their origin. In this animal, the crossed temperoammonic and temperodentate projections to medial regions are reportedly as dense as the projections to the ipsilateral side but are restricted to the septal pole (Hjorth-Simonsen and Zimmer, 1975); within these regions the projections from medial and lateral entorhinal cortex are topographically distributed as in the rat. In the monkey, the contralateral projections are also restricted to the septal pole of hippocampus (which lies posterior in primates) but arise solely from the medial entorhinal cortex and are denser to the dentate gyrus than to region CA1 (Amaral *et al.*, 1984); relative densities which are opposite to those reported for the rat (Goldowitz *et al.*, 1975; Fig. 8).

The issue of how the different subdivisions of entorhinal cortex distribute their projections across the septotemporal axis of hippocampus has been the subject of a number of recent investigations and it is not yet clear whether there are comparative differences in these topographies. This uncertainty is largely due to the lack of a consistent scheme for the identification of anatomically distinct subfields within rat entorhinal cortex. Early work on the rat considered the entorhinal cortex to be composed of simple medial and lateral subdivisions. In an autoradiographic study based on this scheme, Wyss (1981) found the projections from the medial entorhinal cortex to be loosely topographic across the long axis of hippocampus with dorsal aspects of the medial entorhinal cortex projecting to the septal pole of the dentate gyrus, and progressively more ventral and ventroanterior medial entorhinal cortex innervating progressively more temporal dentate gyrus. In contrast, projections from lateral entorhinal cortex were found to be rather diffuse such that a given region of the lateral field might project across the full septotemporal extent of hippocampus (Wyss, 1981; Pohle and Ott, 1984).

More recent work has indicated that the topography of the entorhinal projection system is better appreciated in the rat, as in the cat, as originating from more numerous distinct subfields of entorhinal cortex and that the distributions of the perforant path projections are rather more complex. In studies which exploit the relatively large and well-defined cytoarchitectonic subfields of entorhinal cortex in the cat, Witter and Groenewegen (1984) found that projections from the medial entorhinal, lateral entorhinal, and perirhinal cortices are differ-

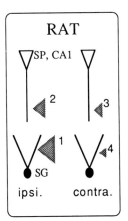 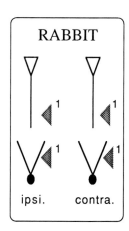 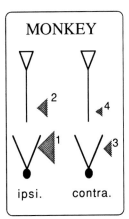

Figure 8. Diagram illustrating comparative differences in the relative density of entorhinal afferent innervation of the dentate gyrus granule cells and CA1 pyramidal cells in the septal regions of ipsilateral and contralateral hippocampus of the rat, rabbit, and monkey. The relative innervation densities across the four fields in each animal are indicated by the size of the shaded arrowhead and have been ranked by number.

entially distributed along the septotemporal axis of hippocampus. They observed that the lateral portions of both medial and lateral entorhinal cortex projected to the septal hippocampus whereas the more medial aspects of entorhinal cortex projected exclusively to temporal hippocampus. Although the cytoarchitectonic subdivisions of the entorhinal area of the rat are more poorly defined, and the subject of much confusion of nomenclature (Haug, 1976; Krettek and Price, 1977), the work of Ruth *et al.* (1982, 1988) indicates that similar topographic distributions are present in the rat. Using retrograde transport techniques, these authors have found that the septotemporal axis of rat hippocampus receives innervation which originates across the posterodorsolateral to anteroventromedial axis of entorhinal cortex. In particular, projections from four separate subdivisions of the lateral entorhinal cortex were found to be differentially distributed across the septotemporal axis of the dentate gyrus such that the dorsolateral division gave rise to afferents to the more septal dentate gyrus and the medial aspects of the ventromedial and ventrolateral subdivisions projected to the ventral dentate gyrus (Ruth *et al.*, 1988).

Clearly, further analysis is needed to define more precisely the topographies of the medial and lateral entorhinal afferents to hippocampus in the rat, and eventually in primates, before statements can be made as to phylogenetic stability. In particular, it will be important to determine whether the topography of the entorhinal afferents to hippocampus of the cat is typical of other mammals. As pointed out by Witter and Groenewegen, this perforant path topography might effect functional differences across the longitudinal dimension of hippocampus which would not have been anticipated from the earlier analyses of these systems in the rat. For example, the lateral entorhinal cortex receives direct input from the olfactory bulb whereas the medial entorhinal cortex does not. As a consequence of stronger olfactory representation within the lateral field, the septal pole of hippocampus which it innervates might also be more strongly influenced by olfactory processes than is the more temporal hippocampus.

4.3. Lack of Exclusive Afferent Lamination in the Hamster Dentate Gyrus

As is evident in the descriptions above, the most characteristic feature of hippocampal anatomy is lamination. Neuronal perikarya, dendritic fields, and major afferent systems define relatively homogeneous lamina in both the hippocampal formation and the dentate gyrus. Light and electron microscopic studies have demonstrated that in rat dentate gyrus molecular layer there is virtually no overlap in the laminae occupied by the commissural/associational and entorhinal afferent systems (Fig. 6). Although the relative distributions of these two systems have not been so thoroughly studied in other mammals, the sharp proximal boundary to the field of medial entorhinal innervation within the middle molecular layer of the rhesus monkey (Van Hoesen and Pandya, 1975), cat (Habets *et al.*, 1980), mouse (Stanfield and Cowan, 1979), and hamster (Fig. 9A), as well as the restricted inner molecular layer termination of commissural/associational afferents in the rabbit (Hjorth-Simonsen and Zimmer, 1975), mouse (West *et al.*, 1979), cat, guinea pig, and monkey (Van Groen and Wyss, 1988; Amaral *et al.*, 1984), have encouraged the conclusion that the adjacent but nonoverlapping termination of these afferents is a consistent, well-regulated feature of hippocampal anatomy.

Experimental work indicates that the entorhinal projections in some way inhibit coextensive growth of the commissural/associational afferents during development, thereby providing an explanation of the afferent lamination seen in the adult. Following removal of entorhinal cortex in young rats, the commissural/associational axons rapidly invade and functionally innervate the full dentate gyrus molecular layer with even density (Zimmer, 1973; Gall *et al.*, 1979, 1980, 1986b; Lynch *et al.*, 1973). This suggests that under normal conditions it is the presence of entorhinal afferents which prevents the growth of commissural axons into the more distal aspects of the granule cell dendritic field. In the genetic mutant mouse "reeler," the commissural and entorhinal afferents remain segregated despite the absence of normal cellular lamination within the fascia dentata (Stanfield and Cowan, 1979; Stanfield *et al.*, 1979), suggesting again that

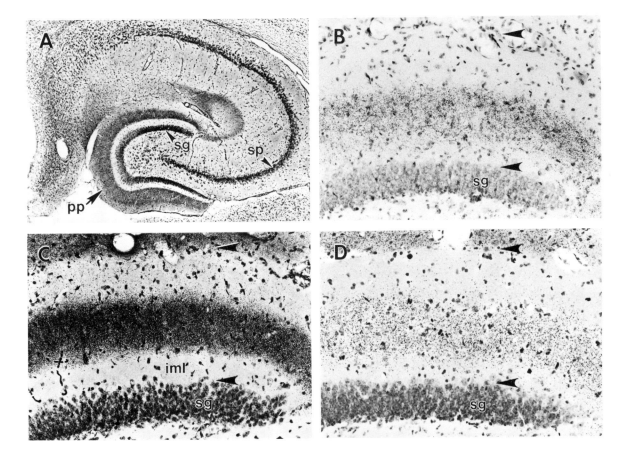

Figure 9. Photomicrographs illustrating the distribution of major afferent systems within the hamster hippocampus. Panels A and C show silver-impregnated terminal degeneration within (A) a full horizontal section through hippocampus and (C) the internal blade of the dentate gyrus following lesion placement in the ipsilateral entorhinal cortex (Fink–Heimer technique). Note the sharply defined proximal limit to the field of entorhinal innervation. Panels B and D show the equivalent distribution of (B) ipsilateral associational and (D) commissural afferents within the internal blade of the dentate gyrus as seen by anterograde transport of tritiated leucine and emulsion autoradiography in B, and by the distribution of silver-impregnated terminal degeneration following the aspiration removal of the contralateral hippocampus in D.

the ordering of these afferents is dictated by some, possibly competitive, interaction between the two axonal systems rather than by environmental cues such as surface characteristics of the postsynaptic dendrites.

In this context, the absence of lamination of the major afferents to the hamster dentate gyrus molecular layer is quite surprising (Gall, unpublished observations). As mentioned above, and illustrated in Figs. 9 and 10, the entorhinal afferents to the hamster dentate gyrus are sharply laminated. Following ablation of entorhinal cortex, dense terminal degeneration is seen throughout the distal molecular layer; the proximal boundary of this field is very abrupt leaving the inner 50 μm of the molecular layer free of degenerating debris. As in the rat, entorhinal projections to contralateral hippocampus are most dense in region CA1 stratum lacunosum-moleculare and only quite sparse in the dentate gyrus and regio inferior of the more septal hippocampus.

In contrast, as seen both in the distribution of terminal degeneration following aspiration removal of an entire hippocampus and in autoradiographic analyses of the transport of tritiated leucine injected into the dentate gyrus hilus, the commissural and associational projections to the hamster dentate gyrus molecular layer are quite diffuse (Figs. 9 and 10). This is particularly evident in the external (infrapyramidal) blade of the septal dentate gyrus where commissural innervation spans the full depth of the granule cell dendritic field. In the internal (suprapyramidal) molecular layer, as well as throughout the molecular layer at more temporal planes, the commissural projection becomes more shallow and is somewhat offset from the granule cell layer. Nevertheless, at all levels the commissural and associational projections both overlap the field of entorhinal innervation and in no way reflect the proximal boundary of the entorhinal afferent field.

Interestingly, the distribution of commissural afferents to the hamster dentate gyrus was not found to correspond to the distribution of heavy metals as has

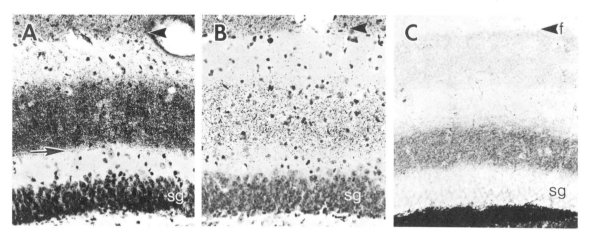

Figure 10. Photomicrographs illustrating the relative placement of (A) entorhinal and (B) commissural afferent systems within the hamster dentate gyrus molecular layer as seen by silver impregnation of terminal degeneration following (A) ablation of the ipsilateral entorhinal cortex (lateral regions spared) and (B) contralateral hippocampus. Panel C shows the distribution of heavy metals within the hamster molecular layer in tissue processed by Timm's technique. Arrowheads indicate the position of the hippocampal fissure at the top of each micrograph. Arrow in A indicates the proximal limit to the field of entorhinal afferent degeneration. Note the extensive overlap of entorhinal and commissural terminal degeneration and the lack of correspondence between the field of commissural afferent termination and the pattern of Timm's staining within the molecular layer.

been observed in the rat (Haug, 1974; Zimmer, 1973; see Figs. 6 and 10). In the rat, the proximal zone of commissural/associational innervation stains moderately densely in Timm's preparations. This has been interpreted as metal accumulation within the commissural and associational afferent axons. In the hamster, moderate Timm's staining is also observed within the proximal molecular layer; this staining is evenly dense for 50 μm from the granule cells bodies and diminishes in density thereafter. Clearly, in the hamster the Timm's-stained band does not correspond with the zone of commissural innervation alone as described above. Possibly a complete understanding of the dentate associational system as well as probable afferents from the supramammillary hypothalamus (Haglund *et al.*, 1984; Wyss *et al.*, 1979) might aid in the interpretation of the locus of heavy metal deposition in the molecular layer of the hamster.

4.4. Summary

In discussing the organization of hippocampus it is sometimes useful to consider it as composed of three principal cell types (granule cell, CA3 pyramidal cell, CA1 pyramidal cell), each of which contains a small number of dendritic subfields defined by the laminated termination of major afferent systems (Fig. 11). The outermost zone in each case constitutes the target of the entorhinal afferents (ipsilateral and contralateral), while the more proximal and basal laminae are innervated by hippocampal commissural and associational fibers. The

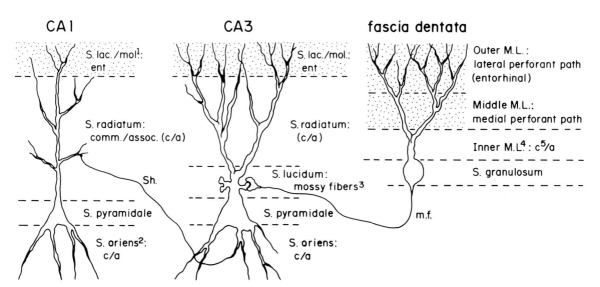

Figure 11. Schematic illustration of the principal afferent laminae within the fields of the CA1 pyramidal cells, the CA3 pyramidal cells, and the dentate gyrus granule cells of the rat. For each lamina, the principal source of innervation is indicated; stippling marks fields of entorhinal afferent termination. Superscripts indicate features which can be seen to vary between animals: (1) There are between-animal differences in the balance of ipsilateral to contralateral entorhinal innervation of stratum lacunosum-moleculare. (2) Stratum oriens is obscured by the scattered distribution of pyramidal cells in region CA1 in primates. (3) The mossy fiber system extends into region CA1 in the cat and hedgehog. (4) The entorhinal and commissural/associational (c/a) afferents are not exclusively laminated at the inner to middle molecular layer (M.L.) boundary in the hamster. (5) Commissural afferents are absent from all but the uncal region of the dentate gyrus inner molecular layer in the monkey.

pyramidal cell dendritic field of CA3 contains an additional thin subfield (stratum lucidum), immediately adjacent to the pyramidal cell bodies, that is occupied by the strictly ipsilateral mossy fiber axons and terminals. This schematic provides a useful device for summarizing the comparative differences so far noted.

1. The most dramatic variations involve the relative magnitude of the crossed projections. For the afferents from entorhinal cortex, extreme differences are found in the septal pole of hippocampus. In the rat, the order of densities across dendritic fields would be ipsilateral dentate > ipsilateral pyramidal cells > contralateral pyramidal cells > contralateral dentate. In some species, such as the rabbit, the contralateral projections are nearly as dense as those on the ipsilateral side, while in others they are greater in the dentate gyrus than in the pyramidal cell fields. The granule cells of the dentate gyrus have a peculiarly prolonged developmental period (in the rat most undergo mitosis after birth) (Bayer, 1980) and, between animals, exhibit considerable differences in the degree to which they approach the midline at the septal pole. It is tempting to speculate that the comparative differences in the distribution and densities of the crossed entorhinal projections reflect these two factors.

The massive hippocampal commissural system also proves to be more variable across species than once suspected. Interesting differences in its contributions to apical versus basal dendrites have been noted (Van Groen and Wyss, 1988), but more remarkable is the great reduction in hippocampal commissural projections in primates (Amaral *et al.,* 1984). It is of interest in this regard that field CA3, the source of the commissural projections to pyramidal cell fields, does decrease in size in proportion to CA1 in bigger-brained animals. However, the dentate gyrus commissural system is also severely reduced in the primate and these projections arise from cells quite distinct in location and type from those of CA3 (i.e., the hilar polymorph neurons). It appears then that some factor other than a change in proportional size of subfields across species effects a kind of separation of the hippocampi in the primate.

2. Lamination itself, often considered as a hallmark of hippocampus, has proven to be somewhat variable. The CA1 cell bodies form a compact sharply defined layer in most rodents but are sufficiently scattered in at least some primates, including man, to make difficult the definition of stratum oriens. Perhaps more surprising still is the finding that the hippocampal commissural and associational afferents to the dentate gyrus are not restricted to what might be considered their "appropriate" lamina in hamster. These observations raise the point that the functional significance of lamination is not well understood. As has been noted by a number of authors, the exquisitely precise lamination of dentate gyrus in the rat can be traced back to the timing of the growth of the components (afferents and granule cell targets) of the structure (Bayer, 1980; Gottlieb and Cowan, 1972). Lamination could be a by-product rather than a "reason" for these developmental rules. There is, however, evidence suggesting that there is more to lamination than this. The pyramidal cell dendritic trees exhibit quite different morphologies in the zones innervated by commissural–associational versus entorhinal afferents (Lorente de Nó, 1934) and these may be associated with pronounced functional differences (Andersen *et al.,* 1980). It is of interest in this regard that the disturbance of afferent lamination found in the hamster occurs in the dentate gyrus, where the dendritic tree is not sharply differentiated, and not in the pyramidal cell fields.

5. Comparative Differences in the Distribution of Neuroactive
Peptides within Hippocampal Circuitry

187

**COMPARATIVE
ANATOMY OF THE
HIPPOCAMPUS**

A large number of neuroactive substances have been localized within the circuitry of the hippocampal formation (Walaas, 1983; Amaral and Campbell, 1986). In a review of this literature one finds that the intrahippocampal distributions of some neuroactive peptides are very consistent across species, whereas clear and rather major interspecies differences in the distributions of other neuroactive substances have been reported. For example, no species differences have been detected in the hippocampal distribution of somatostatin, neuropeptide Y (NPY), or dynorphin. In the rat, Old World monkey, New World monkey, cat (for somatostatin), and man, immunoreactivities for somatostatin and NPY have been localized within neuronal perikarya most densely distributed in the dentate gyrus hilus and stratum oriens and within axons fairly densely distributed in the outer two thirds of the dentate gyrus molecular layer and stratum lacunosum-moleculare (Chan-Palay, 1987; Walaas, 1983; Köhler and Chan-Palay, 1982; Bakst *et al.*, 1985, 1986; Chan-Palay *et al.*, 1985; Köhler *et al.*, 1986; Smith *et al.*, 1985). Similarly, the distribution of dynorphin immunoreactivity appears unchanged in hippocampus of the rat, mouse, squirrel, guinea pig, hamster, and Old World monkey; in each, dynorphin is localized within the mossy fiber axons of the dentate gyrus granule cells and in but a few perikarya and axonal fragments within the fascia dentata and hippocampus proper, respectively (Gall, 1988b; McGinty *et al.*, 1983; McLean *et al.*, 1987). In contrast, work in this laboratory and elsewhere has demonstrated the presence of clear interspecies differences in the hippocampal distribution of immunoreactivities for enkephalin, cholecystokinin octapeptide (CCK), and substance P as will be discussed in the following paragraphs.

5.1. Enkephalin

In the rat, the opioid peptide enkephalin has been immunohistochemically localized within sparsely scattered neuronal perikarya throughout the hippocampal formation, including morphologically characteristic dentate gyrus granule cells, and within three distinct axonal systems: the mossy fibers, axons which line the stratum radiatum/stratum lacunosum-moleculare interface of region CA1, and a component of the lateral perforant path (Fig. 12). The latter axons arise from the most lateral entorhinal and perirhinal cortices and are distributed to stratum lacunosum-moleculare and the outer dentate gyrus molecular layer with increasing density from mid-septotemporal to most temporal hippocampus (Fredens *et al.*, 1984; Gall *et al.*, 1981). These immunocytochemical staining patterns have been replicated using antisera to methionine enkephalin-ArgGlyLeu (McLean *et al.*, 1987) and BAM 22 (McGinty *et al.*, 1984), and a non-dynorphin-reactive antiserum to methionine enkephalin (Gall, 1984b). Moreover, biochemical studies have verified that the dentate gyrus granule cells synthesize, and the mossy fiber axons contain, chromatographically identified methionine enkephalin, methionine enkephalin-ArgGlyLeu, BAM 18, and BAM 22 (White *et al.*, 1986, 1987).

In further support of the original immunocytochemical descriptions, recent *in situ* hybridization analyses have demonstrated the presence of preproenkephalin A mRNA in a small number of dentate gyrus granule cells, as well as within scattered neurons in the hippocampus proper, of the untreated rat (Gall and White, 1989; Gall *et al.*, 1987b). Moreover, following recurrent seizure activity, which has been found to stimulate a large increase in enkephalin synthesis by the dentate gyrus granule cells (White *et al.*, 1987), virtually all of these neurons exhibit high levels of hybridization for preproenkephalin A mRNA (Gall and White, 1989; Fig. 13). Therefore, it is now quite clear that the synthetically unrelated opioid peptides methionine enkephalin and dynorphin are both present within the mossy fiber system. Although the *in situ* hybridization studies argue against there being distinct populations of granule cells which invariably synthesize enkephalin or dynorphin, it is noteworthy that in normal rat hippocampus dynorphin-immunoreactive mossy fiber boutons are far more numerous (Gall, 1988a,b).

Like dynorphin, enkephalin immunoreactivity (ENK-I) has been localized within the mossy fibers of all experimental animals thus far examined including the rat, mouse, hamster, vole, European hedgehog, guinea pig, squirrel, cat, tree shrew, and monkey (Gall, 1984a, 1988b; Gall *et al.*, 1981; Fitzpatrick and Johnson, 1981; Zimmer and Sunde, 1984; McLean *et al.*, 1987; Stengaard-Pedersen *et al.*, 1983; Tielen *et al.*, 1982) (Table I). There are, however, species differences in the presence of ENK-I within the perforant path afferents to hippocampus (Fig.

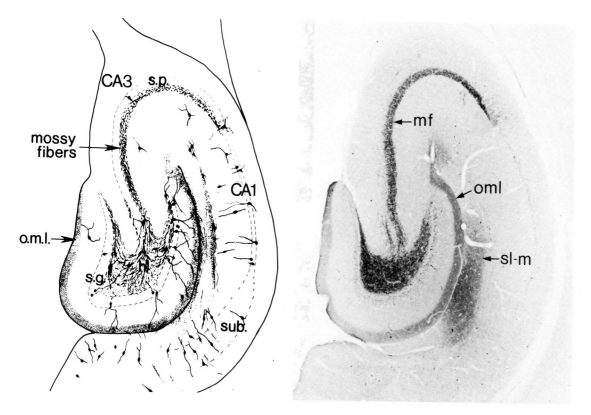

Figure 12. Schematic illustration and low-magnification photomicrograph illustrating the distribution of ENK-I in a horizontal section through the rat hippocampus (as described in the text).

14). In rat stratum lacunosum-moleculare, the distribution of ENK-I follows the topography previously described for projections from the lateral entorhinal cortex: that is, in CA1 axonal ENK-I is most dense and spans the depth of the lamina near the subicular/CA1 border whereas in regio inferior ENK-I occupies a distal field continuous with the dentate gyrus outer molecular layer. The distribution of ENK-I in hippocampus of the monkey (*Macaca fascicularis*) is basically the same as seen in the rat except that immunostaining is much more faint. In monkey dentate gyrus, immunoreactive processes and extremely fine puncta are scattered within a poorly defined field in the outer half of the molecular layer with increasing density toward the hippocampal fissure (Fig. 14E). In hamster, there is dense ENK-I within stratum lacunosum-moleculare at the CA2 limit of CA1, little immunostaining in the distal dendritic fields of CA3, and only a very narrow band of ENK-I in the most distal dentate gyrus molecular layer (McLean *et al.*, 1987). In the guinea pig, ENK-I is only present at the temporal extreme of CA3 stratum lacunosum-moleculare and the dentate outer molecular layer (Tielen *et al.*, 1982), while in the European hedgehog and tree shrew no ENK-I has been observed in either area (Fitzpatrick and Johnson, 1981; Stengaard-Pedersen *et al.*, 1983). As such, it seems that in the latter animals enkephalin may not be present within the perforant path.

Highly unusual patterns of ENK-I are observed in the ground squirrel and cat. In the squirrel, McLean *et al.* (1987) report a supragranular plexus of ENK-I axons which follow the distribution of afferents from the supramammillary hypothalamus as they appear in the rat (Haglund *et al.*, 1984; Wyss *et al.*, 1979) and guinea pig (Gall and Selawski, 1984). In the cat, two distinct bands of dense ENK-I fill the middle and outer dentate gyrus molecular layers, thus occupying the fields of both medial and lateral entorhinal innervation (Habets *et al.*, 1980; Fig. 14D). In addition, it is noteworthy that in the cat, unlike all other animals studied, there is a band of finely punctate ENK-I overlying stratum pyramidale and the adjacent stratum oriens in region CA1 (Call, 1988a). Opiate ligand

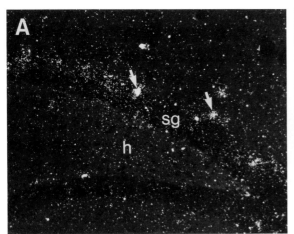
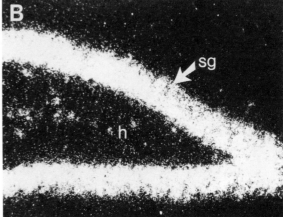

Figure 13. Darkfield photomicrographs of equivalent fields through rat dentate gyrus showing the autoradiographic localization of hybridization of an ^{35}S-labeled riboprobe to preproenkephalin A mRNA in dentate gyrus stratum granulosum of (A) a control rat and (B) a rat sacrificed 24 hr following limbic seizure induction by contralateral lesion placement. Although only a few dentate gyrus granule cells can be seen to contain mRNA for enkephalin in the normal rat (indicated by arrows in A), seemingly all cells in this layer are labeled following seizure activity.

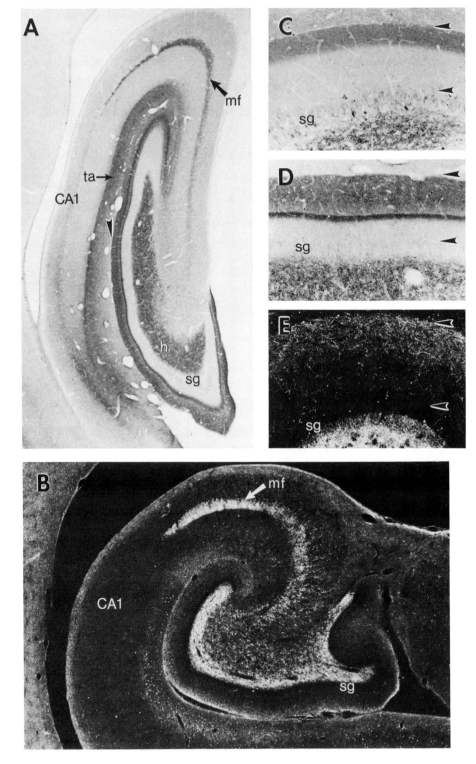

Figure 14. Photomicrographs illustrating comparative differences in the localization of ENK-I in hippocampus of the rat, cat, and monkey. The lightfield photomicrograph of panel A and the darkfield photomicrograph of panel B show full coronal cross sections through temporal hippocam-

binding studies have consistently found high opiate receptor densities in this area (Crain *et al.*, 1986; McLean *et al.*, 1987) but the cat is, to our knowledge, the only animal in which an opioid peptide has been correspondingly localized in this field.

A continuing puzzle in the consideration of the endogenous opioid systems in hippocampus has been the implications of the considerable mismatch between the distributions of the opioid peptides and opioid ligand binding. In general, autoradiographic studies have observed that in the rat the binding of ligands for the three principal receptor subtypes (mu, delta, and kappa) is greatest overlying stratum pyramidale whereas, as described above, the opioids are localized within synaptic systems distributed within the hilus, stratum lucidum, and the distal dentate gyrus molecular layer. In a recent study, McLean *et al.* (1987) compared the localization of mu, delta, and kappa ligand binding in the rat, guinea pig, squirrel, and hamster and found poor correspondence between peptide distribution and ligand binding in these animals as well. Although in some instances dense ligand binding was observed in areas of peptide immunoreactivity (e.g., dense binding to kappa receptors in stratum lucidum of the squirrel, hamster, and guinea pig), the opioid receptor distributions were found to be both much more diffuse and more variable between animals than the distributions of the opioid peptides.

5.2. Cholecystokinin

Like enkephalin, cholecystokinin immunoreactivity (CCK-I) has been localized within a number of distinct cell types and axonal systems within the hippocampal formation (Table II). Some features of the distribution of CCK-I within hippocampus appear to be conserved across species. As first observed in the rat (Greenwood *et al.*, 1981) and later reported for the mouse (Gall *et al.*, 1986a), guinea pig (Gall, 1984a; Stengaard-Pedersen *et al.*, 1983), hedgehog (Stengaard-Pedersen *et al.*, 1983), Old World monkey (C. Gall and J. Lauterborn, unpublished observations), and human (Lotstra and Vanderhaeghen, 1987), CCK-I is localized within a heterogeneity of neuronal types sparsely scattered across the cellular and molecular layers of the hippocampus proper and within the hilus of the dentate gyrus. The numerous CCK-I neurons in the latter area include both pyramidal basket-type cells and polymorph neurons which are most readily seen following colchicine treatment. In all of these animals plus cat,

---

pus of cat (A) and mid-septotemporal hippocampus of monkey (*Macaca fascicularis*) (B) processed for the localization of ENK-I by the peroxidase–antiperoxidase technique. In both of these animals, as in the rat (Fig. 12), ENK-I is localized within the mossy fiber system. However, clear differences can be seen in the localization of ENK-I in the fields of entorhinal afferent innervation. In the cat (A), dense ENK-I is seen associated with the temperoammonic projection throughout the hippocampus proper and within the outer two thirds of the dentate gyrus molecular layer, whereas in the monkey (B) only very sparse ENK-I is seen in either field. The distribution of ENK-I in the dentate gyrus molecular layer of the rat, cat, and monkey can be seen at higher magnification in panels C, D, and E, respectively (arrowheads bracket the molecular layer in each). In these micrographs, ENK-I can be seen within one band in the outer molecular layer in the rat (C), within two bands which occupy the outer and middle molecular layers in the cat (D), and within a poorly defined field in the outer half of the molecular layer in the monkey (E).

Table I. Localization of Axonal ENK-I in Hippocampal Subfields of Different Animals[a]

	Insectivore	Rodents					Carnivore	Primate
	Hedgehog	Rat	Mouse	Hamster	Guinea pig	Squirrel[b]	Cat	Monkey
Dentate gyrus								
oml	−	++t>s	+t[c]	+	+t[c]	−	++	+t
mml	−	−	−	−	+t[c,d]	−	++	−
iml	−	−	−	−	−	−	−	−
sgp	−	−	−	−	−	+	−	−
Mossy fibers	++	++	++	++	++	++	++	++
Regio superior								
sl-m	−	++	++	++	+	?	++	+t
Regio inferior								
sl-m	−	+	+t[c]	+	+	+	++	+t

[a]Symbols for Tables I–III (indicate label presence and intensity): −, no immunoreactive elements; +/−, light immunostaining in some animals; +, immunoreactivity reliably detected; ++, dense immunostaining reliably present; t, temporal hippocampus; s, septal hippocampus; rs, regio superior; ri, regio inferior; ri, regio inferior>regio superior; ?, not determined.
[b]McLean et al. (1987); data from septal pole of hippocampus only.
[c]ENK-I present in extremely temporal regions only.
[d]Reported by Tielen et al. (1982).

Table II. Localization of Axonal CCK-I within Hippocampal Subfields in Different Animals

| | Insectivore | Rodents | | | Lagomorph | Carnivore | Primates | |
	Hedgehog[a]	Mouse	Rat	Guinea pig	Rabbit	Cat	Monkey	Human[b]
Dentate gyrus								
oml	−	−/+	−	−	−	−/+	−/+	−
mml	−	++	+t	+t	+	++,t>s	+,t>s	+t
iml	−	++	+t	−	−/+	++t	−/+[c]	+
sgp	−	?	+	+	−	+	++	++
Mossy fibers	++	++	−	++	−	−	++	?
sp	++	++	++	++	++	++	+	++[ri]
sl-m	−	++[rs]	++	++	++	++	+[rs]	+

[a]Stengaard-Pedersen *et al.* (1983).
[b]Lotstra and Vanderhaeghen (1987).
[c]CCK-I axons from supragranular zone scatter into the inner molecular layer at temporal planes.

gerbil, and rabbit, coarsely varicose CCK-I axons arborize within and loosely around stratum pyramidale of the hippocampus proper. These axons presumably represent innervation to the pyramidal cells from nearby CCK-I local circuit neurons (Hendry and Jones, 1985).

There is considerable interspecies variability in the localization of CCK-I within longer axonal systems in hippocampus. Specifically, the mossy fibers, the dentate gyrus commissural/associational system, and the medial perforant path have each been observed to contain CCK-I in some, but not all, animals examined (Table II, Fig. 15).

The combined use of retrograde axonal transport and immunocytochemistry has demonstrated that the dentate gyrus commissural, and therefore presumably also the ipsilateral associational, afferents contain CCK-I in the mouse (Gall *et al.*, 1986a) and rat (Fredens *et al.*, 1987). In the mouse, terminal-like CCK-I puncta densely fill the full septotemporal extent of the dentate gyrus inner molecular layer, whereas in the rat there is much less inner molecular layer CCK-I which increases in density from mid-septotemporal to temporal dentate gyrus. As such, it seems likely that CCK-I is only present within a temporal component of the commissural system in rat. CCK-I is also present within the dentate gyrus inner molecular layer and, therefore, presumably within the dentate commissural and/or associational afferents of the gerbil and cat but not European hedgehog, guinea pig, or monkey (Gall *et al.*, 1986a; Stengaard-Pedersen *et al.*, 1983; Fig. 15). Rather, in the guinea pig, and more densely in the monkey and human (Lotstra and Vanderhaeghen, 1987; Gall, unpublished observations), CCK-I axons are distributed within the supragranular molecular layer and superficial stratum granulosum which is suggestive of CCK localization within supramammillary afferents in these animals as has been reported for the rat (Haglund *et al.*, 1984).

CCK-I is localized within the middle molecular layer of the rat, gerbil, rabbit, guinea pig, cat, Old World monkey, and human (Gall, 1984a; Lotstra and Vanderhaeghen, 1987; Zimmer and Sunde, 1984) and in the outer molecular layer of the cat (Fig. 15C). Lesion studies have verified that in rat middle molecular layer CCK-I is localized within the afferents from entorhinal cortex (Fredens *et al.*, 1984). As with CCK-I in the rat commissural system, CCK-I in the middle molecular layer is densest in the temporal hippocampus in the rat, gerbil, and guinea pig. In the latter case, CCK-I is only evident at the extreme temporal extent of the field. As such, in all of these animals only a portion of the medial perforant path appears to contain CCK. In the mouse, CCK-I is barely detectable in the middle molecular layer and regio inferior despite a robust system of CCK-I axons with stratum lacunosum-moleculare of region CA1 (Fig. 15D) (Gall *et al.*, 1986a). CCK-I has not been detected in perforant path afferents in the European hedgehog (Stengaard-Pedersen *et al.*, 1983).

Finally, there are very definite species differences in the presence of CCK within the mossy fiber axonal system. CCK-I has been localized within the mossy fibers in the mouse, gerbil, guinea pig, European hedgehog, and monkey (*M. fascicularis* and *Saimiri sciureus*), but not rat, rabbit, cat, or human (Gall, 1984a; Lotstra and Vanderhaeghen, 1987; Gall *et al.*, 1986a; Greenwood *et al.*, 1981; Stengaard-Pedersen *et al.*, 1983; Sloviter *et al.*, 1987). Where present, CCK-I is quite dense within the mossy fiber system and is localized within numerous terminal boutons that fill the central hilus and stratum lucidum.

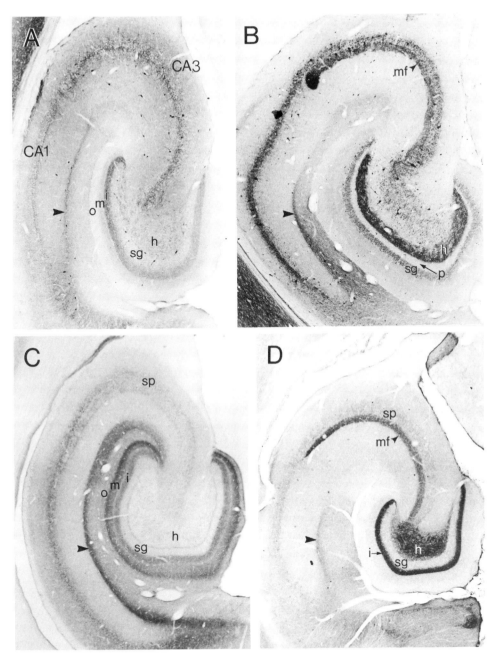

Figure 15. Low-magnification photomicrographs illustrating the distribution of CCK-I in horizontal tissue sections through hippocampus of the rat (A), guinea pig (B), cat (C), and mouse (D). Major differences can be seen in the localization of CCK-I within the inner (i), middle (m), and outer (o) molecular layers of the dentate gyrus and within the mossy fiber axonal system in the hilus and region CA3. Arrowheads indicate CCK-I at the stratum radiatum/stratum lacunosum-moleculare interface of region CA1 in each panel. In panel B, the CCK-I mossy fibers of the guinea pig can be seen to conform to the cytoarchitectonic stratification of the hilar region in this animal, being offset from stratum granulosum by the intervening plexiform zone of Ramón y Cajal (p).

5.3. Tachykinin

The distribution of tachykinin-immunoreactive (T-I) elements within the hippocampal formation has been analyzed in the rat, mouse, guinea pig, cat, squirrel, New World monkey, Old World monkey, and human (Table III). In all of these studies, antisera to the carboxyl terminus of substance P was used. It has recently become appreciated that in the mammalian brain the tachykinin family of peptides includes substance P, substance K (or neurokinin A), and neuromedin K (or neurokinin B) (Maggio and Hunter, 1985), all of which share the same carboxyl terminus. As such, the immunocytochemical staining patterns to be described must be considered indicative of the distribution of T-I with potential contribution from each tachykinin species. However, biochemical studies have demonstrated that both substance P and substance K are encoded by a single gene (Nawa *et al.*, 1983) and the distribution of at least these two tachykinins has proven to be indistinguishable in the ventral tegmental area (Kalivas *et al.*, 1985) and cerebral cortex (Jones *et al.*, 1988). Moreover, preliminary observations in our laboratory indicate that identical immunocytochemical staining patterns are obtained in guinea pig hippocampus using either the carboxyl terminus-directed antisubstance P or a specific antiserum to substance K. As such, the elements described here as containing T-I most probably contain both substance P and substance K.

Very little T-I is observed in the hippocampus of the rat or mouse. As reported by Davies and Köhler (1985), and as seen in our own immunocytochemical material, a few T-I perikarya are observed within the hilus and stratum oriens with the incidence in the latter region being highest toward the subicular and CA3c limits of the lamina. Very sparsely distributed T-I axons are seen in these same regions and occasionally crossing stratum pyramidale into stratum radiatum in the vicinity of CA2. The number of immunoreactive axons is greatest in the temporal extreme of hippocampus. In the rat, and more strikingly in other animals to be described below, two types of T-I axons are seen: larger-caliber axons with densely immunoreactive, irregularly spaced varicosities that are most frequently distributed within the dentate gyrus hilus, and finer axons which predominate within the molecular layers.

The distribution of perikarya containing T-I in rat hippocampus is in agreement with the distribution of cells containing mRNA from the single gene which encodes both substance P and substance K (neurokinin A), but not cells containing mRNA which encodes the tachykinin neurokinin B as identified in the recent *in situ* hybridization study of Warden and Young (1988). The latter cells were, in fact, found to be much more numerous in hippocampus and were distributed both subjacent to stratum granulosum in the hilar region and across stratum radiatum of the regio superior.

In striking contrast to the rat, there is a complex pattern of T-I within perikarya and axons in the guinea pig hippocampus (Fig. 16) and the basic pattern observed in the guinea pig is retained with elaboration and a few additions in the cat, squirrel, monkey, and human. Although small-caliber T-I axons are scattered across all fields of guinea pig hippocampus, fascia dentata, and fimbria, the greatest density of axonal T-I is observed within the supragranular dentate gyrus molecular layer and cascading down from this field into the superficial granule cell layer (Fig. 17B). T-I axons are also present at moderate densities within stratum oriens and surrounding stratum pyramidale of region CA3c.

Table III. Localization of Axonal T-I in Hippocampal Subfields in Different Animals

| | Rodents | | | Lagomorph | Carnivore | Primates | |
	Rat	Guinea pig	Squirrel	Rabbit	Cat	Monkey	Human[a]
Dentate gyrus							
oml	−	−	−	−	−	+s	+
mml	−	+t	+t	−	+t	−/+s	+
iml	−	−	++	−	+t>s[b]	−/+s	−
sgp	−	++	++	−	++	+s	++
Hilus[c]	+	+	+	+	+t>s	+	+
Regio inferior							
so	+	+	+	+	++	++	?. +
sp	−	+t>s	+	−	++t>s	++	+
sl	−	−	+	−	+	+	?. ?. ?
sr	−	+	+	+t	−/+	++	
sl-m	−	++	++	−	+	++	
Regio superior							
so	−/+[d]	+	+	+t	++	+	?. +
sp	−/+[d]	−/+	++	−	++	+	+
sr	−	−/+	+	−	−/+	+	−
sl-m	−	−/+	+	+t	++	++	+

[a]Sakamoto et al. (1987) and Del Fiacco et al. (1987).
[b]Represents scatter of immunoreactive axons from the supragranular plexus.
[c]Coarse varicose axons.
[d]Scattered axons crossing so and sp at the CA1/CA2 border

Finally, a thin band of finely punctate T-I is seen within the middle molecular layer of the most temporal dentate gyrus.

The distribution of axonal T-I within region CA2 and the supragranular dentate gyrus molecular layer is reminiscent of the distribution of hippocampal afferents from the supramammillary hypothalamus (Haglund *et al.*, 1984; Wyss *et al.*, 1979), and lesion and retrograde transport studies have demonstrated that most, but probably not all, of the axonal T-I within guinea pig hippocampus is indeed localized within this afferent system (Gall and Selawski, 1984). Unilateral transection of the fimbria eliminates the great majority of axonal T-I within the ipsilateral hippocampus, demonstrating these axons to be extrinsic afferents which enter hippocampus at the septal pole. In the guinea pig, only those axons which arborize within and around stratum pyramidale of temporal region CA3c

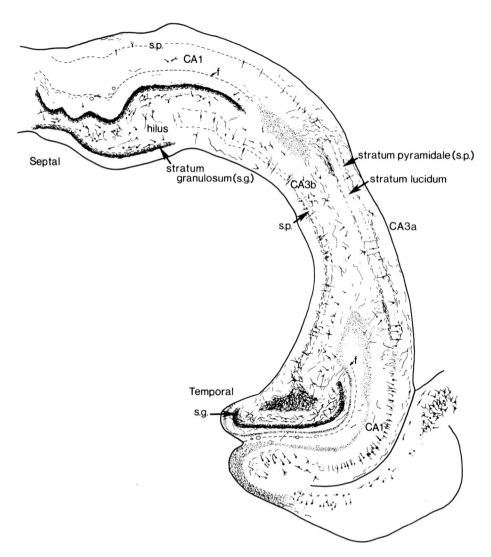

Figure 16. Schematic illustration of the distribution of tachykinin immunoreactivity in a coronal tissue section through guinea pig hippocampus.

appear unaffected by fimbrial transection, suggesting that these axons either arise from within hippocampus or enter the structure from the temporal pole.

With colchicine treatment, T-I perikarya are observed within stratum oriens and, more densely, within the hilus across the full septotemporal extent of guinea pig hippocampus. In addition, T-I is localized within the pathologically swollen proximal axon fragments of neurons within regio superior stratum pyramidale. [A similar pathological immunostaining pattern has been observed for enkephalin (Gall *et al.*, 1981)-, dynorphin (McGinty *et al.*, 1984)-, and cholecystokinin (Gall *et al.*, 1987a)-immunoreactive neurons in other areas following colchicine treatment.] In regard to hippocampal T-I, the large number of immunoreactive proximal axon fragments seen in CA1 suggests that some proportion of the pyramidal neurons which give rise to extrinsic hippocampal efferents contain tachykinin.

Of the species thus far examined, the cat has been found to exhibit the most strikingly dense and regionally differentiated distribution of T-I (Fig. 18). The description that follows derives from our own material, obtained using a mono-

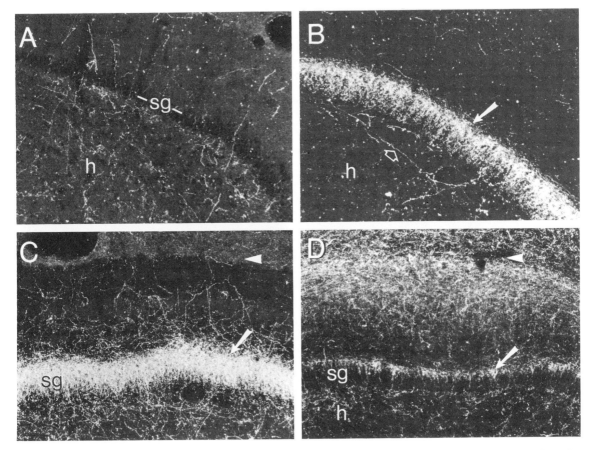

Figure 17. Darkfield photomicrographs illustrating the distribution of tachykinin-immunoreactive axons in the dentate gyrus of the rabbit (A), guinea pig (B), cat (C), and monkey (D). Note that the rabbit, like the rat, lacks the supragranular plexus of tachykinin-immunoreactive axons seen in the other animals (indicated by arrows in B, C, and D). Open arrow in B indicates a coarsely varicose immunoreactive axon in guinea pig hilus; such axons appear morphologically distinct from the finer axons of the supragranular plexus and have been observed in all animals thus far examined.

clonal antibody to substance P (Cuello *et al.*, 1979), and agrees with and extends the report by Vincent *et al.* (1981). As mentioned above, the distribution of axonal T-I observed in cat hippocampus is basically the same as observed in the guinea pig. As such, T-I axons are most densely distributed within the supragranular dentate gyrus molecular layer and cascade down from this plexus to encircle granule cells of the fascia dentata (Fig. 17C). A recent lesion study has

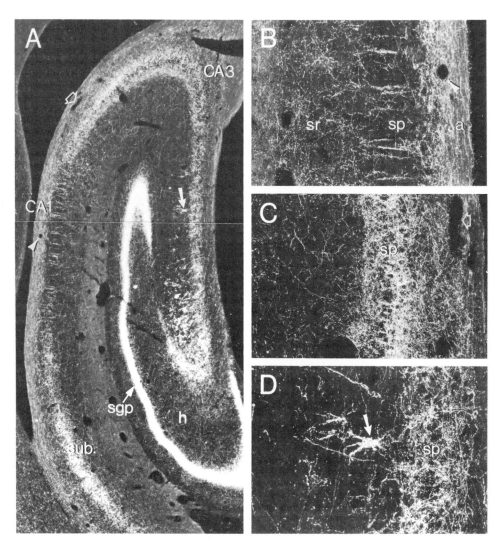

Figure 18. Darkfield photomicrographs illustrating the distribution of tachykinin immunoreactivity in temporal hippocampus of the cat (peroxidase–antiperoxidase technique). In the low-magnification photomicrograph of panel A, tachykinin-immunoreactive axons can be seen to form a dense supragranular plexus in the dentate gyrus and to arborize within and around stratum pyramidale of the hippocampus proper in a regionally differentiated manner. These regional differences can be seen at higher magnification in panels B, C, and D which show regions CA1, CA3a, and CA3b, respectively. Identifying landmarks are indicated by an arrowhead for CA1 (A and B), an open arrow for CA3a (A and C), and a solid arrow for CA3b (A and D).

demonstrated that in the cat, as in the guinea pig, the supragranular axons containing T-I arise from supramammillary hypothalamus (Ino *et al.*, 1988). However, in the cat many of these axons extend from the supragranular zone well into the molecular layer. This distal spread is greater in the infrapyramidal than the suprapyramidal dentate and much greater at temporal than at more septal planes. No T-I perikarya were seen in our material which was from cats sacrificed without colchicine treatment.

In the cat, and similarly but more subtly in the California ground squirrel and human (Del Fiacco *et al.*, 1987; Sakamoto *et al*, 1987), there are regional differences in the distribution of T-I axons within stratum pyramidale (Fig. 18). In region CA3b and c, immunoreactive axons tightly encapsulate the apical dendrites and/or apical halves of select nonimmunoreactive perikarya whereas in region CA3a, labeled axons are profusely distributed within and loosely around the pyramidal cell layer. In further contrast, varicose T-I axons in region CA1 form scattered tube-shaped ghosts suggestive of dense tachykinin innervation of select proximal apical dendrites. As in the guinea pig, there is a strong septotemporal increase in the amount of T-I in cat hippocampus. This is particularly evident in increased numbers of coarsely varicose hilar axons, in the abundance of finer axons distributed diffusely amid the pyramidal cells of CA4, and in the presence of a light band of T-I puncta in the middle molecular layer of the temporal dentate gyrus.

In the Old World monkey (*M. fascicularis*) T-I axons exhibit some of the same distribution observed in the guinea pig, but are both much more diffusely distributed within the hippocampus proper and exhibit unexpected septotemporal gradients within the fascia dentata. In monkey hippocampus, numerous labeled axons are scattered across all laminae of both regio superior and, at slightly less density, regio inferior with little indication of laminar organization except for somewhat reduced density within stratum lucidum (Fig. 19). The one exception is the presence of a system of T-I axons which course through stratum moleculare of both regio inferior and regio superior and within the outer half of the dentate gyrus molecular layer.

Throughout the body of the monkey fascia dentata, T-I axons are distributed within the supragranular molecular layer and superficial stratum granulosum and, as cited above, within the distal molecular layer. Axons within the latter group are not sharply laminated but gradually increase in density with proximity to the hippocampal fissure. Furthermore, in both the supragranular and distal dentate gyrus molecular layer T-I axons *decrease* in density toward the temporal pole of hippocampus and are completely absent within uncal regions. This gradient was unexpected in that the uncal region of monkey hippocampus is homologous to the most temporal region of hippocampus in the guinea pig and cat, and T-I is greatest in the temporal pole of hippocampus in these animals. In the monkey, as in the guinea pig, T-I is localized within neuronal perikarya in the dentate gyrus hilus and hippocampal stratum oriens.

Reports of the distribution of T-I in human hippocampus are consistent with the above description of the monkey. Del Fiacco *et al.* (1987) have reported substance P-like immunoreactivity within perikarya of stratum oriens and the hilus, and within axons most densely distributed in the distal and supragranular aspects of the dentate gyrus molecular layer and stratum pyramidale of region CA2.

5.4. Consideration of Differences in Peptide Localization

In comparative analyses of hippocampal neurochemistry we find that some neurochemical characters are extremely stable phylogenetically. As noted above, the intrahippocampal distributions of a number of neuropeptides including dynorphin, somatostatin, and NPY are conserved with very little modification across the mammals that have been studied. Similarly, aspects of the hippocampal distributions of the neuropeptides considered here appear stable. As described above, CCK-I is present in local circuit neurons and their pericellular arbors within the hippocampus proper in all animals thus far studied. Similarly, ENK-I has been consistently observed within the mossy fiber axonal system. In contrast, we have seen that there is substantial variability in the localization of ENK-I, CCK-I, and T-I within major, anatomically well-documented, and phylogenetically conserved axonal systems. For example, the supramammillary projection to the supragranular dentate gyrus in the rat is well described and exhibits approximately the same distribution in the rat (Haglund *et al.*, 1984) as in the guinea pig. However, this projection contains a great density of T-I axons in the guinea pig but not in the rat. Similarly, the mossy fiber projection of the dentate gyrus granule cells exhibits a relatively consistent morphology in the rat, mouse, guinea pig, and monkey as can be seen in material processed for the localization of heavy metals or for the immunocytochemical localization of enkephalin or dynorphin. However, CCK-I is clearly localized within the mossy fiber system in some animals (mouse, guinea pig, monkey) but has not been detected in others (rat, cat). Although differences in peptide localization such as this raise concern

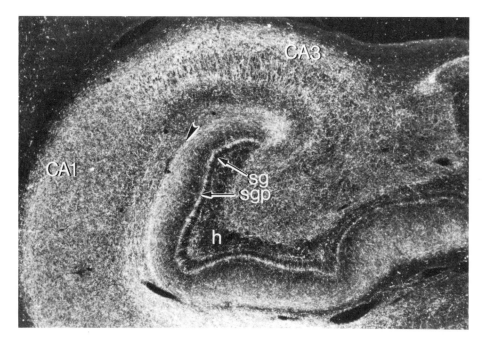

Figure 19. Darkfield photomicrograph of a coronal section through mid-septotemporal hippocampus of *Macaca fascicularis* processed for the localization of tachykinin immunoreactivity by the peroxidase–antiperoxidase technique. As in the guinea pig and cat, a supragranular plexus of tachykinin-immunoreactive axons is seen but, in contrast to these animals, abundant immunoreactive axons are seen throughout all laminae of the hippocampus proper.

as to the sensitivity and specificity of the antisera in use which cannot be discounted, it is noteworthy that species differences in the distribution of all three peptides discussed have been faithfully observed in a number of laboratories using an even greater number of antisera and that these same antisera reliably detect the conserved immunoreactive systems across species.

In many instances reviewed above, the presence or absence of the antigen within a particular system was not so absolute and, indeed, served to reveal that within some of the previously documented projection systems there are neurochemically distinct components which exhibit restricted, and in some instances unanticipated, topographies. An example of this point is provided by the distribution of ENK-I within entorhinal afferents to the dentate gyrus outer molecular layer. ENK-I neurons in the entorhinal area of the rat are most numerous in deep layer II and layer III of the anterolateral extreme of the entorhinal and perirhinal cortices (Gall *et al.*, 1981). Recent transport studies indicate that cells in this area would project to the more septal aspects of both the outer molecular layer and CA1 stratum lacunosum-moleculare (Ruth *et al.*, 1988; Witter *et al.*, 1988). It is, therefore, surprising that ENK-I is virtually absent in the septal dentate gyrus molecular layer and increases in density across the middle to caudal thirds of the structure.

Other density gradients are less surprising but still highlight the point that within the projection systems that have been described for large populations of neurons, the "occult" projections of neuronal subpopulations might exhibit more restricted distributions. These subsystems, selectively viewed with immunocytochemistry, may or may not be representative of the fine topography of the fields of nonimmunoreactive neurons in which they are embedded but nevertheless provide clues as to levels of organization which may be of considerable value in the design of further, more appropriately focused analyses of circuitry.

As has been noted by others (Witter, 1986), one reliably encountered and noteworthy feature of neuropeptide localization within hippocampus is the presence of clear septotemporal gradients. In some instances, these density gradients are very broad, as in the gradual septotemporal increase in ENK-I and CCK-I in outer and inner molecular layers of the rat dentate gyrus, respectively. In other cases, such gradients are more narrow and acute as in the abrupt increase in ENK-I and CCK-I in the outer and middle molecular layers of the most temporal dentate gyrus in the guinea pig. In only one instance was a "reverse" density gradient seen; in the monkey dentate gyrus molecular layer there is a septotemporal decrease in T-I. Despite this exception, the temporal hippocampus is generally quite "peptide rich" relative to the more septal regions. As discussed below, depending upon the functional role of these putative messenger molecules in hippocampal circuitry, the septotemporal gradients described might confer profound regional differences upon hippocampal synaptic physiology.

The functional roles of enkephalin, CCK, and the tachykinins in hippocampal physiology are at present very poorly understood. All three peptides are "neuroactive" when applied to hippocampus but it appears likely that the responses to exogenous peptide application are poor predictors of endogenous peptide function. The limited data on the responses of hippocampal neurons to exogenous CCK are rather contradictory. CCK has been reported to excite hippocampal pyramidal cells when iontophoresed into region CA1 (Dodd and Kelly, 1981), whereas, upon bath application to hippocampal slices *in vitro*, the same concentrations of sulfated CCK-8 have been reported by one group to inhibit

(MacVicar *et al.*, 1987) and by another group to augment (Jaffe *et al.*, 1987) the response of the CA1 pyramidal cells to stimulation of the non-CCK-containing Schaffer collaterals. Immunocytochemical studies have demonstrated that perikaryal CCK-I within rat hippocampus and dentate gyrus is largely colocalized with immunoreactivity to GABA (Kosaka *et al.*, 1985) and electron microscopic analyses have localized CCK-I within terminals forming asymmetric synapses in region CA1 (Hendry and Jones, 1985). As such, it seems quite probable that in these regions CCK is coreleased with GABA and is modulatory to GABA-based transmission. However, CCK-I is also localized in the excitatory mossy fiber and perforant path projection systems which are both thought to use a glutamatelike acidic amino acid as principal neurotransmitter (Crawford and Connor, 1973; Watkins and Evans, 1981; Altschuler *et al.*, 1985). As such, it seems that CCK might modulate the excitatory influences of glutamate, or a related compound, at these synapses. We have as yet no direct evidence for the role of endogenous CCK at either of these loci.

Although there has been a great deal more work on the responses of hippocampal neurons to opioid peptides, similarly little resolution has been reached as to the endogenous action of enkephalin in hippocampus (see Chavkin *et al.*, 1988, and Henriksen *et al.*, 1988, for reviews). Enkephalin is generally considered to increase the excitability of hippocampal neurons. Iontophoretic application of enkephalin or its analogues leads to increased firing of pyramidal cells (Nicoll *et al.*, 1977). Moreover, both *in vivo* (Wiesner and Henriksen, 1987; Henriksen *et al.*, 1988) and *in vitro* (Dingledine, 1981; Chavkin *et al.*, 1988; Lynch *et al.*, 1981) studies have observed that exogenously applied enkephalin has an *indirect* excitatory effect on the dentate gyrus granule and hippocampal pyramidal cells which augments the responsiveness of these neurons to stimulation of nonopioid afferent systems. The results of some studies suggest that this phenomenon is due to an inhibition of the inhibitory interneurons by the opioid which leads, in turn, to a disinhibition of the principal projection neurons (Nicoll *et al.*, 1980; Zieglgansberger *et al.*, 1979). Other studies have found no evidence for disinhibition and have led to speculation as to potential opioid-induced alterations in dendrosomatic coupling (Dingledine, 1981; Lynch *et al.*, 1981). Neither interpretation of these experimental results holds much promise for providing direct information on the role of the endogenous opioid in hippocampal circuitry. Enkephalin is localized within the mossy fibers and the lateral perforant path and, like CCK, would be expected to be released from these excitatory systems at synapses which primarily innervate the principal hippocampal projection neurons. However, the opioid antagonist naloxone has not been found to block or significantly alter the postsynaptic response to stimulation of the mossy fibers (Chavkin and Bloom, 1986; Gall, unpublished observations). As such, the opioid contribution to synaptic transmission in this system has not been convincingly identified.

There has been much less work on the influence of the tachykinins on hippocampal neurons. Dodd and Kelly reported in 1981 that substance P had no effect of the firing of hippocampal pyramidal cells when iontophoresed into region CA1 of the rat. More recently, Dreifuss and Raggenbass (1986) reported that bath application of substance P to rat hippocampal slices *in vitro* causes an increase in the rate of firing of nonpyramidal cells in region CA1 which is not dependent upon synaptic transmission (suggesting direct activation as opposed to disinhibition). As yet, the influence of substance P upon neurons which receive even moderate substance P-containing innervation, such as the dentate gyrus granule cells in the guinea pig or hippocampal pyramidal cells in the cat, has not been examined.

Clearly, definite hypotheses as to the consequence of species differences in the presence of these neuropeptides in hippocampal circuitry must await advances in our understanding of their endogenous actions. However, by analogy with data from other systems, we might anticipate potential physiological consequences of the colocalization of modulatory peptides with classical neurotransmitters in hippocampus. As reviewed by Lundberg and Hökfelt (1986), it has been observed that colocalized substances may exhibit differential frequency-dependent release characteristics. In particular, Lundberg and Hökfelt have obtained evidence in two separate systems that, in contrast to the classical neurotransmitter substances (noradrenaline in one case, acetylcholine in another), colocalized modulatory peptides are preferentially released with high-frequency stimulation. As such, the neuropeptide was only seen to contribute to the postsynaptic response with activity in the high-frequency range. Second, many neuropeptides have been found to have slow onset and long duration effects (Nicoll, 1982; Jan and Jan, 1983; Tokimasa *et al.*, 1981; Womack *et al.*, 1988). Should this be the case for the hippocampal neuropeptides discussed, one would anticipate that the peptide might influence the frequency responsiveness (e.g., duration of depolarization, and/or refractory periods) of the synapses, and target cells, involved. Finally, a number of recent studies have demonstrated that in many central systems, including hippocampus, the synthesis and resting levels of neuroactive peptides are regulated to a large extent by extrinsic influences including changes in the levels of physiological activity. Recent work in this laboratory and elsewhere has demonstrated that in both the rat and mouse, brief episodes of epileptiform activity lead to an increase in the synthesis of enkephalin pentapeptide both within the entorhinal cortex and the dentate gyrus granule cells (Fig. 13) which, in turn, leads to dramatic elevations in the amount of enkephalin in both the mossy fiber axons and the perforant path innervation of the dentate gyrus (Gall, 1988a; Gall and White, 1989; Hong *et al.*, 1988; White *et al.*, 1987). The seizure-induced increases in enkephalin content last well over 1 week. In these same paradigms the levels of CCK-I and DYN-I within the mossy fibers are dramatically reduced (Gall, 1988b). These observations, in combination with those of others, lead to the conclusion that the amounts of enkephalin, CCK, and dynorphin within hippocampal pathways reflect the recent physiological activity of the system; as a corollary, one would then anticipate that the contribution of these neuropeptides to synaptic physiology might also vary over time as a function of changes in recent activity and in the releasable peptide pool.

These features of neuropeptide action and regulation suggest that the presence of a modulatory peptide with a classical neurotransmitter might influence both the frequency responsiveness of a system and the plasticity of these physiological characteristics over time. As such, the regional and comparative differences seen in the localization of neuropeptides within major components of hippocampal circuitry might give rise to peptide-dependent differences in the frequency coding characteristics and in certain forms of physiological plasticity both between septal and temporal hippocampus of a given animal and in a comparison of these properties for a given system between animals.

6. Concluding Comments

The material reviewed indicates that although the most conspicuous features of hippocampal cytoarchitectonis and circuitry are relatively consistent across a number of mammalian species, there are several comparative differences in the organization and neurochemistry of hippocampus which could be of great functional consequence. In allometric analyses, the relationship of the size of the three major hippocampal subfields (CA1, CA3, dentate gyrus) proved to be extremely well correlated with the absolute size of hippocampus in two orders of mammals. However, the exponents of the curves relating the size of the part to the size of the whole differed slightly for CA3, CA1, and dentate gyrus and these variations in allometric relationships were different for primates as compared to insectivores. These observations suggest two conclusions. First, the basic plan of hippocampus is relatively conservative in that individual species do not deviate greatly from a general pattern that holds for the order as a group. Second, a change in this basic plan occurred at some point after the divergence of the primates and insectivores and was retained over the subsequent course of evolutionary history of each order. It should be noted that the allometric relationships of the three hippocampal subdivisions change the relative proportions of these subdivisions as a function of brain and hippocampal size. Thus, as an example, human hippocampus is quite different from that of a small primate for reasons that are unrelated to evolutionary adaptations acting at the species level. The functional significance of this remains to be investigated.

The distribution of fiber projections within hipppocampus has proven to be somewhat more variable than the relative size of the various subdivisions. This is particularly true for the "crossed" projection systems. Considerable variability has been observed in the relative density of afferents from entorhinal cortex to the contralateral hippocampus and dentate gyrus between animals; in distinction from other animals, such crossed projections in the Old World monkey are very sparse and originate from medial, as opposed to both medial and lateral, entorhinal cortex. Still more dramatic are the variations in the size of the hippocampal commissural projections. In particular, the absence of commissural projections to the major portion of the dentate gyrus and hippocampus proper of the Old World monkey suggests there may be a trend toward hemispheric isolation of hippocampus in primates. As noted by others (Amaral *et al.*, 1984; Demeter *et al.*, 1985), such a trend would be quite intriguing in that it might provide an anatomical basis for the lateralization of hippocampal function indicated by behavioral deficits observed following unilateral hippocampal damage in humans. However, further work is needed before this conclusion can be confirmed. In particular, examination of the hippocampal commissural projections in prosimians and New World monkeys would indicate whether limited interhemispheric associations are typical of all primates, suggesting a specialization which has been present during the full history of the order, or are more specifically characteristic of the simians, or possibly of larger-brained primates.

The recent immunocytochemical studies reviewed demonstrate that within hippocampus the distributions of some of the neuroactive peptides differ greatly between groups, and notable variations are observed between even closely related species. Although some neurochemical characters appear to be conserved, the comparative differences reported here, together with reports of interspecies variability in the distribution of acetylcholine esterase (Geneser, 1987; Bakst and Amaral, 1984; Rosene and Van Hoesen, 1987), give the impression of surprisingly large differences in hippocampal neurochemistry that might be of direct consequence to properties of neurotransmission. It is intriguing that the expression of some of the same neuropeptides which vary in localization between animals can be profoundly altered by intense physiological activity in the adult. As the functional consequences of these alterations become understood, it may be possible to further interpret the significance of the comparative differences in peptide localization.

7. Abbreviations

f	Hippocampal fissure	pp	Perforant path
h	Dentate gyrus hilus	sg, SG	Stratum granulosum
i,iml	Dentate gyrus inner molecular layer	sgp	Supragranular plexus
		sh	Schaffer collaterals
ia	Ipsilateral dentate gyrus associational system	sl	Stratum lucidum
		sl-m	Stratum lacunosum-moleculare
m,mml	Dentate gyrus middle molecular layer	so	Stratum oriens
		sp,SP	Stratum pyramidale
mf	Mossy fibers	sr	Stratum radiatum
o,oml	Dentate gyrus outer molecular layer	sub.	Subiculum
		ta	Temperoammonic system
p	Plexiform zone of Ramón y Cajal		

ACKNOWLEDGMENTS. I thank Gary Lynch for his collaboration in the allometric analyses and comments on the manuscript and Julie Lauterborn for her contributions to much of the work described here. The support of NSF Grant BNS8417098 and Research Career Development Award NS00915 is gratefully acknowledged.

8. References

Altschuler, R. A., Monaghan, D. T., Hasser, W. G., Wenthold, R. J., Curthoys, N. P., and Cotman, C. W., 1985, Immunocytochemical localization of glutaminase-like and aspartate aminotransferase-like immunoreactivities in the rat and guinea pig hippocampus, *Brain Res.* **330**:225–233.

Amaral, D. G., 1978, A Golgi study of cell types in the hilar region of the hippocampus in the rat, *J. Comp. Neurol.* **182**:851–914.

Amaral, D. G., and Campbell, M. J., 1986, Transmitter systems in the primate dentate gyrus, *Hum. Neurobiol.* **5**:169–180.

Amaral, D. G., Insausti, R., and Cowan, W. M., 1984, The commissural connections of the monkey hippocampal formation, *J. Comp. Neurol.* **224**:307–336.

Andersen, P., Bliss, T. V. P., and Skrede, K. K., 1971, Lamellar organization of hippocampal excitatory pathways, *Exp. Brain Res.* **13**:222–238.

Andersen, P., Silfvenius, H., Sundberg, S. H., and Sveen, O., 1980, A comparison of distal and proximal dendritic synapses on CA1 pyramids in hippocampal slices *in vitro, J. Physiol. (London)* **307**:273–299.

Armstrong, E., 1982, A look at relative brain size in mammals, *Neurosci. Lett.* **34**:101–104.

Bakst, I., and Amaral, D. G., 1984, The distribution of acetylcholinesterase in the hippocampal formation of the monkey, *J. Comp. Neurol.* **225**:344–371.

Bakst, I., Morrison, J. H., and Amaral, D. G., 1985, The distribution of somatostatin-like immunoreactivity in the monkey hippocampal formation, *J. Comp. Neurol.* **236:**423–442.

Bakst, I., Avendano, C., Morrison, J. H., and Amaral, D. G., 1986, An experimental analysis of the origins of somatostatin-like immunoreactivity in the dentate gyrus of the rat, *J. Neurosci.* **6:**1452–1463.

Barber, R. P., Vaughn, J. E., Wimer, R. E., and Wimer, C. C., 1974, Genetically-associated variations in the distribution of dentate granule cell synapses upon the pyramidal dendrites in mouse hippocampus, *J. Comp. Neurol.* **156:**417–434.

Bayer, S., 1980, Development of the hippocampal region in the rat: I. Neurogenesis examined with ³H-thymidine autoradiography, *J. Comp. Neurol.* **190:**87–114.

Blackstad, T. W., 1956, Commissural connections of the hippocampal region of the rat with special reference to their mode of termination, *J. Comp. Neurol.* **105:**417–538.

Blackstad, T. W., and Kjaerheim, A., 1961, Special axo-dendritic synapses in the hippocampal cortex: Electron and light microscopic studies on the layer of mossy fibers, *J. Comp. Neurol.* **117:**133–159.

Blackstad, T. W., Brink, K., Hem, J., and Jeune, B., 1970, Distribution of hippocampal mossy fibers in the rat. An experimental study with silver impregnation methods, *J. Comp. Neurol.* **138:**443–450.

Chan-Palay, V., 1987, Somatostatin immunoreactive neurons in the human hippocampus and cortex shown by immunogold/silver intensification on vibratome sections: Coexistence with neuropeptide Y neurons, and effects in Alzheimer-type dementia, *J. Comp. Neurol.* **260:**201–223.

Chan-Palay, V., Köhler, C., Haesler, U., Lang, W., and Yasargil, G., 1985, Distribution of neurons and axons immunoreactive with antisera against neuropeptide Y in the normal human hippocampus, *J. Comp. Neurol.* **248:**360–375.

Chavkin, C., and Bloom, F., 1986, Opiate antagonists do not alter neuronal responses to stimulation of opioid-containing pathways in rat hippocampus, *Neuropeptides* **7:**19–22.

Chavkin, C., Neumaier, J. F., and Swearengen, E., 1988, Opioid receptor mechanisms in the rat hippocampus, in: *Opioids in the Hippocampus*, NIDA Research Monograph No. 82 (J. F. McGinty and D. P. Friedman, eds.), pp. 94–117.

Crain, B. J., Chang, K.-J., and McNamara, J. O., 1986, Quantitative autoradiographic analysis of mu and delta opioid binding sites in the rat hippocampal formation, *J. Comp. Neurol.* **246:**170–180.

Crawford, I. L., and Connor, J. D., 1973, Localization and release of glutamic acid in relation to the hippocampal mossy fibre pathway, *Nature* **244:**442–443.

Cuello, A. C., Galfre, G., and Milstein, C., 1979, Detection of substance P in the central nervous system by a monoclonal antibody, *Proc. Natl. Acad. Sci. USA* **76:**3532–3536.

Davies, S., and Köhler, C., 1985, The substance P innervation of the rat hippocampal region, *Anat. Embryol.* **173:**45–52.

Del Fiacco, M., Levanti, M. C., Dessi, M. L., and Zucca, G., 1987, The human hippocampal formation and parahippocampal gyrus: Localization of substance P-like immunoreactivity in newborn and adult post-mortem tissue, *Neuroscience* **21:**141–150.

Demeter, S., Rosene, D. L., and Van Hoesen, G., 1985, Interhemispheric pathways of the hippocampal formation, presubiculum, and entorhinal and posterior parahippocampal cortices in the rhesus monkey: The structure and organization of the hippocampal commissures, *J. Comp. Neurol.* **233:**30–47.

Dingledine, R., 1981, Possible mechanisms of enkephalin action on hippocampal CA1 pyramidal neurons, *J. Neurosci.* **1:**1022–1035.

Dodd, J., and Kelly, J. S., 1981, The actions of cholecystokinin and related peptides on pyramidal neurons of the mammalian hippocampus, *Brain Res.* **205:**337–350.

Dreifuss, J. J., and Raggenbass, M., 1986, Tachykinins and bombesin excite non-pyramidal neurones in rat hippocampus, *J. Physiol. (London)* **379:**417–428.

Fitzpatrick, D., and Johnson, R. P., 1981, Enkephalin-like immunoreactivity in the mossy fiber pathway of the hippocampal formation of the tree shrew (*Tupaia glis*), *Neuroscience* **6:**2485–2494.

Fredens, K., Stengaard-Pedersen, K., and Larsson, L.-I., 1984, Localization of enkephalin and cholecystokinin immunoreactivities in the perforant path terminal fields of the rat hippocampal formation, *Brain Res.* **304:**255–263.

Fredens, K., Stengaard-Pedersen, K., and Wallace, M. N., 1987, Localization of cholecystokinin in the dentate commissural–associational system of the mouse and rat, *Brain Res.* **401:**68–78.

Fricke, R., and Cowan, W. M., 1978, An autoradiographic study of the commissural and ipsilateral hippocampo-dentate projections in the adult rat, *J. Comp. Neurol.* **181:**253–270.

Gaarskjaer, F. B., 1978, Organization of the mossy fiber system of the rat studied in extended hippocampi. II. Experimental analysis of fiber distribution with silver impregnation methods, *J. Comp. Neurol.* **178**:73–88.

Gaarskjaer, F. B., Danscher, G., and West, M. J., 1982, Hippocampal mossy fibers in the regio superior of the European hedgehog, *Brain Res.* **237**:79–90.

Gall, C., 1984a, The distribution of cholecystokinin-like immunoreactivity in the hippocampal formation of the guinea pig: Localization in the mossy fibers, *Brain Res.* **306**:73–83.

Gall, C., 1984b, Ontogeny of dynorphin-like immunoreactivity in the hippocampal formation of the rat, *Brain Res.* **307**:327–331.

Gall, C., 1988a, Localization and seizure-induced alterations of opioid peptides and CCK in the hippocampus, in: *Opioids in the Hippocampus*, NIDA Research Monograph No. 82 (J. F. McGinty and D. P. Friedman, eds.), pp. 12–32.

Gall, C., 1988b, Seizures induce dramatic and distinctly different changes in enkephalin, dynorphin, and cholecystokinin immunoreactivities in mouse hippocampal mossy fibers, *J. Neurosci.* **8**:1852–1862.

Gall, C., and Selawski, L., 1984, Supramammillary afferents to guinea pig hippocampus contain substance P-like immunoreactivity, *J. Comp. Neurol.* **51**:171–176.

Gall, C., and White, J. D., 1989, Studies on the expression of opioid peptides and their respective mRNAs in hippocampal seizure, in: *The Hippocampus: New Vistas* (V. Chan-Palay and C. Kohler, Alan Liss, New York, pp. 153–170.

Gall, C., McWilliams, R., and Lynch, G., 1979, The effect of collateral sprouting on the density of innervation of normal target sites: Implications for theories on the regulation of the size of developing synaptic domains, *Brain Res.* **175**:37–47.

Gall, C., McWilliams, R., and Lynch, G., 1980, Accelerated rates of synaptogenesis by 'sprouting' afferents in the immature hippocampal formation, *J. Comp. Neurol.* **193**:1047–1063.

Gall, C., Brecha, N., Karten, H. J., and Chang, K.-J., 1981, Localization of enkephalin-like immunoreactivity to identified axonal and neuronal populations of the rat hippocampus, *J. Comp. Neurol.* **198**:335–350.

Gall, C., Berry, L. M., and Hodgson, L. A., 1986a, Cholecystokinin in the mouse hippocampus: Localization in the mossy fiber and dentate commissural systems, *Exp. Brain Res.* **62**:431–437.

Gall, C., Ivy, G., and Lynch, G., 1986b, Neuroanatomical plasticity: Its role in organizing and reorganizing the central nervous system, in: *Human Growth*, Volume 2 (F. Falkner and J. M. Tanner, eds.), Plenum Press, New York, pp. 411–436.

Gall, C., Lauterborn, J., Burks, D., and Seroogy, K., 1987a, Colocalization of enkephalin and cholecystokinin in discrete areas of rat brain, *Brain Res.* **403**:403–408.

Gall, C., White, J. D., and Lauterborn, J. C., 1987b, In situ hybridization analyses of increased preproenkephalin mRNA following seizures, *Soc. Neurosci. Abstr.* **13**:1277.

Geneser, F. A., 1987, Distribution of acetylcholinesterase in the hippocampal region of the rabbit: III. The dentate area, *J. Comp. Neurol.* **262**:594–606.

Geneser-Jensen, F. A., Haug, F.-M. S., and Danscher, G., 1974, Distribution of heavy metals in the hippocampal region of the guinea pig. A light microscope study with Timm's sulfide silver method, *Z. Zellforsch.* **147**:441–478.

Goldowitz, D., White, W. F., Steward, O., Lynch, G., and Cotman, C., 1975, Anatomical evidence for a projection from the entorhinal cortex to the contralateral dentate gyrus of the rat, *Exp. Neurol.* **47**:433–441.

Gottlieb, D. I., and Cowan, W. M., 1972, Evidence for a temporal factor in the occupation of available synaptic sites during the development of the dentate gyrus, *Brain Res.* **41**:452–456.

Gottlieb, D. I., and Cowan, W. M., 1973, Autoradiographic studies of the commissural and ipsilateral association connections of the hippocampus and dentate gyrus of the rat. I. The commissural connections, *J. Comp. Neurol.* **149**:393–422.

Greenwood, R. S., Godar, S., Reaves, T. A., Jr., and Hayward, J., 1981, Cholecystokinin in hippocampal pathways, *J. Comp. Neurol.* **203**:335–350.

Habets, A. M. M. C., Lopes da Silva, F. H., and de Quartel, F. W., 1980, Autoradiography of an olfactory hippocampal pathway in the cat with special reference to the perforant path, *Exp. Brain Res.* **38**:257–265.

Haglund, L., Swanson, L. W., and Köhler, C., 1984, The projection of the supramammillary nucleus to the hippocampal formation: An immunohistochemical and anterograde transport study with the lectin PHA-L in the rat, *J. Comp. Neurol.* **229**:171–185.

Haug, F.-M. S., 1974, Light microscopical mapping of the hippocampal region, the pyriform cortex and the corticomedial amygdaloid nuclei of the rat with Timm's sulphide silver method. I. Area dentata, hippocampus, and subiculum, *Z. Anat. Entwicklungsgesch.* **145**:1–27.

Haug. F.-M. S., 1976, Sulphide silver pattern and cytoarchitectonics of parahippocampal areas in the rat, *Adv. Anat. Embryol. Cell Bio.* **52**:1–73.

Haug, F. M., Blackstad, T., Hjorth-Simonsen, A., and Zimmer, J., 1971, Timm's sulfide silver reaction for zinc during experimental anterograde degeneration of hippocampal mossy fibers, *J. Comp. Neurol.* **142**:23–32.

Hendry, S. H. C., and Jones, E. G., 1985, Morphology of synapses formed by cholecystokinin-immunoreactive axon terminals in regio superior of rat hippocampus, *Neuroscience* **16**:57–68.

Henriksen, S. J., Wiesner, J. B., and Chouvet, G., 1988, Opioids in the hippocampus: Progress obtained from *in vivo* electrophysiological analyses, in: *Opioids in the Hippocampus*, NIDA Research Monograph No. 82 (J. F. McGinty and D. P. Friedman, eds.), pp. 67–93.

Hjorth-Simonsen, A., 1972a, Some intrinsic connections of the hippocampus in the rat: An experimental analysis, *J. Comp. Neurol.* **147**:145–161.

Hjorth-Simonsen, A., 1972b, Projection of the lateral part of the entorhinal area to the hippocampus and fascia dentata, *J. Comp. Neurol.* **146**:219–232.

Hjorth-Simonsen, A., 1977, Distribution of commissural afferents to the hippocampus of the rabbit, *J. Comp. Neurol.* **176**:495–514.

Hjorth-Simonsen, A., and Jeune, B., 1972, Origin and termination of the hippocampal perforant path in the rat studied by silver impregnation, *J. Comp. Neurol.* **144**:215–232.

Hjorth-Simonsen, A., and Laurberg, S., 1977, Commissural connections of the dentate area in the rat, *J. Comp. Neurol.* **174**:591–606.

Hjorth-Simonsen, A., and Zimmer, J., 1975, Crossed pathways from the entorhinal area to the fascia dentata: I. Normal in rabbits, *J. Comp. Neurol.* **161**:57–70.

Hong, J.-S., McGinty, J. F., Grimes, L., Kanamatsu, T., Obie, J., and Mitchell, C. L., 1988, Seizure-induced alterations in the metabolism of hippocampal opioid peptides suggest opioid modulation of seizure-related behaviors, in: *Opioids in the Hippocampus*, NIDA Research Monograph No. 82 (J. F. McGinty and D. P. Friedman, eds.), pp. 48–66.

Ino, T., Itoh, K., Sugimoto, T., Kaneko, T., Kamiya, H., and Mizuno, N., 1988, The supramammillary region of the cat sends substance P-like immunoreactive axons to the hippocampal formation and the entorhinal cortex, *Neurosci. Lett.* **90**:259–264.

Jaffe, D. B., Aitken, P. G., and Nadler, J. V., 1987, The effects of cholecystokinin and cholecystokinin antagonists on synaptic function in the CA1 region of the rat hippocampal slice, *Brain Res.* **415**:197–203.

Jan, Y. N., and Jan, L. Y., 1983, Co-existence and co-release of cholinergic and peptidergic transmitters in frog sympathetic ganglia, *Fed. Proc.* **42**:2929–2933.

Jerison, H. J., 1973, *Evolution of the Brain and Intelligence*, Academic Press, New York.

Jones, E. G., DeFelipe, J., Hendry, S. H. C., and Maggio, J. E., 1988, A study of tachykinin immunoreactive neurons in monkey cerebral cortex, *J. Neurosci.* **8**:1206–1224.

Kalivas, P. W., Deutch, A. Y., Maggio, J. E., Mantyh, P. W., and Roth, R. H., 1985, Substance K and substance P in the ventral tegmental area, *Neurosci. Lett.* **57**:241–246.

Köhler, C., and Chan-Palay, V., 1982, Somatostatin-like immunoreactive neurons in the hippocampus: An immunocytochemical study in the rat, *Neurosci. Lett.* **34**:259–264.

Köhler, C., Eriksson, L., Davies, S., and Chan-Palay, V., 1986, Neuropeptide Y innervation of the hippocampal region in the rat and monkey brain, *J. Comp. Neurol.* **244**:384–444.

Kosaka, T., Kosaka, K., Tateishi, K., Hamaoka, Y., Yanaihara, N., Wu, J.-Y., and Hama, K., 1985, Gabaergic neurons containing CCK-8-like and/or VIP-like immunoreactivities in the rat hippocampus and dentate gyrus, *J. Comp. Neurol.* **239**:420–430.

Krettek, J. E., and Price, J. L., 1977, Projections from the amygdaloid complex and adjacent olfactory structures to the entorhinal cortex and to the subiculum in the rat and cat, *J. Comp. Neurol.* **172**:723–752.

Laatsch, R. H., and Cowan, W. M., 1965, Electron microscopic studies of the dentate gyrus of the rat. I. Normal structure with special reference to synaptic organization, *J. Comp. Neurol.* **128**:359–396.

Laurberg, S., and Sørensen, K. E., 1981, Associational and commissural collaterals of neurons in the hippocampal formation (hilus fasciae dentatae and subfield CA3), *Brain Res.* **212**:287–300.

Laurberg, S., and Zimmer, J., 1980, Aberrant hippocampal mossy fibers in cats, *Brain Res.* **188**:555–559.

Lorente de Nó, R., 1934, Studies on the structure of the cerebral cortex. II. Continuation of the study of the ammonic system, *J. Psychol. Neurol.* **46**:113–177.

Lotstra, F., and Vanderhaeghen, J.-J., 1987, Distribution of immunoreactive cholecystokinin in the human hippocampus, *Peptides* **8**:911–920.

Lundberg, J. M., and Hökfelt, T., 1986, Multiple co-existence of peptides and classical transmitters in peripheral autonomic and sensory neurons—Functional and pharmacological implications, *Prog. Brain Res.* **68:**241–262.

Lynch, G., Mosko, S., Parks, T., and Cotman, C., 1973, Relocation and hyperdevelopment of the dentate gyrus commissural system after entorhinal lesions in immature rats, *Brain Res.* **50:**174–178.

Lynch, G. S., Jensen, R. A., McGaugh, J., Davila, K., and Oliver, M. W., 1981, Effects of enkephalin, morphine and naloxone on the electrical activity of the in vitro hippocampal slice preparation, *Exp. Neurol.* **71:**527–540.

McGinty, J. F., Henriksen, S., Goldstein, A., Terenius, L., and Bloom, F. E., 1983, Dynorphin is contained within hippocampal mossy fibers: Immunochemical alterations after kainic acid administration and colchicine induced neurotoxicity, *Proc. Natl. Acad. Sci. USA* **80:**589–593.

McGinty, J. F., Van Der Kooy, D., and Bloom, F. E., 1984, The distribution and morphology of opioid peptide immunoreactive neurons in the cerebral cortex of rats, *J. Neurosci.* **4:**1104–1117.

McLean, S., Rothman, R. B., Jacobson, A. E., Rice, K. C., and Herkenham, M., 1987, Distribution of opiate receptor subtypes and enkephalin and dynorphin immunoreactivity in the hippocampus of squirrel, guinea pig, rat, and hamster, *J. Comp. Neurol.* **255:**497–510.

MacVicar, B. A., Kerrin, J. P., and Davison, J. S., 1987, Inhibition of synaptic transmission in the hippocampus by cholecystokinin (CCK) and its antagonism by a CCK analog (CCK 27-33), *Brain Res.* **406:**130–135.

Maggio, J. E., and Hunter, J. C., 1985, "Kassinin" in mammals: The newest tachykinin, *Peptides* **6:**(Suppl. 3):237–243.

Nawa, H., Hirose, T., Takashima, H., Inayaka, S., and Nakanishi, S., 1983, Nucleotide sequences of cloned cDNAs for two types of bovine brain substance P precursor, *Nature* **306:**32–36.

Nicoll, R. A., 1982, Neurotransmitters can say more than just "yes" and "no," *Trends Neurosci.* **5:**369–374.

Nicoll, R. A., Siggins, G. R., Ling, N., Bloom, F. E., and Guillemin, R., 1977, Neuronal actions of endorphins and enkephalins among brain regions: A comparative microiontophoretic study, *Proc. Natl. Acad. Sci. USA* **74:**2584–2588.

Nicoll, R., Alger, B., and Jahr, C., 1980, Enkephalin blocks inhibitory pathways in the vertebrate CNS, *Nature* **287:**22–25.

Pohle, W., and Ott, T., 1984, Localization of entorhinal cortex neurons projecting to the dorsal hippocampal formation. A stereotaxic tool in three dimensions, *J. Hirnforsch.* **25:**661–669.

Ramón y Cajal, S., 1911, *Histologie due Système Nerveux de l'Homme et des Vertébrés*, Volume II, Maloine, Paris.

Ramón y Cajal, S., 1968, *The Structure of Ammon's Horn*, Thomas, Springfield, Ill.

Rawlins, J. N. P., and Green, K. F., 1977, Lamellar organisation in the rat hippocampus, *Exp. Brain Res.* **28:**335–344.

Ribak, C. E., and Seress, L., 1983, Five types of basket cell in the hippocampal dentate gyrus. A combined Golgi and electron microscopic study, *J. Neurocytol.* **12:**577–597.

Rosene, D. L., and Van Hoesen, G. W., 1987, The hippocampal formation of the primate brain: A review of some comparative aspects of cytoarchitecture and connections, in: *Cerebral Cortex*, Volume 6 (E. G. Jones and A. Peters, eds.), Plenum Press, New York, pp. 345–356.

Ruth, R. E., Collier, T. J., and Routtenberg, A., 1982, Topography between the entorhinal cortex and the dentate septotemporal axis in rats: I. Medial and intermediate entorhinal projecting cells, *J. Comp. Neurol.* **209:**69–78.

Ruth, R. E., Collier, T. J., and Routtenberg, A., 1988, Topographical relationship between the entorhinal cortex and the septotemporal axis of the dentate gyrus in rats: II. Cells projecting from lateral entorhinal subdivisions, *J. Comp. Neurol.* **270:**506–516.

Sakamoto, N., Michel, J.-P., Kopp, N., Tohyama, M., and Pearson, J., 1987, Substance P and enkephalin-immunoreactive neurons in the hippocampus and related areas of the human infant brain, *Neuroscience* **22:**801–811.

Schwerdtfeger, W. K., and Buhl, E., 1986, Various types of non-pyramidal hippocampal neurons project to the septum and contralateral hippocampus, *Brain Res.* **386:**146–154.

Seress, L., and Mrzljak, L., 1987, Basal dendrites of granule cells are normal features of the fetal and adult dentate gyrus of both monkey and human hippocampal formations, *Brain Res.* **405:**169–174.

Sloviter, R. S., and Nilaver, G., 1987, Immunocytochemical localization of GABA-, cholecystokinin-, vasoactive intestinal polypeptide- and somatostatin-like immunoreactivity in the area dentata and hippocampus of the rat, *J. Comp. Neurol.* **256:**42–60.

Smith, Y., Parent, A., Kerkerian, L., and Pelletire, G., 1985, Distribution of neuropeptide Y immunoreactivity in the basal forebrain and upper brainstem of the squirrel monkey (*Saimiri sciureus*), *J. Comp. Neurol.* **236:**71–89.

Stanfield, B. B., and Cowan, W. M., 1979, The morphology of the hippocampus and dentate gyrus in normal and reeler mice, *J. Comp. Neurol.* **185:**393–422.

Stanfield, B. B., Caviness, V. S., Jr., and Cowan, W. M., 1979, The organization of certain afferents to the hippocampus and dentate gyrus in normal and reeler mice, *J. Comp. Neurol.* **185:**461–484.

Stengaard-Pedersen, K., Fredens, K., and Larsson, L. I., 1983, Comparative localization of enkephalin, cholecystokinin and heavy metals in the hippocampus, *Brain Res.* **273:**81–96.

Stephan, H., and Manolescu, J., 1980, Comparative investigations on hippocampus in insectivores and primates, *Z. Mikrosk. Anat. Forsch.* **94:**1025–1050.

Stephan, H., Frahm, H., and Baron, G., 1981, New and revised data on volumes of brain structures in insectivores and primates, *Folia Primatol.* **35:**1–29.

Steward, O., 1976, Topographic organization of the projections from the entorhinal area to the hippocampal formation of the rat, *J. Comp. Neurol.* **167:**285–314.

Swanson, L. W., Wyss, J. M., and Cowan, W. M., 1978, An autoradiographic study of the organization of the intrahippocampal association pathways in the rat, *J. Comp. Neurol.* **181:**681–716.

Swanson, L. W., Sawchenko, P. E., and Cowan, W. M., 1981, Evidence for collateral projections by neurons in Ammon's horn, the dentate gyrus and the subiculum: A multiple retrograde labeling study in the rat, *J. Neurosci.* **1:**548–559.

Tielen, A. M., van Leeuwen, F. W., and Lopes da Silva, F. H., 1982, The localization of leucine-enkephalin immunoreactivity within guinea pig hippocampus, *Exp. Brain Res.* **48:**288–295.

Tokimasa, T., Morita, K., and North, A., 1981, Opiates and clonidine prolong calcium-dependent after-hyperpolarizations, *Nature* **294:**162–163.

Van Groen, T., and Wyss, J. M., 1988, Species differences in hippocampal commissural connections: Studies in rat, guinea pig, rabbit, and cat, *J. Comp. Neurol.* **267:**322–334.

Van Hoesen, G. W., and Pandya, D. N., 1975, Some connections of the entorhinal (area 28) and perirhinal (area 35) cortices of the rhesus monkey. III. Efferent connections, *Brain Res.* **95:**39–59.

Vincent, S. R., Kimura, H., and McGeer, E., 1981, Organization of substance P fibers within the hippocampal formation demonstrated with a biotin–avidin immunoperoxidase technique, *J. Comp. Neurol.* **199:**113–123.

Walaas, I., 1983, The hippocampus, in: *Chemical Neuroanatomy* (P. C. Emson, ed.), Raven Press, New York, pp. 337–358.

Warden, M. K., and Young, W. S., III, 1988, Distribution of cells containing mRNAs encoding substance P and neurokinin B in the rat central nervous system, *J. Comp. Neurol.* **272:**90–113.

Watkins, J. C., and Evans, R. H., 1981, Excitatory amino acid transmitters, *Annu. Rev. Pharmacol. Toxicol.* **21:**165–204.

West, J. R., 1983, Distal infrapyramidal and longitudinal mossy fibers at a midtemporal hippocampal level, *Brain Res. Bull.* **10:**137–146.

West, J. R., Nornes, H. O., Barnes, C. L., and Bronfenbrenner, M., 1979, The cells of origin of the commissural afferents to the area dentata in the mouse, *Brain Res.* **160:**203–215.

West, J. R., Van Hoesen, G. W., and Kosel, K. C., 1982, A demonstration of hippocampal mossy fiber axon morphology using anterograde transport of horseradish peroxidase, *Exp. Brain Res.* **48:**209–216.

West, M. J., and Andersen, A. H., 1980, An allometric study of the area dentata in the rat and mouse, *Brain Res. Rev.* **2:**317–348.

West, M. J., and Schwerdtfeger, W. K., 1985, An allometric study of hippocampal components: A comparative study of the brains of the European hedgehog (*Erinaceus europaeus*), the tree shrew (*Tupaia glis*), and the marmoset monkey (*Callithrix jacchus*), *Brain Behav. Evol.* **27:**93–105.

White, J. D., Gall, C. M., and McKelvy, J. F., 1986, Evidence for projection-specific processing of proenkephalin in the rat central nervous system, *Proc. Natl. Acad. Sci. USA* **83:**7099–7103.

White, J. D., Gall, C. M., and McKelvy, J. F., 1987, Enkephalin biosynthesis and enkephalin gene expression are increased in hippocampal mossy fibers following a unilateral lesion of the hilus, *J. Neurosci.* **7:**753–759.

Wiesner, J. B., and Henriksen, S. J., 1987, Enkephalin enhances responsiveness to perforant path input while decreasing spontaneous activity in the dentate gyrus, *Neurosci. Lett.* **74:**95–101.

Witter, M. P., 1986, A survey of the anatomy of the hippocampal formation, with emphasis on the septotemporal organization of its intrinsic and extrinsic connections, in: *Excitatory Amino Acids and Epilepsy* (R. Schwarz and Y. Ben-Ari, eds.), Plenum Press, New York, pp. 67–82.

Witter, M. P., and Groenewegen, H. J., 1984, Laminar origin and septotemporal distribution of entorhinal and perirhinal projections to the hippocampus in the cat, *J. Comp. Neurol.* **224:**371–385.

Witter, M. P., Griffioen, A. W., Jorritsma-Byham, B., and Krijnen, J. L. M., 1988, Entorhinal projections to the hippocampal CA1 region in the rat: An underestimated pathway, *Neurosci. Lett.* **85:**193–198.

Womack, M. D., MacDermott, A. B., and Jessel, T. M., 1988, Sensory transmitters regulate intracellular calcium in dorsal horn neurons, *Nature* **334:**351–353.

Wyss, J. M., 1981, An autoradiographic study of the efferent connections of the entorhinal cortex in the rat, *J. Comp. Neurol.* **199:**495–512.

Wyss, J. M., Swanson, L. W., and Cowan, W. M., 1979, Evidence for an input to the molecular layer and the *stratum granulosum* of the dentate gyrus from the supramammillary region of the hypothalamus, *Anat. Embryol.* **156:**165–176.

Zieglgansberger, W., French, E. D., Siggins, G. R., and Bloom, F. E., 1979, Opioid peptides may excite hippocampal pyramidal neurons by inhibiting adjacent inhibitory interneurons, *Science* **205:**415–417.

Zimmer, J., 1971, Ipsilateral afferents to the commissural zone of the fascia dentata, demonstrated in de-commissurated rats by silver impregnation, *J. Comp. Neurol.* **142:**393–409.

Zimmer, J., 1973, Extended commissural and ipsilateral projections in postnatally deentorhinated hippocampus and fascia dentata demonstrated in rats by silver impregnation, *Brain Res.* **64:**293–311.

Zimmer, J., and Sunde, N., 1984, Neuropeptides and astroglia in intracerebral hippocampal transplants: An immunohistochemical study in the rat, *J. Comp. Neurol.* **227:**331–347.

13

Comparative and Evolutionary Anatomy of the Visual Cortex of the Dolphin

PETER J. MORGANE, ILYA I. GLEZER, and
MYRON S. JACOBS

1. Introduction

The cetaceans (great whales, dolphins, and porpoises) are known to have descended back to the sea more than 50 million years ago and thus are considered as secondary aquatic mammals (Kesarev *et al.,* 1977a,b; Gaskin, 1982; Gingerich *et al.,* 1983). They completely adapted themselves to the new conditions, not only in terms of changes in body shape, but also in the structure and function of their neuromuscular apparatus and internal organs and, especially, in regard to development of the brain. They appear to have preserved characteristic features of the original structure of the brain of primitive mammals in far greater measure than have more advanced land animals. At the same time the cetaceans were in a position in this new environment to develop specific features of adaptation not characteristic of land mammals. Thus, studies of the cetacean brain structure

PETER J. MORGANE • Laboratory of Neurobiology, Worcester Foundation for Experimental Biology, Shrewsbury, Massachusetts 01545. ILYA I. GLEZER • Neuroscience Program, The City College of New York Medical School, New York, New York 10031; and Osborn Laboratories of Marine Sciences, New York Aquarium, Brooklyn, New York 11224. MYRON S. JACOBS • New York University Dental Center, New York University, New York, New York 10010, and Osborn Laboratories of Marine Sciences, New York Aquarium, Brooklyn, New York 11224.

may make it possible to move closer to unraveling some important problems of evolution of the mammalian brain. Genetically related to terrestrial mammals, whales are of particular evolutionary value and uniqueness since they have adapted themselves to activity in an aqueous medium according to laws characteristic of this Order alone and, in so doing, have made evident the potential possibilities of the structural adaptations of the brain and, in particular, the great adaptability of the cerebral cortex (Nikitenko, 1965; Tomilin, 1968; Ladygina and Supin, 1974; Zvorykin, 1963, 1977; Kesarev *et al.*, 1977a; Mehedlidze, 1984; Morgane *et al.*, 1986a,b).

Cetaceans differ from most other mammals in being fully adapted to an aquatic environment through specializations of practically every system in the body (Kellogg, 1928, 1938; Howell, 1930; Slijper, 1962, 1979). While their precise ancestry is still uncertain, their progenitors were terrestrial animals (Gaskin, 1976, 1982; Barnes *et al.*, 1985) possibly related to primitive insectivore or carnivore stock with brains displaying generalized mammalian characters (Morgane and Jacobs, 1972; Zvorykin, 1977; Kesarev *et al.*, 1977a; Morgane *et al.*, 1985, 1986a,b; Morgane and Glezer, 1990). McKenna (1975) proposed an ungulate ancestor for whales though this matter is still the subject of continued debate. In any event, a study of the cetacean neocortex might be expected to yield valuable information concerning the influence of particular specializations on mammalian cortical morphology, and, in addition, knowledge relating to somatotopic localization in parts of the cerebral cortex capable of application to mammals generally might emerge.

The telencephalon of cetaceans is characterized by a number of specific macroscopic features which markedly differentiate it from that of representatives of all other orders of mammals. Among these features are the considerable transverse dimension of the forebrain which greatly exceeds its length, an abundance of fissures along with great variability of their pattern even in each hemisphere of the same forebrain, a large number of transitional convolutions, an almost vertical position of the Sylvian fissure, and very considerable dimensions of the temporal lobes (Breathnach, 1960; McFarland *et al.*, 1969; Morgane and Jacobs, 1972; Morgane *et al.*, 1980). Of special interest is the brain of representatives of the suborder Odontoceti (toothed whales), which differ from the suborder Mysticeti (baleen whales) by the complete absence of the olfactory bulb and olfactory tract (Filimonoff, 1965; Jacobs *et al.*, 1971; Morgane *et al.*, 1980). As noted, the globular shape of the cerebral hemispheres and thus lack of frontal and occipital poles, along with their large size and the great extent of highly convoluted cortex are noteworthy features of the cetacean brain (Morgane and Jacobs, 1972; Hammelbo, 1972; Morgane *et al.*, 1980). Figures 1 and 2 show the gyral arrangement is one of great arcuate or circumferential cortical tiers surmounting the almost vertically oriented Sylvian fissure. In general, the first-order sulci tend to resemble the arcuate arrangement of sulci in carnivores and ungulates. The analysis of these features in terms of functional mapping is of special interest and the basic studies in this regard have been carried out by Lende and Akdikmen (1968), Lende and Welker (1972), and by Russian investigators (Sokolov *et al.*, 1972; Avksent'Eva *et al.*, 1972; Ladygina *et al.*, 1978; Supin *et al.*, 1978; Popov *et al.*, 1986). The attention of earlier investigators, such as Beauregard (1883), Guldberg (1885), Kükenthal and Ziehen (1889), and others, was largely directed toward elucidation of the sulcal and gyral patterns in an effort to identify the various cortical convolutions and their homologies. More detailed attempts were made in this regard in a variety of whale species by Elliot Smith (1902), Pettit (1905), Rawitz (1910), Anthony (1925), and Wilson (1933) and, later, by Kojima (1951), Friant (1953, 1955, 1958), Pilleri (1962, 1964, 1966a–c), Morgane and Jacobs (1972), and Morgane *et al.* (1980). These various studies demonstrated that the sulcal pattern in cetaceans bears general resemblance to that found in carnivores and ungulates. They provide some topographical basis for comparison with other mammals, though they shed only limited light on fundamental problems of homologies of the fissures and sulci and on the localization and extent of specific functional areas.

Earlier cytoarchitectonic studies of the whale brain likewise contributed little to our knowledge of functional localization in the cetacean cortex. Studies in circumscribed cortical areas by Major (1879), Kükenthal and Ziehen (1889), Bianchi (1905), Riese (1925), and Rawitz (1927) led to general conclusions that a low density of neurons, weak differentiation of laminae, and a lack of regional variations in neuron type and lamination are characteristic of the entire cetacean cortex and that its organization is considerably different from that of other mammals. Rose (1926) questioned these earlier findings and claimed to identify

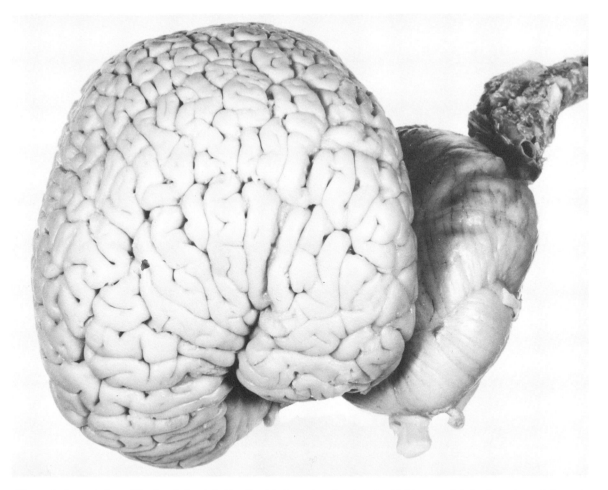

Figure 1. Lateral view of brain of the dolphin, *Tursiops truncatus*, showing the highly convoluted, circumferentially positioned gyri and sulci surmounting the vertically oriented Sylvian fissure.

seven cortical layers in Weigert preparations of *Delphinus delphis*. However, his figures are of inferior quality and provide inadequate justification for the subdivisions made. Grünthal (1942) emphasized a "primate character" of the dolphin cortex, though largely on inadequate histological grounds. Langworthy (1931a,b, 1932, 1935) and Reis and Langworthy (1937) studied Nissl sections from various regions of the neocortex of *Tursiops truncatus* and concluded that the histological structure was overall markedly "primitive." Langworthy distinguished only four layers, namely, zonal, supragranular pyramidal, granular, and polymorph layers and reported that large areas of the cortex show a markedly undifferentiated structure which he considered to be "correlation" cortex. These identifications, it should be stressed, were based on morphological criteria only, namely recognition of a true granular layer, which, though discussed, is not apparent in Langworthy's published figures. Kojima (1951) examined over 30 areas of neocortex from the sperm whale and also emphasized the scarcity of neurons and a relative lack of laminar differentiation, though he claimed to distinguish five layers in most of the cortical areas studied. So-called "giant" pyramidal cells were reported to be extensively distributed among different areas of the hemisphere and granular cells were reported to occupy the occipital region.

    Kraus and Pilleri (1969), Pilleri and Kraus (1969), Kesarev (1969, 1970), Kesarev and Malofeeva (1969), Entin (1973), Kesarev *et al.* (1977a,b), Morgane *et al.* (1980), Jacobs *et al.* (1984), Garey *et al.* (1985), Garey and Leuba (1986), and Morgane *et al.* (1986a,b, 1988) have all added new and more definitive data in regard to the cellular organization of the neocortex in whales, including Golgi analyses. The latter are absolutely essential for establishing the neuronal organi-

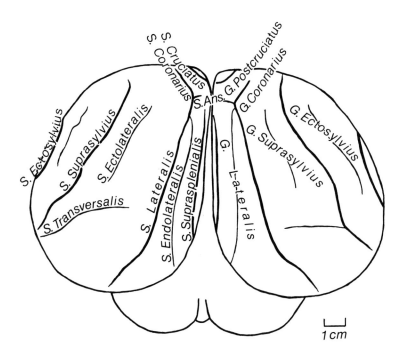

Figure 2. Schematic dorsal view of brain of the dolphin, *Tursiops truncatus*, showing major gyri and sulci of cerebral cortex.

zation of the cortex and provide critical data for interpreting the status of the cerebral cortex in whales. In assessing the findings from all these studies, including our own recent evolutionary interpretations regarding cortical organization in whales (Morgane *et al.*, 1985, 1986a,b, 1988; Glezer *et al.*, 1988; Morgane and Glezer, 1990), it appears that in the neocortex of the dolphin we are still seeing the early developments which originated when thalamic afferent fibers entered a primitive cortical matter and began to shape a population of new pyramidal-type neocortical cells and interneurons. In progressive evolution, the association circuitry of local cortical axons becomes increasingly more complicated whereas in the cetacean brain this development still remains relatively weak. In this feature and others reviewed below, the neocortex in cetaceans retains many features of its ancestral character.

We find that the chief structural distinction of the cerebral neocortex in cetaceans is its low degree of granularity and a relatively poor neuronal differentiation with transitional imprecisely formed types of neurons being dominant (Morgane *et al.*, 1986a,b, 1988; Morgane and Glezer, 1990). In all whale neocortex we have examined, there is a marked thickness of the phylogenetically older layers I and VI. These various characteristics evidently reflect a phylogenetically earlier isolation of the cetaceans on an independent evolutionary branch in which development of the nervous system proceeded chiefly along the path of an increase in the number of nerve cells (associated with great cortical expansion) with retention of their relatively primitive structure. Thus, we see a marked quantitative expansion of neocortex in whales but without any substantial reorganization of the prototypic or "initial" six-layer stratification plan. As pointed out by Zvorykin (1977) and Glezer *et al.* (1988), this mode of cortical evolution can be considered to be the most ancient type among present-day mammals. At this point, it is well to observe that, heretofore, studies of the organization of the cerebral cortical formations in the brains of whales, including smaller species such as dolphins and porpoises and, especially, the great whales, have been hindered by a lack of suitable material, particularly material that is well preserved by perfusion fixation or immediate immersion fixation of small cortical blocks immediately at death. Hence, in the past most studies of the cerebral cortex have been limited in extent and, in most instances, have largely been cytoarchitectural analyses or extremely limited Golgi studies. In addition to our three well-perfused brains of the dolphin *T. truncatus* cut in three planes and stained by the Loyez myelin and Nissl methods, we have three additional *Tursiops* brains that were perfusion fixed and some 95 cortical areas blocked and stained by the Golgi procedure. We have in the past 4 years also been able to obtain and fix brains of the blue dolphin *Stenella coeruleoalba* and the pilot whale *Globicephala melaena* immediately at death. These specimens have proven quite adequate for ultrastructural analysis of the cerebral cortex as well as for Golgi studies of neuronal form and dendritic architecture and, in most sections, for axonal analysis. Recently we have applied image analysis procedures and ultrastructural studies to the convexity cortex of the *Stenella* and *Globicephala* brains (Morgane *et al.*, 1988; Glezer and Morgane, 1990). We have concentrated our recent studies on the lateral gyrus which represents the areas from which the Russian investigators have obtained both short- and long-latency visual evoked responses (Figs. 3 and 4).

In our studies during the past 15 years we have examined the structural organization of the cetacean cerebral cortex in relation to that of various terrestrial and semiaquatic mammals and have recently described and elucidated some principles of organization of the cetacean neocortex (Morgane *et al.*,

1986a,b, 1988; Morgane and Glezer, 1990). In general, as is well known (see Valverde, 1983; Valverde and Facal-Valverde, 1986), there are two fundamental characteristics which basically define neocortical organization in all mammals: (1) the existence of pyramidal cells, in the restricted sense, i.e., the true neocortical pyramids and (2) the existence of a complex, topographically organized, sensory-modulated set of thalamocortical afferents which arborize consistently at middle neocortical levels. In contrast, the remaining allocortex shows no concomitant type pyramidal cells and its major afferent system is formed through a strong input in the plexiform or first layer. In this regard, we have recently reported that the convexity neocortex of the dolphin shows elements of both types of cortical organization (Morgane *et al.*, 1988; Morgane and Glezer, 1990) which is a pattern similar to that described in the hedgehog cortex by Valverde (1983, 1986), Valverde and Facal-Valverde (1986), and Valverde and López-Mascaraque (1981).

Our general objectives in analyzing the neocortex of whales can be grouped under four main categories: First, we have sought to establish a neuronal typology of dolphin convexity neocortex, particularly the visual cortical areas physiologically mapped by the Russian investigators (Sokolov *et al.*, 1972; Ladygina *et al.*, 1978; Supin *et al.*, 1978). Obviously, classification of neurons into various morphological types has played an important part in the investigation of

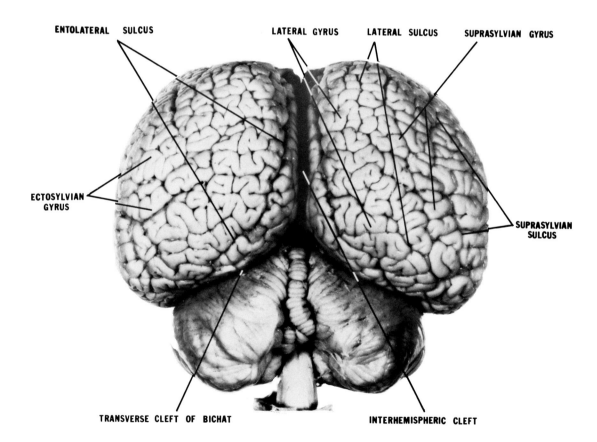

Figure 3. Dorsal view of brain of the dolphin, *Tursiops truncatus,* showing the lateral gyrus which is the area from which visual evoked responses were obtained by the Russian investigators (see text).

the structural and functional organization of the cerebral cortex. A clear-cut picture of neuronal morphology and both areal and laminar distribution of cell types has been sorely needed in the whale cortex. Heretofore, systematic classification of neurons in the whale neocortex has not been done and no previous studies have attempted to elucidate the numbers and types of pyramidal and nonpyramidal neurons. With respect to dendritic architecture of neocortical neurons as examined in Golgi material, we have considered dendritic characteristics, alone or in combination with other histological properties, as valid criteria in conceptualizing neuronal organization in the evolutionary sense. Thus, it is well known that in lower vertebrates the more generalized dendritic pattern is the prevalent one (Poliakov, 1959, 1964; Zhukova and Leontovich, 1964). In the case of the vertebrate CNS, it appears that the degree of dendritic complexity and differentiation is one of the clearest histological manifestations of the ascent in phylogeny (Ramón-Moliner, 1968, 1975). In this regard, the second major objective has been to characterize on the basis of cellular architecture and neuronal morphology the cortical areas in the dolphin shown by the Russian investigators to respond to visual stimuli. The third major aim has been to test our premise that the dolphin cerebral cortex has only reached the parinsular/paralimbic stage of evolutionary development in terms of the growth ring concepts of Sanides (1970, 1972). In recent studies using Golgi material we find that the great mass of convexity neocortex in the dolphin brain, in addition to showing an allocortical type of organization of layers I and II, is also dominated by paralimbic and parinsular traits. Our neuronal and cytoarchitectonic analyses show clearly that there is also a lack of koniocortices and gigantopyramidal areas in the dolphin cortex which, combined with poor lamination and a low degree of granularization, along with dramatic accentuation of layer II, indicate that the last stage of sensory and motor cortex differentiation, as defined by Sanides (1970, 1972), has not been attained in whales. On these and other grounds we have argued that the brain of the dolphin has only reached the paralimbic/ parinsular stage of neocortical evolution (Morgane *et al.*, 1985, 1986a,b, 1988). We have postulated that the whale brain may, therefore, represent a prototypic mammalian brain of special interest since whales returned to water some 50 million years ago before terrestrial mammalian forms specialized and gran-

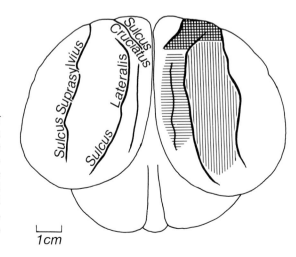

Figure 4. Schematic dorsal view of major gyri and sulci of cerebral cortex in the dolphin, *Tursiops truncatus*. The visual cortex occupies largely the lateral gyrus in and on both banks of the entolateral sulcus. The auditory and somatosensory cortices, as mapped physiologically, are also indicated. ▥, Auditory cortex; ▤, visual cortex; ▦, somatosensory cortex.

ularized their cortices, representing a time well before the rise of koniocortical foci of stellarization, i.e., prior to the development of hypergranular cores of cortical specialization. According to Sanides (1970, 1972), the latest step in sensory and motor cortex evolution occurred in somewhat advanced mammals about 50 million years ago in the Eocene period. Interestingly, Sanides pointed out that the hedgehogs, whose CNS serves as a key model of the so-called "initial" brain of mammals (see Glezer *et al.*, 1988), are survivors of the Paleocene, a period dominated by archaic mammals who had not reached the stage of highest sensory and motor cortex evolution, i.e., they have no hyperspecialized cortices such as koniocortices or area gigantopyramidalis. This is of particular interest since we have found remarkable resemblances between the basic structural plan of the hedgehog neocortex and that of the dolphin (Morgane *et al.*, 1985, 1986a,b, 1988; Morgane and Glezer, 1990). Hedgehogs are apparently the only known placental mammals which were present during the Cretaceous period (approximately 120 to 70 million years ago) and thus represent archetypal mammals that are thought to have first showed the multilayered cellular pattern typical of the mammalian neocortex (Ebner, 1969). Finally, a fourth major aspect of our studies has been to develop lines of evidence relating to whether the whale brain can itself serve as a useful model of the brain of the "initial" ancestor of mammals (see Glezer *et al.*, 1988). This involves drawing parallels between the basic laminar and cellular organization of the whale neocortex and that of the hedgehog and other basal insectivores considered to represent a prime model of the "initial" brain. It is obvious that there has occurred extremely vigorous quantitative expansion of the neocortex in whales and, in considering the various modes of structural evolution of the neocortex as defined by Zvorykin (1977), our data indicate that in the cetacean brain there is a marked increase in territory occupied by neocortex but it remains relatively simple in plan and thus appears to be without substantial reorganization of the initial organizational plan seen in the earliest mammals.

2. Cerebral Cortex: Evolutionary Aspects

Based on its six-layered structure in all mammals, Brodmann (1909) defined the basic structural principles of organization of the neocortex. This hexalaminar stratification plan can be considered as the ancestral stratification Bauplan for the further evolution of the neocortex over the course of approximately the last 100 million years. Over this period the six-layered neocortex has changed in each of the orders of mammals in entirely independent fashion, both cytoarchitectonically, i.e., in the form and interrelationship of its constituent nerve cells, as well as quantitatively. Hence, the cetacean neocortex has changed in its own peculiar way in adapting to marine life and no other brains have developed under these same environmental situations, for no other mammalian forms have gone to an aquatic environment as rapid-moving, deep-diving mammals totally adapted to water.

2.1. General Phylogenetic Considerations

We may assume that the whales, having left terrestrial life many millions of years ago, at about the same time as the Chiroptera became aerially adapted, reflect in their present neocortical structure the primitive features of those early mammalian stages that were preserved because of the decisive lack of further somatic sensory experience of land life (Zvorykin, 1977; Kesarev *et al.*, 1977b). Using the "initial" type of cortical organization as a starting point and lacking terrestrial stimuli for higher neocortical differentiation, neocortical evolution in whales has taken an obviously different path, leading to the enormous surface spread of the neocortex, compensating or even hypercompensating for the reduced level of cortical differentiation found in all neocortical areas. Cetacea, then, represent still another line of evolution of the mammalian brain which cannot fail to add to our information on general principles of neocortical development. Further, the study of the whale cortex may help us in classifying similarities among advanced mammals as either homologous or the result of convergent evolution and, further, may assist in understanding differences among advanced mammals as modifications of a basic or "initial" plan.

As is well known, the mammalian neocortex shows similarities with regard to the topographical relations of the main cytoarchitectonic sensory formations throughout the comparative anatomical series extending from the hypothetical common ancestor (Fig. 5). However, the developmental level as well as the relative dimensions of those formations appear to be very different in members of different orders. These differences are due, on the one hand, to the phylogenetic features of a given order and, on the other, to the ecological–functional loads on the sensory apparatus whose central parts form the main sensory zones of the cortex (Nikitenko, 1970). General correlations can be made between the anatomical features which have been found in the neocortex and the mode of existence of cetaceans in an aqueous environment, which, in many ways, is simpler than an aerial environment with regard to regulation of the constancy of the internal milieu of the body. Also to be taken into consideration is the fact that in the aqueous environment the cetaceans have practically no competitors at or even near the same level of development of the CNS.

2.2. The "Initial" Brain Concept

Basic to a consideration of the status and evolutionary position of the dolphin cerebral cortex in phylogeny is an understanding of the so-called "initial" or archetypal brain concept. We have elaborated on this precursory type of cerebral cortical organization in a recent review (Glezer *et al.*, 1988) and will here only touch on the principal aspects of the concept and note the utility of such a concept in interpreting the evolutionary status of whale brains. Initially, we point out that there are extant mammalian species that reflect little morphological evolution since their divergence from their closest relatives and, in most cases, they have been found to be sole survivors of their lineages. These have been referred to as "living fossils," which generally describes them well (Sanides, 1970, 1972). Because such living fossils retain many "primitive" characters, i.e., characters of the putative mammalian progenitor brain, morphologists have often found it difficult to ascertain their phylogenetic position as, for example, in the tarsiers, aardvarks, and hedgehogs, among others. Fossil evidence suggests that both the marsupial opossum and placental insectivores existed in the Cretaceous period approximately 100 million years ago (Ebner, 1969). In fact, the insectivores are the only known extant placental mammals thought to have been present during the Cretaceous. In our studies (Morgane *et al.*, 1985, 1986a,b,

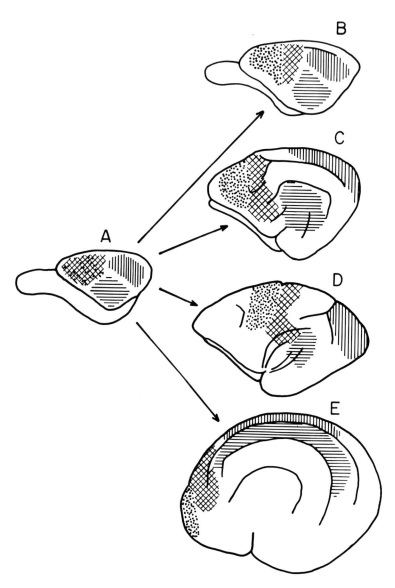

1988; Morgane and Glezer, 1990) we have pointed out the many resemblances in the fundamental neocortical organizational plan in the dolphin and hedgehog as well as in the so-called "flying insectivores," the bats. Comparison of the neocortical organization of insectivores and highly specialized mammalian forms such as whales and bats is of special interest since insectivores are as close as any living form to archetypal mammals that first showed the multilayered cell pattern typical of the mammalian neocortex. Such comparisons thus represent useful approaches for clarifying the origin and development of neocortical structural specializations. The absence of ancestral-type brains prohibits complete answers

Figure 5. Schema showing the position of major motor and sensory projectional areas in the cerebral cortex of the hypothetical "initial" brain mammal (A) and the relative location of these same areas in the cortices of the rabbit (B), cat (C), rhesus monkey (D), and dolphin (E). Only the first-order sulci are shown. (Modified from Supin *et al.*, 1978). ▤, Auditory; ⦚, visual; ⬗, somatosensory; ▨, motor.

so that organization of extant neocortices in mammals has to be assessed relative to a hypothetical mammalian archetypal neocortex. We have already pointed out many features of similarity of basic neocortical organization in the dolphin, hedgehog, and bat and have provided several lines of evidence for considering the dolphin neocortical organization, in terms of its fundamental cortical modular units (see below), as archetypal in nature (Morgane *et al.*, 1986a,b, 1988; Glezer *et al.*, 1988). The fact that whales have also become aquatic, and primarily marine, and thus removed from further terrestrial-type stresses and challenges, also makes the dolphin cortex of special interest in terms of assessing possible additional aquatic adaptations and specializations freed from terrestrial demands. Or, perhaps the aquatic medium has stiffled further cortical internal organization during evolution of the basic cortical units or modules. These basic units may continue to grow in size and number, but not in terms of internal cellular differentiation and, particularly, local circuit organization. If that is so, then we are dealing with a very unique situation of a massive cerebral cortex, in many cases considerably larger than in the human brain, but one in which the fundamental cortical structural plan is similar to that of smaller, more conservatively organized brains such as seen in basal insectivores and bats. Computationally, such a cortex is of special interest in that the total number of functional cortical modules may be very great but the fundamental organization is one of relative simplicity compared to those of more progressive terrestrial mammalian forms.

In studies of the cetacean neocortex from a comparative and evolutionary point of view, there are some basic considerations to keep in mind. Thus, we must reconstruct, largely by retrospective inference, an "initial" type of mammalian neocortex and study potential pathways of derivation from this hypothetical "initial" type of cortex. The cetaceans, in entering water, adapted completely to a medium that was unfamiliar to other mammals and were better able, to a greater extent than most terrestrial forms extant at that time, to preserve signs of the initial brain structure of primitive terrestrial mammals. In modern terrestrial forms, especially in primates, the general initial features of the neocortex are excessively variable and are overgrown by acquisitions that are specific only for the phylogenesis of each particular order in question. The brains of basal insectivores appear to have changed little from the ancestral prototypical brain and possess some basic organizational features in their cerebral cortex that are present, though highly modified in being dominated by recent acquisitions, in higher mammals. Our assumption of similarity of the structural organization of the cetacean neocortex to the presumed "original" architectonics of the neocortex of primitive mammals discussed below makes it possible to suggest that granularity of the neocortex of terrestrial mammals developed long after the ancestors of the whales descended into the sea. The incipient granularization of the whale neocortex that Kesarev *et al.* (1977b) and we (Morgane *et al.*, 1985, 1986a,b, 1988; Morgane and Glezer, 1990) previously described tends to lend credence to this point of view. While it is agreed that modern basal insectivores such as the hedgehog are themselves considerably removed from the true ancestral mammalian condition, it is certainly clear that the neocortices of extant hedgehogs and the dolphin are sufficiently generalized to serve as useful *models* of the so-called "initial" brain. In these considerations, we recognize, of course, that it can never be established absolutely that any extant group of mammals is totally representative of the ancestral condition of mammals.

CHAPTER 13

3. Neocortex of Hedgehog as Model of "Initial" Brain Compared to Dolphin Neocortex

We have found in our comparative studies that the hedgehog model of the "initial" brain has many similarities to what we have described in our analyses of the dolphin neocortex and we will briefly summarize these here. The neocortex of the hedgehog is as a whole poorly laminated and weakly granularized and nowhere reaches the stage of true hypergranular koniocortex. Moreover, there is in the convexity neocortex of the hedgehog a conservative feature which in other placentals is characteristic of neocortical growth rings I and II of Sanides (1970, 1972). This is the accentuated layer II which, in the hemisphere of the rat, covers the periallocortex and proisocortex from the hippocampal and from the paleocortical borders, whereas the bulk of the convexity cortex, i.e., the mature isocortex, is free of this densely packed, medium-sized cell layer and shows the inconspicuous so-called granuloid layer II characteristic of the fundamental isocortical scheme. In the hedgehog, however, this layer II accentuation can be clearly recognized over the entire convexity neocortex. We stress again that, among the insectivores, the hedgehog *Erinaceus europaeus* is regarded as one of the most direct modern descendants of the primitive placentals (Romer, 1966). It has retained, apparently with minor variation, some basic characteristics of its early ancestors so that it is a good reference for the study of what might be considered a prototype of neocortical organization and a valid, though not unique, model of neocortical phylogenetic development. Since our Golgi typological studies of neurons in the dolphin neocortex (see below) have so far revealed numerous neuronal types similar to those seen in the hedgehog neocortex, including presence of a host of immature, transitional-type neurons and long radiator, isodendritic type neurons, we consider the whale cortex as another important model of the cortex of the initial ancestor of mammals, not in terms of its size but in terms of its basic internal organizational plan. To this end, our studies in the dolphin have been designed to unravel cytoarchitectural and neuronal details in the neocortex with the aim of characterizing types of pyramidal cells as well as local circuit neurons of the stellate family that might be present in this cortex. In addition, we have studied the dendritic architecture and, to a lesser extent, the form and distribution of axonal plexuses in different neocortical layers as well as the specificity versus the nonspecificity of particular neuronal representatives in relation to homologous types described in other species, particularly those in the hedgehog neocortex. Ultimately a cell classification scheme based on morphology is only useful if it can segregate functionally different groups of neurons and our studies comprise a first step in this direction in the dolphin. Though we report below our findings to date in this regard, it is clear that more quantitative data are needed in the dolphin concerning the number and distribution of cortical neurons, the extent of their dendritic fields, as well as types, location, and number of synapses, and so forth, in order to establish an appropriate morphological foundation for further neurophysiological investigations. Until our recent studies in the dolphin, the comparative morphology and physiology of the mammalian CNS were supported by adequately detailed studies of its representatives only in two basic branches of mammalian evolution, i.e., from the "initial" forms, which clearly were close to the insectivores, rodents, lagomorphs, and also the lower primates, on the one hand, and the carnivores and ungulates to the higher primates, on the other. Our studies of the cetacean brain make it possible to add to these previous studies additional material relating to still another line of development of the mammalian cortex, which cannot fail to add additional information on some general principles of neocortical development. The phylogenetically earlier isolation of cetaceans on an independent evolutionary branch makes them of special interest in this regard.

One of the approaches that makes it possible to establish some stages of evolution of the cerebral cortex is a comparison of the distribution and relative development of various cortical regions, including, especially, the projection sensory areas. Higher sensory analysis is one of the basic functions of the cerebral cortex and the projection sensory areas of some species, such as the hedgehog, occupy a considerable area of the neocortex. In addition to the projection areas, however, regions that have more limited connections with specific sensory zones also arise in the cerebral cortex. These so-called nonprojection areas may be connected with more complex, polymodal forms of sensory analysis and with other higher functions connected with the formation of complex behaviors. Comparative studies of the neocortex in a number of mammals can show which areas of the cortex are common to all groups of mammals and which have arisen and developed in the evolutionary process in individual animal groups. In this connection, it is important to establish the relation between the development of the neocortex and the phylogenetic position of each mammalian group, inasmuch as this may provide clues to the various directions of deviations from a postulated initial ancestor of modern mammals, i.e., the directions of evolution of the neocortex. Therefore, studies of specialized mammalian groups such as whales are of particular interest. It is of interest that for such phylogenetically rather distant groups of mammals as the carnivores and higher primates, there is the same general tendency for development of the neocortex in the direction of a decrease in the relative magnitude of the sensory projection zones of the cortex and a substantial development of the nonprojection zones. In the case of cetaceans, considerable further physiological mapping is needed to determine if there are wide areas not responsive to sensory stimuli given that the whole concept of "association" cortex needs reassessment in light of the newer mapping studies (Kaas, 1987, 1989).

In our studies, various principles governing the structural organization of the dolphin neocortex have been derived. In considering the concept of cortical growth rings described by Sanides (1968, 1970, 1972), we have examined cortices such as the limbic (Morgane *et al.*, 1982) and insular cortex (Jacobs *et al.*, 1984) and followed these transitional cortical territories outward from archicortical and paleocortical formations to neocortical structures. The basic characteristics of organization of the convexity cortex are easier to derive by analysis of these sequential steps in cortical development. Using Golgi material, we have extended these analyses onto the convexity neocortex with emphasis on the visual cortical areas mapped electrophysiologically by the Russian investigators. These mapping studies have shown that the projectional regions of the cortex in cetaceans directly interlock with each other and are not clearly separated by associative regions as is seen in higher mammals. Projectional areas of the cortex in cetaceans are arranged in the very same order as in the hypothetical ancestor of mammals (Fig. 5). Thus, the visual region is retromedial, the auditory region is lateral, and the somatosensory-motor region is rostral. However, there is obvious displacement of areas in dolphin cortex such that the position of the projection zones of the sensory systems are considerably different compared to the presumed "initial" pattern of their distribution. As shown in Fig. 4, the visual area is displaced to the upper parietal part of the hemisphere occupying the depths of the lateral sulcus and cortical areas lateral and medial to this sulcus. The auditory zone is also displaced considerably and occupies a rather broad area of a first-order gyrus adjoining the visual zone. A similarity to that of many terrestrial mammals is observed only in the distribution of the somatosensory and motor zones in the anterior part of the hemisphere (Fig. 5). Thus, neither the occipital nor the temporal "pole" of the hemisphere in the dolphin has any direct connection with the visual and auditory cortical areas, though further electrophysiological mapping of these regions needs to be done. Although great cortical expansion has occurred in whales, it is noteworthy that these cortical relationships of adjacency are not violated. Where adjacent localization is maintained, it presumably represents a functional requirement. For example, the relationships of neighborhood seen among receptors or effectors peripherally are essentially preserved cortically despite considerable distortion of patterns.

Overall, our studies clearly indicate that the dolphin neocortex is sufficiently generalized to serve as a useful model of the status of neocortex some 50–60 million years ago and thus helps provide initial insights into the evolutionary or adaptive significance of variations in cortical organization seen in various mammalian species. Our architectonic studies of convexity cortex show that there is very little evidence of intensification of certain layers other than layer II in the neocortex of the dolphin and also little evidence of specialization of laminae, such as thickening or sublamination due to splitting of layers. There is, in fact, considerable attenuation of particular layers, e.g., layer III, and even an almost complete effacement of the entire layer IV. Before we can begin to understand how neurons are organized in the neocortex of the dolphin and how they interact with each other and form functional groups, we need to know how many neurons of each type are present in particular cortical areas as well as what percentages of the different types of neurons are contained within the population and how they are apportioned to the different layers. This has been one of our continuing goals and findings to date are summarized below.

4. Studies of Neuronal Typology in Dolphin Neocortex

Our examination of neurons in the visual cortices of the lateral gyrus of the dolphin in subareas mapped by the Russian investigators indicates many marked differences in cortical structure compared to higher mammalian forms, namely in the ratios of the width of layers and in the cellular composition and cell types in different layers. These analyses have led us to the view that the cetacean neocortex is organized in a fashion remarkably similar to that of the hedgehog and bat, particularly in regards to the presence of a powerfully accentuated layer II, presence of "extraverted" neurons in layer II (see below), absence or incipience of layer IV, and presence of numerous types of transitional, imprecisely shaped neuronal forms as well as presence in all layers of giant stellate, isodendritic-type neurons.

In considering progressive and conservative features of cortical neuronal evolution, there are two opposite groups of neurons from the point of view of their dendritic geometry, namely, generalized and specialized. They are extremes of a spectrum made out of intermediary-type neurons. Dendroarchitectonic analysis reveals a number of well-characterized neuronal families. Using dendritic parameters for classification of neurons is in no sense a mere inventory but, rather, it suggests the existence of certain correlations between morphology and function. More importantly, it has evolutionary meaning in terms of primitive or specialized neuronal types and in providing data on where dendrites end and how they establish contacts with incoming axonal systems. It should be kept in mind that the term "primitivity" in referring to neurons is defined by what neurons are considered closest to the general radiate or prototype neuron. Thus, dendrites radiating in all directions with branches occurring dichotomously and with daughter branches longer than the mother branch may be considered as the prototype from which all other dendritic patterns are derived (Ramón-Moliner, 1975). The radiate dendritic pattern is likely related to an input of heterogeneous origin and/or to the presence of relatively widely spaced afferent terminal fibers. In our morphological studies of dendroarchitecture in the dolphin neocortex, particular attention has been paid to the phylogenetic modification of the dendritic pattern of neurons considered in relation to more evolutionarily conservative mammalian lines such as hedgehogs and bats. Ramón-Moliner and co-workers (Ramón-Moliner and Nauta, 1966; Ramón-Moliner, 1962, 1967, 1968, 1969, 1975), examining the morphological complexity of dendrites in medulla and thalamus, suggested that dendritic organization becomes more complex as the type of information received by neurons becomes more restricted and specialized. Further, examination of a number of vertebrate taxa has led to the suggestion of an evolutionary framework for dendroarchitectonic changes (Ramón-Moliner, 1968, 1975). This work suggests, in considering the shape and spatial arrangements of neurons, that a morphofunctional shift in evolution leads from generalized isodendritic neurons toward highly specialized idiodendritic cells. Generalized neurons or long radiator neurons are characteristic of the lower vertebrate brain, but are preserved in the so-called "isodendritic core" of mammals and in its extensions into the forebrain, including allocortical and, in particular species such as the hedgehog and dolphin, even in the neocortical formations. Long radiator neurons resemble the most generalized reticular neurons of the phylogenetically old core of the brain stem as pointed out initially by Leontovich and Zhukova (1963) and later by Ramón-Moliner and Nauta (1966). The insectivore group of mammals stands out by having a particularly high share of the generalized type of long radiator neurons which actually reach more than 60% in some basal species. The generalized neuron or reticular isodendritic type is found only in layer VI of the neocortex in most mammals whereas in hedgehogs this long radiator-type cell is found in all cortical layers. Interestingly, we have similarly identified this same type of neuron in all layers of the dolphin visual neocortex. On the other hand, we have found that short radiator neurons are few in number in the dolphin neocortex and are generally larger in size than found in rodents and rabbits. We have pointed out that this clearly indicates a lack of a trend toward granularization of the stellate cells in dolphin neocortex (Morgane *et al.*, 1988; Morgane and Glezer, 1990). Large stellate cells with nonspinous dendrites intercalated between input neurons and layer V pyramidal cell axons form a basic circuit in the hedgehog and mouse brain and we have recently demonstrated this essentially same pattern in the dolphin visual neocortex (Fig. 6). But in the mouse and cat,

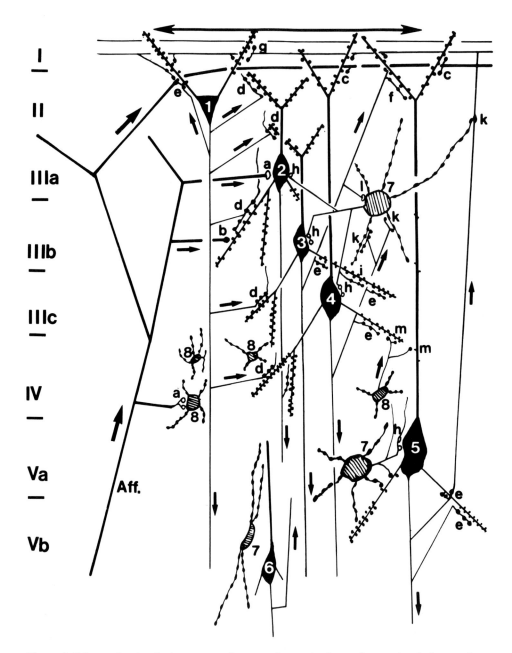

I

II

IIIa

IIIb

IIIc

IV

Va

Vb

Aff.

Figure 6. Schema showing basic patterns of neuronal organization and synaptic relations we have observed in layers of posterior heterolaminar visual cortex of lateral gyrus of the dolphins, *Stenella coeruleoalba* and *Tursiops truncatus*. This scheme was prepared from analysis of our Golgi sections as well as from electron microscopic and combined Golgi–electron microscopic studies of this cortical formation and represents a preliminary view of the microcircuitry, especially of the upper layers of the cortex. In general, the following characteristics of the intracortical relations are seen: (1) Subcortical afferents (Aff.) divide dichotomously in all cortical layers sending collaterals to each layer and establish axosomatic (a) and axodendritic (b) synaptic connections with pyramidal neurons. These collaterals are especially rich in layers III and V. The main termination of these afferents is in layer I where they establish *en passage* type synapses (c), primarily with apical dendrites of neurons in layers II and III which branch profusely in this layer. (2) Extraverted neurons of layer II (1) send their axons down into the white matter though almost all their axon collaterals project in an ascending direction to form synapses, as we have verified in electron microscopic studies, with basal and,

smaller multipolar cells develop with spinous dendrites located in layer IV which are only rarely found in the hedgehog and dolphin and these may represent a new cell variety which apparently substitutes for the large multipolar cells, thus resulting in an increasing "granularization" of the neocortex in more derived mammals. As is well known, such small spinous stellate cells are the principal recipients of thalamic fibers in the cat and monkey.

Overall, progressive differentiation of the neocortex in advanced mammals involves essentially the following: thickening of the cortex, accentuation of lamination, and, eventually, the appearance of granular cells. Layer IV, containing star cells or granules, makes its first appearance in the proisocortices, i.e., in the limbic and insular cortices. Stellarization is a powerful trend in higher neocortical evolution extending to extreme granularization (konicortices) in the higher primates. This packing of star cells in layer IV, a stellarization or granularization process, also has a strong effect on lamination. In this regard, it is interesting to compare long radiators and double bouquet cells of the hedgehog and guinea pig, which appear to have functional importance. In each case the insectivore stellates possess a much larger cell body in spite of the same dendritic spread. With increasing complexity in advanced mammals, several types of intrinsic neurons with local axons, barely present in the hedgehog, appear intercalated in

---

especially, apical dendrites of pyramidal neurons of layers II and III (d). (3) Transitional type pyramidal neurons of layer III (2, 3, 4) and V (5, 6) also have a descending axon with numerous ascending collaterals which form synapses on apical and basal dendrites of the neuron of origin (e) as well as on pyramidal neurons of the upper cortical levels (f). These ascending collaterals eventually reach layer I and form numerous axodendritic synapses *en passage* (g), which are all of the asymmetric type, and with apical dendrites of both layer II and layer III pyramidal neurons. (4) Large- and medium-sized stellate neurons (7) of the isodendritic type usually show a very complicated netlike axon which establishes axosomatic synapses (h) with the perikarya of pyramidal neurons and their basilar dendrites (i). Ascending varicose collaterals of pyramidal neurons form synapses (k) on varicose dendrites of stellate neurons. Our preliminary Golgi–electron microscopic studies show that perikarya of large- and medium-sized stellate cells receive symmetric synapses presumably from collaterals of ascending pyramidal cell axons (l). Small aspinous stellate cells are found in incipient layer IV of heterolaminar cortex (8) and their axons extend into layers IIIa and Va and make synaptic contacts on dendrites of neurons in these layers (m). (5) Our electron microscopic findings indicate that all axosomatic synapses (open circles) found in visual cortex of the dolphin are of the symmetric type with flat synaptic vesicles, whereas all axodendritic synapses (solid circles) are of the asymmetric type and contain polymorphic vesicles of different sizes and types, including small round light, large round light, and large and small granular types. (6) A great majority of synapses found in the dolphin neocortex are of the *en passage* type. This has been demonstrated in our electron microscopic and Golgi–electron microscopic studies and are indicated in the figure by the drawings of varicose axons (a, b, c, etc.). We have found that even axosomatic synapses have certain *en passage* characteristics (e.g., serial varicose axons on neuron 5). Overall, this preliminary schema represents the first attempts to work out the local circuitry in the neocortex of the dolphin. Basically, the principal findings are that the main afferent inputs from the subcortex reach an extremely thick layer I and these form synapses on extremely rich branchlets of the many apical dendrites of pyramids in layer II and, to a lesser extent, in layers III and IV. Axons of extraverted and nonextraverted pyramids form numerous feedback connections which are predominantly directed upward to layer I. The prevalence of synapses *en passage* is strongly suggestive of more mass-action type of neuron activity, i.e., operations occur across large numbers of neurons simultaneously rather than in a point-to-point manner. Since this is a well-known characteristic of allocortices and periallocortices, this reinforces our view that the upper cortical layers in the dolphin show largely an allocortical type of organization which is superimposed on lower cortical layers that exhibit a more typical neocortical type of organization. In this respect, the neocortex of the dolphin shows a pattern similar to that of the hedgehog brain described by Valverde (1983, 1986), Valverde and López-Mascaraque (1981), and Valverde and Facal-Valverde (1986).

the local circuits to become a rather elaborate target system of new cell types. In this regard, type II neurons (stellate family) form the major central integrating circuits and relate to the complexity of central analyzing and processing functions whereas type I neurons form the early hard-wiring of the cortex and show a remarkably conservative evolution. We stress again that small neurons rich in spines and without a clear pyramidal character scarcely occur in the insectivores, rodents, or lagomorphs and, interestingly, we have not yet found such spiny stellate elements in the convexity neocortex of the dolphin either in incipient layer IV or elsewhere. The distribution of the three types of stellate neurons as defined by their dendritic patterns lends further support to the generalized type of cortical organization seen in insectivores. Particularly the presence of long radiators in this mammalian group is significant. This means that the stellate cell type which most clearly resembles the generalized neuron of the phylogenetically oldest formations of the vertebrate brain stem, i.e., the reticular formation and central gray, is the leading neuron type among the stellates of the neocortex of the primitive insectivorous species (Poliakov, 1959, 1964; Leontovich and Zhukova, 1963). We have, similarly, found this same type of neuron in dolphin neocortex as the dominant cell type among the stellate neurons (Fig. 7). As Sanides (1970, 1972) pointed out, the differential distribution of these cells in mammalian brains implies a significant species difference in intracortical synaptic circuitry.

We have found that most neurons in the dolphin neocortex are of a pyramidal type and of imprecisely-shaped, transitional intermediate form (Figs. 7 and 8). Thus, we have identified in the dolphin visual neocortex a considerable number of pyramids of triangular, club-shaped, or clavate type indicating a low degree of differentiation of these types of neurons. Transitional type neurons represent a weak development of neuronal elements and are considered evidence of poor differentiation of the cortex.

As indicated, stellarization, or more properly granularization, is also a strong lamination-affecting factor. A poorly differentiated layer IV along with the presence of largely agranular-type modified pyramidal cells in the cortex, combine to make cytoarchitectural isolation of projection sensory zones especially difficult in the dolphin neocortex. The absence or incipience of layer IV can be considered a sign of intermediate-type cortex which is defined primarily as being of transitional character (Filimonoff, 1949, 1965). Hence, the dolphin convexity neocortex appears to be intermediate in type and, in this regard, retains many features of its ancestral character. The principle of intermediate cortical formations can be regarded as one of the leading principles in the process of cerebral cortex organization and, correspondingly, it serves as the basis of division of the cortex into its basic areas and subareas. In this regard, our studies of the convexity visual neocortex of the dolphin reveal, especially in the upper layers, a remarkable similarity of structure with the intermediate cortical formations such as the periarchicortex and peripaleocortex and even with the allocortices. Interestingly, the dolphin cortex combines the features of both conservative and progressive brains when we compare the upper cortical laminae with the lower cortical laminae. Thus, in the dolphin the upper laminae, particularly layers I and II, are organized more as intermediate cortex and allocortex and this type of organization appears to be superimposed on a more advanced type cortex forming the lower cortical layers. Thus in some ways the dolphin neocortex corresponds, in one sense, to the "original architectonics" of the neocortex of the earliest mammals. As is well known, one of the main criteria of neocortical differentiation is stepwise granularization, or more exactly designated, stellarization (Sanides, 1970). Granularity, which is markedly attenuated in the dolphin cortex (Morgane *et al.*, 1985, 1986a,b, 1988; Glezer and Morgane, 1990), is a later sign of differentiation of the neocortex in terrestrial mammals, considered to have developed some 50 million years ago after the cetacean ancestors had already made the transition from the terrestrial to the aquatic milieu. Of course, progress in cortical differentiation is also characterized by an increase in size of the efferent pyramids of layer V and by a stepwise increase of layer III which is still weakly developed in the limbic and insular proisocortices. In dolphin visual neocortex, layer III continues to be weak in differentiation and, furthermore, we do not see an increase in size of efferent pyramids of layer V.

Our findings indicate that the basic mammalian plan of a six-layered neocortical scheme is not completely valid in the dolphin brain since the organization of the first two layers is different from that of most other placental mammals, excluding the hedgehog and bat, and layer IV is either incipient or totally absent (Fig. 7A). In the composition of the neocortical gray there is a remarkable relative reduction in the molecular layer (lamina I) from about 32% in the basal insectivores to about 12% in the higher primates. In convexity neocortex of the dolphin, we calculate layer I to average 34% of the entire cortical thickness. According to Sanides's (1970, 1972) measurements, the molecular layer is about one-third of the total thickness of the cortical gray in the Tenrecidae and about one-eighth in the higher primates. It is noteworthy that an especially thick molecular layer is found in those cortices which are transitional to the various parts of the allocortex and in the allocortex itself (Economo and Koskinas, 1925) and, in that sense, as well as in the internal organization, the convexity neocortex in the dolphin is clearly of transitional or intermediate character. In the allocortical regions of mammalian brains there is also a strong superposition of myelinated fibers. These superposed myelinated fibers appear to be long and come from other cortical regions in contrast to the short tangential fibers of the molecular layer of the true neocortex which have their origin in deeper cells of the same or adjacent cortical columns or fields.

Ramón-Moliner (1967) long ago pointed out in the brain of lower vertebrates two main types of nerve cells which are present. The first are types of neurons with subpial tufts (lophodendritic) with a dendritic configuration reminiscent of that of the neurons of the dentate gyrus. The term *lophodendritic* emphasizes the dense, tufted character of these subpial dendrites. In this type of cell structure the decisive character is the emphasis on zonal arborization which has obvious functional meaning, as opposed to basal dendritic arborization. Tufted cortical neurons have their extreme in mammals in the granule cells of the fascia dentata, the zonal layer in allocortex and periallocortex still representing the main afferent and association plexus of the cortex. It is often viewed that the endbrain has arisen in evolution as an olfactory brain and only the olfactory input has, therefore, the unique structural quality to be, and to remain, surface bound, and thus reaches its sites of cortical representation as striae olfactoriae through the zonal layer of the paleocortex. This primitive arrangement of a functional overemphasis of the zonal layer is valid not only for paleocortex (prepyriform cortex, periamygdalar cortex) and archicortex (fascia dentata, cornu ammonis, subiculum), but also for the periallocortex and, to a lesser extent, for the proisocortex. In these latter intermediate cortices there are also cells which have much stronger apical dendritic arborization into the zonal layer than into the cortical plate by basal dendrites. In the archicortex the zonal layer is the principal collector of afferent fibers as well as ascending branches of the long axons of efferent neurons coming from other parts of the archicortex. Ths so-called "extraversion" of the neurons composing layer II points to a greater significance of the zonal layer in intercortical interactions via the tangential connections in the zonal layer. For all neurons with predominant zonal (subpial) dendritic arborization, the term *extraverted neurons* was originally proposed by Sanides (1970, 1972) and Sanides and Sanides (1972). They defined the extraverted telencephalic neurons as comprising all neurons which border the subpial zonal layer and preserve clear predominance of subpial dendrites over basal dendrites. From the classic investigations of Ramón y Cajal (1909–1911) and more recent studies of Ramón-Moliner (1962), it was shown that the neurons of

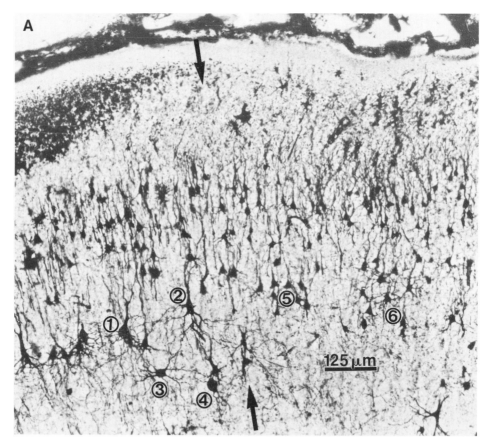

Figure 7. (A) General view of Golgi section showing neuroarchitectonics of both hetero- and homo-laminar cortices of lateral gyrus of the dolphin, *Stenella coeruleoalba*. There is a clear distinction between two cortical areas shown in this figure, which illustrates heterolaminar cortex on the left side and homolaminar cortex on the right. The limiting border between these two areas is quite sharp and labeled by arrows. In heterolaminar cortex there is a distinctly less cellular band between layers IIIc and Va, corresponding to incipient layer IV. In this particular section, two nonspinous stellate cells in this band are impregnated. Note also in heterolaminar cortex the presence of large atypical pyramidal neurons in layer Va (1, 2), which are larger than neurons in layer IIIc. Also in layer V, there are large stellate cells of the isodendritic type (3, 4). In homolaminar cortex (right side of

the older cortices show this type of zonal arborization along with poorly developed basal dendrites. On the other hand, the average layer II neuron of the isocortex of advanced mammals is a small pyramidal cell with a short or no apical shaft and having approximately the same range of apical bouquet as basal skirt dendrites. In the scheme of cortical growth rings developed by Sanides (1968, 1970, 1972), the first wave of mammalian neocortex is a two-cell-stratum cortex with emphasis on the larger-celled inner stratum. In this primary neocortex there are condensations of medium-sized tufted cells at the surface and their dendritic tufts in the zonal layer receive synaptic contacts from the fibers of the surface-bound olfactory system and from the thalamic afferents. A lamina dissecans separates the two strata of this cortex. In the next wave of neocortical differentiation, i.e., proisocortex, the thalamic input switches from axodendritic synaptic contacts in the zonal layer and outer stratum to axosomatic synapses in

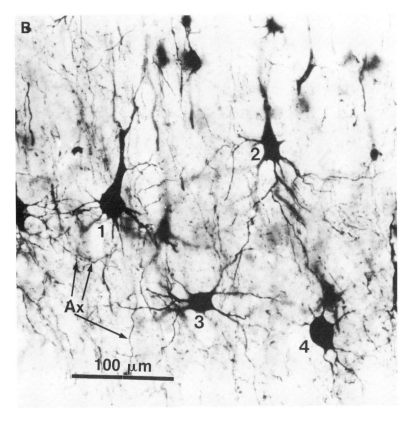

Figure 7. (*Continued*)
figure), layers IIIc and Va are fused, no obvious layer IV being present. The size of the pyramidal neurons in layers IIIc and Va (5, 6) in this cortex is of the same order. Silver deposits are seen as a darkened area in layer I of heterolaminar cortex. Rapid Golgi impregnation. (B) Higher magnification showing neurons in layer Va of heterolaminar cortex. The large atypical pyramids (1, 2) have club- or pear-shaped perikarya. The apical dendrites of both pyramidal neurons are bifurcated at the level of layers IIIc or IV or IIIc (panel A). Giant multipolar stellate cells (3, 4) are seen below the large pyramids and are of the isodendritic type. Some ascending oblique and vertical branches of axons (Ax) of other neurons are also shown. Rapid Golgi impregnation.

the star-celled lamina IV. This is reflected in myeloarchitectonics as a decrease in the zonal afferent plexus and the development of the outer stripe of Baillarger afferent plexus (Sanides, 1972). All of these points are important in assessing our findings pertaining to the status of these upper layers of the dolphin neocortex.

Neurons of layer II of the convexity neocortex of the hedgehog brain and the older cortices of more progressive mammalian brains are provided with numerous spreading dendritic branches entering the wide layer I. As noted, this type of cell arrangement is highly typical of allocortical formations where a dense row of cell bodies stands out clearly with notable external and internal dendritic spreads (Valverde, 1986). In the hedgehog convexity neocortex, more typical pyramidal cells populate the underlying cortical layers which would suggest an overlapping of two types of cortical formations, one consisting of neurons with marked dendritic extensions toward a broader layer I with strong fiber input, and a second type of cortex comprising the lower cortical layers in which pyramidal cells share with local circuit neurons a more elaborate type of architecture. The first type is obviously very similar to that found in cortical olfactory centers and thus defines a cortical organization as more allocortical or periallocortical in nature. The darkly staining dense layer II that we have found

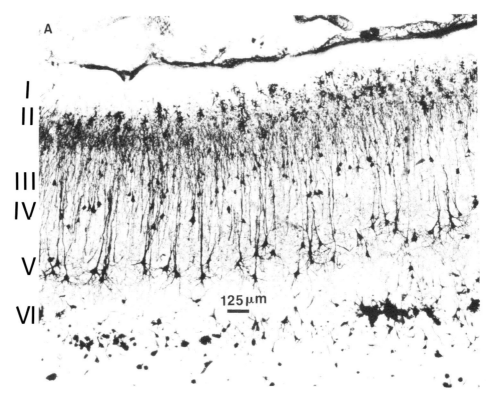

Figure 8. (A) General view of impregnated heterolaminar cortex in the posterior part of the lateral gyrus of the dolphin, *Stenella coeruleoalba,* showing transitional types of pyramidal neurons and the rather regular distribution of vertically oriented cellular and acellular strips of cortex. This figure illustrates the presence of "columnar"-type vertical organization in the dolphin cortex. We have in quantitative image analysis studies termed these vertically oriented chains of neurons *cytoarchitectonic columns* (Morgane *et al.,* 1988). Rapid Golgi impregnation. (B) A higher magnification showing the imprecise or transitional shapes of pyramidal neurons.

throughout the convexity neocortical fields is one of the most distinguishing features of the neocortical formations of the dolphin (Morgane *et al.*, 1986a,b, 1988; Morgane and Glezer, 1990). In some instances in the dolphin convexity neocortex we have found extraverted neurons of layer II appearing along with neurons having more progressive or advanced dendritic patterns approaching those of pyramidal neurons with well-balanced outer and inner dendrites. The Golgi picture reveals the peculiar nature of the neurons which form these superficial cell condensations (Figs. 9 and 10). The significance of these "extraverted" neurons of the older cortices, including those in convexity cortex of the hedgehog and dolphin, appears rather obvious. Thus, in the older cortices their extraverted dendrites aim to the surface-bound olfactory input of first and second order, and in the first neocortical growth ring (periallocortex) even thalamic input to the zonal layer is known (Domesick, 1969). In the hedgehog a thalamic input to the zonal layer has also been shown for the convexity neocortex (Ebner, 1969), while in the dolphin (*Phocoena phocoena*) Krasnoshchekova and Figurina

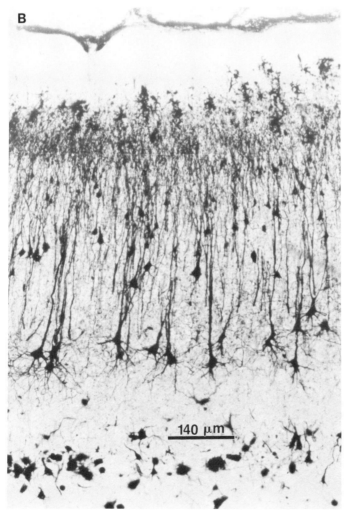

Figure 8. (*Continued*)

(1980) traced a heavy contingent of degenerating fibers to layer I following medial geniculate lesions.

The extraversion of the neurons of accentuated layer II toward layer I in the neocortex of the insectivorous placentals as well as findings of a major thalamic input aiming at this layer (Ebner, 1969) in these mammals indicate a persisting major significance of this layer in this conservative group of mammals. This is a conservative expression or ancient functional organizational pattern in neocortical evolution being a protoneocortical mark indicating the originally prevailing layer I input of the axodendritic type. Such axodendritic contact through the zonal layer is a general feature of organization of the older cortices and this type of contact appears common in the dolphin (Figs. 11 and 12). Dendritic extraversion is thus a neuronal and architectonic feature of obvious evolutionary value. It marks the periallocortical and proisocortical stage and, partly, the paralimbic stage of cortical evolution. The isocortex in advanced mammals has an accentuated layer II extending only to the level of the insular and limbic cortices. Extreme extraversion goes back to the amphibian level of brain evolution before a cerebral neocortex has developed. The zonal layer, the original synaptic site in the cerebral cortex, which plays an ontogenetically and phylogenetically ancient role, thus apparently continues to play such a role in both the hedgehog and dolphin brains. Thus, the extraversion of the neurons composing layer II points to a greater functional significance of the zonal layer in evolutionarily conservative mammals such as the hedgehog and dolphin which is also in line with its ancient role in phylogenesis and ontogenesis prior to higher cortical development. The shape of layer II pyramidal cells and their

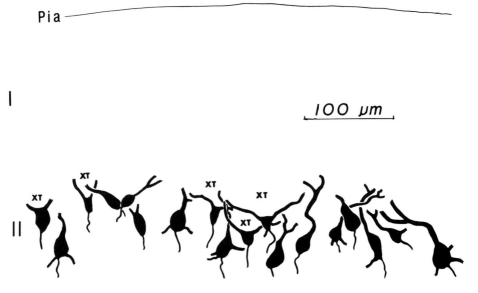

Figure 9. Camera lucida drawing of perikarya, primary dendrites, and axons of pyramidal cells in layer II in heterolaminar cortex of posterior part of lateral gyrus in the dolphin, *Tursiops truncatus*. The extension of the apical dendrites into layer I and their dendritic spines are omitted for simplicity. This figure shows an abundance of extraverted neurons in layer II, these cells being characterized by extreme separation of their "hornlike" dendrites which extend widely into layer I. Other layer II pyramidal cells drawn are largely of the modified or transitional type and thus not of the typical pyramidal shape. XT, extraverted neurons.

dendritic patterns also help disclose their evolutionary origins from the oldest type of telencephalic neurons with subpial tufts which, as noted, are types of cells found in lower vertebrates where they actually precede formation of a superficial cortex. Accentuated layer II is a common characteristic only of the older cortical growth rings in most of the recent placental mammals whereas it also dominates the convexity neocortex in insectivores and bats and, as we have recently shown, in dolphins.

Summarizing the organization of the dolphin neocortex, one of the most distinctive features we have found is the organization of layers I and II which appear almost as a derivative of a paleocortical or archicortical structure. Layer I is exceedingly thick and contains a dense palisade of peripheral highly spinous dendrites extending from nearly all the neurons located in layer II. It also contains the ascending superficial ramifications of apical dendrites of deeper pyramidal cells as well as a large number of tangential fibers derived from the ascending axons of Martinotti cells located in layer VI, from bipolar cells in layers III and V, and from collateral branches of the large multipolar cells of layer III with smooth dendrites which run horizontally for extremely long distances. However, as further described below, the main axonal inputs to layer I are the ascending collaterals of descending axons of pyramidal cells of layers II, III, and V. These collaterals in most cases ascend to layer I and form multiple contacts *en passage* with apical and basal dendrites of cells in all layers which they are crossing. In layer I these collaterals make contacts with terminal dendritic

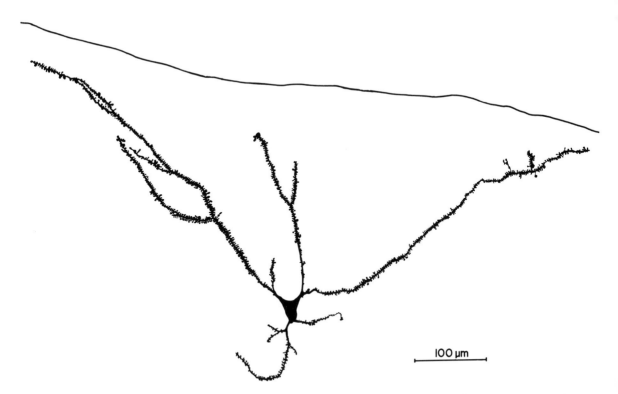

100 μm

Figure 10. Camera lucida drawing of a maximally "extraverted" neuron of layer II of lateral gyrus (visual cortex) of the dolphin, *Tursiops truncatus*. Note the widespread diverging, highly spinous apical dendrites extending into layer I and the relative weakness of development of the basilar dendrites.

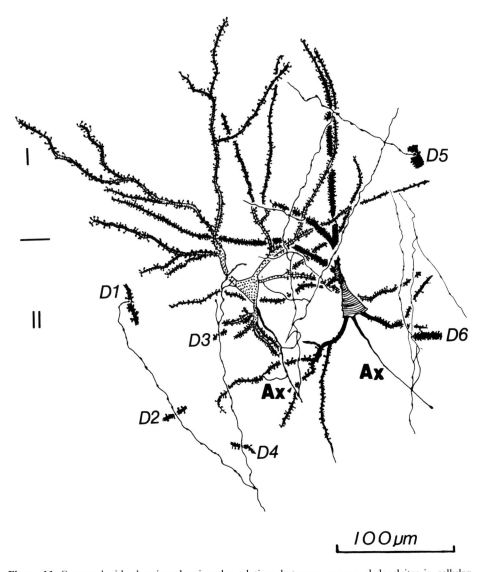

I

II

D5

D1

D3

D6

D2

Ax

D4

Ax

100μm

Figure 11. Camera lucida drawing showing the relations between axons and dendrites in cellular groups of layer II of posterior homolaminar cortex (lateral gyrus) of the dolphin, *Tursiops truncatus*. Note that almost all recurrent collaterals of the axons of the extraverted neuron (stippling) and small pyramidal neuron (cross-hatching) ascend to layer I. These recurrent collaterals make presumptive synaptic contacts with both apical and basal dendrites of the two illustrated neurons which, in electron microscopic studies, we have demonstrated to be mostly of *en passage* type. Axon collaterals from both cells shown provide a source of many of the *en passage* synapses that are so abundant in layer II and, especially, in layer I of the cetacean cortex. Such collaterals form the morphological basis for widespread activation of the neurons in dense layer II via dendrites in layer I. Small portions of dendrites from a number of neurons other than those shown are labeled D1–D6. Dendrite D1 is a secondary branch of a layer II pyramidal cell that receives a presumptive terminal synapse from a recurrent branch of the axon of a small pyramidal cell located at a superficial level of layer III. Dendrite D2 is a secondary branch from the apical tree of a layer II pyramidal cell receiving *en passage* fibers from the same neuron as D1. Dendrite D3 is a secondary branch from the apical tree of a layer III pyramid, also receiving an *en passage* synapse from the same neuron as D1. Dendrite D4 is a secondary branch from the apical tree of another layer III neuron receiving an *en passage* synapse from the same neuron as does D1. Dendrite D5 is a portion of the apical dendrite of a small layer II pyramid that appears to receive a terminal synapse from a fiber connected to the recurrent branch of

arborizations of apical dendrites of pyramidal cells of layers II and III. These contacts are mostly axospinous in nature and thus most synapses are formed on the heads of dendritic spines.

Relative to the special organization of layer I in the dolphin, we might assume, from a functional point of view, that such an arrangement relates to a more "massive action" in layer I in the dolphin. In this regard, Valverde (1983, 1986) and Valverde and Facal-Valverde (1986) have shown that apical dendrites of pyramidal neurons in the hedgehog convexity neocortex all go to layer I. On the other hand, Poliakov (1949) has pointed out that in phylogenetically progressive neocortices some pyramidal neurons do not have apical dendrites extending into layer I. This type of evidence again indicates that brains showing a more conservative type of organization have a neocortical layer I that appears to be a prime site of integrative activity.

With regard to dendritic patterns of organization, our studies also indicate that the overall lack of neuronal specialization we observed in the dolphin convexity neocortex may be one manifestation of pluripotentiality. If, in neurons, heterogeneity of connections is regarded as a particular example of multiplicity of potential attributes, it may be possible to account for the apparent rule that generalized dendritic patterns are associated with diversified connections which are afferent, efferent, or both. The "density specificity gradient" expressed by the terms *isodendritic, allodendritic,* and *idiodentritic* (Ramón-Moliner, 1968) could in that case be considered to reflect a gradual decrease in the number of potential connections and, hence, of functional properties. Thus, it appears clear that differences in the geometrical patterns of dendrites observed in various types of neurons are of particular evolutionary interest and it is these differences that determine the spatial interaction of postsynaptic events taking place on the membrane of dendritic branches. Observations by various workers, including Sanides (1970, 1972), in both mammals and lower vertebrates fully confirm the findings of Ramón-Moliner (1968) that the shape of the dendritic tree characterizes not only the degree of functional specialization of the neuron, but also its degree of phyletic complexity.

As pointed out by Sanides (1970, 1972), the paralimbic and parinsular belt of fields represent an intermediate stage on the way from limbic and insular proisocortex to the individual fields of the convexity. Presumably the paralimbic and parinsular cortical belts contain the supplementary motor and prokoniocortical sensory representations. The higher stages of sensory-motor organization, with the classical precentral motor and precentral somatic regions flanked medially by paralimbic supplementary motor and ventrolaterally by parinsular second sensory-motor areas, are, according to the studies of Sanides (1970, 1972), preceded in evolution by a stage where the paralimbic and parinsular representations are still contiguous. This may well be the situation in the dolphin brain, though from our findings to date definitive answers are not possible. In this

---

the axon of the pictured extraverted neuron. Dendrite D6 is a basal dendrite of a layer II cell receiving an *en passage* synapse from the recurrent branch arising from the axon of the layer II pyramidal neuron shown in the drawing. Numerous ascending axon collaterals to layer I from deeper cortical neurons, including layer II neurons, are a feature of organization of convexity neocortex in the dolphin. In electron microscopic studies we have shown these numerous ascending collaterals to make axodendritic synapses *en passage* with upper-level neurons (see also Figs. 13 and 14).

regard, our cytoarchitectonic and recent Golgi studies of the convexity neo-cortex in the dolphin have not revealed the presence of any hypergranular cortices. Thus, there are really no highly differentiated areas of the dolphin neocortex such as striate or acoustic koniocortical areas that are seen in most progressive mammalian species. To date we have not been able to identify any emerging cores of hypergranular development between the paralimbic and par-insular areas in the dolphin cortex. Accordingly, from this point of view the highest degree of cytoarchitectonic specialization, as defined by Sanides (1970,

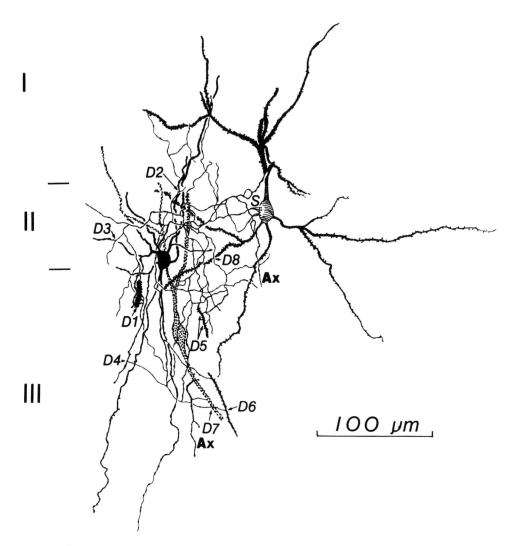

Figure 12. Camera lucida drawing showing a group of three neurons in layers II and IIIa of posterior homolaminar cortex of lateral gyrus in the dolphin, *Tursiops truncatus.* Not the rich mesh-like net of axons of the nonpyramidal (stellate) cell (solid black). Multiple axon collaterals of this cell are shown crossing dendrites of the bipolar (stippling) neuron and atypical club-shaped pyramidal (cross-hatched) neuron. Most of the axons form presumptive axodendritic *en passage* synapses, though some terminal-type contacts (axosomatic) are found on the perikaryon of the pyramidal cell (S). These types of synaptic contacts of the axodendritic and axosomatic type, respectively, have been verified by us in electron microscopic studies (see Figs. 14 and 16). D_1–D_8: number of axonal crossings of dendrites of neurons not shown in the drawing. Ax, axon.

1972), is nowhere to be found in the neocortex of the dolphin. Therefore, a true "belt–core" pattern (Rose and Woolsey, 1949) of structural differentiation of the neocortex is not seen in the dolphin. The lack of distinct koniocortex and gigantopyramidal neurons, combined with poor lamination and weak granularization, might be interpreted to indicate that, as in the insectivores and bats (Sanides, 1970, 1972), the latest stage of sensory and motor cortical differentiation has not been reached in the whale brain.

5. Image Analysis of Dolphin Visual Cortex

One of the quantitative techniques we have recently applied to analysis of the visual neocortex of the dolphin is computerized image analysis. In these studies (Morgane *et al.*, 1988) we have obtained considerable quantitative data, including information on density profiles of the cortical areas for vision in the lateral gyrus representing total cell density and laminar distribution of density across the thickness of the cortex. Thus, we established a more objective basis for subdividing the cortical laminae and different cytoarchitectonic subareas of the lateral gyrus in the dolphin. We also identified a "columnar" type of organization of the dolphin cortex and determined the sizes of cytoarchitectonic columns and number of cytoarchitectonic columns per unit of cortical area (Fig. 8). Whether these cytoarchitectonic columns are in any way equivalent to the functional orientation and dominance columns mapped for visual cortex is still unknown, but the data do indicate that this fundamental plan of vertical organization of the cortex in the form of translaminar cords of neurons or columnar parcellation also holds for the dolphin neocortex. This radial type of cortical organization has apparently remained basically unchanged over considerable periods of mammalian evolution.

6. Ultrastructural Analysis of Dolphin Visual Cortex

In our electron microscopic analyses of the lateral gyrus (visual cortex) of the dolphin brain we have placed special emphasis on the ultrastructural features of synaptic organization in this area (Glezer and Morgane, 1990). We will summarize some of the features of synaptology and synaptic relations in both pyramidal and nonpyramidal neurons in this cortex.

In all layers of the dolphin visual cortex we found typical axodendritic asymmetrical synapses (type I synapses of Gray, presumably excitatory) and symmetrical axosomatic synapses (type II synapses of Gray, presumably inhibitory). Though the overall characteristics of pre- and postsynaptic axodendritic synaptic structures are, as expected, similar in dolphin visual neocortex to those in other mammals (presence of presynaptic boutons, multiple synaptic vesicles of different types, asymmetric postsynaptic density, and the presence of spine apparatus, neurotubules, and mitochondria in presynaptic boutons), there are some prominent peculiarities of the axodendritic synaptology in the dolphin neocortex on which we will focus our attention and which are well correlated with our light microscopic findings in Golgi material. The first of these is the great dominance of synapses *en passage* which we have found in all cortical laminae but especially in layer I where multiple axons form axodendritic synaptic contacts with subpial terminal branches of apical dendrites. Thus, most of the synaptic contacts that are found in layer I of dolphin visual cortex are not end-feet or terminal-type contacts but rather are passing contacts between heads of the presynaptic spines and chainlike presynaptic varicosities of axons (Figs. 13 and 14). These synapses *en passage* are found between different types of axons (specific thalamocortical, intracortical collaterals, and nonspecific thalamocortical axons) and different types of dendrites, both apical and basilar. The dominance of these types of contacts, which simultaneously activate large neuronal groups with each axon contacting many postsynaptic structures (spines), is suggestive of an overall mass action of neurons in the dolphin neocortex. In a functional sense, according to Marr (1969, 1970), this type of synaptic organization permits obtaining information as to the context of the event and consequently puts it into memory. As noted by Marr, however, this type of organization of synapses would appear to have more limited ability for classification of events. It is especially interesting that this type of predominant neocortical synaptic organization of the *en passage* type in the dolphin neocortex is similar to that seen in the archicortex and paleocortex of terrestrial mammals. Thus, we stress that these additional indicators of conservative neocortical organization of the dolphin neocortex, i.e., the synaptic relations, especially in the upper cortical layers, are similar to the allocortical-type organization rather than the neocortical. The other interesting feature of most synaptic contacts of axodendritic synapses of the *en passage* type

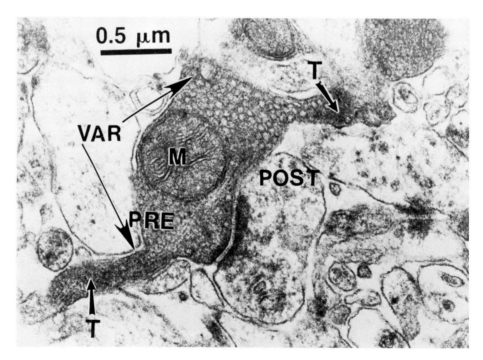

Figure 13. Electron micrograph showing a varicosity (VAR) of an axonal branch (T) filled with round light synaptic vesicles in layer I of the posterior heterolaminar cortex of the dolphin, *Stenella coeruleoalba*. This varicosity is the presynaptic part (PRE) of a synapse *en passage* contacting the head of the dendritic spine (POST). This type of synapse is characteristically seen in all cortical layers in the dolphin neocortex and is especially prominent in layer I.

is the presence of multiform synaptic vesicles in the same terminal areas. Most, if not all, presynaptic profiles in our material contain round, transparent, small vesicles along with flat and granular (dense core) vesicles (Figs. 13–15). This finding is in general agreement with contemporary views of multiple transmitters (cotransmission) in neurons in several mammalian species studied to date. This is a dominant feature in nearly all axodendritic synapses we have so far examined in the dolphin visual neocortex.

Relative to axosomatic synapses, we have been especially interested in the structure of synaptic endings of various neuronal types, pyramidal and nonpyramidal, particularly on small aspinous stellate cells in incipient layer IV of heterolaminar cortex. We have so far not found spiny stellate neurons in any layer of dolphin neocortex, including incipient layer IV. Not unexpectedly, all axosomatic synapses that we have examined in the dolphin, including those on stellate neurons of layer IV, are of the symmetric type with short pre- and postsynaptic symmetric densities (Fig. 16). In these synapses the thick regions of membranes are never over 35% of the apposed total membrane surface. The vesicles in the presynaptic boutons in this type of synapse are predominantly of the flat type (Fig. 16). This feature, along with the symmetric type of synapse, is suggestive of the presence of inhibitory-type synapses. One of the main problems, obviously, is establishing from which type of neurons these axon terminals originate and, to this end, we have carried out some preliminary combined Golgi–electron microscopic studies in dolphin visual neocortex. In light microscopic (Golgi) sections we found that end-feet terminals of small nonpyramidal neurons come in close approximation to the cell bodies of neighboring pyramidal neurons (Figs. 11 and 12). Also we have seen this type of relation between terminals of ascending axon collaterals of pyramidal neurons and cell bodies of stellate neurons located in the same or upper cortical layers.

Among the most powerful techniques available to neuromorphologists are the Golgi method and electron microscopy. The feasibility of combining these two techniques to permit electron microscopic analysis of Golgi-impregnated tissue and the potential importance of such a combination in studies of cellular and synaptic organization in the CNS were recognized long ago (Stell, 1964; Blackstad, 1965) and have been exploited to great advantage by a variety of workers providing data on the types, numbers, and placement of synapses for modeling the integrative processes of the cerebral cortex (Fairén *et al.*, 1977; Peters, 1981). We have similarly carried out combined Golgi–electron microscopic studies in limited areas of the dolphin visual cortex. Figure 17 shows a combined Golgi–electron microscopic preparation indicating a stellate neuron of layer V which we deimpregnated and thin-sectioned for ultrastructural analysis. In this instance we see a symmetric synapse on this neuron body which contains mitochondria and multiple flat and round vesicles. To date we have shown, pending further combined Golgi–electron microscopic studies, that all of the axodendritic synapses *en passage* are asymmetric in type and that there are symmetric axosomatic synapses on both pyramidal and nonpyramidal neurons in the dolphin neocortex. From our preliminary studies of the organization of the visual cortex, we have devloped a preliminary schema (Fig. 6) showing some of the synaptic relationships we have seen so far in the dolphin visual cortex. To date, the cytological features and synaptic relations of a number of types of neurons, both pyramidal and nonpyramidal, in dolphin visual cortex have been examined. Additionally, our Golgi studies of axons have now unraveled some of the characteristics of neural circuits involving some of these neurons. Further advances in understanding the organization of the visual cortex in the dolphin depend on additional studies now in progress on the synaptic relations of various types of neurons and deriving morphometric data on the numbers of neurons of various types present in the different laminae as well as the distribution of synapses in which these neurons are involved in both a presynaptic and a postsy-

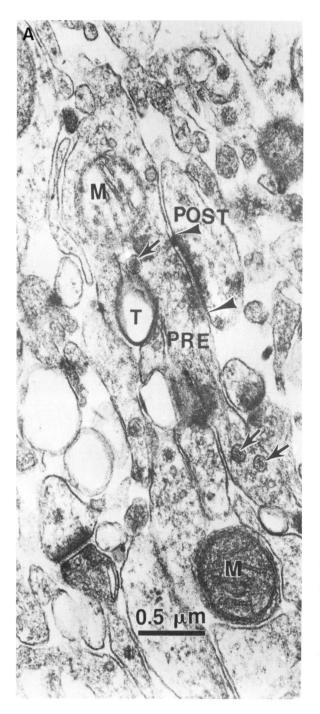

Figure 14. Electron micrograph showing ultrastructure of synapses *en passage*. (A) Neuropil of layer I. The figure shows a part of a thin axonal terminal which is presynaptic (PRE) to the head of a dendritic spine (POST). Note an asymmetric type of synapse (arrowheads) and polymorphism of synaptic vesicles, most of the latter being of the round, light type. Some large granular vesicles are also present (arrows). (B) (Opposite page) Neuropil of layer III of posterior heterolaminar cortex of the lateral gyrus of the dolphin, *Stenella coeruleoalba*. The axon terminal (T) is filled with a variety of types of vesicles and makes a synapse *en passage* with a dendritic spine. The structure of the postsynaptic density shows the asymmetry of the contact (arrowheads). Polymorphism of vesicles is also shown in neighboring presynaptic structure (SV). Note flat and round vesicles of different sizes in the same synapse.

naptic capacity. These further studies of axonal plexuses and synaptic relations should provide additional information of comparative and evolutionary value.

Additionally, we have recently carried out immunocytochemical studies of dolphin visual cortex and identified several types of neurons, in particular cholecystokinin, neuropeptide-Y, and tyrosine hydroxylase-positive perikarya in this cortex (Glezer *et al.*, 1990). The cholecystokinin (Fig. 18A) and tyrosine hydroxlase-positive perikarya are concentrated largely in layers I and II while the neuropeptide-Y-positive perikarya are scattered throughout the entire cortical plate with higher densities in layers III and V (Fig. 18B). The cholecystokinin-positive neurons form some 70% of the total perikarya in layer I and are fusiform-shaped and vertically oriented. In our comparative studies we have found these same features of distribution and orientation of immunoreactive neurons in the convexity neocortices of the hedgehog and bat brain. Further studies of these immunoreactive neurons, as well as GABAergic neurons, are now in progress. This type of analysis, combined with out other analyses, should provide new information about the functional organization of the cetacean convexity neocortex.

7. Concluding Remarks

The brains of species serving as valid and useful models of the "initial" mammalian brain appear more generalized in organization and not overgrown

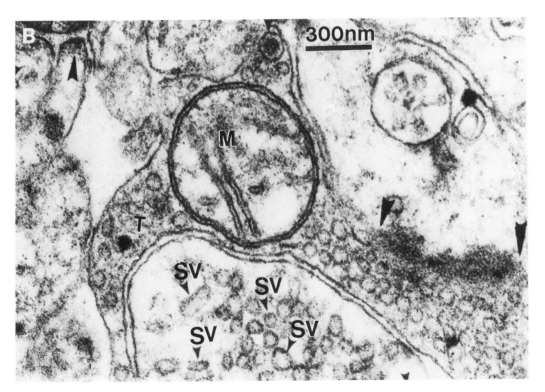

Figure 14. (*Continued*)

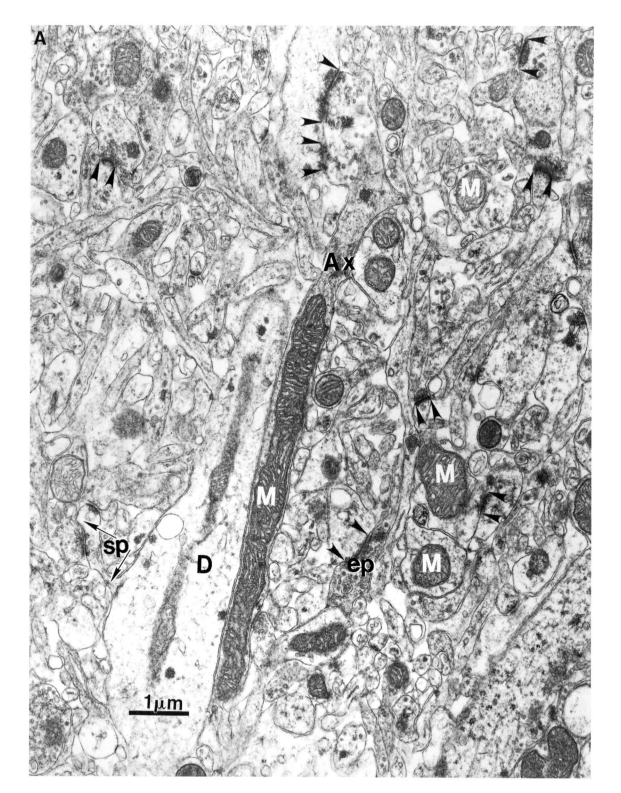

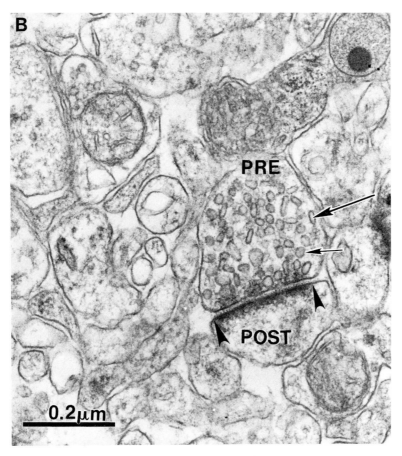

Figure 15. (*Continued*)

by more recent phylogenetic acquisitions and such brains are likely to reveal themselves more clearly as reliquaries of their past. The concept of the "initial" brain is of special value in examining the status of the whale brain since they went to water some 50–70 million years ago when primitive terrestrial mammals were dominant. Thus, the phylogenetically earlier isolation of cetaceans on an independent evolutionary branch makes a study of their neocortices of special interest.

Our studies have revealed that the neocortex of the dolphin brain shows

Figure 15. Ultrastructural features of the neuropil in layer I of the lateral gyrus (visual cortex) in the dolphin, *Tursiops truncatus*. (A) Photomicrograph showing a net of axonal collaterals and fine dendritic branches. Several asymmetric axodendritic synapses are present and their postsynaptic densities are indicated by the arrowheads. Most of them are synapses *en passage*. The most conspicuous example of the latter is in the lower right part of the micrograph (ep). Branches of the apical pyramidal dendrites (D) have typical spines (sp). Both dendritic branches and axonal collaterals (Ax) contain large, darkly stained mitochondria (M). (B) Photomicrograph showing a typical synapse between terminal bouton (PRE) and the head of a dendritic spine (POST). The postsynaptic density is indicated by the arrowheads. Flat (large arrow) and round (small arrow) clear vesicles are present in the synaptic bouton (PRE). Extreme degrees of pleomorphism of synaptic vesicles is one of the characteristic features of synapses in the dolphin neocortex. Presynaptic density is indicated by the arrowheads.

generally a single structural design and is characterized as (1) being basically five-layered, considered in terms of an absence of or incipience of layer IV; (2) being predominantly agranular or, at best, showing rudimentary granularization, with a predominance among nonpyramidal neurons of large isodendritic stellate cells; (3) possessing well-developed phylogenetically old layers I and VI; (4) having an accentuated layer II containing large numbers of primitive-type pyramidal neurons organized similar to those in allocortical formations; (5) hav-

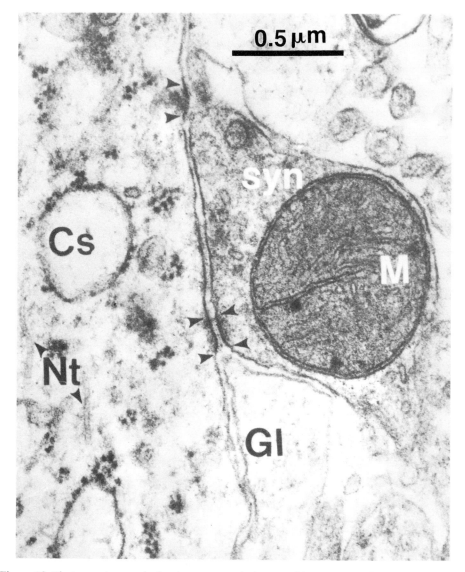

Figure 16. Electron micrograph showing axosomatic (symmetric) synapse on the perikaryal membrane of a pyramidal neuron in layer IIIc of posterior heterolaminar cortex of lateral gyrus of the dolphin, *Stenella coeruleoalba.* In presynaptic bouton (syn) there is a large mitochondrion (M) and synaptic vesicles mostly of the flat type. Both the pre- and postsynaptic densities are of the same length and thickness as indicated by arrowheads. In the postsynaptic area there are cisterns of endoplasmic reticulum (Cs), as well as numerous polysomes and neurotubules (Nt).

ing a largely pyramidal composition of neurons in all layers, (6) having an abundance of transitional or undifferentiated imprecisely shaped pyramidal neurons, dendrites with relatively few branches, and a high degree of return collaterals of axons of the larger pyramids to layer I, (7) having an internal circuitry organized synaptically through a predominance of fibers of *en passage*-type connectivity; and (8) lacking hypergranular "cores" of cortical specialization (koniocortices) and lacking giant pyramidal cells (area gigantopyramidalis).

In our studies we have found that the greater number of neurons in the dolphin convexity neocortex of the lateral gyrus (visual cortex) are pyramidal in type, most of which are of the transitional, intermediate type with highly imprecise shapes. In general, the transitional shape of neurons is considered evidence of weak differentiation of the cortex. The presence of retrogressive collaterals of axons of the larger pyramids, in addition to nonreturning collaterals of axons from the same neuron, may also represent one sign of conservative evolution in showing a lack of differentiation of neurons of the pyramidal family into projectional versus associative neurons, i.e., the same neuron may retain elements of both functions in the dolphin.

Layer II is particularly distinctive or accentuated in the dolphin in terms of its highly compact and dark staining character. This layer contains primitive (transitional or intermediate type) pyramidal neurons ranging from semilunar to stellate in form many of which are strongly "extraverted" in that they send their highly spinous dendrites in a widely diverging manner into layer I. Accentuated layer II is typical of cortical growth rings I and II of Sanides (1970, 1972) in having primarily a zonal dendritic arborization. Most of the layer II pyramids in the dolphin neocortex appear to be at an intermediary stage of pyramidal cell evolution. Such a neuronal structure, almost indistinguishable from pyramidal cells of the olfactory cortices, in many ways resembles the superficial neurons of the allocortical formations, especially those of piriform cortex, hippocampal formation (including pyramids of hippocampus proper and dentate "granule" cells), and the paleocortical–olfactory forebrain areas. This major feature reflects the retention of a conservative character in neocortical evolution. The structure and connections, especially of layers I and II, of convexity neocortex of the dolphin differ significantly from the neocortical formations of more advanced mammalian species. It is important to note, even with the powerful development of extraverted neurons in accentuated layer II, that there is no doubt that this convexity cortex of the lateral gyrus is true neocortex in that there are large numbers of pyramidal cells in deeper layers III and V, albeit transitional or immature in shape and form, which have long apical dendrites extending upward to the upper cortical layers. There seems little question of the continuing functional importance of the first and second layers in the dolphin neocortex in comparison to other mammals, owing to the strong input these layers receive from subjacent layers and subcortical formations. The functional significance of dendritic extraversion is that this type of protoneocortical organization represents axodendritic contact through the zonal layer which is a well-known feature of organization in the allocortices and intermediate cortical formations. It would appear, just as in the hedgehog cortex, that layers I and II represent the most important level of neocortical integration in the dolphin. We would stress that layer I appears to be the main excitatory input layer in dolphin convexity neocortex and layer II serves as a distributor of this excitation into other cortical layers via an extensive collateral system and these *en passage*-type

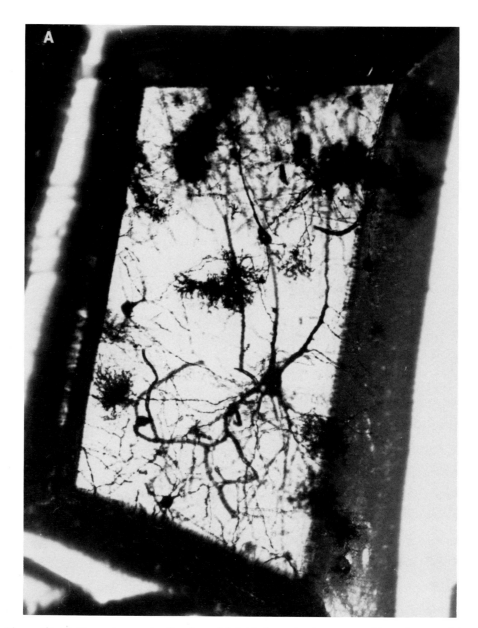

Figure 17. (A) Photomicrograph of surface of dolphin heterolaminar cortex of lateral gyrus of the dolphin *Stenella coeruleoalba*, showing the structure of several neurons in layer V. The block was impregnated with silver nitrate (rapid Golgi method) and embedded in araldite–Epon. Note well-impregnated pyramidal and nonpyramidal neurons, as well as glial cells and vessels. Artifacts shown are related to deimpregnation and often seen in combined Golgi–electron microscopic preparations. × 75. (B) Same surface at higher magnification showing the giant stellate cell with well-impregnated axon and its collaterals (Ax). Note that the cell is of a lesser spinous type. The box indicates the area of the initial part of the dendrite shown at the electron microscopic level in photomicrograph Fig. 17C. (C) Structure of the axosomatic synapse on the plasma membrane of the perikaryon of the identified nonpyramidal neuron (NP) shown in A and B. Almost the entire synaptic bouton is occupied by the mitochondrion (M) and contains tightly packed synaptic vesicles obscured by the gold deposits. Note that this synapse has symmetric pre- and postsynaptic densities (arrowheads) and is of the *en passage* type. The latter feature is indicated by the presence of axonal processes protruding from the side of the bouton (Ax). (D) Structure of the axodendritic asymmetric synapses (arrowheads) on the initial part of the primary dendrite (D) of the identified nonpyramidal neuron shown in Figs. 17A, B, and C. The area shown in the photomicrograph is indicated by the box in Fig. 17B. Synaptic boutons (Pre) contain numerous vesicles whose structure is obscured by the gold deposits.

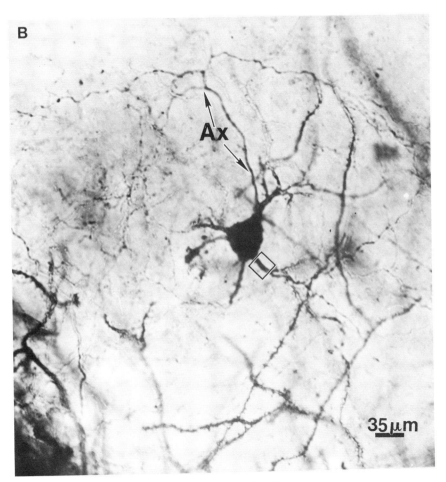

Figure 17. (*Continued*)

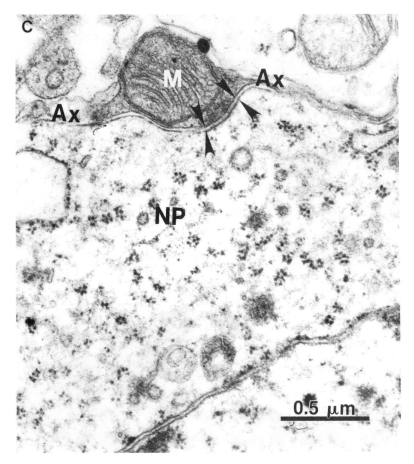

Figure 17. (*Continued*)

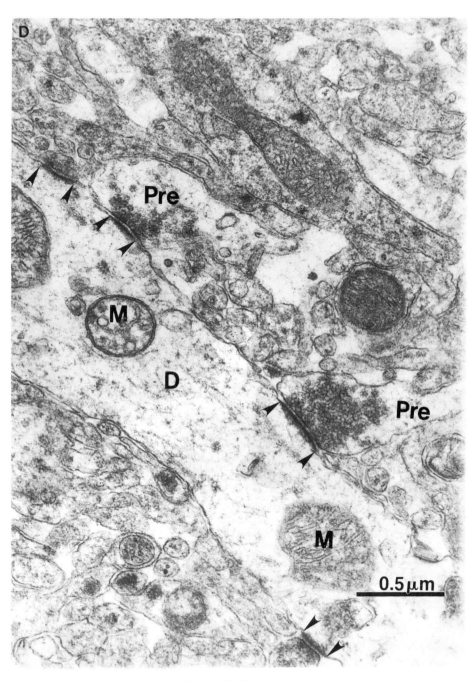

Figure 17. (*Continued*)

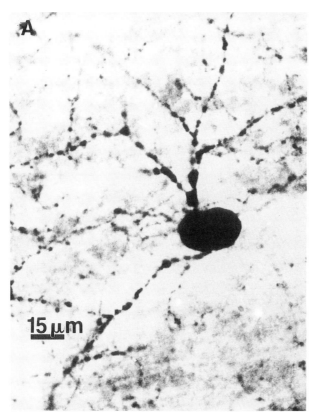

Figure 18. Photomicrographs showing neuropeptide Y (NPY) and cholecystokinin-containing (CCK) neurons in visual heterolaminar cortex. (A) Immunostained ovoid stellate NPY cell with long rectilinear dendrites in layer IIIb of Pilot whale (*Globicephala melaena*). Note numerous varicosities along the dendrites of the immunostained neuron. (B) Immunostained large CCK-containing fusiform neuron in layer I of dolphin (*Tursiops truncatus*). The neuron is oriented radially, i.e., along the vertical cortical axis and perpendicular to the pia.

turn, return to layer I to close the loop very much resembling some type of reverberating circuit.

Since there are no hypergranular cores of specialization in the dolphin neocortex, there is also no "belt–core" pattern of structural differentiation of the neocortex so common in most higher mammals which, again, indicates a conservative type of cortical evolution. Retention of the large or giant stellate neurons of the isodendritic type in dolphin convexity neocortex implies also a lack of granularity as earlier noted in the hedgehog by Sanides (1970, 1972). Diminution in size of the stellate elements in rodents can be interpreted as the beginning of a trend which leads eventually to full granularization of the stellate cells in advanced mammals culminating in higher primates. In general, the dolphin cortex shows fewer and much less diversified types of stellate neurons in the cortical local circuits. This is further evidence of a more conservative type of cortical organization in that the types of interneurons concerned with "fine tuning" activities are not well expressed.

The absence or marked incipience of layer IV is also a clear sign seen in transitional- or intermediate-type cortices. Hence, the entire convexity neocortex of the dolphin appears to show features of this transitional type of organization which, in Sanides's terms, is evidence of development of the neocortex only to the level of paralimbic/parinsular type of neocortical organization similar to that seen in basal insectivores and bats. We have found this same feature in the dolphin neocortex of the lateral gyrus (visual cortex) in that their upper cortical

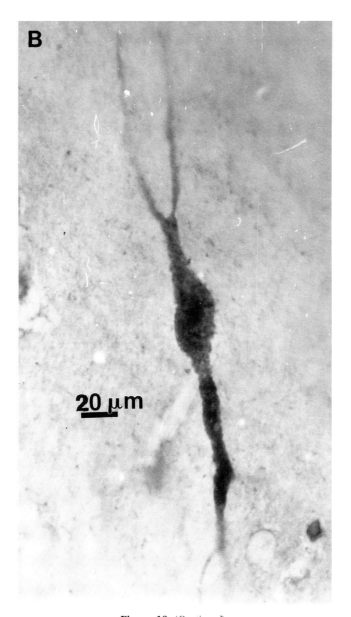

Figure 18. (*Continued*)

layers are organized in remarkably similar patterns to the paleocortical, archicortical, and transitional cortical type of organization. These allocortical features of the upper neocortical layers in dolphins are further evidence of a conservative type of neocortical organization. Until our studies of the dolphin neocortex, the hedgehog had been considered unique among the recent eutheria in keeping the paralimbic/parinsular stage as the highest leading stage in cortical differentiation.

In terms of the basic cortical modules or architectonic columns which we have described in the dolphin neocortex (Morgane *et al.*, 1988), these appear to be organized rather simply in terms of degree of complexity. Computationally the whale neocortex then appears to have many such conservatively organized cytoarchitectonic columns with minimal variation between them. It would appear overall that there is a vast increase in the territory of the neocortex in the dolphin but without substantial reorganization of the basic "initial" stratification plan that first appeared in the common ancestors of present-day mammals.

ACKNOWLEDGMENTS. This research was supported by National Science Foundation Grants BNS 84-14523, BNS 85-45732, BNS 87-42032, NIH Grant HD 06364-13 and the New York Zoological Society. We are indebted to the late Dr. George Ruggieri, Director of the New York Aquarium, for making facilities of the Osborn Laboratories of Marine Sciences, New York Aquarium, Brooklyn, New York, available to this project. We thank the present director, Dr. Louis Garibaldi, for his continued help and assistance in this project.

8. References

Anthony, M. R., 1925, Sur un cerveau de foetus de Mégaptère, *C.R. Acad. Sci.* **181**:681–683.

Avksent'eva, L. I., Ladygina, T. F., and Supin, A. Ya., 1972, Morphology and physiology of marine mammals: Morphophysiologic characteristics of cerebrocortical organization in the dolphin *Tursiops truncatus* and *Phocaena phocaena*, Thesis presented at the Fifth All-Union Conference on Study of Marine Mammals, *Makhachkala*, Chapter II, pp. 3–5.

Barnes, L. G., Domning, D. P., and Ray, C. E., 1985, Status of studies on fossil marine mammals, *Mar. Mammal Sci.* **1**:15–53.

Beauregard, H., 1883, Recherches sur l'encéphale des Balaenides, *J. Anat. Physiol.* **19**:481–516.

Bianchi, V., 1905, Il mantello cerebrale del delfino (*Delphinus delphis*), *R. Accad. Sci. Fis. Mat. (Napoli)* **12**:1–18.

Blackstad, T. W., 1965, Mapping of experimental axon degeneration for the study of neuronal relations, *Z. Zellforsch. Mikrosk. Anat.* **67**:818–834.

Breathnach, A. S., 1960, The cetacean central nervous system, *Biol. Rev.* **35**:187–230.

Brodmann, K., 1909, *Vergleichende Lokalisationslehre der Grosshirnrinde in ihren Prinzipien Dargestellt auf Grund des Zellenbaues*, Barth, Leipzig.

Domesick, V., 1969, Projections from the cingulate cortex in the rat, *Brain Res.* **12**:296–320.

Ebner, F. F., 1969, A comparison of primitive forebrain organization in metatherian and eutherian mammals, *Ann. N.Y. Acad. Sci.* **167**:241–257.

Economo, C., von, and Koskinas, G. N., 1925, *Die Cytoarchitektonik der Hirnrinde des erwachsenen Menschen*, Springer, Berlin.

Elliot Smith, G., 1902, Order Cetacea, in: *Descriptive and Illustrated Catalogue of the Physiological Series of Comparative Anatomy Contained in the Museum of the Royal College of Surgeons of England*, Volume 2, 2nd ed., Taylor & Francis, London, pp. 348–359.

Entin, T. I., 1973, Histologic studies of the occipital cortex of the dolphin brain, *Arkh. Anat. Gistol. Embriol.* **65**:92–100.

Fairén, A., Peters, A., and Saldanha, J., 1977, A new procedure for examining Golgi impregnated neurons by light and electron microscopy, *J. Neurocytol.* **6**:311–337.

Filimonoff, I. N., 1949, *Comparative Anatomy of the Cerebral Cortex of Mammals: Paleocortex, Archicortex, and Intermediate Cortex*, Publ. Acad. Med. Sci., Moscow.

Filimonoff, I. N., 1965, On the so-called rhinencephalon in the dolphin, *J. Hirnforsch.* **8**:1–23.

Flower, W. H., 1883, On whales, past and present, and their probable origin, *Nature* **28**:199–202, 226–230.

Friant, M., 1953, Le cerveau du marsouin (*Phocaena communis Cuv.*) et les caracteristiques fondamentales du cerveau des Cétacés, *Acta Anat.* **17**:61–71.

Friant, M., 1955, Le cerveau du Baleinoptere (*Balaeonoptera* sp.), *Acta Anat.* **23**:242–250.

Friant, M., 1958, Un stade de l'évolution cérébrale du rorqual (*Balaenoptera musculus L.*), *Hvalradets Skr.* **42**:4–15.

Friant, M., 1974, Sur les sillons palleaux de la face cerebrale externe des Cétacés, *Acta Anat.* **89:**145–148.

Garey, L. J., and Leuba, G., 1986, A quantitative study of neuronal and glial numerical density in the visual cortex of the bottlenose dolphin: Evidence for a specialized subarea and changes with age, *J. Comp. Neurol.* **247:**491–496.

Garey, L. J., Winkelmann, E., and Brauer, K., 1985, Golgi and Nissl studies of the visual cortex of the bottlenose dolphin, *J. Comp. Neurol.* **240:**305–321.

Gaskin, D. E., 1976, The evolution, zoogeography and ecology of Cetacea, *Oceanogr. Marine Biol. Ann. Rev.* **14:**247–346.

Gaskin, D. E., 1982, Evolution of Cetacea, in: *The Ecology of Whales and Dolphins* (D. E. Gaskin, ed.), Heinemann, London, pp. 159–199.

Gingerich, P. D., Wells, N. D., Russell, D. E., and Shail, S. M. L., 1983, Origin of whales in epicontinental remnant seas: New evidence from the early Eocene of Pakistan, *Science* **220:**403–406.

Glezer, I. I., and Morgane, P. J., 1990, Ultrastructure of synapses and Golgi analysis of neurons in the neocortex of the lateral gyrus (visual cortex) of the dolphin and pilot whale, *Brain Res. Bull.,* **24:**401–427.

Glezer, I., Jacobs, M. S., and Morgane, P. J., 1988, The "initial" brain concept and its implications for brain evolution in Cetacea, *Behav. Brain Sci.* **11:**75–116.

Glezer, I., Morgane, P. J., and Leranth, C., 1990, Immunocytochemistry of neurotransmitters in visual neocortex of toothed whales: Light and electron microscopic studies, in: *Sensory Abilities of Cetaceans: Laboratory and Field Evidence* (NATO Advanced Research Workshop, Rome, Italy, Aug. 1989) (J. Thomas and Kastelein, eds.), Plenum Press, New York, in press.

Grünthal, E. von, 1942, Über den Primatencharakter des Gehirns von *Delphinus delphis, Monatsschr. Psychiatr. Neurol.* **105:**249–274.

Guldberg, G. A., 1885, Über das Centralnervensystem der Bartenwale, *Forhand. Vidensk. Selsk. Christiania* **4:**1–154.

Hammelbo, T., 1972, On the development of the cerebral fissures in Cetacea, *Acta Anat.* **82:**606–618.

Howell, A. B., 1930, *Aquatic Mammals,* Thomas, Springfield, Ill.

Jacobs, M. S., Morgane, P. J., and McFarland, W. L., 1971, The anatomy of the brain of the bottlenose dolphin (*Tursiops truncatus*). Rhinic lobe (rhinencephalon). I. The paleocortex, *J. Comp. Neurol.* **141:**205–272.

Jacobs, M. S., McFarland, W. L., and Morgane, P. J., 1979, The anatomy of the brain of the bottlenose dolphin (*Tursiops truncatus*). Rhinic lobe (*rhinencephalon*): The archicortex, *Brain Res. Bull.* **4**(Suppl. 1):1–108.

Jacobs, M. S., Galaburda, A., McFarland, W. L., and Morgane, P. J., 1984, The insular formations of the dolphin brain. Cytoarchitectonics of the insular component of the limbic lobe, *J. Comp. Neurol.* **225:**396–432.

Kaas, J. H., 1987, The organization and evolution of neocortex, in: *Higher Brain Functions. Recent Explorations of Brains' Emergent Properties* (S. P. Wise, ed.), Wiley, New York, pp. 347–371.

Kaas, J. H., 1989, The evolution of complex sensory systems in mammals, *J. Exp. Biol.* **146:**165–176.

Kellogg, R., 1928, The history of whales—Their adaptation to life in water, *Q. Rev. Biol.* **3:**29–76, 174–208.

Kellogg, R., 1938, Cooperation in research: Adaptation of structure to function in whales, *Publ. Carnegie Inst.* **501:**649–682.

Kesarev, V. S., 1969, Structural organization of the limbic cortex in dolphins, *Arkh. Anat. Gistol. Embriol.* **56:**28–35.

Kesarev, V. S., 1970, Certain data on neuronal organization of the neocortex in the dolphin brain, *Arkh. Anat. Gistol. Embriol.* **59:**71–77.

Kesarev, V. S., and Malofeeva, L. I., 1969, Structural organization of the dolphin motor cortex, *Arkh. Anat. Gistol. Embriol.* **56:**48–55.

Kesarev, V. S., Malofeeva, L. I., and Trykova, O. V., 1977a, Structural organization of the cerebral neocortex in cetaceans, *Arkh. Anat. Gistol. Embriol.* **73:**23–30.

Kesarev, V. S., Malofeeva, L. I., and Trykova, O. V., 1977b, Ecological specificity of cetacean neocortex, *J. Hirnforsch.* **18:**447–460.

Kojima, T., 1951, On the brain of the sperm whale (*Physeter catodon L.*), *Sci. Rep. Whales Res. Inst. (Tokyo)* **6:**49–72.

Krasnoshchekova, E. I., and Figurina, I. I., 1980, The cortical projection of the medial geniculate body of the dolphin brain, *Arkh. Anat. Gistol. Embriol.* **78:**19–24.

Kraus, C., and Pilleri, G., 1969, Zur Feinstruktur der grossen Pyramidenzellen in der V. Cortexschicht der Cetaceen (*Delphinus delphis* und *Balaenoptera borealis*), *Z. Mikrosk. Anat. Forsch.* **80:**89–99.

Kükenthal, W., and Ziehen, T., 1889, Ueber das Centralnervensystem der Cetaceen, *Denkschr. Med. Naturwiss. Ges. Jena* **3:**80–200.

Ladygina, T. F., and Supin, A. Ya., 1974, Evolution of cortical areas in terrestrial and aquatic mammals, in: *Morphology, Physiology, and Accoustics of Marine Mammals*, Nauka, Moscow, pp. 6–15.

Ladygina, T. F., Mass, A. M., and Supin, A. Y., 1978, Multiple sensory projections in the dolphin cerebral cortex, *Zh. Vyssh. Nerv. Deyat. im I. P. Pavlova* **18:**1047–1054.

Langworthy, O. R., 1931a, Factors determining the differentiation of the cerebral cortex in sea-living mammals (the Cetacea). A study of the brain of the porpoise, *Tursiops truncatus, Brain* **54:**225–236.

Langworthy, O. R., 1931b, Central nervous system of the porpoise, *Tursiops truncatus, J. Mammal.* **12:**381–389.

Langworthy, O. R., 1932, A description of the central nervous system of the porpoise *(Tursiops truncatus), J. Comp. Neurol.* **54:**437–499.

Langworthy, O. R., 1935, The brain of the whalebone whale, *Balaenoptera physalus, Johns Hopkins Hosp. Bull.* **57:**143–147.

Lende, R. A., and Akdikmen, S., 1968, Motor field in cerebral cortex of the bottlenose dolphin, *J. Neurosurg.* **29:**495–499.

Lende, R. A., and Welker, W. I., 1972, An unusual sensory area in the cerebral neocortex of the bottlenose dolphin, *Tursiops truncatus, Brain Res.* **45:**555–560.

Leontovich, T. A., and Zhukova, G. P., 1963, The specificity of the neuronal structure and topography of the reticular formation in the brain and spinal cord of Carnivora, *J. Comp. Neurol.* **121:**347–381.

McFarland, W. L., Morgane, P. J., and Jacobs, M. S., 1969, Ventricular system of the brain of the dolphin, *Tursiops truncatus*, with comparative anatomical observations and relations to brain specializations, *J. Comp. Neurol.* **135:**275–368.

Mc Kenna, M. C., 1975, Toward a phylogenetic classification of the Mammalia, in: *Phylogeny of the Primates* (W. P. Luckett and F. S. Szalay, eds.), Plenum Press, New York, pp. 21–46.

Major, H. C., 1879, Observations on the structure of the brain of the white whale *(Delphinapterus leucas), J. Anat. Physiol.* **13:**127–138.

Marr, D., 1969, A theory of cerebellar cortex, *J. Physiol. (London)* **202:**437–470.

Marr, D., 1970, A theory for cerebral neocortex, *Proc. R. Soc. London Ser. B* **176:**161–234.

Mehedlidze, G. A., 1984, General features of the paleobiological evolution of Cetacea, Pub. for *Smithsonian Institution Libraries and National Science Foundation* (TT78-52026), Amerind Publ. Co., New Delhi.

Morgane, P. J., 1965, Lamination characteristics and areal differentiation in the cerebral cortex of the bottlenose dolphin *(Tursiops truncatus), Anat. Rec.* **151:**390–391.

Morgane, P. J., and Glezer, I., 1990, Sensory neocortex in dolphin brain, in: *Sensory Abilities of Cetaceans: Laboratory and Field Evidence* (NATO Advanced Research Workshop, Rome, Italy, Aug. 1989) (J. Thomas and R. Kastelein, eds.), Plenum Press, New York, in press.

Morgane, P. J., and Jacobs, M. S., 1972, Comparative anatomy of the cetacean nervous system, in: *Functional Anatomy of Marine Mammals*, Volume I (R. J. Harrison, ed.), Academic Press, New York, pp. 117–244.

Morgane, P. J., and Jacobs, M. S., 1986, A morphometric Golgi and cytoarchitectonic study of the hippocampal formation of the bottlenose dolphin, *Tursiops truncatus*, in: *The Hippocampus*, Volume 3 (R. L. Isaacson and K. H. Pribram, eds.), Plenum Press, New York, pp. 369–432.

Morgane, P. J., Jacobs, M. S., and McFarland, W. L., 1980, The anatomy of the brain of the bottlenose dolphin *(Tursiops truncatus)*. Surface configurations of the telencephalon of the bottlenose dolphin with comparative anatomical observations in four other cetacean species, *Brain Res. Bull* **5:**(Suppl. 3):1–107.

Morgane, P. J., McFarland, W. L., and Jacobs, M. S., 1982, The limbic lobe of the dolphin brain: A quantitative cytoarchitectonic study, *J. Hirnforsch.* **23:**465–552.

Morgane, P. J., Jacobs, M. S., and Galaburda, A., 1985, Conservative features of neocortical evolution in dolphin brain, *Brain Behav. Evol.* **23:**276–284.

Morgane, P. J., Jacobs, M. S., and Galaburda, A., 1986a, Evolutionary aspects of cortical organization in the dolphin brain, in: *Research on Dolphins* (M. Bryden and R. J. Harrison, eds.), Oxford University Press, Oxford, pp. 71–89.

Morgane, P. J., Jacobs, M. S., and Galaburda, A., 1986b, Evolutionary morphology of the dolphin brain, in: *Dolphin Cognition and Behavior: A Comparative Approach* (R. Schusterman, J. Thomas, and F. Wood, eds.), Erlbaum, Hillsdale, N.J., pp. 5–29.

Morgane, P. J., Glezer, I., and Jacobs, M. S., 1988, The visual cortex of the dolphin: An image analysis study, *J. Comp. Neurol.* **273**:3–25.

Nikitenko, M. F., 1965, Concerning the paths of adaptation to and of specialization for aquatic mode of life in different mammals, in: *Contributions of the All-Union Conference of "Intraspecies Variability of Land Living Vertebrate Animals and Microevolution,"* pp. 109–117.

Nikitenko, M. F., 1970, Evolutionary and ecological characterization of neocortical formation in mammals in: *IX Int. Congr. Anat.*, Leningrad, pp. 1–5.

Peters, A., 1981, Neuronal organization in rat visual cortex, in: *Progress in Anatomy*, Volume 1 (R. J. Harrison and R. L. Holmes, eds.), Cambridge University Press, London, pp. 95–121.

Pettit, A., 1905, Description des encéphales de *Grampus griseus Cuv.,* de *Steno frontatus Cuv.,* et de *Globiocephalus melas Traill,* provenant des campagnes du yacht Princesse-Alice, *Result. Camp. Sci. Monaco* **31**:1–58.

Pilleri, G., 1962, Die Zentralnervöse Rangordnung der Cetacea (Mammalia), *Acta Anat.* **51**:241–258.

Pilleri, G., 1964, Morphologie des Gehirnes des "Southern Right Whale," *Eubalaena australis Desmoulins* 1822 *(Cetacea, Mysticeti, Balaenidae),* *Acta Zool.* **46**:245–272.

Pilleri, G., 1966a, Über die Anatomie des Gehirnes des Gangesdelphins, *Platanista gangetica, Rev. Suisse Zool.* **73**:113–118.

Pilleri, G., 1966b, Morphologie des Gehirnes des Seiwals, *Balaenoptera borealis* Lesson *(Cetacea, Mysticeti, Balaenopteridae),* *J. Hirnforsch.* **8**:221–267.

Pilleri, G., 1966c, Morphologie des Gehirnes des Buckewals *Megaptera novaeangliae Borowski (Cetacea, Mysticeti, Balaenopteridae),* *J. Hirnforsch.* **8**:437–491.

Pilleri, G., and Kraus, C., 1969, Zum aufbau des cortex bei "Cetaceen," *Rev. Suisse Zool.* **76**:760–767.

Pilleri, G., Kraus, C., and Gihr, M., 1968, The structure of the cerebral cortex of the ganges dolphin *Susu (Platanista) gangetica* Le Beck 1801, *Z. Mikrosk. Anat. Forsch.* **79**:373–388.

Poliakov, G. I., 1949, Structural organization of the human cerebral cortex during ontogenetic development, in: *Cytoarchitectonics of the Cerebral Cortex in Man* (S. A. Sarkisov, I. N. Filimonoff, and N. S. Preobrazenskaya, eds.), Medgiz, Moscow, pp. 1–46.

Poliakov, G. I., 1959, Progressive differentiation of the neurons of the cerebral cortex in man during ontogenesis, in: *Development of the Central Nervous System: Onto- and Phylogenesis of the Cortex and Subcortical Formations* (S. A. Sarkisov and N. S. Preobrazenskaya, eds.), Medgiz, Moscow, pp. 11–26.

Poliakov, G. I., 1964, Development and complication of the cortical part of the coupling mechanism in the evolution of vertebrates, *J. Hirnforsch.* **7**:253–273.

Popov, V. V., Ladygina, T. F., and Supin, A. Y., 1986, Evoked potentials of the auditory cortex of the porpoise, *Phocaena phocaena, J. Comp. Physiol. A* **158**:705–711.

Ramón-Moliner, E., 1962, An attempt at classifying nerve cells on the basis of their dendritic patterns, *J. Comp. Neurol.* **119**:211–227.

Ramón-Moliner, E., 1967, La differentiation morphologique des neurones, *Arch. Ital. Biol.* **105**:149–188.

Ramón-Moliner, E., 1968, The morphology of dendrites, in: *The Structure and Function of Nervous Tissue* (G. F. Bourne, ed.), Academic Press, New York, pp. 205–267.

Ramón-Moliner, E., 1969, The leptodendritic neuron: its distribution and significance, *Ann. N.Y. Acad. Sci.* **167**:65–70.

Ramón-Moliner, E., 1975, Specialized and generalized dendritic patterns, in: *Golgi Centennial Symp. Proc.* (M. Santini, ed.), Raven Press, New York, pp. 87–100.

Ramón-Moliner, E., and Nauta, W. J. H., 1966, The isodendritic core of the brain stem, *J. Comp. Neurol.* **126**:311–335.

Ramón y Cajal, S., 1909–1911, *Histologie du Système Nerveux de l'Homme et des Vertébrés* (translated by L. Azoulay), Volumes I and II, Maloine, Paris.

Rawitz, B., 1910, Das Zentralnervensystem der Cetaceen. III. Die Furchen und Windungen des Grosshirns von *Balaenoptera rostrata Fabr., Arch. Mikrosk. Anat.* **75**:225–239.

Rawitz, B., 1927, Aus Kenntniss der Architektonik der Grosshirnrinde des Menschen und Einiger Saügetiere. III. Die Hirnrinde von Schwein, Schaf, Pferd, Zahnwal, Bartenwal, Beutelratte. IV. Allgemeine Betrachtungen, *Zeit. Gesamte Anat. Anat. Entwicklungsgesch.* **82**:122–141.

Rehkämper, G., 1981, Vergleichende Architektonik des neocortex der Insectivora, *Z. Zool. Syst. Evolutionsforsch.* **19**:233–263.

Reis, E. A., and Langworthy, O. R., 1937, A study of the surface structure of the brain of the whale, *Balaenoptera physalus* and *Physeter catodon, J. Comp. Neurol.* **68**:1–47.

Riese, W., 1925, Formprobleme des Gehirns. Uber die Hirnrinde der Wale, *J. Psychol. Neurol.* **31**:275–280.

Romer, A. S., 1960, *The Vertebrate Body*, 3rd ed., Saunders, Philadelphia.

Romer, A. S., 1966, *Vertebrate Paleontology*, 3rd ed., University of Chicago Press, Chicago.

Rose, J., and Woolsey, C., 1949, The relation of thalamic connections, cellular structure and evokable activity in the auditory region of the cat, *J. Comp. Neurol.* **91**:441–466.

Rose, M., 1926, Der Grundplan der Cortextektonic beim Delphin, *J. Psychol. Neurol.* **32**:161–169.

Sanides, F., 1968, The architecture of the cortical taste nerve areas in squirrel monkey *Saimiri sciureus* and their relationships to insular, sensorimotor and prefrontal regions, *Brain Res.* **8**:97–124.

Sanides, F., 1970, Functional architecture of motor and sensory cortices in primates in the light of a new concept of neocortex evolution, in: *The Primate Brain* (C. Noback and W. Montagna, eds.), Appleton–Century–Crofts, New York, pp. 137–208.

Sanides, F., 1972, Representation in the cerebral cortex and its areal lamination patterns, in: *The Structure and Function of Nervous Tissue*, Volume V (G. Bourne, ed.), Academic Press, New York, pp. 329–453.

Sanides, F., and Sanides, D., 1972, The "extraverted neurons" of the mammalian cerebral cortex, *Zeit. Anat. Entwickl.-Gesch.* **136**:272–293.

Slijper, E. J., 1962, *Whales*, Hutchinson, London, pp. 226–252.

Slijper, E. J., 1979, *Whales*, Cornell University Press, Ithaca, N.Y.

Sokolov, V. E., Ladygina, T. F., and Supin, A. Y., 1972, Localization of the sensory zones in the cerebral cortex of the dolphin, *Dokl. Akad. Nauk SSSR* **202**:490–493.

Stell, W. K., 1964, Correlated light and electron microscopy observations on Golgi preparations of goldfish retina, *J. Cell Biol.* **23**:89a.

Supin, A. Y., Mukhametov, L. M., Ladygina, T. F., Popov, V. V., Mass, A. M., and Polyakova, I. G., 1978, Neurophysiologic characteristics of the cerebral cortex in dolphins, in: *Electrophysiological Study of Dolphin Brain*, Academy of Sciences of the USSR, Moscow, pp. 29–85.

Tomilin, A. G., 1968, Factor promoting powerful development of the brain in Odontoceti, *Sov. Stud. Cetaceans* **31**:191–200.

Valverde, F., 1983, A comparative approach to neocortical organization based on the study of the brain of the hedgehog *Erinaceus europaeus*, in: *Ramón y Cajal's Contribution to the Neurosciences* (S. Grisolia, C. Guerri, F. Sampson, S. Norton, and F. Reinoso-Suarez, eds.), Elsevier, Amsterdam, pp. 149–170.

Valverde, F., 1986, Instrinsic neocortical organization: Some comparative aspects, *Neuroscience* **18**:1–23.

Valverde, F., and Facal-Valverde, M. V., 1986, Neocortical layers I and II of the hedgehog *Erinaceus europaeus*. I. Intrinsic organization, *Anat. Embryol.* **173**:413–430.

Valverde, F., and López-Mascaraque, L., 1981, Neocortical endeavor: Basic neuronal organization in the cortex of the hedgehog, in: *Glial and Neuronal Cell Biology* (E. A. Vidrio and S. Fedoroff, eds.), Liss, New York, pp. 281–290.

Wilson, R. B., 1933, The anatomy of the brain of the whale (*Balaenoptera sulfurea*), *J. Comp. Neurol.* **58**:419–480.

Zhukova, G. P., and Leontovich, T. A., 1964, Special features of neuronal structure and of topography of the reticular formation in Carnivora, *J. Higher Nerv. Act.* **14**:122–146.

Zvorykin, V. P., 1963, Morphological bases of ultrasonic and locational properties of the dolphin, *Arkh. Anat. Gistol. Embriol.* **45**:3–17.

Zvorykin, V. P., 1977, Principles of structural organization of the cetacean neocortex, *Arkh. Anat. Gistol. Embriol.* **72**:5–22.

14

Organization of the Cerebral Cortex in Monotremes and Marsupials

MARK ROWE

1. Evolutionary Relations of Marsupial, Monotreme, and Eutherian Mammals: Historical Aspects

The view that monotreme, marsupial, and placental orders of mammals formed an orderly progression in mammalian evolution arose in the 19th century. Monotremes were designated the Prototheria, or first mammals, based largely on their reptilian-like reproductive practice of laying eggs, while the marsupials were designated the Metatheria, or changed mammals, and were thought to form the next stage of mammalian evolution toward placental mammals—the Eutheria or complete mammals. However, these notions of a simple hierarchy in mammalian evolution are misguided in that each of the three orders has undergone its independent evolutionary development with perhaps major transformations having taken place within each order from the earliest forebears of that order (for reviews, see Tyndale-Biscoe, 1973; Clemens, 1977, 1979a,b; Griffiths, 1978; Archer, 1982; Dawson, 1983; Tyndale-Biscoe and Renfree, 1987). Furthermore, the reptilian-like precursors of these three mammalian orders may bear

MARK ROWE • School of Physiology and Pharmacology, University of New South Wales, Sydney, Australia 2033.

little resemblance to surviving reptiles as both the reptilian and the mammalian lines have evolved over independent courses for approximately 300 million years since the Carboniferous period (Dawson, 1983). The evolutionary line that was to lead to mammals probably underwent a reptilian-to-mammalian transition about 200 million years ago in the late Triassic Period (Fig. 1). The monotreme ancestors formed a separate line of mammalian evolution at about that time or, even earlier, emerged through the reptile-to-mammal barrier on a separate path from the therian mammals. Thus, mammalian evolutionary progress may have come from two broad stem lines, the therian mammals, from which placental and marsupial species have arisen, and the nontherian mammals that are now represented by present-day monotremes (Fig. 1). A more detailed representation of the marsupial radiation is given in Fig. 2 from Kirsch (1977).

The formation of distinct marsupial and placental lines in therian evolution took place only in the Cretaceous period between 136 and 64 million years ago (Fig. 1). Thus, the grouping of monotreme and marsupial orders in this chapter is not so much a reflection of their evolutionary proximity as it is their sharing of

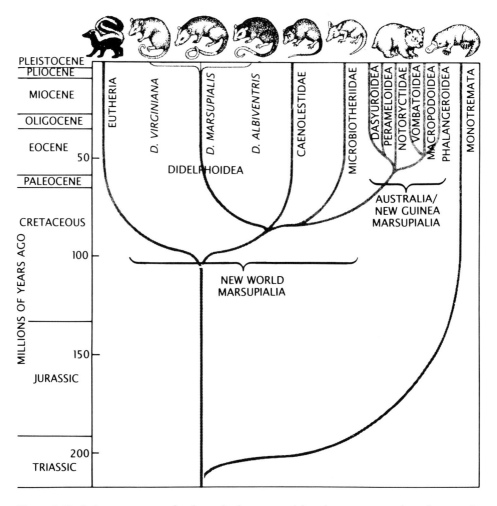

Figure 1. Evolutionary sequence for the eutherian, marsupial, and monotreme orders of mammals. (From Austad, 1988.)

the historical exclusion from the ranks of eutherian or *true* mammals. Indeed, there are probably fewer similarities between these two orders of noneutherian mammals than between marsupials and eutherians (Dawson, 1983).

2. Brain Studies in Marsupial and Monotreme Species

Studies of the brain and, in particular, the cerebral cortex in representatives from the marsupial and monotreme orders have been undertaken for three major reasons. First, comparative neurological analysis, at either an organizational or a functional level, may be of evolutionary importance in elucidating the archetypal features of the mammalian cerebral cortex and the transformations that have taken place in the course of evolution. Second, the analysis within individual species is of interest for the anatomical and functional specializations in the brain that can be correlated with the behavioral or ecological adaptations of individual species. Third, the noneutherian species offer enormous advantages for the experimental investigation of brain development. As birth takes place at a very primitive phase of ontogeny, many of the developmental stages that would occur within the relatively inaccessible uterus of the placental mammal take place within the maternal pouch and are therefore accessible for observation and manipulation (see Section 11).

The Cerebral Cortex in Relation to the Evolution of the Monotremata

The expectation that present-day monotremes may provide a window on the earliest forms of mammalian evolution was based, first, on their status as the oldest surviving order of mammals and, second, on their retention of reproductive mechanisms resembling their reptilian forebears. However, their retention of phylogenetically ancient mechanisms for reproduction need not mean that other body systems have been constrained in their evolutionary adaptability. Indeed, the marked differences between *Ornithorhynchus* and *Tachyglossus* in cortical surface anatomy (Figs. 3 and 4) suggest that, in this attribute at least, these two species of monotreme have developed in very different ways since taking their separate evolutionary paths about 30–50 million years ago in the Eocene or early Oligocene epoch of the Tertiary (Griffiths, 1978; Dawson, 1983). Thus, instead of sharing cortical attributes that distinguish them from marsupial and placental species, the platypus and echidna are distinguished from one another on account of the lissencephalic form of the platypus cortex compared with the elaborately fissured cortex of the echidna.

3. Indices of Brain and Cerebral Cortical Development

Many attempts have been made to quantify the extent of brain and cerebral cortical development in different mammals. These are based, for example, on measures of brain size, the degree of cortical folding, and measures of regional development within the cerebral cortex. Each of these is considered briefly in

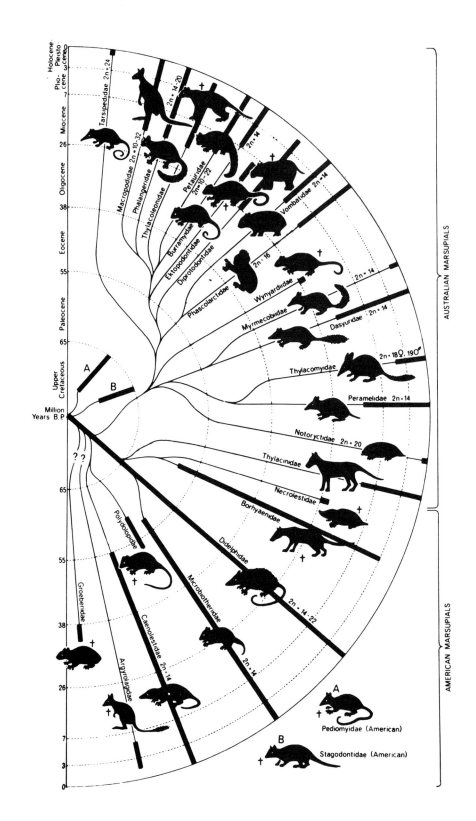

Tarsipedidae 2n = 24

2n = 14-20

†

2n = 14

Macropodidae 2n = 10-32

Phalangeridae

Petauridae 2n = 10-22

Thylacoleonidae

Burramyidae

Vombatidae 2n = 14

Ektopodontidae

†

Diprotodontidae

2n = 16

†

Phascolarctidae

Wynyardiidae

2n = 14

Myrmecobiidae

Dasyuridae 2n = 14

Thylacomyidae

2n = 18♀, 19♂

Peramelidae 2n = 14

Notoryctidae 2n = 20

Thylacinidae

Necrolestidae

Borhyaenidae

†

A

B

Million
Years B.P.

? ?

Polydolopidae

†

Didelphidae

Groeberidae

Microbiotheriidae

2n = 14-22

†

Caenolestidae 2n = 14

2n = 14

Argyrolagidae

†

A

†

Pediomyidae (American)

B

† Stagodontidae (American)

AUSTRALIAN MARSUPIALS

AMERICAN MARSUPIALS

Holocene
Pleisto-
cene
Plio-
cene
3
7
Miocene
26
Oligocene
38
Eocene
55
Paleocene
65
Upper
Cretaceous
65
55
38
26
7
3
0

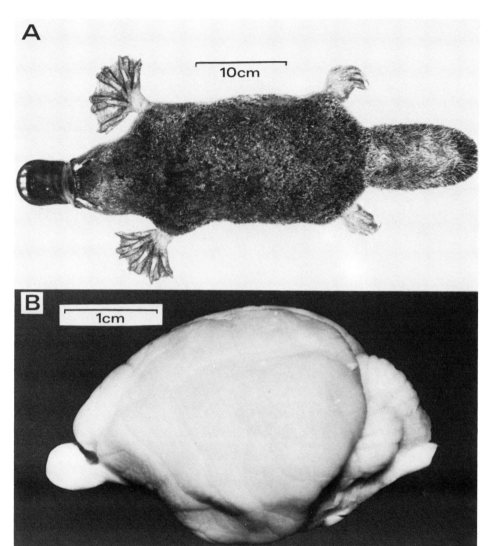

Figure 3. (A) Dorsal view of an adult female platypus (*Ornithorhynchus anatinus*) weighing 1.18 kg. (B) Lateral view of the lissencephalic brain of a platypus. The shallow surface markings do not represent a sulcal pattern but the impressions left on the cortical surface by large blood vessels; frontal pole of brain to the left. (From Bohringer and Rowe, 1977.)

Figure 2. Phylogeny of Marsupialia according to Kirsch (1977), incorporating serological, karyological, morphological, and paleontological data. In general, relative amounts of divergence from a radius indicate the degree of departure from primitive characters where this can be assessed. Wholly extinct families are indicated by a dagger, and the period for which fossils are known is shown by the thickened portion of each lineage. The range of chromosome numbers for each family is indicated, when known. All families listed as "American" are South American, except for Stagodontidae, which is only known from North America; Pediomyidae, which is North and possibly South American; and Didelphidae, which occurs in North America and was also present in Europe from Eocene to Miocene. Fossil data collated from several sources given in Kirsch's paper. The time intervals are not shown in exact proportion in order to preserve clarity in the branching pattern, nor the silhouettes drawn to scale. (Drawing by Frank Knight; figure and legend from Kirsch, 1977.)

this section before dealing with more detailed aspects of sensory and motor organization within the cerebral cortex of monotreme and marsupial species.

3.1. Brain Size and the Encephalization Index

Some quantitative indices of brain development have been based on the ratio of brain mass to total body mass, or on some closely related measures. These indices have been justified, in part, on the grounds that fossil data derived from endocast studies can then be included in the comparative analysis of brain development. Jerison (1973), a prominent advocate of these measures, has reviewed the historical background to these studies based on the contributions of Snell (1891), Dubois (1897), von Bonin (1937), and others, and has derived an encephalization quotient (EQ) which is the ratio of actual brain mass (E_i) for a given species, divided by the *expected* brain mass, E_e, for a mammalian species of a given body mass, P_i. The value of E_e is obtained from the equation $E_e = kP_i^{2/3}$,

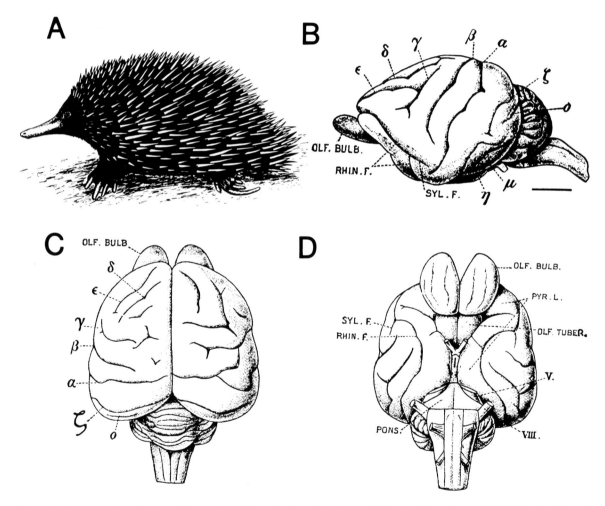

Figure 4. (A) Drawing of the echidna; the adult animal weighs about 3–5 kg; the rigid spines on the dorsal surface are firmly embedded; the nostrils and mouth are at the tip of the immobile beak. (From Lyne, 1967.) (B–D) Brain of the echida drawn from lateral, dorsal, and ventral views, respectively. (From Elliot Smith, 1902.) Bar = 1 cm.

which is derived from the overall relation between brain mass and body mass in living mammals (Jerison, 1973). The value of ⅔ for the exponent in this relation and the value for k (0.12) are based on the average values for living mammals.

On this EQ scale, Jerison estimates a value of 1 for the average living placental mammal with the range extending from about 0.25 for basal insectivores such as the hedgehog (*Erinaceus europaeus*) and the Madagascan tenrecs, through to values of about 6 or 7 for man and some cetaceans, such as the bottlenose dolphin (*Tursiops truncatus*).

Jerison concluded that the monotremes are relatively large-brained compared with most "primitive" living mammals. EQ values for echidnas were in the range 0.5–0.75 which places them in the range of values for "progressive" marsupials such as the kangaroo rather than "primitive" marsupials (e.g., opossum) or basal insectivores which have EQ values from about 0.25 to 0.4 (Jerison, 1973, p. 354).

Jerison (1961) has argued that marsupial species have smaller brains relative to body size than do placental mammals. However, this conclusion has been questioned by Meyer (1981) on the grounds that Jerison's observations were based principally on the *primitive* marsupial, the opossum.

Comparative measures of brain development within 89 Australian representatives of the order Marsupialia are summarized in Table I based on data from Nelson and Stephan (1982). As a basis for comparison, these authors assigned an encephalization index of 100 to the dasyurids based on the brain and body weight relations for 21 species excluding the Planigale species. Among the highest values found were those for the Macropodidae in which 31 species were examined. Within this group the Potoroinae had an average index of 166 and the Macropodinae 142. Another with a high index (over 200) is *Dactylopsila trivirgata,* a striped possum from northern Australia and New Guinea whose digital function in the forelimb is well developed for searching for ants and extracting them from crevices or holes in the bark of trees (Dawson, 1983).

Eutherian values of the encephalization index calculated by Nelson and Stephan (1982) for comparison with their marsupial indices, give an average

Table I. Encephalization Indices of Some Marsupials with Dasyuridae (100) as a Base[a]

Group	Encephalization index	Comments
Didelphidae	116 (75–137)	*Didelphis* spp. 75
Dasyuridae	100 (85–120)	Planigale species (39–61) omitted
Thylacinidae	148	
Peramelidae	99 (84–122)	
Thylacomyidae	128	*Macrotis* only
Phalangeridae	130 (120–140)	
Burramyidae	98 (89–105)	
Petauridae		
Petaurus-group	156 (139–171)	Including *Gymnobelideus* sp.
Pseudocheirus-group	83 (69–105)	Including *Schoinobates* sp.
Dactylopsila	224	From a single specimen
Macropodidae		
Potoroinae	166 (149–182)	*Hypsiprymnodon* sp. 176
Macropodinae	142 (104–176)	*Petrogale* spp. up to 176

[a]From Dawson (1983) based on the data of Nelson and Stephan (1982).

index of 60 for basal insectivorans and a value of about 100 for the Insectivora as a whole. Prosimians had average indices of 256 (based on 29 species) and simians 543. Nelson and Stephan concluded, based on their encephalization index as one indicator of evolutionary development, that the Australian marsupials are "above the grade of basal insectivorans, about the grade of progressive insectivorans and lower prosimians, but below higher prosimians and all simians."

As the EQ and similar measures permit comparisons of brain development only in terms of overall brain size, it has been argued by Meyer (1981) and others that quite different conclusions about comparative brain development may be reached if alternative measures are used, particularly measures of the extent of neocortical development, or measures based on nerve cell numbers or densities.

3.2. Regional Brain Development: Extent of the Neocortex in Monotremes and Marsupials

Although neocortical expansion distinguishes mammals from other vertebrates, measures of the extent of neocortex in the different mammalian orders fail to identify the Monotremata or Marsupialia as distinctly primitive relatives of placental mammals. Of the three major divisions of cortex, the neocortical component is larger than either the paleocortex or archicortex in the monotremes. In the platypus it represents about 48% of the cortex and in the echidna about 43% (Pirlot and Nelson, 1978).

In marsupial species, the proportion of neocortex is never as high as in some placental groups such as the primates and cetaceans where, for example, it occupies more than 95% of the cortex in man and the dolphin. However, surveys of marsupial representatives reviewed by Johnson (1977) have shown that those with the most extensive neocortex, such as the kangaroo with about 70% of cortex as neocortex, fall in the middle range of placental mammals (e.g., see Harman, 1947; Moeller, 1973). These surveys show that some marsupial species, for example, the opossum (*Didelphis virginiana*), have a less extensive neocortex (Harman, 1947). More recent observations (Meyer, 1981) show that in the Australian possum (*Trichosurus vulpecula*) and quokka wallaby (*Setonix brachyurus*) the neocortex forms 30–35% of total brain weight, which is similar to that found in the rat and rabbit—placental species of roughly similar size, and exceeds the proportion seen for neocortex in all placental species examined within the Insectivora by Stephan *et al.* (1970). Thus, it is not possible to identify monotremes and marsupials as being systematically less advanced than eutherian mammals either on grounds of overall brain size or on measures of neocortical development.

3.3. Cortical Folding as an Index of Brain Development

Although the acquisition of convolutions (i.e., gyrencephaly) within the cerebral cortex enables a greater area of cortex to be accommodated within the available cranial space, the presence or absence of convolutions may not be a reliable index of brain development. For example, the platypus brain is relatively large based on measures such as the encephalization index despite having a lissencephalic cortex. Furthermore, examples of an unfolded, or lissencephalic cortex are not confined to the monotreme ranks but are also present in marsupial and eutherian species, including primate representatives such as the marmoset (*Callithrix jacchus*). Other eutherians with a lissencephalic cortex include the rat, tree shrew, squirrel, and hedgehog, while marsupial examples include Dasyuridae such as the marsupial mole (*Notoryctes typhlops*), several Antechinus species, and the opossum (except for a small indentation forming the orbital sulcus or sulcus α; Johnson, 1977). In strict terms, no mammalian cerebral cortex is lissencephalic as all appear to have an infolding or indentation corresponding to the rhinal sulcus which marks the lateral boundary of neocortex with the paleocortex. Beyond this border the pyriform cortex shows a dense outermost layer of cells in both monotreme and marsupial species as it does in placental mammals (Abbie, 1940a; Johnson, 1977; Bohringer and Rowe, 1977).

As a general rule it seems that the degree of convolution in the cortex is related to body size rather than to any systematic differences among the three orders of mammals. Thus, the largest marsupials such as the kangaroos, the large wallabies, and the wombat all have prominent patterns of convolution (Fig. 5) as do the larger species of eutherian mammals (Johnson, 1977; Haight and Murray, 1981). Furthermore, within the monotremes, the echidnas are bigger than the platypus and have elaborate patterns of infolding in the cortex (Figs. 3 and 4).

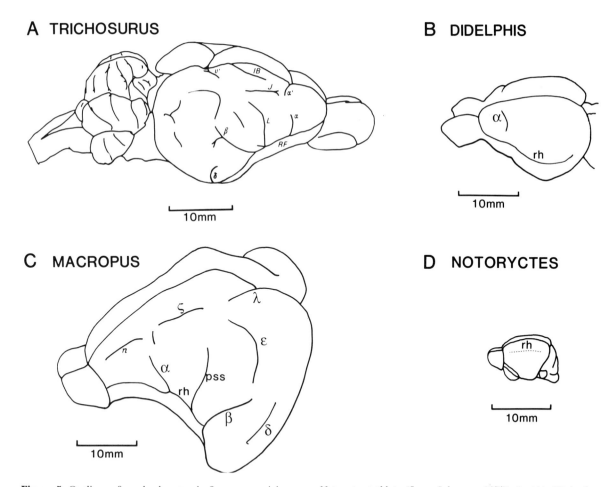

Figure 5. Outlines of cerebral cortex in four marsupial species. (A) *Trichosurus vulpecula* (from Haight and Neylon, 1978b). (B) *Didelphis virginiana* (from Cabana and Martin, 1984). (C) *Macropus eugenii* (from Johnson, 1977). (D) *Notoryctes typhlops* (from Johnson, 1977). In (A), IB is the interbrachial sulcus; J, jugular sulcus; L, labial sulcus; RF, rhinal fissure. In (B–D) rh is rhinal sulcus. In (C), pss is pseudosylvian sulcus.

4. Sulcal and Laminar Patterns within the Cerebral Cortex of Marsupial and Monotreme Species

4.1. The Marsupial Cerebral Cortex

As part of his comprehensive review of the marsupial central nervous system, Johnson (1977) has outlined some of the confusion surrounding the identification of sulci in the marsupial cerebral cortex. As the sulcal patterns have evolved separately within each of the three orders of mammals, Johnson has argued for the adoption of distinctive designations for each order. In the Marsupialia, he advocates the Greek letter nomenclature used by Ziehen (1897) for sulci other than the rhinal—the most consistent sulcal boundary, being present in almost all members of the three orders—and the inappropriately designated Sylvian sulcus. As Johnson observes, the latter term is properly applied only to primates. A detailed description of sulcal charcteristics in different groups of Australian marsupials may be found in the analysis by Haight and Murray (1981).

Apart from the rhinal sulcus, the most consistent sulcal landmark in masupials is sulcus α (Ziehen, 1897) seen for three species in Fig. 5. Sulcus α, also called the orbital sulcus by Elliot Smith (1902), is present in all marsupials except the smaller species (Fig. 5D) of Dasyuridae, Didelphidae, Antechinus, and Sminthopsis (Johnson, 1977). In larger marsupials including *Macropus*, other sulci appear as seen in Fig. 5A,C.

Although Johnson (1977) has commented on the "remarkable consistency in the infoldings that develop in the brains of all marsupials," others (Haight and Neylon, 1978a) have described an "unusual variability" from animal to animal in sulcal depths in the possum (*Trichosurus vulpecula*). These authors felt that the variability exceeded any they had seen in placental mammals or in the American didelphid marsupials. However, Hassler and Muhs-Clement (1964) in their detailed studies on the cat cerebral cortex have reported striking variability in sulcal patterns in this placental animal, and even between hemispheres in a single animal. It therefore remains uncertain whether there are systematic differences in sulcal variability from one gyrencephalic species to another.

4.2. The Monotreme Cerebral Cortex

In the Monotremata, the platypus has only the rhinal sulcus (Elliot Smith, 1902) whereas the echidna has an elaborate pattern of sulci, differing from those of other mammals and designated by Elliot Smith using Greek characters (see Fig. 4). The most consistent are sulci α, ζ, and β (Elliot Smith, 1902; Hines, 1929; Burkitt, 1934; Lende, 1964) each of which runs mediolaterally with ζ located in the posterior half of the hemisphere and β located more rostrally. Other sulci are less consistent. In some cases the sulci mark boundaries between cytoarchitectonically different regions; for example, in the echidna, sulcus α separates a posterior granular or koniocortex, from an anterior agranular one (Schuster, 1910; Abbie, 1938, 1940a; see also Section 5.3.2).

Abbie (1940a) has argued on the basis of cytoarchitectural analysis that in both species of monotreme the neocortex has evolved from expansion of the two older cortical regions—the hippocampus and the pyriform cortex. He concluded that the parahippocampal contribution is the more substantial in the platypus but that roughly equal contributions are made in the echidna.

5. The Somatosensory Cortex

5.1. Electrophysiological Studies of Somatosensory Cortex: Historical Aspects

The development of methods in the 1930s and 1940s for recording cortical potentials evoked by peripheral stimuli introduced a powerful technique for identifying the regions of representation of particular sensory inputs to the cortex and for revealing the organizational pattern within these areas (Gerard *et al.*, 1936; Penfield and Boldrey, 1937; Adrian, 1940, 1941; Marshall *et al.*, 1941). The recognition that a given sensory modality may have dual or multiple representation in the cortex arose from the early evoked potential studies which demonstrated two spatially separate areas of somatosensory representation identified as the primary and secondary somatosensory areas (SI and SII) which in the cat are in the postcruciate gyrus and the anterior ectosylvian gyrus, respectively (Adrian, 1940, 1941; Woolsey and Fairman, 1946). It also became apparent that the representation area for a particular sensory modality coincided with a specific cytoarchitectural region within the cortex.

The evoked potential mapping studies were pursued by Woolsey in a variety of placental mammals and showed that the somatosensory areas in different species had an ordered pattern of representation reflecting the point-to-point relations on the body surface. This somatotopic pattern was identified in all species studied and suggests that the preservation of topographic order is important for sensory function, in particular for the localization of stimuli on the body surface and for the resolution of spatial detail in objects felt or contacted by the body surface. This pattern has its equivalent in the retinotopic and cochleotopic organization of the visual and auditory cortex respectively as well as in the somatotopic organization of the motor cortex.

One of the striking findings in the cortical somatosensory maps was the apparently disproportionate allocation of cortical space to the representation of different body parts. For example, in the rat and rabbit, the cortical map has a greatly magnified representation of the face (Woolsey, 1952, 1958). The face also has a prominent representation in the cat and monkey cerebral cortex but increasingly large areas of cortex are allocated to the distal limbs, in particular the forelimb in the case of the monkey. In all species studied the trunk and proximal regions of the limbs occupy much smaller areas of the cortical map than their body size would suggest. However, these patterns of somatosensory representation are consistent with the behavioral specialization of individual species and are based on the innervation density of the different body parts rather than the actual size of those parts.

5.2. Organization of Somatosensory Cortex in Marsupials

The extension of sensory mapping studies to nonplacental mammals commenced in the 1950s with the somatosensory mapping in the Australian possum (*Trichosurus vulpecula*) by Adey and Kerr (1954; Fig. 6) and was followed by

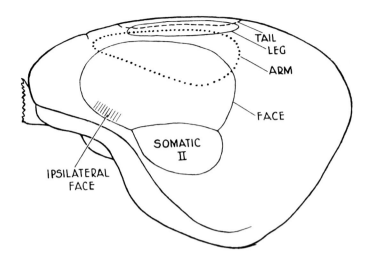

Figure 6. Map of deep somatic representation in *Trichosurus vulpecula*. The shaded portion of the face region of somatic area I yielded only ipsilateral responses. (From Adey and Kerr, 1954.)

sensorimotor maps for the opossum and the wallaby (Bodemer and Towe, 1963; Lende, 1963a–c). The primary somatosensory area of cortex in these species occupies relatively much more of the cortex than is the case, for example, in the rabbit, extending mediolaterally from the medial surface of the hemisphere almost to the rhinal sulcus (Figs. 6 and 7). The maps display the same somatotopic pattern identified in placental species, namely tail and lower leg representation located dorsomedially in the hemisphere with a progressive shift to more rostral body parts in more lateral locations (Figs. 6–8). The rostrocaudal orientation of the body representation was also reported to correspond with the placental plan with trunk and upper limbs represented caudally and the apices of the limbs more rostrally (Figs. 7 and 8). Lende (1963b,c) also concluded that the motor map in the opossum and the wallaby was coincident with the somatosensory one (Fig. 8) forming a sensorimotor amalgam (see Section 9.2).

The SI map for all three species included a large face and substantial distal limb representation. In the opossum the face area was predominantly a maxillary representation but in the wallaby both maxillary and mandibular regions occupied very large cortical areas (Fig. 8; Lende, 1963a,c). Although the tail and hindlimbs are prominent structures in the wallaby their representations occupy only small areas of SI. In contrast, the tail in both *Trichosurus* and *Didelphis* had a substantial representation, which probably reflects a high peripheral innervation density associated with the tail's prehensile function in these species (Adey and Kerr, 1954; Lende, 1963a,c).

Substantial bilateral representation was reported for the SI map in *Trichosurus* (Adey and Kerr, 1954) in contrast to the predominantly or exclusively contralateral representation found for placental mammals and for the opossum and wallaby. This may be related to the *Trichosurus* map being based mainly on electrical stimulation of subcutaneous structures. Although it was found that the bilateral representation survived a curarizing block of reflex contractions elicited *bilaterally* by the electrical stimuli, there were nevertheless, local muscle twitches at the site of electrical stimulation (Adey and Kerr, 1954). It is therefore possible that the mechanical disturbances associated with these twitches may have spread

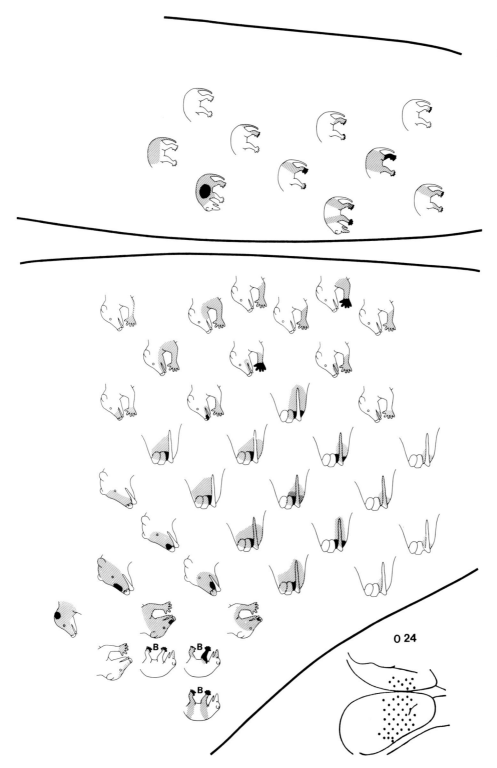

Figure 7. Tactile representation in *Didelphis virginiana*. Results of tactile stimulation in one opossum showing the extension of representation onto the medial wall of the hemisphere. Medial wall pictured above lateral wall. The shading on each figurine indicates the area of skin from which cortical potentials were evoked at each recording site indicated by the dots in the inset. Black areas signify maximal responses and cross-hatch signifies lesser responses. Label B indicates bilateral response. Points generally 2 mm apart in horizontal and vertical lines. 0 24 refers to experiment number. (From Lende, 1963a.)

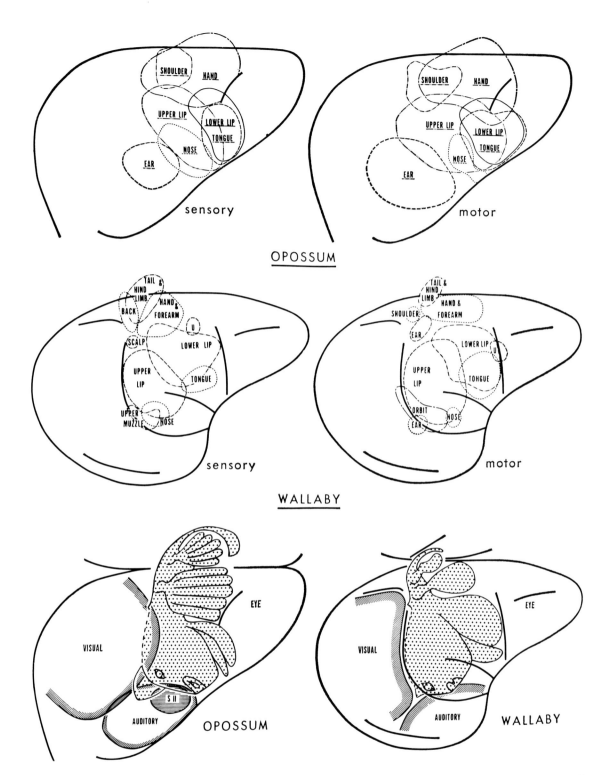

Figure 8. Sensory and motor representation in the cerebral cortex of the opossum and the wallaby. Drawings show the neocortical surface of the right cerebral hemisphere with the frontal pole to the right. Fissures are indicated by heavier lines. The inferior border of the hemisphere sloping down from the frontal pole is the rhinal sulcus in each case. (Top) Opossum. Sensory centers for selected body parts shown on the left, and motor centers shown on the right. Note correspondence of locations. (Middle) Wallaby. Note correspondence of sensory and motor centers. Upper muzzle means the dorsal portion of the snout between the nose proper and the eyes. Orbit refers to eye closure. U indicates a small "upper lip area" separate from the main area. (Bottom) Homunculus-like pictures of sensorimotor body representation in the opossum and the wallaby. Above the lateral aspect of each hemisphere is a partial outline of the adjacent medial aspect which contains tail and hindlimb representations. The borders of visual and auditory areas are indicated. The small second somatic sensory area in the opossum is labeled S II. Stimulation in the region labeled "EYE" gave responses from the eye. (Figure and legend from Lende, 1963c.)

through the experimental table to the opposite side of the body exciting the exquisitely sensitive Pacinian corpuscle receptors that could give rise to the *apparently* ipsilateral cortical evoked potentials (see Bennett *et al.*, 1980; Section 5.2.2). It is of interest that when Adey and Kerr used only light tactile stimuli, mainly hair deflection, they found only a contralateral representation in agreement with the organization in opossum, wallaby, and placental mammals.

The SI pattern of representation identified in the opossum, wallaby, and possum studies has been reported to apply also in the Australian marsupial wombat, *Vombatus ursinus* (Johnson *et al.*, 1973), and the South American opossum, *Didelphis azarae azarae*, (Magalhães-Castro and Saraiva, 1971). Furthermore, detailed histological examination within the SI face area in *Trichosurus vulpecula* suggests that the barrel-like aggregations of lamina IV cells identified in certain placental rodents (Woolsey and Van der Loos, 1970; Van der Loos and Welker, 1985) are also present in this marsupial species (Fig. 9; Weller, 1972; Weller and Haight, 1973), although they are apparently not present in the opossum (Weller, 1972; Pubols *et al.*, 1976). In the mouse and rat the barrels are arranged in rows in the cortex that correspond to the rows of vibrissal follicles on the whisker pad of the upper lip. Furthermore, each barrel is related to a single vibrissal follicle, an arrangement that appears to apply at a functional level as well (Welker, 1976; Simons, 1978). However, although the barrel-like cellular aggregations are found in the area of whisker representation in the possum cortex there is a marked discrepancy between the number of barrels and the number of vibrissal follicles (Weller and Haight, 1973).

5.2.1. Microelectrode Mapping of Marsupial Somatosensory Cortex

Further details of the marsupial somatosensory cortex, in particular for the area of face representation in the opossum, were studied with microelectrode mapping by Pubols *et al.* (1976) who found a double representation of the contralateral mystacial vibrissae and rhinarium (Figs. 10 and 11). The two areas which were adjacent, mirror images were designated the medial and lateral trigeminal areas, MTA and LTA, respectively (Pubols *et al.*, 1976). The LTA occupied 2.5 times the MTA and both fell within the area of projection of the opossum ventrobasal (VB) thalamic nuclei (Pubols, 1968; Killackey and Ebner, 1972, 1973; Pubols *et al.*, 1976). In both MTA and LTA the receptive fields were contralateral. Furthermore, within the vibrissal area, responses were elicited by deflection of only a single vibrissa at almost half of the recording sites. At other sites deflection of two to five vibrissae was effective. In the rhinarial representation areas of MTA and LTA the receptive fields were on average 3.3 mm^2, or ten times larger than those of primary rhinarial afferents (Pubols *et al.*, 1973). No difference in neuronal receptive field size was found between the MTA and LTA, although within the vibrissal area there was greater specificity in MTA than LTA for the direction of vibrissal deflection. The eutherian equivalents of these two face areas, and an additional more laterally placed area of somatic representation (Pubols *et al.*, 1976; Pubols, 1977), are considered in the next section.

5.2.2. The Second Somatosensory Area (SII) in the Marsupial Cerebral Cortex

A small area, identified as an SII area, was found lateral to the SI map in both the possum and opossum (Figs. 6–8 and 11; Adey and Kerr, 1954; Lende,

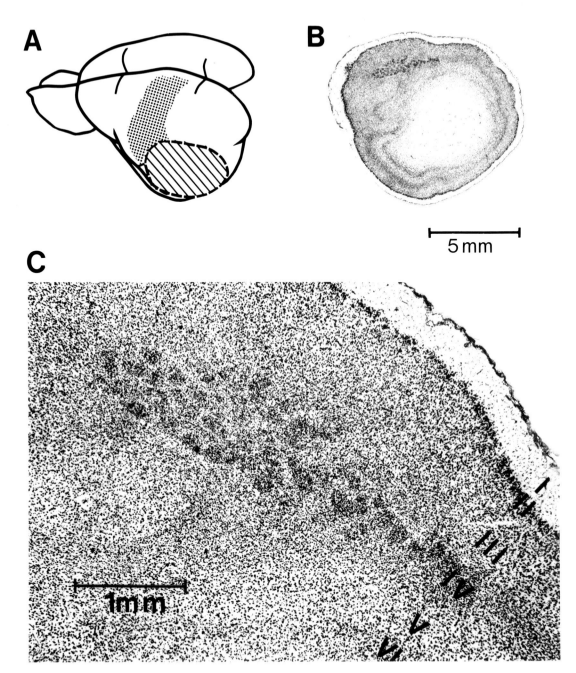

Figure 9. Barrel-like aggregation of cells in marsupial sensory cortex. (A) Dorsolateral view of the cortex of *Trichosurus vulpecula* showing the position of the section shown in B (light shading) in relation to the position of the entire cytoarchitectonic field (stippling). (B) Photomicrograph of parasagittal, Nissl-stained section showing clumps of Nissl-stained cells in layer IV. (C) Enlarged view of the cell clumps seen in B. At the right of the photomicrograph the plane of section is nearly perpendicular to layer IV: at the left, the plane of section is nearly tangential to layer IV. Neocortical laminae are identified by roman numerals at the right. Thionin, 30 μm. (From Weller, 1972.)

1963a; Pubols *et al.*, 1976; Pubols, 1977). Although SII was not found in the wallaby, Lende (1963c, 1969) concluded that it may lie within the unexplored fissure bordering the primary sensorimotor area in this animal. In the opossum, in which Lende also mapped visual and auditory areas, it was found that SII overlapped the auditory area, as seen in Fig. 8, from Lende (1963c). Adey and Kerr (1954) reported that for the possum SII area, all parts of the body are represented; that considerable overlap of different body areas is found, and that the representation is bilateral. Similar observations were made for the opossum (Pubols *et al.*, 1976; Pubols, 1977) using microelectrode mapping in the small area of bilateral representation lateral to and segregated from the topographically organized region of body representation (Fig. 11).

Pubols *et al.* (1976) speculated on whether this small lateral area was an SII area and on the identity of the medial trigeminal area (MTA) and lateral trigeminal area (LTA) of the opossum cortex, in particular in relation to their homologies in placental mammals. One possibility they suggested was that the area of bilateral representation was a part of SII and that the MTA was the SI area for head and face representation. LTA, they proposed, may represent a separate area from SI, unique to the Virginia opossum, that was neither an SII nor an SIII area. However, one of their alternative proposals was that MTA was an SI face area, while LTA was the opossum equivalent of the face component of the *rostral* SII area of the cat and monkey (Carreras and Anderson, 1963; Whitsel *et al.*, 1969) and the bilateral area was a homologue of the *caudal* SII area of the cat and monkey. Although Pubols (1977) later favored the view that the bilateral area constituted the whole of the opossum SII area, this earlier interpretation (Pubols *et al.*, 1976) recognizes the heterogeneity of the area originally designated SII. Furthermore, it is consistent with the increasingly recognized view that the core area of SII, often identified as the *rostral* area of SII in cat and monkey, receives thalamic VB input, has a well-organized topography, little or no ipsilateral input, and no auditory input (Carreras and Anderson, 1963; Bennett *et al.*, 1980; Robinson and Burton, 1980; Fisher *et al.*, 1983; Burton, 1986). In contrast, areas caudal to the topographically organized area of

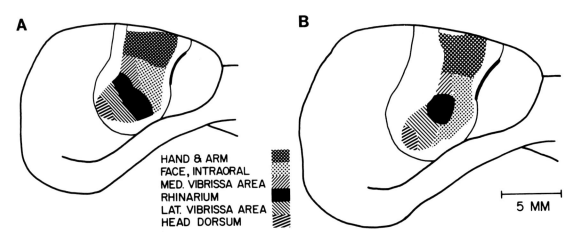

Figure 10. General organization of right opossum cortical somatic sensory receiving area for contralateral cutaneous surfaces as revealed by (A) the evoked potential technique and (B) microelectrode recording. Solid line represents boundaries as originally defined by Lende (1963a). Shaded areas in A include only those recording loci yielding large "focal" evoked potentials. (From Pubols *et al.*, 1976.)

SII have thalamic input from nuclei other than VB, have poor topographic precision, and evidence of both bilateral somatosensory inputs and auditory inputs (Carreras and Anderson, 1963; Burton, 1986). The absence of bilateral convergence on neurons of the topographically organized area of SII in the cat was identified by Bennett *et al.* (1980), but only after taking precautions to minimize direct spread of mechanical stimuli from one side of the body to the

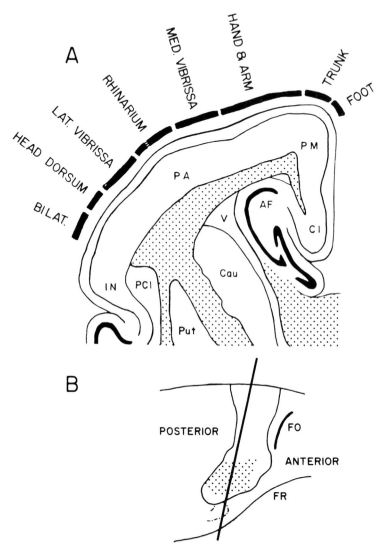

Figure 11. Somatosensory representation in the opossum cortex. (A) A near-transverse section through dorsal half of one hemisphere of opossum somatic sensory cortex, showing (thick lines above cortex) the "sensory sequence" of body representation, and their approximate linear extent on the dorsolateral cortical surface. The interruption in the rhinarium segment separates MTA from LTA, and the segment labeled "BILAT." corresponds to the region of bilateral representation (see text). (B) Dorsolateral view of right neocortex. The heavy line passing through the cortex indicates the plane of section in A. In B, the thin solid line depicts the border of the contralateral tactile receiving area, the area filled with dots is LTA, and the dot–dash line represents the border of the area of bilateral representation. AF, Ammon's formation; Cau, caudate nucleus; CI, cingulate cortex; FO, orbital fissure; FR, rhinal fissure; IN, insular cortex; PA, parietal cortex; PCl, paraclaustrum; PM, parietomarginal cortex; Put, putamen; V, lateral ventricle. (From Pubols *et al.*, 1976.)

other. Unless this was done, in this case by placing the animal and its limbs on a foam rubber pad, it was commonly found that neurons responded to mechanical stimulation of the ipsilateral as well as the contralateral limb. In large part the possible artifactual identification of a bilateral input to this area of SII may be a consequence of the prominent representation of Pacinian corpuscle inputs in SII (Bennett *et al.*, 1980; Ferrington and Rowe, 1980; Fisher *et al.*, 1983; Rowe *et al.*, 1985). Without precautions, the exquisite sensitivity of these receptors enables them to respond to mechanical disturbances spreading through the experimental table to the opposite side of the body.

If the LTA does represent a topographically organized region of SII in the opossum it may mean that there is an incomplete representation of the body in the topographically organized area of SII, or that other body parts have a rather inconspicuous representation as limb and trunk areas were only identified outside SI in the small lateral area of bilateral representation (Pubols *et al.*, 1976). However, another possibility is that the bilateral input and poorer topography in the small lateral area might be a consequence of mechanical spread of stimuli. It is perhaps relevant in this regard that Pubols *et al.* (1976) noted that more intense mechanical stimuli were needed to activate neurons in this area than in the SI area.

5.3. Organization of Somatosensory Cortex in Monotremes

Although there are only three surviving monotreme species, all studies of cortical sensorimotor function have been confined to the two Australian species—*Ornithorhynchus anatinus*, the platypus, and *Tachyglossus aculeatus*, the echidna. The third species is also an echidna, *Zaglossus bruijni*, but it is rare and confined in its distribution to the remote mountain forests of New Guinea (Griffiths, 1978). The remarkable contrast between the platypus with its lissencephalic cerebral cortex and the echidna with its large and elaborately fissured cortex has intrigued comparative neurologists from the earliest studies (Elliot Smith, 1902; Burkitt, 1934). However, systematic electrophysiological analysis of sensory cortex in these species was not undertaken until the 1960s and 1970s with the studies in the echidna by Lende (1964, 1969) and Allison and Goff (1972), and in the platypus by Bohringer and Rowe (1977).

5.3.1. Functional Organization of Somatosensory Cortex in the Echidna

The somatosensory area in the echidna was found (Lende, 1964) in a most unusual cortical location relative to both placental and marsupial species. It occupies a lateral position in the posterior region of the hemisphere which, for the most part, lies between the prominent sulcus α which formed an anterior boundary, and sulcus ζ which formed a posterior boundary (Fig. 12; see also Fig. 4). At its lateral margin the somatosensory area extended to the rhinal sulcus. However, the most striking departure from placental and marsupial precedent was seen with the medial boundary which was found on the midlateral surface of the cortex directly abutting the lateral border of the visual cortex. The location of this border between somatosensory and visual cortex approximated the backward bend often seen in sulcus α (see Figs. 12 and 13) and identified as the genu of α (Lende, 1964). At its posterior border the somatosensory area abuts the auditory cortex (Figs. 12 and 13).

The tight grouping of somatosensory, auditory, and visual areas in the posterior region of the hemisphere leaves no unidentified intervening areas that might be termed association cortex, although there is a very large expanse of frontal cortex that is free of somatosensory, visual, auditory, and motor function (Lende, 1964; Allison and Goff, 1972; Section 10). Lende (1964) described the

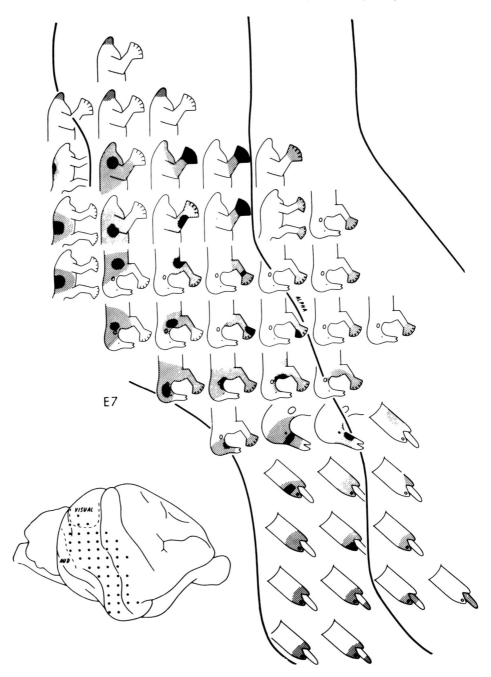

Figure 12. Somatic sensory field in one echidna. Key shows straight right lateral view of brain, frontal pole to the right. Format as in Fig. 7. Visual and auditory borders in this animal are indicated by dashed lines. Dots in key 2 mm apart. (From Lende, 1964.)

arrangement of the three major sensory areas of the echidna cortex as a rotational dislocation of the areal relations found in placental species. Thus, the somatosensory area is displaced downward and backward, the auditory area upward, and the visual area upward and forward.

Despite its unusual location, the somatosensory cortex of the echidna had the common mammalian internal organization for SI, with the tail represented uppermost and areas for hindlimb, trunk, forelimb, and face represented at progressively more lateral positions (Fig. 12). Furthermore, the rostrocaudal pattern of representation illustrated in Fig. 12 shows that the limb apices are represented anterior to the axial regions of the body, again in conformity with the orientation reported to apply generally in placental mammals (Woolsey, 1958). Lende (1964) commented on the large allocation of cortical space to the snout and tongue representations in the echidna which reflects the behavioral importance of these parts in the ant-eating habits of the animal (Griffiths, 1978). Tongue representation consistently extended in front of sulcus α but this was not the case for the forelimb although instances of this were found as seen in Fig. 12. Lende (1964) concluded that the area in front of sulcus α was predominantly a motor area separate from the motor area that overlies the somatosensory area behind sulcus α (see Section 9.3.1).

Although Lende was unable to decide whether the area behind sulcus α was principally a somatosensory or a motor area, its somatosensory attributes were in accord with it being the SI area for the echidna. However, in contrast to placental and marsupial species, no evidence was found for an SII area, although it was sought specifically in a number of experiments (Lende, 1969). Although Lende acknowledged the possibility of an SII area being present in the less accessible region of cortex behind the identified SI area, he felt that this was unlikely.

In more recent observations on the sensory cortex of the echidna, Allison

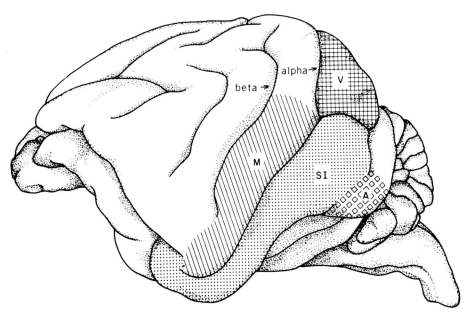

Figure 13. Diagram of the left side of the echidna brain showing locations of motor and sensory areas defined by Lende (1964). M, motor area (MI); SI, first somatic sensory area; V, visual area; A, auditory area. Sulci alpha and beta are indicated. (From Lende and Welker, 1980.)

and Goff (1972) reported that the configuration of both early and late components of the evoked potentials recorded over somatosensory, auditory, and visual cortical areas were very similar to those of placental mammals. These observations imply that similar intracortical mechanisms underlie these evoked potentials in monotremes and eutherians.

5.3.2. Cytoarchitecture and Thalamic Connections of Somatosensory Cortex in the Echidna

The region of cortex in which the somatosensory and motor areas were identified in the echidna comprise three cytoarchitectonic fields (Fig. 14; Ulinski, 1984). In the region of somatosensory and motor overlap there are two fields, a caudal one (labeled c in Fig. 14A) which includes the exposed region of the post-α-gyrus and the caudal wall of sulcus α, and a rostral field (labeled r in Fig. 14A), extending from near the base of sulcus α up the anterior wall of sulcus α where it meets the purely motor area of representation. The latter (Fig. 14B) is characterized by a thin lamina IV and a lamina V populated with large pyramidal cells, and corresponds with part of the agranular PH4 area of Abbie (1940a). Of the two fields in the somatosensory area (Fig. 14C,D), Ulinski (1984) found that both had a well-developed lamina IV but differed in lamina V, where the caudal field had a small number of medium-sized pyramidal cells while the rostral area had large numbers of large pyramidal cells. The caudal field probably corresponds to the PPy3 area of Abbie (1940a) whereas the rostral field is in Abbie's PH4.

The caudal and rostral fields of somatosensory cortex received thalamic input selectively from the ventroposterior nucleus. Ulinski (1984) suggested that, moving rostrocaudally, the three cytoarchitectonic areas identified in the somatosensorimotor cortex may be the monotreme equivalent of the placental cytoarchitectonic areas 4, 3a, and 3b, respectively. He speculated that their presence in a monotreme representative means that they constitute a basic characteristic of the mammalian neocortex.

Lende's comparative analysis of cortical organization led to his hypothesis (Lende, 1969) that the three great divisions of living mammals have evolved from a primordial form with a pattern of cortical organization in which somatic sensorimotor as well as visual and auditory areas were largely superimposed. His hypothesis was based on observations on species that have been considered close to archetypal mammalian forms, namely, the hedgehog from the order Insectivora, as a representative of placental mammals (Lende and Sadler, 1967); the opossum and wallaby from the marsupial order (Lende, 1963a–c), and the echidna from the order Monotremata (Lende, 1964). The extent of sensory and motor overlap in cortex for these three groups was greater for the insectivoran and marsupial representatives than for the echidna (Lende, 1969). However, it is not known whether the elaborately fissured cortex of the echidna represents a greater degree of evolutionary change from the hypothetical primordial cortex than is the case in the cortex of the hedgehog, the opossum, or indeed in the lissencephalic cortex of the platypus. Therefore, we are still unable to say whether the platypus conforms more closely than the echidna to an archetypal mammalian cortical pattern that is assumed to have evolved from the lissencephalic dorsal pallium of reptiles during the Triassic period (Goldby and Gamble, 1957).

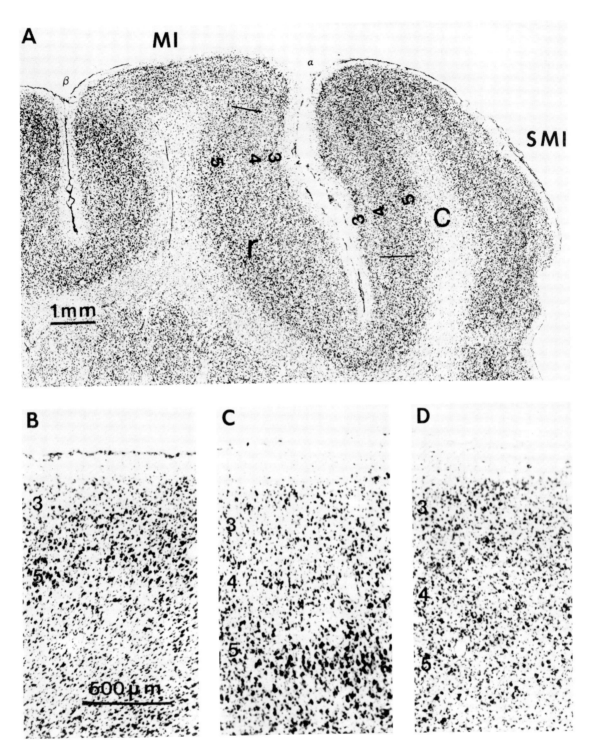

Figure 14. Cytoarchitecture of somatosensory motor cortex in *Tachyglossus*. (A) A coronal section through sulcus alpha and beta shows the cytoarchitecture of the cortex that surrounds sulcus alpha. The physiologically defined somatosensory cortex (SMI) contains two cytoarchitectonic fields. The caudal field (c) comprises most of the postalpha gyrus. The rostral field (r) extends from the floor of sulcus alpha onto the caudal bank of the prealpha gyrus. (B–D) Higher magnification views of the three cortical fields. (B) The cortex in the physiologically defined motor area (MI). (C) The cortex in the rostral field of SMI. (D) The cortex in the caudal field of SMI. (From Ulinski, 1984.)

5.3.3. Functional Organization of Somatosensory Cortex in the Platypus

With electrophysiological mapping of the platypus cerebral cortex, Bohringer and Rowe (1977) found that somatosensory and motor areas were not coincident (see Section 9.3.2), and that visual and auditory areas lay predominantly separate from the somatosensory area (see Sections 6.2 and 7.2). However, based on evoked potential methods, some overlap was found between auditory and visual areas (see Sections 6.2 and 7.2 and Fig. 28).

The somatosensory mapping in the platypus cortex was carried out using evoked potential and microelectrode recording procedures, while peripheral stimulation was based on electrical or mechanical stimuli applied to both sides of the body in order to test systematically for the presence of bilateral representation within the somatosensory cortex (Bohringer, 1977; Bohringer and Rowe, 1977).

Somatosensory evoked potentials had the usual biphasic configuration, consisting of an initial positive-going deflection followed by a larger negative-going component (Fig. 15). The latency of the initial positive wave following electrical stimulation of contralateral body sites was 5 msec for inputs from the animal's bill, 7 msec for forelimb, and 11 msec for hindlimb. The representation was purely contralateral as no responses could be evoked from ipsilateral stimulus

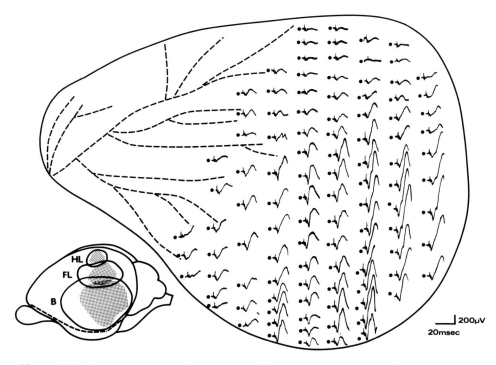

Figure 15. Evoked potentials (positivity downwards) recorded from the cortical surface of the platypus following bipolar stimulation of the anterolateral margin of the contralateral bill (1 V, 100 μsec pulse). Each recording was made from the position indicated by the dot at the left of the trace. Dotted lines indicate positions of large blood vessels in frontal region of hemisphere; view of hemisphere and whole brain (inset) from dorsolateral aspect. Stippled area in inset represent focal projection sites and include sites at which positive-going responses exceed 100 μV for bill (B), 30 μV for forelimb (FL) and 10 μV for hindlimb (HL). Zones between stippling and continuous lines include sites from which smaller responses could be recorded. (From Bohringer and Rowe, 1977.)

sites including the anterolateral margin of the ipsilateral bill (Bohringer and Rowe, 1977). As seen in Fig. 15, the responses to stimulation of the bill could be recorded over a very large area of the dorsolateral surface of the hemisphere. At each of the surface points indicated by the dots in Fig. 15, recordings were made following bill, forelimb, and hindlimb stimulation, but only responses to bill stimulation have been illustrated in the figure. Isopotential contour maps based on the amplitude of the positive-going evoked potential were constructed for the three stimulus sites as indicated in the inset in Fig. 15. The stippled areas indicate the focal projection sites and the zone between the stippling and the surrounding continuous line represents a region from which small evoked potentials could be recorded.

The somatosensory area was found (Bohringer and Rowe, 1977) with both evoked potential (Fig. 15) and unitary recording (Figs. 16–18) to lie predominantly within the posterior half of the hemisphere as was the case in the echidna (Lende, 1964). However, in contrast to the echidna, the area of representation extended from the midline over the whole mediolateral extent of the hemisphere to the region of the rhinal sulcus (Figs. 16–18). The mediolateral sequence of body representation agreed with the classical SI organization in placental and marsupial species, with the hindlimb representation medial and forelimb and face progressively more lateral (Figs. 16–18 and 28).

5.3.4. Is the Second Somatosensory Area (SII) Present in Monotremes?

As no evidence was found for an SII area in the exposed dorsolateral region of the platypus cortex (Fig. 17), we explored the buried ventral regions of the hemisphere by driving microelectrodes through from the dorsal surface as seen in Fig. 18 for the reconstructed electrode tracks in three anteroposterior planes (A–C) each separated by 2 mm. The most anterior plane, A, was almost three quarters of the way back from the frontal pole of the hemisphere. In the course of each track, neurons were examined for their responsiveness to tactile stimulation of the body surface and, in addition, electrical stimuli were applied to the distal forelimb every 2 sec in order to facilitate the detection, by means of either evoked potential or unitary responses, of an SII locus of forelimb representation. Bill stimulation is less satisfactory for identifying an SII area as cranial inputs to SI and SII show some overlap in most species examined (Woolsey and Fairman, 1946; Darian-Smith et al., 1966; Pubols et al., 1976). Within each plane of penetration, neurons with tactile receptive fields were encountered within the dorsal regions of the cerebral cortex, and at depths of 5–10 mm below the surface in the thalamus (Fig. 18). In the ventral regions of cortex, spontaneously active neurons were isolated; however, no peripheral receptive field could be found except in ventrolateral regions near the rhinal sulcus where neurons with receptive fields on the bill were found in penetrations 6 and 7 in plane C (Fig. 18). Penetrations through lateral cortical regions in other experiments demonstrated a continuous representation of the bill from the dorsal part of the hemisphere around to the region of the rhinal sulcus (Bohringer and Rowe, 1977). These investigations revealed no evidence for an SII area. As this was also the case in Lende's (1964) study on the echidna, it appears that the somatosensory cortex in monotremes may differ from mammals of both placental and marsupial orders in lacking an SII area. However, it should be emphasized that our attempts to demonstrate an SII area in the platypus were based principally on investigations of forelimb inputs. Although we think it unlikely, the possibility remains that a forelimb SII area may exist in the ventral region of cortex if it is small enough (< 1–2 mm across) to fall in the spacings between electrode tracks such as those in Fig. 18. We also cannot exclude the possibility that the overall region occupied by bill representation could constitute overlapping SI–SII areas for the bill. Of course, if there is an SII area it may contain only an incomplete body representation.

The suggestion has been made that SII may represent a phylogenetically older somatosensory region than SI (Woolsey and Fairman, 1946; Sanides, 1972). However, it is the SI area which is present in all those species of placental (Lende and Sadler, 1967), marsupial (Lende, 1963a), and monotreme (Lende,

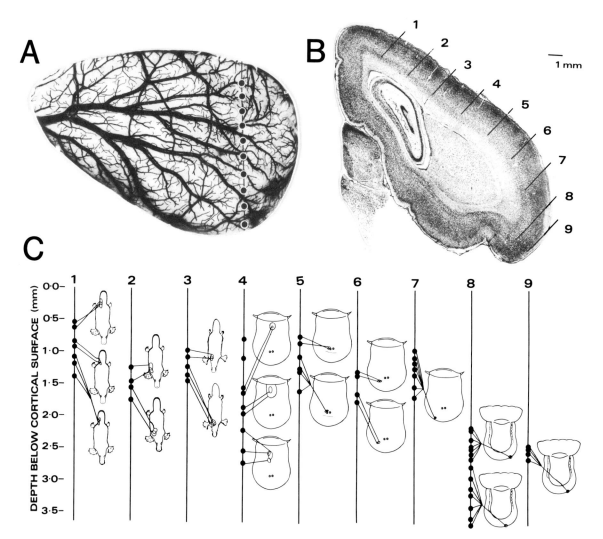

Figure 16. Tactile representation in the platypus cerebral cortex. (A) Photograph of cortical surface from dorsolateral aspect indicating a plane in which nine penetrations were made. (B) Coronal section through hemisphere at the plane indicated in A, showing the course of the nine penetrations. (C) Reconstruction of penetrations 1–9 indicating location of each neuron studied (filled circles) and its peripheral receptive field. No fields could be found for the first two neurons in penetration 4. Receptive fields for all neurons in each of penetrations 7–9 were confined to the shaded areas on each of the associated figurines. (From Bohringer and Rowe, 1977.)

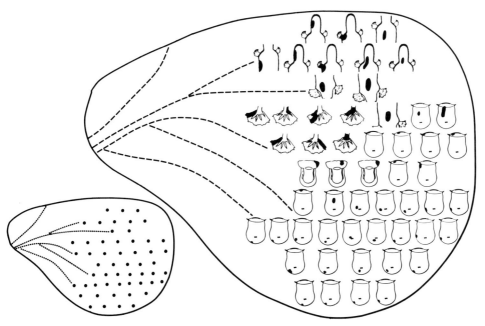

Figure 17. Tactile representation in the platypus cerebral cortex. Inset shows entry points (filled circles) for 54 microelectrode penetrations into the cortex. The black areas on figurines show the combined receptive field areas for all neurons (up to 15) sampled in each of the penetrations. Dotted lines represent positions of large blood vessels in frontal region of hemisphere; view of hemisphere from dorsolateral aspect. (From Bohringer and Rowe, 1977.)

1964; Bohringer and Rowe, 1977) mammals that are considered to approximate the archetypal mammalian form. The presence or absence of either SI or SII may simply reflect a particular specialization in certain species. For example, SI appears to be largely dispensed with in the neocortex of the sheep where an elaborate SII area predominates (Johnson *et al.*, 1974).

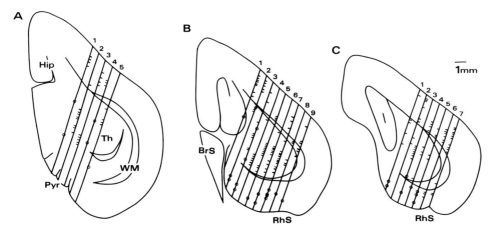

Figure 18. Reconstructions of three coronal planes (A–C) of microelectrode penetrations through the posterior region of the platypus cerebral hemisphere. Neurons with receptive fields on bill and forelimb are indicated by bars to the left and right respectively of each penetration line. Neurons for which no peripheral receptive fields could be found are indicated by the circles. Labeled anatomical features include Hip (hippocampus), Pyr (pyriform cortex), Th (thalamus), WM (subcortical white matter), BrS (brain stem), RhS (rhinal sulcus). (From Bohringer and Rowe, 1977.)

5.3.5. Functional Specialization in the Platypus Somatosensory Cortex

The enormous area of cortex associated with bill inputs, in particular from the margins of the upper bill (Figs. 16, 17, and 19), is consistent with the animal's reliance on this source of sensory information for underwater navigation and feeding. In these circumstances, the eyes, nose, and external auditory meatuses remain closed (Burrell, 1927; Barrett, 1941; Griffiths, 1978; Grant, 1984). The cortical prominence given to sensory inputs from the bill of the platypus provides another case in which behavioral specialization is associated with an enlarged cortical representation; other examples are the enlarged somatosensory cortical areas for the snout in the pig (Woolsey and Fairman, 1946) and hedgehog (Lende and Sadler, 1967), perioral areas in sheep (Woolsey and Fairman, 1946; Johnson *et al.*, 1974), forelimb extremities in the raccoon (Welker and Seidenstein, 1959) and the sloth (Saraiva and Magalhães-Castro, 1975), and the tail in the spider monkey (Pubols and Pubols, 1971).

The part of the somatosensory cortex concerned mainly with bill inputs occupies the highly granulous parapyriform 3 area (PPy3) of Abbie (1940a) and extends ventrally through PPy2, PPy1, and just beyond the rhinal sulcus into the posterior pyriform cortex (PyP) (Figs. 18 and 19; Bohringer, 1977; Bohringer and Rowe, 1977).

The areas of representation for more caudal bodyparts appeared to correspond (Fig. 19) with the agranular parahippocampal 3 and 4 areas, PH3 and PH4 of Abbie (1940a). The foci of visual and auditory projection fell mainly in the posterior region of PPy3, while areas from which motor responses were elicited lay partly in PPy3, but predominantly in the agranular frontal areas of PH4 and PH3 (Fig. 19).

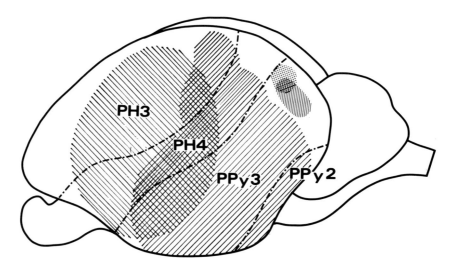

Figure 19. Cortical somatosensory (S), motor (M), visual (VIS), and auditory (AUD) areas in the platypus shown in relation to the cytoarchitectonic regions of Abbie (1940a) on the dorsolateral aspects of the hemisphere. PH3, parahippocampal area 3; PH4, parahippocampal area 4; PPy3, parapyriform area 3; PPy2, parapyriform area 2. (From Bohringer, 1977.) ▨, S; ▧, M; ▦, Vis; ▥, Aud.

5.3.6. Columnar Organization of Somatosensory Cortex in Monotremes

Within individual electrode tracks, responsive neurons were isolated most commonly at depths of 0.75–1.75 mm below the somatosensory cortical surface (Fig. 16; Bohringer and Rowe, 1977). However, they were also found in some cases within 200–300 μm of the immediately overlying surface (penetration 9 in Fig. 16). This wide distribution of responsive neurons within various layers of cortex is in agreement with findings in placental species, with the exception of the sheep in which Johnson *et al.* (1974) found that responsive neurons were strictly confined to a single cortical layer—the outer strip of Baillarger.

In individual experiments using microelectrode recording, the tactile receptive fields were characterized by Bohringer and Rowe (1977) for up to 250 individual neurons sampled in as many as 67 electrode tracks. This *fine grain* analysis of somatosensory cortex revealed a distinct columnar grouping of neurons reminiscent of the organizational pattern in placental mammals (e.g., Mountcastle, 1957; Hubel and Wiesel, 1962). This can be seen in Fig. 16 where neurons encountered within individual electrode penetrations normal to the cortical surface displayed very similar receptive field sizes and locations. For these experiments the platypus's head had been rotated to ensure that penetrations (1–7) entering the dorsal surface of the hemisphere were normal to the surface. Where electrode tracks were made in more lateral positions so that they passed obliquely through the cortex in the area of bill representation there was a remarkably orderly and progressive shift observed in the representation of the bill surface (Fig. 20). Thus, in Fig. 20D, a systematic, medially directed change is seen in the location of receptive fields for 14 neurons isolated for study in a single penetration. This track has an approximately tangential line through the cortex and would therefore have traversed successive radially oriented columns. The lower parts (B and D) of Fig. 20 are enlargements of the indicated areas on the coronal cortical section and the bill in A and C, respectively (Bohringer and Rowe, 1977).

5.3.7. Receptive Fields and Response Properties of Somatosensory Cortical Neurons in the Platypus

For individual cortical neurons, the tactile receptive fields on axial regions of the platypus such as the tail and trunk were up to ~ 15 cm^2 in area (Fig. 16C; penetrations 1–3) and were invariably larger than those toward the limb extremities. Receptive fields on the distal, glabrous skin of the limb were usually 0.5–1.0 cm^2 in area, while those on the bill, in particular on its anterior and lateral margins, consisted of extremely small, punctate areas, usually no more than 1 mm in diameter (Figs. 16 and 20; Bohringer and Rowe, 1977). Within penetration 7 in Fig. 16, all seven neurons studied had receptive fields within the small area indicated on the dorsal surface of the bill, and in penetrations 8 and 9 all fields were confined to the small shaded areas on the anterior margins of the bill, represented here from the ventral side. The tactile receptive fields shown in Fig. 20 on the anterior margin of the bill for 14 neurons isolated in one electrode penetration illustrate the *fine grain* spatial resolution available within the area of bill representation in the platypus cortex. These constitute the smallest tactile receptive fields described at the cortical level whether in placental species

(Mountcastle, 1957; Werner and Whitsel, 1973) or in marsupials, as they are even smaller than those for rhinarial inputs in the opossum cortex (Pubols *et al.*, 1976).

The mechanosensitivity of 25 cortical neurons from the projection focus of the bill was examined by Bohringer and Rowe (1977) using controlled, reproducible mechanical stimulation. All but 2 had spontaneous activity, usually between 2 and 5 impulses/sec. In response to steady indentation of their receptive fields with a 1-mm-diameter probe, *all* 25 displayed rapidly adapting re-

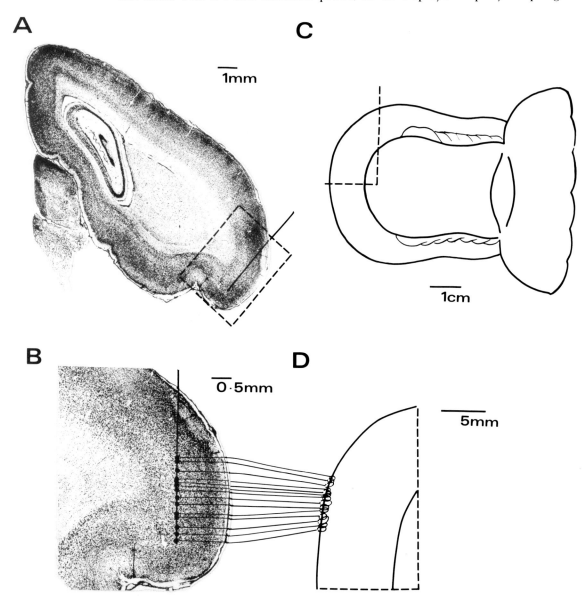

Figure 20. Tactile representation for the bill in the platypus cerebral cortex. (A) Coronal section showing position of a microelectrode penetration made obliquely to the cortical surface. The area contained within the rectangle in A is enlarged in B to indicate (filled circles) the locations of the 14 neurons studied. The receptive field for each neuron is indicated in D, which is an enlargement of the area on the ventral surface of the bill indicated by the broken lines in C. (From Bohringer and Rowe, 1977.)

sponses as seen in Fig. 21A for a neuron responding to just the dynamic components (*on* and *off* phases) of the indentation. The dynamic sensitivity of these cortical tactile neurons was studied using trains of sinusoidal vibration up to 1 sec in duration applied to their receptive fields. One group was insensitive at all vibration frequencies up to the maximum tested, 300 Hz, at amplitudes up to 250 μm (Fig. 21B,C). Neurons of the other group were responsive to low-frequency sinusoidal vibration (Fig. 21D). The responsiveness of these neurons to different frequencies was tested by constructing poststimulus time histograms from responses to a series of repetitions of the vibration train (Fig. 22). As seen in Fig. 22, neurons of this group were most sensitive at frequencies of 10–20 Hz and their impulse activity was tightly phase-locked to the applied vibration stimulus. At higher vibration frequencies, such as 60 Hz, there was a response to the first cycle of vibration but no subsequent response.

Although cortical neurons responsive to bill inputs were sensitive to just the changing components of tactile stimuli, these attributes are consistent with the platypus's behavior during swimming and feeding when the bill is kept moving from side to side so that steady, maintained tactile stimulation would rarely arise (Burrell, 1927; Griffiths, 1978).

There was no indication from the Bohringer and Rowe (1977) study, nor indeed is it likely, that *individually* these cortical neurons whose receptive fields are punctate and often less than 1 mm in diameter, could signal the *direction* of tactile stimuli moving across the bill surface. However, the highly ordered somatotopic progression within the bill area (see Fig. 20) suggests that the direction of moving tactile stimuli could be coded by a *population response* based on the sequence in which adjacent cortical cell columns underwent peripheral-induced activation. The speed as well as the direction of the moving stimulus could be encoded by the rate at which neural activation proceeded through successive columnar arrays (Bohringer and Rowe, 1977). These coding mechanisms may also operate in other species, including the monkey, even though there is evi-

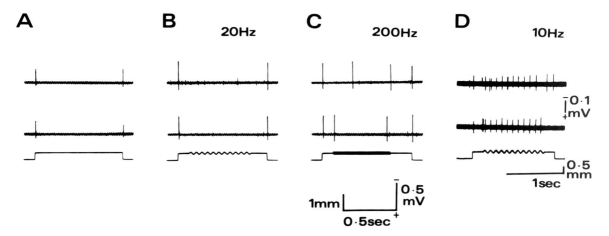

Figure 21. Responses of cerebral cortical neurons in the platypus to controlled mechanical stimulation of the bill. Stimuli delivered by means of a 1-mm-diameter probe. (A) Two traces showing responses to a steady indentation (500-μm amplitude; 0.8-sec duration) the voltage analogue of which is seen in the bottom trace. (B, C) Responses of the same neuron to stimuli in which 0.5-sec trains of sinusoidal vibration at 20 Hz (B) and 200 Hz (C) were superimposed on the steady indentation. (D) Responses of another cortical neuron to 10-Hz vibration. Peak-to-peak vibration amplitudes were 250 μm in B–D. Calibration scales beneath C apply also to A and B. (From Bohringer and Rowe, 1977.)

dence that *individual* neurons in the monkey somatosensory cortex display a selective sensitivity to the direction of stimulus motion across their receptive fields (Werner and Whitsel, 1973).

5.3.8. Cortical Responses to Bill Inputs: Relation to Electroreceptive Mechanisms in the Platypus Bill

Since Bohringer and Rowe's (1977) analysis of the cortical representation of bill inputs there has been behavioral and peripheral neural evidence presented for electroreception in the platypus bill, the first report of the phenomenon in higher vertebrates. The behavioral studies by Scheich *et al.* (1986) reported that the platypus could detect weak electric fields with threshold strengths as low as 50–200 μV/cm. They concluded that this behavioral sensitivity was mediated by the bill, as evoked potentials could be recorded from the somatosensory region of the cortex in response to weak voltage stimuli across the bill. The behavioral observations were followed with an analysis of trigeminal afferent fibers by Gre-

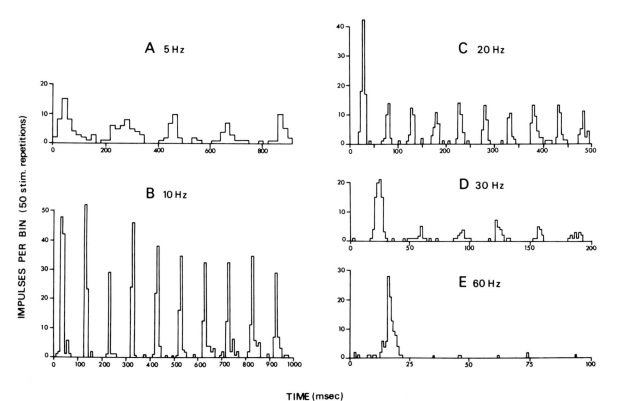

Figure 22. Vibrotactile sensitivity for cerebral cortical neurons responding to bill stimulation in the platypus. Poststimulus time histograms constructed from the accumulated responses of a cortical neuron to 50 repetitions of a 1-sec-duration vibration train at five different frequencies (A–E). Stimuli delivered using a 1-mm-diameter probe. The analyses started at the onset of the sinusoidal vibration train. The analysis period was different for each frequency of vibratory stimulation (see abscissae), but in each case was divided into a number of equally spaced time segments or addresses, the height of each indicating the number of impulses accumulated during the 50 repetitions of the stimulus train. Address or bin widths were 18.18 msec in A, 9.07 msec in B, 4.54 msec in C, 1.83 msec in D, and 0.83 msec in E. (From Bohringer and Rowe, 1977.)

gory *et al.* (1987, 1988) who concluded that myelinated afferents supplying the bill could be readily classified into two broad groups—electroreceptive afferents and mechanoreceptive afferents. Thresholds for the electroreceptive afferents were, at their lowest, 20 mV, when a cathodal electrode was placed over the point of peak sensitivity, which, under the dissecting microscope, corresponded with the pores in the bill that open to ducts associated with the large mucus-secreting glands (Poulton, 1885; Bohringer, 1981; Andres and von Düring, 1984; Gregory *et al.*, 1988). The ducts, at the level of their epidermal border, have an elaborate myelinated innervation from which slender unmyelinated axonal protrusions emerge to make close contact with cells in the wall of the duct. Gregory *et al.* (1988) argue that these protrusions may have a role in the transduction process for electroreception in the bill.

As the electroreceptive afferents were insensitive, or had high thresholds to mechanical stimulation, and as they were reported to be more numerous than mechanosensitive afferents in infraorbital nerve strands supplying the lateral margins of the bill (Gregory *et al.*, 1987, 1988), it is surprising that we encountered few neurons in the cortical area for bill representation that were unresponsive to gentle tactile stimulation (Bohringer and Rowe, 1977). For example, in Fig. 16, only 2 neurons out of the 60 studied in penetrations 1–9 could not be activated by gentle tactile stimuli. Of course, some bias toward tactile-sensitive neurons would have arisen in our cortical study as we were using tactile search stimuli in the course of our microelectrode recording. However, most cortical neurons had spontaneous activity and are therefore identifiable with microelectrode recording even if they fail to respond to peripheral stimuli. Indeed, only 2 of 25 neurons studied with controlled tactile stimuli lacked spontaneous activity. Several hypotheses may be advanced to explain why so few neurons unresponsive to tactile stimuli were found in the bill area of the platypus cortex:

1. Electroreceptive inputs project to areas outside the cortical region of bill representation identified in the Bohringer and Rowe study.
2. Electroreceptive neurons in the bill area of the somatosensory cortex differ from tactile-sensitive neurons in having no spontaneous activity and were therefore not detected as unresponsive neurons in the cortical study by Bohringer and Rowe.
3. Electroreceptive and tactile inputs converge onto common cells within the central pathways and thus, the cortical cells studied by Bohringer and Rowe may have shown a combined tactile and electroreceptive responsiveness had they been tested for both.

In relation to the first of these hypotheses, Scheich *et al.* (1986) reported that their electroreceptive-induced cortical evoked potentials were found in the posterolateral region of the hemisphere, *next to* the map of bill mechanoreceptor input. However, no tactile mapping for the bill was reported in their study and, from our work, it is clear that the area concerned with tactile representation of the bill occupies almost the whole of the posterolateral region (see Fig. 17). If, as Gregory *et al.* (1987) suggest, the electroreceptive afferents are more numerous than the tactile afferents from the bill margins, it is hard to see how the electroreceptive representation can be accommodated *next to* the mechanoreceptive representation. However, there is additional evidence against this hypothesis because our cortical mapping study was based on *both* mechanical and electrical stimulation of the bill. The electrical stimuli that were applied to the anterolateral margin of the bill would have activated both mechanosensory afferents and the electroreceptive afferents. However, comparison of the two maps (see Figs. 15 and 17) shows no evidence of a separate area of bill representation in the map based on electrical stimulation from that obtained with mechanical stimulation (Bohringer and Rowe, 1977). Even if the area of bill representation following electrical stimulation is fractionally larger than that seen with mechanical stimulation, and this is by no means certain, this could simply be a consequence of the more synchronous afferent volley created by the electrical stimulus rather than being evidence for a separate representation of electroreceptor input around the periphery of the mechanosensory map (Figs. 15 and 17). On the available evidence it appears, therefore, that electroreceptive inputs must be represented in the bill region of cortex identified in our cortical study (Bohringer and Rowe, 1977). If this is so, then hypotheses 2 and 3 should be considered. The second hypothesis—that electroreceptive cortical neurons differ from tactile neurons in not having spontaneous activity—also seems improbable, however, as the majority of electroreceptive afferent fibers have high levels of spontaneous activity (20–50 impulses/sec) whereas the trigeminal mechanosensitive fibers have no spontaneous activity (Gregory *et al.*, 1988). Finally, it is also difficult to see how the third hypothesis could apply, as convergence of tactile and electroreceptive inputs onto common central neurons may mean that the platypus is unable to discriminate these separate forms of sensory data. However, the behavioral study of Scheich *et al.* (1986) indicates that the platypus has electroreception in the bill, in addition to mechanosensitivity.

In conclusion, it appears that further study of the cortical representation of bill inputs is needed in the platypus to resolve some of these issues. There is also a need for further investigation of the discrepancy between peripheral neural thresholds and behavioral thresholds for electroreception. The electroreceptive afferent fibers prove to be much less sensitive than might have been expected from the behavioral thresholds (Scheich *et al.*, 1986; Gregory *et al.*, 1988). Although it has been suggested that spatial summation, based on convergence of electroreceptive afferents onto central neurons, may mean that the discrepancy is more apparent than real, it is difficult to see that this provides a full explanation when the most sensitive afferent fibers do not start to respond until electrical field strengths exceed behavioral thresholds by about 100 times (Gregory *et al.*, 1988).

5.3.9. Cortical Responses to Bill Inputs: Relation to the Properties of Primary Mechanosensitive Fibers

The second broad class of bill afferents studied by Gregory *et al.* (1988) consisted of mechanosensitive fibers that were divided into three subgroups each of which is probably associated with different mechanoreceptors identified in light and electron microscopy by Bohringer (1977, 1981) and subsequently by Andres and von Düring (1984) at the base of the epidermal rod organs. The rod organs were described originally by Poulton (1885, 1894) and Wilson and Martin (1893) as structures that may serve to direct tactile stimuli to the underlying nerve terminals.

One group of afferent fibers had slowly adapting responses to steady deformation of the bill surface and was thought to be associated with Merkel receptors at the base of the rod organ. The rapidly adapting, vibration-sensitive afferents identified by Gregory *et al.* (1988) are probably associated with the lamellated, or Paciniform receptors also present at the base of the rod organ (Bohringer, 1977, 1981; Andres and von Düring, 1984). For the third group of mechanosensitive afferent fibers, which had intermediate adaptation rates, the peripheral receptor association is less certain.

The behavior of cortical neurons sensitive to gentle tactile stimulation of the bill (Bohringer and Rowe, 1977) suggests that some transformation in mechanosensitive response properties occurs within the central pathways. As indicated above (Figs. 21 and 22), no slowly adapting responses were found in 25 cortical neurons tested with controlled mechanical deformation of the bill surface, and among dynamically sensitive cortical neurons, vibrotactile sensitivity was greatest at low frequencies (10–20 Hz), whereas the primary afferents have much higher best frequencies of 150–250 Hz (Gregory *et al.*, 1988). The differences may reflect a marked susceptibility of cortical responsiveness in the platypus to depressant effects of the general anesthetic (Dial Urethane; Ciba) that was used in this study, or may reflect a marked transformation of peripheral signaling by virtue of the transmission characteristics within the tactile pathways of the platypus. As yet there has been no electrophysiological analysis of the transmission characteristics through subcortical nuclei in the monotreme sensory pathways.

6. The Auditory Cortex

6.1. Organization of Auditory Cortex in Marsupials

Evoked potential recordings by Lende (1963a) identified the posterolateral location of the auditory cortex in the American opossum as seen in Fig. 23 which also shows the region in which visual evoked potentials were obtained for this species.

The auditory field identified electrophysiologically by Gates and Aitkin (1982) in the cortex of the possum, *Trichosurus vulpecula,* was in the area predicted to be auditory cortex from earlier retrograde anatomical tracing experiments which identified it as the cortical target of the thalamic medial geniculate body (Rockel *et al.*, 1972; Haight *et al.*, 1980). The area falls in the temporal region of the cortex lateral and ventral to the shallow sulcus β. The tonotopic pattern of organization was predominantly dorsoventral in its orientation (Fig. 24) in contrast to the more common anteroposterior orientation in placental mammals (Merzenich and Brugge, 1973; Merzenich *et al.*, 1975, 1976; Reale and Imig, 1980). However, as Gates and Aitkin (1982) point out, this orientation—in which high frequencies are represented dorsally and low frequencies progressively more ventrally (Fig. 24)—probably reflects an evolutionary adaptation in the marsupial line leading to *Trichosurus* and cannot be taken as some index of *primitiveness* in the organization of auditory cortex in this species.

Of more fundamental significance, perhaps, is the finding that only one distinct cortical field was discernible. Although Gates and Aitkin speculated that this may represent a distinction between *Trichosurus* and placental mammals, they allow that some of the more ventral regions of cortex in the vicinity of the rhinal sulcus were less accessible to their microelectrode mapping and therefore could contain smaller additional representations. Alternatively, they suggest that if there are dual or multiple areas, they may overlap and share a similar tonotopic pattern. However, Gates and Aitkin also found, around the tonotopically organized area, regions where they could record evoked potentials broadly tuned to high tone frequencies in which labile responses were observed. Perhaps these surrounding areas represent supplementary auditory areas concerned with processing aspects of auditory information other than sound frequency.

6.1.1. Functional Properties of Neurons in the Possum Auditory Cortex

Neurons sampled within the tonotopically organized auditory cortex of *Trichosurus* had best frequencies that ranged from 330 Hz to 39 kHz (Gates and Aitkin, 1982). The most sensitive neurons had best frequencies around 18 kHz which lies close to the most sensitive region of the behavioral audiogram of the American opossum, the only marsupial for which a behavioral audiogram has been obtained (Ravizza *et al.,* 1969). Whether *Trichosurus* proves to have the same behavioral best frequency remains to be seen. Some species, notably bats (Suga

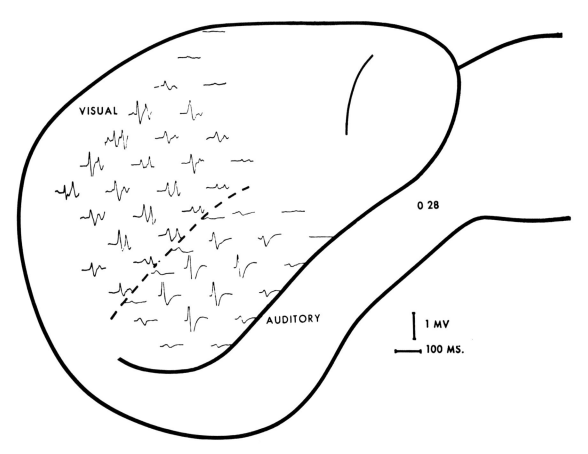

Figure 23. Areas of auditory and visual representation in the cerebral cortex of the opossum revealed by evoked potential studies. Points at 2-mm intervals in horizontal and vertical lines. Dashed line is boundary between the two areas. (From Lende, 1963a.)

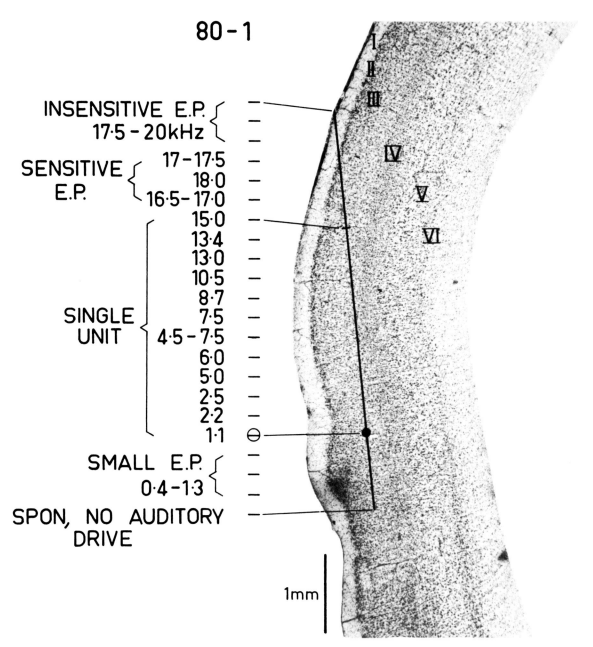

80-1

INSENSITIVE E.P. 17·5 – 20kHz

SENSITIVE E.P.
17 – 17·5
18·0
16·5 – 17·0

SINGLE UNIT
15·0
13·4
13·0
10·5
8·7
7·5
4·5 – 7·5
6·0
5·0
2·5
2·2
1·1

SMALL E.P. 0·4 – 1·3

SPON, NO AUDITORY DRIVE

1mm

Figure 24. Tonotopic representation in the cerebral cortex of *Trichosurus vulpecula*. Reconstruction of a tangential microelectrode penetration through auditory cortex of opossum 80-1. Top of figure, dorsal; bottom, ventral. Numbers to left of section represent best frequencies (BFs) of units, unit cluster, or evoked potentials. Numerals I–VI represent cortical layers on frontal section of cortex. As electrode progressed from dorsal to ventral, BFs fell from higher to lower frequencies in a systematic fashion. Lack of auditory response at end of track suggests ventral boundary of auditory cortex. Calibration bar at bottom of figure represents 1 mm. SPON, spontaneous activity, not driven by auditory stimulation; E.P., evoked potential. (From Gates and Aitkin, 1982.)

and Jen, 1976), have relatively large areas of auditory cortex devoted to specific frequencies that are of particular importance in the animal's behavior. However, no major clustering of units around particular sound frequencies was observed for the possum apart from this clustering of lowest thresholds at frequencies around 18 kHz.

6.1.2. Connections of the Marsupial Auditory Cortex

Connections between the temporal area of the possum cortex and the medial geniculate body of the thalamus were identified first by Rockel *et al.* (1972) and Haight *et al.* (1980). More recently, Aitkin and Gates (1983) have extended these observations by first defining the auditory cortex physiologically and injecting horseradish peroxidase into the functionally identified region. Their tentative suggestion was that the inputs to auditory cortex arise from divisions of the medial geniculate nucleus that may fall into a dorsomedial, a medial, and a lateral division resembling those in the cat (Morest, 1964; Aitkin *et al.*, 1981). In particular, it was the lateral division that projected to the tonotopically organized area of auditory cortex, whereas more medial regions of the medial geniculate nucleus project outside the tonotopic area to the surrounding region of more broadly tuned neurons that displayed a more labile responsiveness.

Input connections to auditory cortex from the opposite hemisphere arose from laminae III and IV and, in the absence of a corpus callosum, traverse the anterior commissure or fasciculus aberrans (Heath and Jones, 1971; Aitkin and Gates, 1983).

Physiological mapping of auditory cortex in other marsupials has been confined to the Australian northern native cat (*Dasyurus hallucatus*) in which Aitkin *et al.* (1986) have also found a tonotopic pattern in the temporal region of cortex above the rhinal sulcus. However, in this animal the orientation of the map (Fig. 25) appears to be intermediate between the placental anteroposterior progression in frequency and the dorsoventral one found in the possum. In *Dasyurus*, the frequency range represented is principally between 1 kHz and about 40 kHz, with the highest frequencies represented in the dorsorostral region of temporal cortex. A progression toward lower frequencies is seen as the recording site is moved in a ventrocaudal direction (Fig. 25). The representation is biased heavily toward frequencies above 10 kHz with little representation at all of frequencies below 1 kHz. About five times more cortical space is allocated to an octave above 10 kHz than to one below this frequency (Fig. 26).

In *Dasyurus* there was evidence of a second auditory cortical field rostral to the main or presumed *primary* area. This was based on the appearance of a reversal in frequency representation beyond the high-frequency limit at the dorsorostral end of the primary map (Fig. 25; Aitkin *et al.*, 1986). It appears improbable therefore that the auditory cortex of nonplacental mammals is distinguished from those of the placental order by the absence of dual or multiple auditory areas in the cerebral cortex.

6.2. Auditory Cortex in Monotremes

The auditory cortex has been mapped in both the echidna (Lende, 1964) and the platypus (Bohringer and Rowe, 1977) using a standard click stimulus, which for the platypus study was 2 msec in duration, delivered every 10 sec from a loudspeaker placed near the opening to the external auditory meatus. In the echidna the auditory area was found in the posterior pole of the hemisphere (Lende, 1964) and was demarcated sharply from the somatosensory and visual areas, which lay immediately anterior to it, by sulcus zeta (Fig. 27).

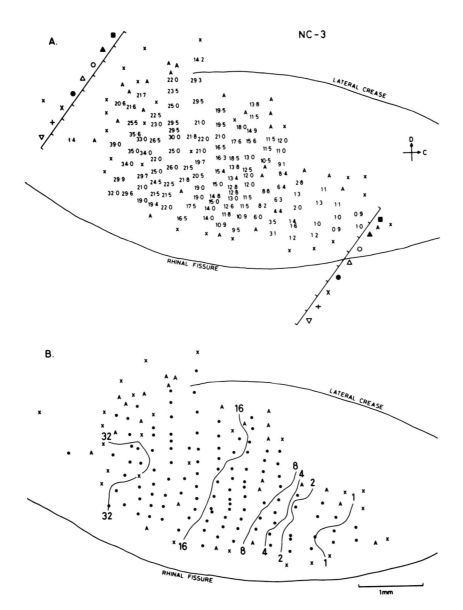

Figure 25. Tonotopic representation in the auditory cortex of *Dasyurus hallucatus*. (A) The distribution of best frequencies of units and clusters across the acoustically responsive gyral surface in native cat 3 (NC-3). Sites marked with "A" responded to auditory stimuli but no best frequency could be defined; those indicated by "X" were unresponsive to tones. The tilted axes at the figure margins mark the dorsorostral (left) and ventrocaudal (right) limits of eight one-third-mm-wide cortical strips from which Aitkin *et al.* (1986) derived the best frequency versus transcortical distance plots of Fig. 26. D and C indicate dorsal and caudal. (B) Estimated isofrequency contours in octave steps for 1, 2, 4, 8, 16, and 32 kHz; each dot relates to a best frequency in A. (From Aitkin *et al.*, 1986.)

In the platypus, the auditory area occupies a more posteromedial region of cortex than in placental species and, in comparison with the echidna, is more medially located, but again in the posterior region of the hemisphere (Fig. 28). The posteromedial displacement of the auditory area may be a consequence of the large expanse of cortex associated with cranial inputs from the bill in this species. The area from which evoked potentials (latency 10 msec) could be recorded partly overlapped the areas from which visual and somatosensory evoked potentials could be recorded (Fig. 28). However, as the mapping of auditory and visual areas was based purely on evoked potentials (Bohringer and Rowe, 1977), it is possible that the overlap between these areas and with the somatosensory area is less than the extent illustrated in Fig. 28 (Bohringer and Rowe, 1977) as Pubols *et al.* (1976) have reported that sensory receiving areas revealed by microelectrode recording are somewhat smaller than those demonstrated by evoked potential methods.

No data were obtained in either of these monotreme species on the internal organization of auditory cortex, in particular, whether there is an orderly representation of sound frequencies indicative of a *place* code for pitch at the cortical level. Another feature for investigation in any future unitary recordings is whether there is an expanded representation of tone frequencies around 5 kHz which were found to be the best frequencies in both echidna and platypus based on cochlear microphonic audiograms (Gates *et al.*, 1974; Griffiths, 1978). Al-

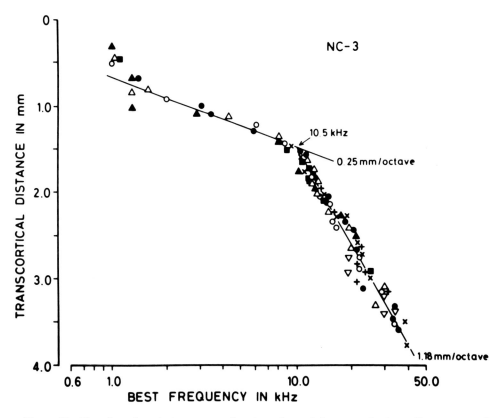

Figure 26. Allocation of cortical space as a function of sound frequency in the auditory cortex of *Dasyurus hallucatus*. Transcortical distance versus best frequency plot derived by Aitkin *et al.* (1986) from the data of Fig. 25, with each symbol relating to a particular cortical strip. Lines have been fitted by eye. (From Aitkin *et al.*, 1986.)

though the peripheral auditory apparatus responded over a broad frequency bandwidth, the sensitivity over most of the range was poor compared with most placental species (Gates *et al.*, 1974). However, Griffiths (1978) has suggested that the 5-kHz *best* frequency may equip the echidna well for detecting the noises emitted by termites or for detecting vibrations transmitted through bone.

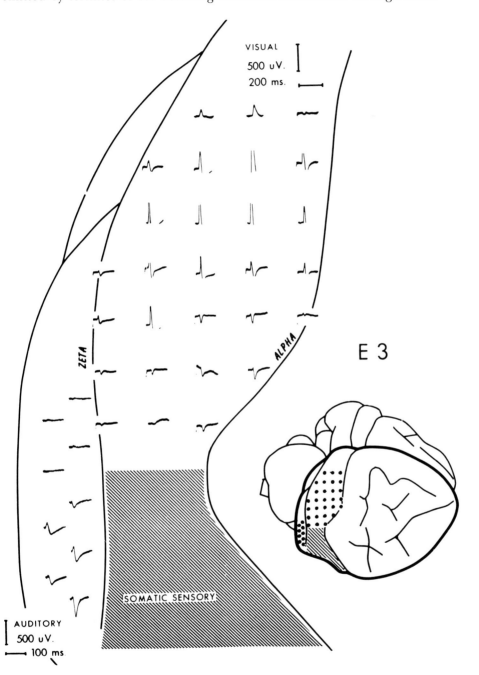

Figure 27. Auditory and visual fields for the echidna cerebral cortex. Key shows right dorsolateral view of brain, frontal pole to right, cerebellum to left, right hemisphere outline in heavier line. Each dot in the key corresponds to an evoked potential. Responses behind zeta are auditory, in front of zeta are visual. The somatosensory field in this animal is indicated by diagonal stripes. (From Lende, 1964.)

It is apparent from Figs. 27 and 28 that the auditory cortex in both species, and the visual cortex in the platypus at least, occupy very small areas of cortex, in particular in comparison with the areas allocated to somatosensory and motor function. However, this is in keeping with the apparently limited extent to which auditory and visual information is used by the platypus during swimming and feeding. In these circumstances the eyes and external auditory meatuses are closed and the animal appears to rely on information derived from the bill (Poulton, 1885; Wilson and Martin, 1893, 1894; Burrell, 1927; Griffiths, 1978). Perhaps the small auditory cortex in the echidna is related to the relative insensitivity of the cochlea except at frequencies of about 5 kHz (Gates *et al.*, 1974).

7. The Visual Cortex

7.1. Organization of Visual Cortex in Marsupials

The visual cortex in marsupials appears to conform more closely than the auditory cortex to the general placental pattern of organization in that multiple areas have been reported within the occipital lobe of both the Australian possum and the American opossum (Benevento and Ebner, 1971a; Kaas, 1980; Haight *et*

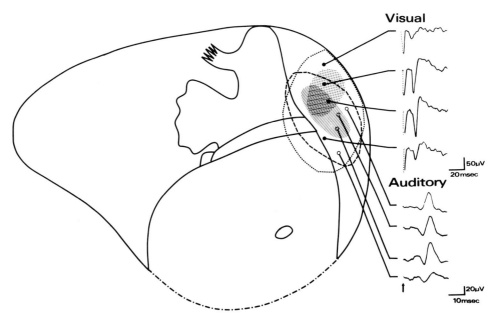

Figure 28. Visual and auditory projection areas in the platypus cerebral cortex and their relation to the somatosensory area (figurine). The broken line on the figurine indicates the continuation of the bill representation to the region of the rhinal sulcus. Positive-going evoked potentials exceeding 60 μV were recorded from the stippled area following visual stimulation using an electronic flash. Auditory responses exceeding 15 μV were evoked following click stimulation (2 msec duration) from the shaded area. Smaller responses to both visual and auditory stimulation were evoked from the zone between the focal projection sites and the corresponding continuous lines. Examples of recorded responses are shown on the right. Visual stimuli were delivered at a point corresponding to the start of the traces (upper records); auditory stimuli at the point indicated by the arrow. (From Bohringer and Rowe, 1977.)

al., 1980; Crewther *et al.,* 1984). These multiple representations in placental mammals have been studied in most detail in the monkey where approximately 12 visual cortical areas have been designated (Van Essen and Maunsell, 1983) and in the cat where the striate cortex has connections with areas 18 and 19 and with approximately nine areas of the suprasylvian sulcus or gyrus (Bullier, 1984). Furthermore, there are some additional extrastriate visual areas that do not receive striate projections.

In both *Trichosurus* and *Didelphis* the primary visual area in the striate region of occipital cortex (Gray, 1924) was identified from its precise reciprocal linkage with the dorsal lateral geniculate nucleus (dLGN) (Packer, 1941; Bodian, 1942; Diamond and Utley, 1963; Benevento and Ebner, 1971b; Haight *et al.,* 1980). Apart from the primary area there are at least four other cytoarchitecturally distinguishable regions identified as putative visual areas of cortex. Descriptions of the histological features of striate and extrastriate areas in *Trichosurus* were given by Heath and Jones (1971) and Haight *et al.* (1980) and in *Didelphis* by Benevento and Ebner (1971a). As none of the extrastriate visual areas has been mapped physiologically in a complete way for *Trichosurus* or *Didelphis,* they were identified principally on account of their anatomical connections with either dLGN or the striate cortex. One of these is the *peristriate* (PS) area which in *Trichosurus* (Fig. 29) has connections with the dLGN that are similar to those of the striate area (Haight *et al.,* 1980; Crewther *et al.,* 1984). It is probable also, as Johnson (1977) points out, that the peristriate area is directly responsive to visual inputs in *Didelphis virginiana* (Lende, 1963a), in *Didelphis azarae azarae* (Magalhães-Castro and Saraiva, 1971), and in the Australian marsupial wallaby, *Thylogale* (or *Macropus*) *eugenii* (Lende, 1963c).

Other areas in *Trichosurus* that have connections with the striate cortex include the *posterior parietal* (PP), *medial temporal* (MT), and *lateral temporal* (LT) areas of cortex (Fig. 29) all of which are the recipients, in laminae III and IV, of inputs from the striate area (Haight *et al.,* 1980; Crewther *et al.,* 1984). In turn, the striate area receives projections from supra- and infragranular layers of the extrastriate visual cortex as in the monkey (Van Essen and Maunsell, 1983). This striate input consists, in the possum, of a major projection from cells in laminae II and III and, to a smaller extent, from laminae V and VI of the PP area, and minor projections from MT, LT, and PS cortex (Crewther *et al.,* 1984).

The PP area also has reciprocal connections with dLGN and with the thalamic lateroposterior nucleus (Haight *et al.,* 1980). A region on the medial (M) surface of the hemisphere in the occipital lobe has also been shown to receive visual input but of monocular origin (Sanderson *et al.,* 1980), and is said to send projections to the superior colliculus. This area M is therefore also a possible visual area (Crewther *et al.,* 1984). As Crewther *et al.* point out, there may be further visual areas that lack connections with the striate area and which, in the absence of physiological mapping, remain unidentified as visual areas. Although the thalamic connections of MT, LT, and M have not been established in *Trichosurus,* it was suggested, on the basis of their connections with the striate area, that each probably functions as a visual area of cortex (Crewther *et al.,* 1984). Similar extrastriate areas of visual cortex appear to be present in the American opossum (Benevento and Ebner, 1971a; Kaas, 1980).

The striate cortex also has reciprocal connections with the claustrum in *Trichosurus* (Crewther *et al.,* 1984), an arrangement that also exists in placental mammals (LeVay and Sherk, 1981; Norita, 1983; Sherk, 1986). The interhemi-

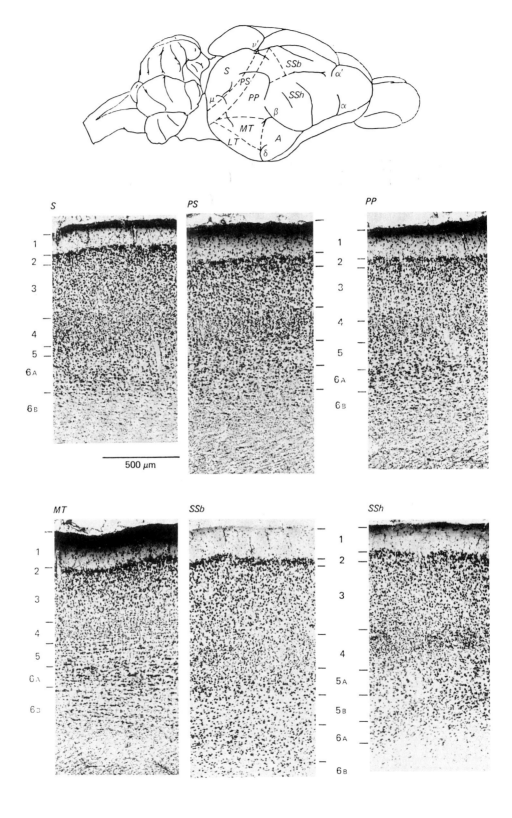

spheric connections in the occipital lobe of *Trichosurus* also resemble those seen in placental mammals in being confined to the striate–peristriate border (Heath and Jones, 1971; Crewther *et al.*, 1984) whereas the polyprotodont opossum, *Didelphis virginiana*, has commissural connections to all parts of the cortex as does the relatively simple placental representative, the hedgehog (Ebner, 1969). In some additional respects the visual system of the opossum may be less developed than that of the possum (see Haight *et al.*, 1980). For example, its dLGN lacks the lamination that is so prominent in *Trichosurus* (Hayhow, 1967; Royce *et al.*, 1976; Sanderson *et al.*, 1978).

Functional Properties of Neurons in the Marsupial Visual Cortex

Two thirds of neurons within the primary visual area in *Trichosurus* responded to binocular inputs and a third of all neurons studied responded equally well to each eye (Crewther *et al.*, 1984). The ocular dominance distribution was similar to that for cat striate cortex (Hubel and Wiesel, 1962) except that greater contralateral dominance was found in the possum. With the use of quantitative stimulation and response procedures, Crewther *et al.* (1984) found that only 30% of cells in possum visual cortex were selective for the orientation of visual stimuli. However, whether this represents a significant difference from the behavior of neurons in the visual cortex of placental mammals is uncertain. The extent to which rigorous quantitative controls on both stimulus and response parameters are employed may vary from study to study where conclusions about orientation selectivity are made. Nevertheless, the percentage of orientation-selective neurons corresponds closely with that found for *Didelphis* (Rocha-Miranda *et al.*, 1976) and for the rabbit (Murphy and Berman, 1979). In the cat visual cortex, neurons are orientation selective in 95% of cases (Kato *et al.*, 1978; Murphy and Berman, 1979). The existence of orientation selectivity and binocular convergence for neurons of the marsupial visual cortex suggests that fundamentally similar mechanisms may operate in the visual cortex for different mammalian orders.

7.2. Visual Cortex in Monotremes

Mapping of visual cortex in the platypus and echidna was carried out using the evoked potential method following stimulation with an electronic flash stimulus (duration < 1 msec) delivered every 2 min (Lende, 1964; Bohringer and Rowe, 1977). In the gyrencephalic echidna cortex the anterior boundary is

Figure 29. Cytoarchitecture of visual and neighboring areas of opossum neocortex. Cytoarchitectural regions in the caudal portions of the cortical mantle together with various landmark sulci, indicated by Greek letters, are shown in the top drawing. The three visual areas are pictured in the top row of sections. From left to right these are striate (S), peristriate (PS), and posterior parietal cortex (PP). Each of these regions displays differing connectivity patterns with other CNS centers. Adjacent, nonvisual, cortical areas are shown in the bottom row. These are from left to right, the medial temporal (MT), somatic sensory, body (SSb), and somatic sensory, head (SSh) regions. The positions of the lateral temporal (LT) and auditory (A) cortical areas are shown on the line drawing but are not otherwise illustrated. The cortical sections shown were taken from celloidin-embedded material cut at 30 μm and stained with aqueous thionin. (Figure and legend from Haight *et al.*, 1980.)

formed by sulcus alpha and the posterior by sulcus zeta (Figs. 13 and 27). Of course, no such borders are identifiable in the lissencephalic platypus cortex.

In the echidna the visual cortex appears to be substantially larger than the auditory area and perhaps little different in area from the somatosensory cortex (Lende, 1964, 1969; Figs. 13 and 27). In contrast, in the platypus, the dorsomedially placed visual area is very small (Fig. 28; Bohringer and Rowe, 1977) as might be expected from the small eye and optic nerve (about 30,000 fibers; Hines, 1929; Griffiths, 1978) and the minor role vision plays in the animal's behavior (see Section 6.2; Poulton, 1885; Wilson and Martin, 1894; Burrell, 1927; Griffiths, 1978). Furthermore, the eyes are unlikely to be of use in the darkness of the animal's burrow.

Any unitary studies in the visual cortex, in particular on ocular dominance or orientation specificity, will need to take account of monotreme visual mechanisms at lower levels of the visual pathway, including, for example, the uncertainty over whether the monotremes possess accommodation in vision and whether, in the platypus, emmetropia exists in air or water (Griffiths, 1978). In both species the optic nerve is almost entirely crossed (Abbie, 1934; Campbell and Hayhow, 1971, 1972), and therefore the incidence of binocularity may be low in visual cortex.

8. Sensory Cortex in Marsupialia and Monotremata: Summary and Concluding Comments

8.1. Location and Organization of Cortical Sensory Areas

Some variation occurs in the position of particular sensory areas and in their relations to one another in the different orders of mammals. However, this variability appears no greater than that seen within a given order. One striking instance of the latter is in the Monotremata where there are marked differences between the echidna and the platypus in the cortical disposition of the sensorimotor areas (see Figs. 13 and 28). Despite these differences, a unifying factor *within* and *across* orders appears to be the internal pattern of organization for particular sensory areas. For example, in all species in which somatosensory cortex has been identified and mapped, it has a recognizable somatotopic plan. Similarly, the auditory cortex in placental and marsupial representatives has a tonotopic pattern of organization although this has yet to be examined in the monotreme cortex.

In the case of the primary visual cortex there is evidence in marsupials of a retinotopic plan of the type seen in placental mammals. This conclusion is based, first, on the ordered topographic pattern of projection that exists between the dLGN and the striate cortex in both *Didelphis virginiana* (Bodian, 1942; Diamond and Utley, 1963; Benevento and Ebner, 1971b) and *Trichosurus vulpecula* (Packer, 1941; Haight *et al.*, 1980; Crewther *et al.*, 1984), and, second, on the electrophysiological mapping in *Didelphis,* which shows an ordered representation of the contralateral visual hemifield in the striate cortex (Sousa *et al.,* 1978; Kaas, 1980). Although visual areas of the cortex have been identified in both echidna and platypus, the internal organization of these areas was not mapped (Lende, 1964;

Bohringer and Rowe, 1977). Furthermore, studies of the thalamocortical connections (Welker and Lende, 1980; Ulinski, 1984) have not concentrated on visual areas. Thus, there is not yet evidence for a retinotopic organization of visual cortex in monotremes.

8.2. Multiple Representation in Cortex for Particular Sensory Modalities

The presence of multiple cortical representations of a given sensory modality is now well established in placental mammals for visual inputs (Hubel and Wiesel, 1965; Van Essen, 1979; Van Essen and Maunsell, 1983), for auditory inputs (Aitkin *et al.*, 1984; Brugge and Reale, 1985), and for somatosensory inputs to cortex (Mountcastle, 1978, 1986; Ferrington and Rowe, 1980; Fisher *et al.*, 1983; Jones, 1985, 1986; Rowe *et al.*, 1985; Burton, 1986). The presence of perhaps just one area of auditory representation in the possum (*Trichosurus vulpecula*) raised the possibility of a distinction between marsupial and placental species in this respect (Gates and Aitkin, 1982), but subsequent observations in another marsupial, the Australian native cat (*Dasyurus hallucatus*), revealed multiple areas (Aitkin *et al.*, 1986), indicating that such differences are as likely to be intraorder variations as variations between orders.

Another form of variability in the cortical representation patterns may be found between sensory modalities within a given species. For example, the possum, despite its single representation of auditory inputs, displays multiple visual cortical areas (as does *Didelphis*) reminiscent of many of the placental species (Benevento and Ebner, 1971a; Heath and Jones, 1971, Haight *et al.*, 1980; Crewther *et al.*, 1984).

Perhaps one instance of a systematic interorder difference in sensory cortical organization is seen with the apparent absence of a second somatosensory area (SII) of cortex in both echidna (Lende, 1964) and platypus (Bohringer and Rowe, 1977). In contrast, SII is consistently found in those placental or marsupial species whose somatosensory cortex has been carefully mapped (Woolsey, 1958; Johnson, 1977; Burton, 1986).

8.3. Interhemispheric and Thalamic Connectivity

Differences between the possum and placental species in visual thalamocortical relations have been reported. For example, Haight *et al.* (1980) found in the possum that the dLGN projects to both striate and extrastriate areas of cortex, whereas the dLGN projection was thought to be confined to the striate area across the range of placental species from hedgehog (Gould *et al.*, 1978) to primates (Ogren and Hendrickson, 1976; Rezak and Benevento, 1979). Once again, however, this appears not to be a systematic interorder difference, first, because cortical projections from dLGN in the polyprotodont opossum are confined to the striate area (Benevento and Ebner, 1971b; Coleman *et al.*, 1977) and, second, it is now increasingly recognized that, in some placentals including the cat and monkey, the dLGN provides input to cortical areas outside the striate area 17 (Stone, 1983).

Distinct anatomical differences exist between placental and nonplacental mammals in the interhemispheric pathways, as neither monotremes nor marsupials possess the placental corpus callosum (Abbie, 1939; Ebner, 1969; Heath and Jones, 1971; Johnson, 1977). However, despite its alternative system of three interhemispheric paths—the hippocampal and anterior commissures and the fasciculus aberrans—the possum has a pattern of interhemispheric connections for visual cortex that are similar to those of most placental species. These connections are confined to the border of the striate and peristriate regions (Heath and Jones, 1971; Crewther *et al.*, 1984) whereas in the opossum (Ebner, 1967) and at least one placental representative, the hedgehog (Ebner, 1969), they are more generalized with no parts of the cortex being devoid of such connections.

9. Localization of Motor Function within the Cerebral Cortex

9.1. Motor Areas in the Marsupial Cerebral Cortex

Studies employing electrical stimulation to map the motor cortex in marsupials started in the late 19th century with investigations by Herrick (1898) and Cunningham (1898) on the opossums, *Didelphis virginiana* and *D. marsupialis*. An account of these and subsequent studies can be found in Johnson (1977). Detailed motor maps constructed for *D. virginiana* and for the wallaby [*Macropus (or Thylogale) eugenii*] by Lende (1963b,c, 1969) confirmed the earlier observations of Vogt and Vogt (1906) that the motor representation, at least for arm, trunk, and leg, lies behind the single sulcus (sulcus α, or the orbital sulcus) present in the anterior, dorsal region of the cortex in several of these marsupial species including the opossum (*D. virginiana*), the wallaby (*M. eugenii*), and the possum (*Trichosurus vulpecula*).

In the Australian brush-tailed possum, *T. vulpecula*, the mappings of motor cortex by Goldby (1939b), Abbie (1940b), and Rees and Hore (1970) have all revealed motor representation for forelimb and hindlimb behind the orbital sulcus in typical granular cortex (Abbie, 1940b) in contrast to the agranular area of placental mammals. No consistent motor representation was found for the head. Nor was there evidence of a supplementary motor area (Rees and Hore, 1970), although this may be located in the less accessible medial surface of the hemisphere.

The behavioral effects of lesions in the motor area of cortex have been variable. Bromiley and Brooks (1940) reported motor impairment with lesions behind, but not in front of sulcus α in the opossum. However, in the same species, Bautista and Matzke (1965) found no motor impairment following motor cortical lesions. Motor cortical ablation in *Trichosurus* (Rees and Hore, 1970) produced no defect in gait or climbing ability or in the animal's posture while it was in the sitting position. However, specific tests involving grasping, holding, and placing revealed temporary motor deficits in the fore- and hindlimbs when large areas of motor cortex were ablated (Rees and Hore, 1970). Furthermore, disruption of the corticospinal fibers at the level of the medullary pyramid (Hore *et al.*, 1973) caused a similar impairment in fine manipulative motor functions to that seen after equivalent lesions in monkeys.

9.2. Lende's Hypothesis: A Sensorimotor Amalgam in Marsupials and Monotremes

Lende (1963c, 1969) concluded that marsupials show a unique plan of overlap of somatosensory and motor cortex (Figs. 8 and 30). For both opossum and wallaby, he demonstrated the same mediolateral sequence in motor and somatosensory representation that is found in placental mammals, namely, representation of hindlimb and caudal body in the medial part of the hemisphere, with a progressive shift to forelimb and face in more lateral locations (Fig. 8). Furthermore, as outlined in Section 5.2, Lende (1963a,c, 1969) concluded that in the somatosensory area, the trunk and upper parts of the limbs were represented caudally and limb extremities were represented rostrally as is found in the primary somatosensory cortex of placental mammals (Woolsey, 1952, 1958, 1964). However, he concluded that the motor representation in these two marsupial species differed from the placental plan in having the trunk representation located behind the limb extremities (Lende, 1963a,c, 1969). In placental species, the motor representation lies rostral to the primary somatosensory cortex; for example, in the primate cortex, it lies in cytoarchitectonic area 4 and is separated from the somatosensory representation in areas 3, 1, and 2 by the central or Rolandic sulcus. The eutherian motor map is described as forming a mirror

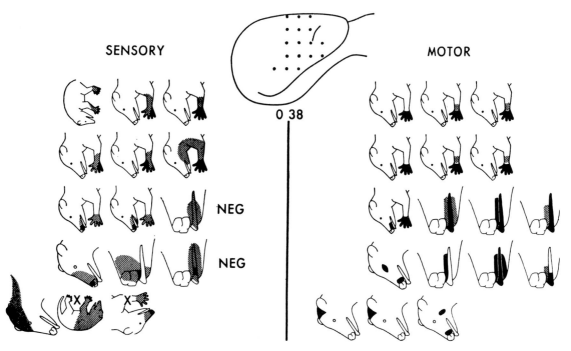

Figure 30. Overlap of somatosensory and motor representation in the cortex of *Didelphis virginiana*. Results of cortical stimulation and evoked potential recording done at the same cortical sites on the lateral wall of the hemisphere in one opossum. Representations on the sensory figurines as in Fig. 7. Points marked "X" showed bilateral representation. Black shading on the motor figurines indicates primary threshold movements. Secondary movements which either had a slightly higher threshold or had their onset slightly later are indicated with cross-hatching. (From Lende, 1963b.)

image of the somatosensory representation. Thus, limb extremities are placed caudal to the trunk representation (Woolsey, 1952, 1958, 1964). The orientation of the motor representation in the rostrocaudal dimension in the two marsupial species studied by Lende results in the somatosensory and motor maps being coincident, or, as Lende has argued, there is a sensorimotor amalgam with no evidence of regional predominance of either sensory or motor function within this combined area of representation (Figs. 8 and 30).

Lende's finding of a sensorimotor amalgam in marsupials, together with his observations on the cortex of the monotreme, *Tachyglossus aculeatus* (Lende, 1964, 1969), and placental insectivores (Lende and Sadler, 1967) led him to the hypothesis that mammalian neocortical organization evolved from a primitive pallium with completely superimposed representation areas for somatosensory and motor function (Lende, 1963c, 1969). Lende argued that mammalian evolution has led to an increasing spatial differentiation of sensory and motor areas to the point where, in particular, in man and higher primates, they may be separated by intervening cortical areas, generally termed association areas (Diamond and Hall, 1969; Lende, 1969). In the hedgehog (*Erinaceus europaeus*), a representative of the placental insectivores—a group thought to represent, in terms of comparative brain development, a placental mammal closer to the archetypal mammalian forms—Lende and Sadler (1967) observed partial overlap of somatosensory and motor areas, consistent with the proposed proximity of this placental group to the hypothetical primordial mammalian form.

9.3. Motor Representation in Monotremes

9.3.1. The Motor Cortex in the Echidna

Lende's observations were extended to the echidna (*Tachyglossus aculeatus*), as a representative of the third mammalian order, the Monotremata. He found (Fig. 31) that motor responses could be elicited not only from the area anterior to sulcus α as described earlier by Abbie (1938), but also from the whole of the identified somatosensory area of cortex in the gyrus located behind sulcus α (Lende, 1964). Within this region of overlap a correspondence in somatotopy was found for motor and sensory representation. Although the motor thresholds and pattern of representation were similar on either side of sulcus α, Lende considered that the motor area anterior to sulcus α was a separate representation from that behind sulcus α. His arguments were, first, that the anterior region contains a "rather complete representation of the body"; second, sulcus α forms a division between the two; third, there are cytoarchitectonic differences between anterior and posterior areas, the area behind sulcus α being granular cortex whereas the area in front is agranular (Schuster, 1910; Abbie, 1940a); and fourth, the anterior area lacked sensory function in contrast to the posterior area. Despite these arguments it remains uncertain whether anterior and pos-

Figure 31. Somatic sensory and motor fields in the cerebral cortex of the echidna. Results of cortical recording following tactile stimulation are shown above, results of bipolar cortical stimulation are below. Keys show right ventrolateral view of brain, frontal pole to the right, right hemisphere outlined in heavier line. Data are illustrated by figurines, each of which corresponds to a dot in the key which indicates the site of the stimulation or recording. (From Lende, 1964.)

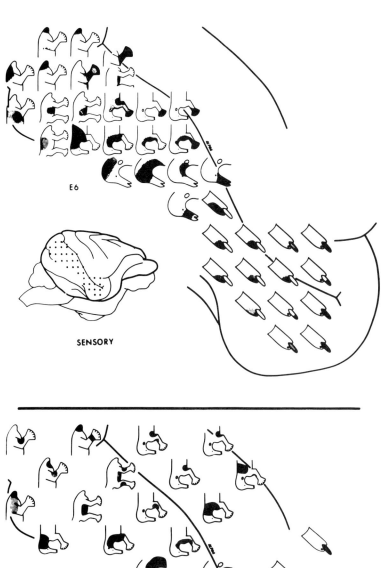

E6

SENSORY

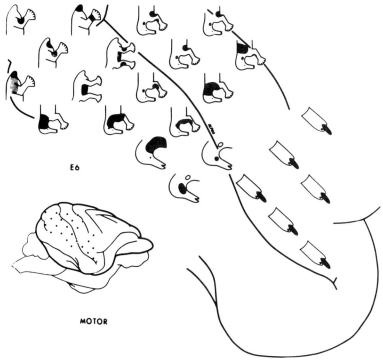

E6

MOTOR

terior areas can be identified legitimately as separate motor areas, in particular in the absence of intracortical stimulation procedures being used in the walls and at the base of sulcus α in order to establish whether any discontinuity exists in the motor representation across the sulcus. Lende (1964, 1969) argued that the region behind sulcus α represented a sensorimotor amalgam of the type he described in the opossum and wallaby.

9.3.2. The Motor Cortex in the Platypus

Our own studies (Bohringer and Rowe, 1977) on the platypus (*Ornithorhynchus anatinus*) do little to reinforce Lende's idea of a sensorimotor amalgam in the order Monotremata. Although substantial overlap of somatosensory and motor representations was found (Fig. 32), the motor cortex in platypus extended farther anterior than the somatosensory cortex and, in contrast to the pattern in the echidna, failed to cover the entire somatosensory area. Although Fig. 32 shows motor representation of the distal forelimb both rostral and caudal to that for the proximal forelimb and shoulder, this pattern was not clear in all

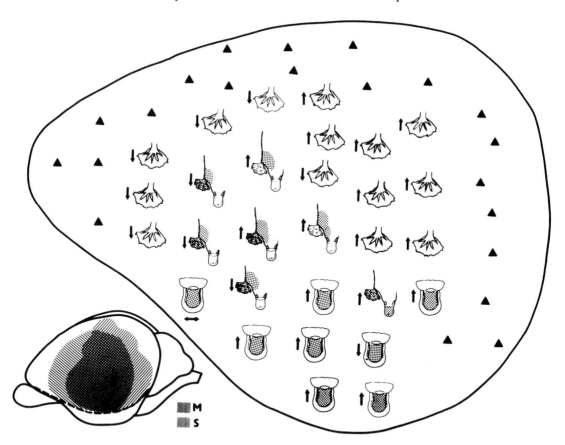

Figure 32. Motor representation in the platypus cerebral cortex. Figurines indicate body areas from which movements were elicited by cortical stimulation. These included the contralateral forelimb and the shaded areas of the body in other sketches. Upgoing arrows denote flexion of forelimb or bill opening; downgoing arrows denote forelimb extension or bill closing. Horizontal arrows denote lateral movements of mandible. Triangles mark points from which no movement could be elicited. The inset shows the relative positions of motor (M) and somatosensory (S) cortical areas. View of hemisphere from dorsolateral aspect. (From Bohringer and Rowe, 1977.)

experiments. Furthermore, as no hindlimb and few trunk responses could be elicited, we were uncertain about the anteroposterior orientation of the body representation in the motor cortex of the platypus, in particular whether the representation is oriented with apices caudal to the trunk representation as in most placental species (Woolsey, 1952, 1958, 1964) or reversed as described for the opossum (Lende, 1963b, 1969), the armadillo (Royce *et al.*, 1975), and the sloth (Saraiva and Magalhães-Castro, 1975).

Observations in two early studies of the *excitable* or motor cortex in platypus (Martin, 1898; Abbie, 1938) were not supported by our observations (Bohringer and Rowe, 1977). Martin found that movements were poorly localized and obtained from patchy areas of cortex whereas Abbie reported that practically the whole dorsolateral surface was diffusely excitable, with head representation anterior, and the forelimb and trunk progressively more posterior. The inconsistencies in the early attempts to map the platypus motor cortex, and our failure to identify a region of motor representation for hindlimb (Fig. 32; Bohringer and Rowe, 1977) may, in part, be attributed to the thickness of platypus cortex which, as Abbie (1938) observed, is almost twice as thick as that of the echidna. The extra thickness may mean that greater current strength is needed to elicit movements with some loss of precision in localization. This may mean that intracortical stimulation procedures are needed to achieve a complete mapping of the motor cortex in the platypus.

The prominent representation demonstrated for the forelimb in our motor map in platypus (Fig. 32) is consistent with the importance of the forelimbs in propulsion during underwater activity. In contrast, the hindlimbs and tail, for which we were unable to demonstrate motor representation, act chiefly as rudders (Burrell, 1927; Griffiths, 1978).

The location of motor cortex in platypus (Fig. 32) leaves a much smaller area of frontal cortex free of somatosensory and motor function than is the case for the echidna (Fig. 13; Lende, 1964; Welker and Lende, 1980) in which the unusually caudal location of the motor cortex leaves an extensive frontal area whose connections and functions have been studied by Welker and Lende (1980) and Divac *et al.* (1987a,b; see Section 10).

9.3.3. Reconsideration of Lende's Hypothesis of a Sensorimotor Amalgam in Cortex

Support for Lende's concept of a sensorimotor amalgam in the opossum has come from the observation in this species by Killackey and Ebner (1973) that the ventroposterior (VP) and ventrolateral (VL) thalamic nuclei (which, in placental mammals, form the major thalamic relays for subcortical input to somatosensory and motor cortex, respectively) converge to a common area of neocortex, thus providing an anatomical correlate for Lende's functional sensorimotor amalgam. Among Australian marsupials, it is clear from the earliest somatosensory map in *Trichosurus vulpecula* (Adey and Kerr, 1954) that there is at least some overlap with the motor area (Rees and Hore, 1970). Nevertheless, it is not possible on the available data in these two papers to suggest that motor and sensory areas might be coincident, thereby constituting an *amalgam* of the kind described by Lende for the opossum and the wallaby.

However, more recent studies in diprotodont marsupials, including the possum, *T. vulpecula,* suggest that motor and somatosensory areas are not coincident. First, the cortical projection fields of the VP and VL nuclei are not congruent (Haight and Neylon, 1978b, 1979). Their extent of overlap varies in different parts of the body map as has been reported for the rat (Hall and Lindholm, 1974). In both the possum and the rat, the overlap of VL and VP projections is greatest for the hindlimb representation in the medial parietal region of the hemisphere, but declines moving laterally to the regions of forelimb and head representation (Hall and Lindholm, 1974; Haight and Neylon, 1978b, 1979). Haight and Neylon (1978b) found that the VP projection area in the possum covered the identified SI projection field. In the case of the VL projection, they concluded (Haight and Neylon, 1979) that it corresponded well with the motor cortex identified in stimulation experiments in the possum by Goldby (1939b), Abbie (1940b), and Rees and Hore (1970).

One of the areas of discrepancy in the sensory and motor maps for the possum was in the region just posterior to sulcus α' which lacks somatosensory representation *and* VP input (Haight and Neylon, 1979), but receives VL input (Ward and Watson, 1973; Haight and Neylon, 1979) and is interpreted by Haight and Neylon (1979) as falling in the motor maps outlined by Abbie (1940b), Goldby (1939b), and Rees and Hore (1970).

Haight and Neylon (1979) have also suggested, on the basis of somatosensory maps, that sensory and motor congruence may not be present either in the wombat, *Vombatus ursinus* (Johnson *et al.*, 1973), or in another wallaby, *Thylogale* (or *Macropus*) *billardierii* (Weller *et al.*, 1977). However, further data are needed to substantiate this suggestion.

The various observations outlined above indicate that the Lende hypothesis (1963c, 1969) of a sensorimotor amalgam for marsupials cannot be sustained for the order as a whole. Furthermore, a recent study by Hummelsheim and Wiesendanger (1985) emphasizes the need for caution in interpreting any claims for a sensorimotor amalgam in cortical organization. They investigated for a particular hindlimb structure, the gastrocnemius muscle, the reported sensorimotor amalgam in the hindlimb region of the rat cortex (Hall and Lindholm, 1974; Sanderson *et al.*, 1984). Using intracortical microstimulation to map the cortical area from which gastrocnemius contractions could be elicited, and a combination of evoked potentials and unitary recording for mapping proprioceptive representation arising from gastrocnemius, they found that, although motor and sensory areas lay within the same cytoarchitectural area of granular cortex, they were largely separate with only a small zone of overlap.

Finally, even in the opossum, the species which gave rise to Lende's hypothesis, it appears that the sensorimotor amalgam hypothesis is no longer sustainable as Pubols *et al.* (1976) have shown, using microelectrode mapping, that the somatosensory cortex is significantly smaller than the area revealed by Lende's evoked potential analysis (see Fig. 10). This means that it would not correspond with the motor area unless, of course, intracortical, microstimulation procedures reveal that the size of the motor area was also overestimated in Lende's original studies (which relied upon surface stimulation of the cortex).

9.4. Corticospinal Projections from Motor Cortex in Marsupials and Monotremes

Direct projections from motor areas of cortex to spinal cord have been demonstrated for both marsupial and monotreme species. Johnson's (1977) review of the marsupial data indicates that corticospinal fibers only project as far as the cervical and thoracic segments of the cord. Although most fibers end within the segments C5 to T1, projections have been described as far caudal as T10–T12 in *Trichosurus* and *Potorous* (Martin *et al.*, 1970, 1972; Rees and Hore, 1970). Johnson (1977) concluded that the absence of corticospinal projections to more caudal levels in marsupials does not permit phylogenetic generalizations among the three mammalian orders as some placental mammals, e.g., the armadillo (*Desypus novemcinctus mexicanus*) of the order Edentata (Fisher *et al.*, 1969), also have corticospinal projections that are limited to cervical and thoracic segments. Furthermore, in the monotremes, the echidna has corticospinal projections to all levels of the cord (Goldby, 1939a) as is the case in primates and carnivores (Petras, 1969).

The corticospinal projection in the possum arises from areas of cortex both anterior and posterior to sulcus α (Porter, 1955) and may therefore slightly exceed the area identified as motor cortex in stimulation experiments (Goldby, 1939b; Abbie, 1940b; Rees and Hore, 1970).

Development of the Corticospinal Tract in Marsupials

The immaturity of marsupials at birth compared with placental mammals, and their subsequent accessibility in the maternal pouch has enabled Martin's group to analyze the development of the corticospinal system in the American opossum (Cabana and Martin, 1984, 1985). This particular species is born after a gestational period of 12 days when the snout-to-rump length of the animal may be no more than 12 mm. Retrograde labeling studies show that direct projections from the cortex to spinal cord are only established by about postnatal day (PND) 30 and that these corticospinal fibers are the last of the major supraspinal descending pathways to reach the spinal cord (Cabana and Martin, 1984, 1985). In comparison, brain-stem axons that contain serotonin are present in the cord at the time of birth (Martin *et al.*, 1978).

Martin's work shows that the first corticospinal connections to be established in the opossum around PND 30 arise from the somatosensory–motor areas of cortex (Fig. 33A). However, there is a subsequent phase starting a week later, during which neurons can be labeled over a much wider area of cortex (Fig. 33B), including regions which do not innervate the spinal cord in the adult animal (Fig. 33C). The period in which this transient, diffuse corticospinal projection is apparent lasts about a month until sometime between PND 62 and 80. During this same period, corticospinal axons are present in the spinal cord beyond the dorsal and lateral funiculi in which they are confined in the adult animal. Furthermore, they are present in apparently greater density in the gray matter than in the adult animal (Cabana and Martin, 1985). However, these additional or transient corticospinal axons do not grow beyond the cervical and upper thoracic cord to more caudal locations than those ordinarily supplied in the adult opossum.

The results of these developmental studies are interpreted by Cabana and Martin (1984, 1985) as evidence for transient corticospinal projections which reach a peak density in the period from about PND 42 to 62. The phenomenon, in which it is assumed that selective elimination of the transient inappropriate projections takes place as a result of neuronal cell death or retraction of particular axon collaterals (Jacobson, 1978; Cowan *et al.*, 1984), has also been described for the developing corticospinal tract in the rat (D'Amato and Hicks, 1978; Ivy and Killackey, 1982; Stanfield *et al.*, 1982). However, as the entire phenomenon, from the earliest evidence of overproduction of corticospinal neurons through to the elimination of the inappropriate neurons, takes place well into postnatal life in the marsupials, these species offer considerable advantages for further study of the factors controlling these processes (see also Section 11).

9.5. Corticocortical Connections of the Marsupial Motor Cortex

Studies of the intracortical connections of the motor cortex have been made in both the American opossum (Ebner, 1967; Foster and Ebner, 1977; Foster and Donoghue, 1979; Foster *et al.*, 1981) and the Australian possum (Heath and Jones, 1971; Joschko and Sanderson, 1987). In each species the motor cortex receives input from the primary and secondary somatosensory areas of the same hemisphere. There is also some evidence in the possum for an input from a parietal area immediately caudal to SI (Joschko and Sanderson, 1987). Interhemispheric inputs come from the primary somatic sensorimotor areas, predominantly from the face and the trunk areas rather than from the limb areas (Heath and Jones, 1971; Joschko and Sanderson, 1987). Thus, the interhemispheric pattern of connections corresponds to that described in primates (Jones and Wise, 1977; Jenny, 1979). They arise mainly from lamina V neurons and travel, in the absence of a corpus callosum, via the cerebral commissures.

It was concluded by Joschko and Sanderson (1987) that, in general, the

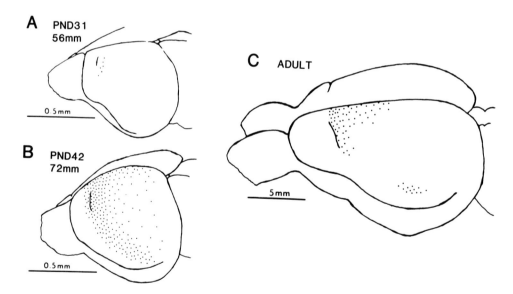

Figure 33. Cortical regions from which corticospinal projections arise during development in the opossum. Summary diagram of the cortical labeling produced by spinal injections of markers at three stages of the opossum's development. In the adult opossum (C), labeled neurons are found in regions corresponding topographically to trunk–limb areas of motor–sensory cortex. The first neurons labeled, at approximately PND 31 (A), are located in areas corresponding to part of the presumptive motor–sensory cortex. There is a subsequent period of development (B) during which neurons can be labeled not only in presumptive motor–sensory cortex, but also in areas outside it. PND, postnatal day; 56 and 72 mm represent the snout-to-rump lengths of the opossum at PND 31 and 42, respectively. (From Cabana and Martin, 1984.)

pattern of cortical connections of the possum motor cortex was similar to that in other mammals. Furthermore, the subcortical structures projecting to motor cortex were similar to those in placental mammals and included the ventrolateral and ventromedial thalamic nuclei, as well as the raphe nucleus of the midbrain, the basal forebrain, and the hypothalamus (Haight and Neylon, 1979; Joschko and Sanderson, 1987). Reciprocal connections were also found between motor cortex and the claustrum as were projections from motor cortex to the caudate nucleus, the putamen, and globus pallidus (Heath and Jones, 1971; Joschko and Sanderson, 1987). However, the projection to the striatum appears more diffuse for the possum than in most placental mammals (Heath and Jones, 1971), both in its cortical origin (most of the neocortex with the exception of visual areas) and in its termination, which covers the whole of the striatum in contrast to the restricted striatal projection described for placental mammals (Carman *et al.*, 1965).

10. Frontal Cortex

The discovery that the echidna has an extensive area of frontal cortex free of specific motor or sensory representation (Abbie, 1938; Goldby, 1939a; Lende, 1964) presented a paradox for students of comparative neurology who felt, first, that monotremes approximated an archetypal mammalian form and, second, that phylogenetic advancement could be measured in terms of the proportion of cerebral cortex taken up by areas not concerned with specific sensory or motor function (see Diamond and Hall, 1969; Section 12). The frontal granular cortex in particular is an area whose relative size has been assumed to increase in ascending the phylogenetic scale (Brodmann, 1909; Diamond and Hall, 1969; Ebner, 1969). The hedgehog has virtually no frontal area beyond the motor cortex, while at the other extreme of the placental range this frontal area makes up about 30% of the human cortex (Fuster, 1980). With the recognition that it makes up about 50% of the echidna neocortex, Welker and Lende (1980) and Divac *et al.* (1987a,b) set out to determine whether the frontal area in the echidna corresponded to the prefrontal cortex of placental mammals, an area defined by Rose and Woolsey (1948) as the cortical projection area of the thalamic mediodorsal nucleus, or whether it represented an equivalent of a combination of the anterior and posterior association areas of placental mammals.

Both groups found that thalamic input arose from a large nuclear mass in the dorsal frontomedial thalamus which, based on an architectonic analysis of the echidna thalamus (Regidor and Divac, 1987), appears to correspond to the mediodorsal nucleus (Welker and Lende, 1980; Divac *et al.*, 1987a) and which may therefore serve in the echidna as the thalamic relay for olfactory information destined for the cerebral cortex as it does in other mammals (Powell *et al.*, 1965; Leonard, 1972; Benjamin and Jackson, 1974; Potter and Nauta, 1979). Within the frontal area, adjacent regions of cortex received input from adjacent regions within the dorsomedial thalamus (Welker and Lende, 1980). Inputs of nonthalamic origin were from sources similar to those in placental mammals and included symmetrical areas of the contralateral hemisphere, the ipsilateral paleocortex, in particular the cortex at the base of sulcus μ (for location see Fig. 4B) and from subcortical structures including mesencephalic tegmentum, the raphe nuclei, and the locus coeruleus. It was concluded from these observations that the prefrontal area in the echidna may be innervated by axons containing dopamine, noradrenaline, serotonin, and acetylcholine as in other mammals, and that the large area of echidna cortex in front of sulcus β (Fig. 13) not only corresponds to the prefrontal cortex of placental mammals but represents a proportionately larger area in the echidna than it does in the human (Divac *et al.*, 1987a; Regidor and Divac, 1987).

The efferent connections of the echidna prefrontal area also show striking similarities to those of placental mammals including primates (Divac *et al.*, 1987b). They involve projections to the symmetrical area of the opposite hemisphere, bilateral projections to the striatum and the paleocortex, the ipsilateral mediodorsal region of thalamus, the hypothalamus, the ventral tegmentum, and the pons. Although no efferent projections were found to the hippocampus, the amygdala, and the mesencephalic central gray, all of which are present in placental mammals, Divac *et al.* (1987b) point out that their study was conducted in only two animals and that further data are needed before these connections can be ruled out for the echidna.

The connections of the frontal area of cortex in the platypus have not been explored. However, the area in front of the specific sensory and motor areas of cortex is very much smaller than the equivalent area in the echidna (Bohringer and Rowe, 1977). This may in part reflect a smaller relative size of the thalamic mediodorsal nucleus in the platypus (Hines, 1929) and a lesser importance of olfaction in the largely aquatic platypus than is the case in the echidna (Burrell, 1927; Barrett, 1941; Griffiths, 1978, 1988).

The suggestion (Divac *et al.*, 1987a) that the frontal area in the platypus may be related to the recently reported electroreception in the bill of the platypus (Scheich *et al.*, 1986) is not tenable for the reasons outlined in Section 5.3.8.

In the case of the frontal area of cortex in marsupials, it appears that connections are similar to those of the echidna and placental mammals, at least for the Australian possum, *Trichosurus vulpecula* (Goldby, 1943; Broomhead, 1974; Joschko and Sanderson, 1987).

11. Marsupials as Models for the Study of Cerebral Cortical Development

As marsupials are born at a very immature stage, they offer advantages for developmental studies, in particular when they remain for a long period readily available in the maternal pouch. The advantages are not simply related to a short gestation period (e.g., 12 days in *Didelphis virginiana*) but to the protracted period over which development may take place. Thus, even in marsupials such as the tammar wallaby, *Macropus eugenii*, with a longer gestation time (27 days), all major phases of cerebral cortical development take place postnatally. These processes are therefore much more amenable to experimental investigation and manipulation than is the case in placental mammals (see also Section 9.4).

At birth, the tammar wallaby weighs approximately 0.5 g, or 1/10,000 its adult weight (Renfree *et al.*, 1982). The developing neocortex is at a two-layered embryonic stage consisting of a marginal layer (or primordial plexiform layer; Reynolds *et al.*, 1985) and a ventricular zone (Fig. 34a) and resembles the stage seen in an early human embryo (Reynolds *et al.*, 1985). Subsequent stages during postnatal life involve, first, the appearance of the cortical plate within the plexiform layer at about 5–6 days after birth (Fig. 34f). The cells forming this plate arise close to the ventricular surface, where the active mitotic region exists, and migrate through the ventricular zone in the inside-to-outside pattern of differentiation that has been described in the fetal placental animal. By PND 10–15 the cortical plate is distinct, and separates an outer marginal layer from an intermediate or subplate zone (Fig. 34g,h). Although little increase takes place in the width of the cortical plate up to PND 75, the intermediate zone—which lies between the cortical plate and the ventricular zone—undergoes substantial development and displays, by PND 20, striking patterns of widely spaced rows of cells aligned parallel to the cortical surface (Reynolds *et al.*, 1985). This arrangement persists until PND 75 when the regularity of these rows disappears.

Thymidine-labeling studies show that the majority of cells forming the primordial plexiform and future marginal layer appear to be generated before the end of the 27-day gestation period. The earliest cells destined for the cortical plate do not arise until the time of birth. Therefore, most cells forming the plate arise postnatally. The earliest are located deeper than cells that are born later and which migrate through to occupy the outer layers of the cortical plate (Reynolds *et al.*, 1985).

In all marsupial species examined by Reynolds and Saunders (1988), the neocortex was at an embryonic stage of differentiation at the time of birth. However, differences are discernible within this metatherian group. Of those studied, the most immature was *Phascogale calura* (the red-tailed phascogale) which had no detectable marginal layer at birth. This zone was also not well defined in *Dasyroides byrnie* (the kowari, or brush-tailed marsupial rat) and *Dasyurus viverrinus* (the western quoll or western native cat). However, this layer is fully established at birth for *Isoodon macrourus* and *Monodelphis domestica*.

The development of the intermediate zone also shows some variability among marsupial species. The highly ordered pattern of differentiation seen for the tammar wallaby, with rows of cells aligned parallel to the cortical surface, is also seen in *Trichosurus vulpecula* between PND 19 and 40, but was not seen in *Monodelphis domestica*.

The differences that are seen at the time of birth emphasize the inappropriateness of using the time of birth as a reference for evaluating brain or cortical development. Nevertheless, the fact that the sequence of neocortical development in marsupials follows the eutherian pattern and occurs at a postnatal rather than the less accessible fetal stage, suggests that the tammar wallaby and other marsupials could prove useful experimental models in which to examine the early events in neocortical development (Reynolds and Saunders, 1988). This could be of importance, for example, in investigating the developmental significance of *plasma* proteins which are now known from immunocytochemical analysis to be present in the immature cerebral cortex of many species including the mouse, sheep, pig, tammar wallaby, and human (Cavanagh and Møllgard, 1985; Saunders, 1985). Although it was originally thought that these proteins were taken up in the brain from blood or cerebrospinal fluid, it has now been reported that labeled plasma proteins do not appear to penetrate from blood into the brain even in very immature fetuses (Saunders, 1985). Furthermore, there is now evidence that some of these proteins are synthesized within the developing brain itself (Saunders, 1985). *Plasma* proteins found within the im-

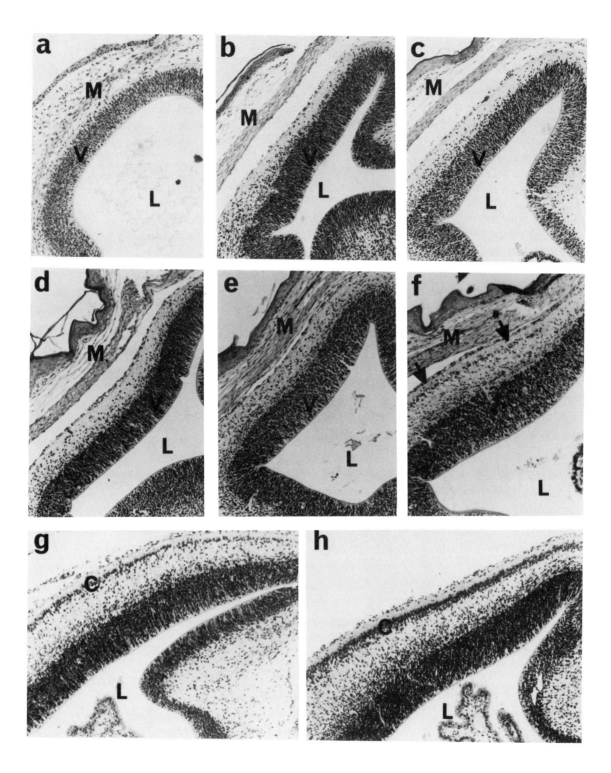

mature cerebral cortex include α-fetoprotein, fetuin, transferrin, and albumin (Benno and Williams, 1978; Cavanagh and Møllgard, 1985; Saunders, 1985; Reynolds and Saunders, 1988).

Albumin staining has been demonstrated for cells of the cortical plate within the pouch-young tammar wallaby at 8 weeks of postnatal age. Although transferrin-positive cells are not detectable in the plate cells at this time, processes within the subplate zone show weakly positive labeling. The fiber plexuses of this subplate zone are largely made up of catecholamine-containing fibers arising from brain-stem and thalamic nuclei (Zecevic and Molliver, 1978). This subplate zone is the site of formation of many synaptic contacts in the developing neocortex (Molliver *et al.*, 1973). Although the functional significance of *plasma* proteins in the developing brain remains unclear, Saunders (1985) has speculated that differential distributions of them between plate cells and incoming fibers may be important in the formation of contacts between these different neuronal populations.

Marsupial representatives such as the tammar wallaby may provide easier access for studying the effects of interfering with one population of neurons (e.g., the brain-stem raphe nuclei) on the development of the cortical plate cells, and for investigating the role of the *plasma* proteins in cortical differentiation (Saunders, 1985; Reynolds and Saunders, 1988). They also allow much earlier study of the effects of afferent input on development and differentiation of mammalian central neural structures, including the cerebral cortex, than is possible in placental mammals. In placentals, for example, it is difficult, because of the requirements for intrauterine surgery, to study the effects of deafferentation before primary afferent connectivity is established with central target neurons. In contrast, in many marsupials, deafferentation can be carried out in postnatal life well before central connections are made. An example of this is seen in the Australian northern native cat (*Dasyurus hallucatus*) which has a birth weight of about 18 mg (Nelson, 1987; Crewther *et al.*, 1988). In this marsupial, the retinal ganglion cell axons do not leave the eye until PND 3. Furthermore, they do not reach the chiasm before PND 6 or reach central target structures before about PND 25. Crewther *et al.* (1988) have shown that enucleation prior to establishment of central connections produces a volume reduction in those parts of the lateral geniculate and superior colliculus that were deprived of input. However, they found, in contrast to reports in placental species, that there was no expan-

---

Figure 34. Development of marsupial cerebral cortex. Development of the dorsolateral wall of the telencephalon in the tammar wallaby (*Macropus eugenii*) from the embryonic stage, which consists of a marginal, or primordial plexiform layer and a ventricular zone, up to the stage when a cortical plate is differentiated throughout. Marginal, intermediate (or subplate zone), and subventricular zones are also present. Coronal sections of the midregion (except e) of the left hemisphere including the ventricle. Brains from 24 days fetal to 6 days postnatal fixed and cut *in situ* in the skull. Older brains removed from the skull after initial fixation by perfusion. Stain: haematoxylin and eosin. × 88. L, lateral ventricle; M, mesenchyme of developing skull; V, ventricular zone underlying the marginal or primordial plexiform layer (a); C, cortical plate throughout dorsolateral wall (g, h). (a) 24 days gestation; (b) newborn day 0; (c) 2 days postnatal. (d–f). 5–6 days postnatal; cortical plate anlage appearing in the midregion. (d) 5 days and (e) 6 days anterior region. (f) 6 days midlateral region; first differentiation of the cortical plate (arrows). (g, h) 10–15 days postnatal; cortical plate differentiated throughout the dorsolateral wall of the telencephalon; marginal, intermediate, and subventricular zones now present. (g) 10 days postnatal; (h) 15 days postnatal. (From Reynolds *et al.*, 1985.)

sion of the zone of termination of surviving optic nerve axons into deafferented areas of the target structures. Preliminary observations at the cortical level indicated that there were differences in thickness of visual cortex between ipsi- and contralateral sides following enucleation, but more detailed analysis has yet to be carried out (Crewther *et al.*, 1988).

12. Functional Localization in the Cerebral Cortex and the Evolutionary Place of the Marsupials and Monotremes: Concluding Comments

Comparative studies of sensorimotor representation within the mammalian neocortex have shown that in certain placental mammals such as the hedgehog, porcupine, tree shrew, and rabbit, the neocortex is taken up almost entirely with specific sensory and motor function (Lende and Woolsey, 1956; Woolsey, 1958; Lende and Sadler, 1967; Diamond and Hall, 1969; Lende, 1969). Species displaying this pattern of cortical organization have often been taken to represent a more *primitive* group of mammals that may reflect a phylogenetically ancient, or less highly evolved stage of cerebral cortical development (Lende, 1969). Furthermore, it has been argued (Lende, 1969) that the starting point in the functional evolution of neocortex was a common, superimposed sensorimotor area of representation, and that, in the course of evolution, there has been a progressive spatial differentiation of the constituent sensory and motor maps until each acquires distinct spatial independence with the emergence of substantial intervening cortical areas generally termed association areas or belt areas (Diamond and Hall, 1969). Thus, in mammals that are often considered more advanced in evolutionary terms, such as the higher primates, but also the cat, there is a much smaller proportion of neocortex allocated to specific sensorimotor representation (Woolsey, 1958, 1964).

These observations and interpretations have been based, for the most part, on the use of evoked potential methods to identify sensory areas and surface stimulation procedures for the identification of motor areas. With these techniques it appears that the neocortical expansion in evolution is related principally to an increase in the association areas. These areas receive intracortical inputs from the specific sensory and motor areas of cortex, and are therefore thought to provide the opportunity for cross-modality integration of a kind that may allow elementary sensory data to be transformed into more complex perceptual recognition.

However, this view of the so-called association cortex may have arisen in part because too little attention was given to the thalamic sources of input to the association areas. These inputs arise from thalamic subnuclei different from those that supply the identified *specific* sensory areas of cortex and include, for example, the mediodorsal nucleus and the pulvinar, a thalamic region which is known to undergo expansion in the course of primate evolution (Diamond, 1979). In giving greater emphasis to these subcortical inputs, Diamond (1979) concluded that the neocortex is made up of just a few fields—somatic sensory and motor, visual and auditory in particular—but that, in the course of evolutionary advancement, each field acquires greater numbers of subdivisions whose inputs reach the cortex over a series of parallel ascending systems that traverse different brain-stem nuclei in their path to the cortex. Not all of the subdivisions within one of the broader sensory fields will necessarily be identified with evoked potential techniques. However, with the more sensitive and detailed analysis of neocortical organization that is possible with microelectrode recording techniques and newer fiber tracing methods it is becoming increasingly clear that in higher mammals larger proportions of neocortex are being identified as visual, auditory, or somatosensory in nature (see Pandya and Yeterian, 1985; Jones, 1986). Multiple representations or maps are being identified for a given sensory modality within areas that were previously designated association cortex. A striking example of this is seen for the visual cortex in the monkey which, it is now argued, occupies the entire posterior half of the hemisphere and may be made up of at least a dozen distinctive areas that are largely or exclusively visual in function (Van Essen and Maunsell, 1983). The identification of these as multiple visual areas is based on the connections, topographic organization, cytoarchitecture, and functional properties of the different areas. They are interrelated in parallel and hierarchical schemes which Van Essen and Maunsell (1983) suggest form two major functional streams, one related to the analysis of motion and the other to the analysis of form and color.

The same trend is apparent in the analysis of auditory and somatosensory areas of cortex. Thus, auditory cortex is traditionally defined as that part of the temporal cortex which receives afferent input from the medial geniculate body and which contains neurons responsive to acoustic stimulation (Brugge and Reale, 1985). However, as Diamond (1979) and Brugge and Reale (1985) point out, the definition of auditory areas of cortex may be expanded to include those areas referred to as *associational* that receive acoustic inputs, but mainly from sources outside those making up the main auditory lemniscal pathway. Within the somatosensory modality the identification of multiple areas of cortical representation has been based on both a fractionation of the originally identified SI and SII areas and the identification of additional areas, such as SIII and SIV, beyond SI and SII (Jones, 1985, 1986; Burton, 1986).

With the identification of multiple cortical fields for different sensory modalities, it is now clear in placental representatives such as the monkey and cat that a much larger proportion of neocortex is occupied by sensory representation than appeared to be the case with evoked potential recordings. In view of these developments in our understanding of neocortical organization, it may no longer be appropriate to attempt to evaluate neocortical evolutionary progress in terms of the extent to which association areas have come to occupy the neocortex. An alternative view might be that evolutionary advancement is more reliably reflected in the extent to which there are multiple representation zones within the cortex for a given sensory modality. However, it may be premature to apply such an index of evolutionary development to species, including those in the marsupial and monotreme orders, in which the analysis of neocortical sensorimotor organization has been less exhaustive than that carried out for the cat and monkey.

However, there is a further reservation. Although the appearance of multiple representation for a particular sensory modality may reflect evolutionary advancement in the neocortex for *some* animal groups, in others it may have been a more appropriate evolutionary course to develop and elaborate the processing mechanisms for that sensory modality within the one representational field in the cortex. This may be the case, for example, in the platypus where its great behavioral reliance upon sensory processing from the bill appears to be consolidated within a single, but vast area of representation within the cortex (see Section 5.3). Nevertheless, examples of multiple representation have been observed in nonplacental species, but the incidence does vary considerably. Multiple visual areas have been reported in both the possum and the opossum (Section 7) and a triple representation of parts of the face was found in the somatosensory cortex of the opossum (Section 5.2). There is also evidence of multiple auditory areas in the marsupial Australian native cat (Section 6.1). However, in species that have multiple cortical ares for one sensory modality, for example the possum, which is reported to have multiple visual areas, there may be only a single auditory area (Sections 6.1 and 7.1). It is therefore possible that within the one species there may be evidence for differential evolutionary advancement in the neocortex from one sensory modality to another.

Only a single area of representation was reported for each of the visual, auditory, and somatosensory modalities in the monotreme studies (Lende, 1964; Bohringer and Rowe, 1977). However, the mappings of visual and auditory areas were based only on evoked potential studies and therefore would not reveal dual or multiple areas unless they were spatially distinct. Further studies with microelectrodes are needed in order to test for multiple representation in these modalities. Perhaps, as Diamond (1979) and others have suggested, the number of parallel ascending pathways which convey information to cortex for a given sensory modality may provide a further index of the evolutionary adaptations in different orders of mammals, or from species to species within the one order. However, much more data are needed, from the monotremes in particular, on the subcortical pathways before any reliable comparisons are possible in this respect.

On present evidence therefore, it is difficult to identify cerebral cortical attributes that may be considered diagnostic of a particular order of mammals, and that identify a particular order as being closer to a hypothetical primordial, or ancestral form of the cerebral cortex. This is true whether one considers gross measures such as brain size or the extent of the neocortex, or electrophysiologically identified features of the sensory and motor areas of the cortex. As the monotremes diverged from the therian mammals about 200 million years ago, and the marsupial and placental mammals themselves diverged about 100 million years ago, the surviving members of each order are the product of independent evolutionary streams and none need necessarily resemble the hypothetical mammalian ancestral form in cerebral cortical organization. Similarities that do exist between orders may reflect parallel evolution rather than the retention of attributes characteristic of an ancestral form of the cerebral cortex.

ACKNOWLEDGMENTS. The author's work is supported by the National Health and Medical Research Council of Australia and the Australian Research Council.

13. References

Abbie, A. A., 1934, The brain stem and cerebellum of *Echidna aculeata*, *Philos. Trans. R. Soc. London Ser. B* **224**:1–74.

Abbie, A. A., 1938, The excitable cortex in the Monotremata, *Aust. J. Exp. Biol. Med. Sci.* **16:**143–152.

Abbie, A. A., 1939, The origin of the corpus callosum and the fate of the structures related to it, *J. Comp. Neurol.* **71:**9–44.

Abbie, A. A., 1940a, Cortical lamination in the Monotremata, *J. Comp. Neurol.* **72:**429–467.

Abbie, A. A., 1940b, The excitable cortex in *Perameles, Sarcophilus, Dasyurus, Trichosurus,* and *Wallabia (Macropus), J. Comp. Neurol.* **72:**469–487.

Adey, W. R., and Kerr, D. I. B., 1954, The cerebral representation of deep somatic sensibility in the marsupial phalanger and rabbit; an evoked potential and histological study, *J. Comp. Neurol.* **100:**597–626.

Adrian, E. D., 1940, Double representation of the feet in the sensory cortex of the cat, *J. Physiol. (London)* **98:**16P–18P.

Adrian, E. D., 1941, Afferent discharges to the cerebral cortex from peripheral sense organs, *J. Physiol. (London)* **100:**159–191.

Aitkin, L. M., and Gates, G. R., 1983, Connections of the auditory cortex of the brush-tailed possum, *Trichosurus vulpecula, Brain Behav. Evol.* **22:**75–88.

Aitkin, L. M., Calford, M. B., Kenyon, C. E., and Webster, W. R., 1981, Some facets of the organization of the principal division of the cat medial geniculate body, in: *Neuronal Mechanisms of Hearing* (J. Syka and L. M. Aitkin, eds.), Plenum Press, New York, pp. 163–181.

Aitkin, L. M., Irvine, D. R. F., and Webster, W. R., 1984, Central neural mechanisms of hearing, in: *Handbook of Physiology,* Section I, Volume III, Part 2 (I. Darian-Smith, ed.), American Physiological Society, Bethesda, pp. 675–737.

Aitkin, L. M., Irvine, D. R. F., Nelson, J. E., Merzenich, M. M., and Clarey, J. C., 1986, Frequency representation in the auditory midbrain and forebrain of a marsupial, the northern native cat (*Dasyurus hallucatus*), *Brain Behav. Evol.* **29:**17–28.

Allison, T., and Goff, W. R., 1972, Electrophysiological studies of the echidna, *Tachyglossus aculeatus* III. Sensory and interhemispheric evoked responses, *Arch. Ital. Biol.* **110:**195–216.

Andres, K. H., and von Düring, M., 1984, The platypus bill. A structural and functional model of a pattern-like arrangement of different cutaneous sensory receptors, in: *Sensory Receptor Mechanisms* (W. Hamann and A. Iggo, eds.), World Scientific Publishers, Singapore, pp. 81–88.

Archer, M., 1982, A review of the origins of radiations of Australian mammals, in: *Ecological Biogeography of Australia* (A. Keast, ed.), Junk, The Hague, pp. 1435–1488.

Austad, S. N., 1988, The adaptable opossum, *Sci. Am.* **258**(2):54–59.

Barrett, C., 1941, *The Platypus,* Robertson & Mullend, Melbourne.

Bautista, N. A., and Matzke, H. A., 1965, A degeneration study of the course and extent of the pyramidal tract of the opossum, *J. Comp. Neurol.* **124:**367–375.

Benevento, L. A., and Ebner, F. F., 1971a, The areas and layers of corticocortical terminations in the visual cortex of the Virginia opossum, *J. Comp. Neurol.* **141:**157–190.

Benevento, L. A., and Ebner, F. F., 1971b, The contribution of the dorsal lateral geniculate nucleus to the total pattern of thalamic terminations in striate cortex of the Virginia opossum, *J. Comp. Neurol.* **143:**243–260.

Benjamin, R. M., and Jackson, J. C., 1974, Unit discharges in the mediodorsal nucleus of the squirrel monkey evoked by electrical stimulation of the olfactory bulb, *Brain Res.* **75:**181–191.

Bennett, R. E., Ferrington, D. G., and Rowe, M. J., 1980, Tactile neuron classes within second somatosensory area (SII) of cat cerebral cortex, *J. Neurophysiol.* **43:**292–309.

Benno, R. H., and Williams, T. H., 1978, Evidence for intracellular localization of alpha-fetoprotein in the developing rat brain, *Brain Res.* **142:**182–186.

Bodemer, C. W., and Towe, A. L., 1963, Cortical localization patterns in the somatic sensory cortex of the opossum, *Exp. Neurol.* **8:**380–394.

Bodian, D., 1942, Studies on the diencephalon of the Virginia opossum. Part III. The thalamocortical projection, *J. Comp. Neurol.* **77:**525–575.

Bohringer, R. C., 1977, The somatosensory system of the platypus (*Ornithorhynchus anatinus*), Ph.D. thesis, University of New South Wales, Sydney.

Bohringer, R. C., 1981, Cutaneous receptors in the bill of the platypus (*Ornithorhynchus anatinus*), *Aust. Mammal.* **4:**93–105.

Bohringer, R. C., and Rowe, M. J., 1977, The organization of the sensory and motor areas of cerebral cortex in the platypus (*Ornithorhynchus anatinus*), *J. Comp. Neurol.* **174:**1–14.

Brodmann, K., 1909, *Vergleichende Lokalissationslehre der Grosshirnrinde,* Barth, Leipzig.

Bromiley, R. B., and Brooks, C. M., 1940, Role of neocortex in regulating postural reactions of the opossum (*Didelphis virginiana*), *J. Neurophysiol.* **3:**339–346.

Broomhead, A., 1974, The mediodorsal thalamic nucleus of the brush-tailed possum, *Trichosurus vulpecula, J. Anat.* **118:**392.

Brugge, J. F., and Reale, R. A., 1985, Auditory cortex, in: *Cerebral Cortex,* Volume 4 (A. Peters and E. G. Jones, eds.), Plenum Press, New York, pp. 229–271.

Bullier, J., 1984, Axonal bifurcation in the afferents to cortical areas of the visual system, in: *Visual Neuroscience* (J. D. Pettigrew, K. J. Sanderson, and W. R. Levick, eds.), Cambridge University Press, London, pp. 239–259.

Burkitt, A. N. S., 1934, The variability of the gyri and sulci in the cerebral hemispheres of *Tachyglossus* (echidna) *aculeata, Psychiatr. Neurol. Bl.* **38:**368–378.

Burrell, H., 1927, *The Platypus: Its Discovery, Zoological Position, Form and Characteristics, Habits, Life History Etc.,* Angus & Robertson, Sydney.

Burton, H., 1986, The second somatosensory cortex and related areas, in: *Cerebral Cortex,* Volume 5 (E. G. Jones and A. Peters, eds.), Plenum Press, New York, pp. 31–98.

Cabana, T., and Martin, G. F., 1984, Developmental sequence in the origin of descending spinal pathways. Studies using retrograde transport techniques in the North American opossum *(Didelphis virginiana), Dev. Brain Res.* **15:**247–263.

Cabana, T., and Martin, G. F., 1985, Corticospinal development in the North-American opossum: Evidence for a sequence in the growth of cortical axons in the spinal cord and for transient projections, *Dev. Brain Res.* **23:**69–80.

Campbell, C. B. G., and Hayhow, W. R., 1971, Primary optic pathways in the echidna *Tachyglossus aculeatus:* An experimental degeneration study, *J. Comp. Neurol.* **143:**119–136.

Campbell, C. B. G., and Hayhow, W. R., 1972, Primary optic pathways in the duckbill platypus *Ornithorynchus anatinus:* An experimental degeneration study, *J. Comp. Neurol.* **145:**195–208.

Carman, J. B., Cowan, W. M., Powell, T. P. S., and Webster, K. E., 1965, A bilateral corticostriate projection, *J. Neurol. Neurosurg. Psychiatry* **28:**71–77.

Carreras, M., and Anderson, S. A., 1963, Functional properties of neurons of the anterior ectosylvian gyrus of the cat, *J. Neurophysiol.* **26:**100–126.

Cavanagh, M. E., and Møllgard, K., 1985, An immunocytochemical study of the distribution of some plasma proteins within the developing forebrain of the pig with reference to the neocortex, *Dev. Brain Res.* **17:**183–194.

Clemens, W. A., 1977, Phylogeny of the marsupials, in: *Biology of Marsupials* (B. Stonehouse and D. Gilmore, eds.), Macmillan & Co., London, pp. 51–68.

Clemens, W. A., 1979a, Marsupialia, in: *Mesozoic Animals* (J. A. Lillegraven, Z. Kielan-Jaworowska, and W. A. Clemens, eds.), University of California Press, Berkeley, pp. 192–220.

Clemens, W. A., 1979b, Marsupialia, in: *Mesozoic Animals* (J. A. Lillegraven, Z. Kielan-Jaworowska, and W. A. Clemens, eds.), University of California Press, Berkeley, pp. 309–311.

Coleman, J., Diamond, I. T., and Winer, J. A., 1977, The visual cortex of the opossum: The retrograde transport of horseradish peroxidase to the lateral geniculate and lateral posterior nuclei, *Brain Res.* **137:**233–252.

Cowan, W. M., Fawcett, J. W., O'Leary, D. D. M., and Stanfield, B. B., 1984, Regressive events in neurogenesis, *Science* **225:**1258–1265.

Crewther, D. P., Crewther, S. G., and Sanderson, K. J., 1984, Primary visual cortex in the brush-tailed possum: Receptive field properties and corticocortical connections, *Brain Behav. Evol.* **24:**184–197.

Crewther, D. P., Nelson, J. E., and Crewther, S. G., 1988, Afferent input for target survival in marsupial visual development, *Neurosci. Lett.* **86:**147–154.

Cunningham, R. H., 1898, The cortical motor centres of the opossum, *Didelphis virginiana, J. Physiol. (London)* **22:**264–269.

D'Amato, C. J., and Hicks, S. P., 1978, Normal development and post-traumatic plasticity of corticospinal neurons in rats, *Exp. Neurol.* **60:**557–569.

Darian-Smith, I., Isbister, J., Mok, H., and Yokota, T., 1966, Somatic sensory cortical projection areas excited by tactile stimulation of the cat: A triple representation, *J. Physiol. (London)* **182:**671–689.

Dawson, T. J., 1983, *Monotremes and Marsupials: The Other Mammals,* Arnold, London, pp. 1–87.

Diamond, I. T., 1979, The subdivisions of neocortex: A proposal to revise the traditional view of sensory, motor and association areas, *Prog. Psychobiol. Physiol. Psychol.* **8:**1–43.

Diamond, I. T., and Hall, W. C., 1969, Evolution of neocortex, *Science* **164:**251–262.

Diamond, I. T., and Utley, J. D., 1963, Thalamic retrograde degeneration study of sensory cortex in opossum, *J. Comp. Neurol.* **120:**129–160.

Divac, I., Holst, M.-C., Nelson, J., and McKenzie, J. S., 1987a, Afferents of the frontal cortex in the echidna *(Tachyglossus aculeatus).* Indication of an outstandingly large prefrontal area, *Brain Behav. Evol.* **30:**303–320.

Divac, I., Pettigrew, J. D., Holst, M.-C., and McKenzie, J. S., 1987b, Efferent connections of the prefrontal cortex of echidna (*Tachyglossus aculeatus*), *Brain Behav. Evol.* **30:**321–327.

Dubois, E., 1897, Sur le rapport du poids de l'encéphale avec la grandeur du corps chez mammifères, *Bull. Soc. Anthropol.* Paris [4] **8:**337–376.

Ebner, F. F., 1967, Afferent connections to neocortex in the opossum (*Didelphis virginiana*), *J. Comp. Neurol.* **129:**241–268.

Ebner, F. F., 1969, A comparison of primitive forebrain organization in metatherian and eutherian mammals, *Ann. N.Y. Acad. Sci.* **167:**241–257.

Elliot Smith, G., 1902, Descriptive and illustrated catalogue of the physiological series of comparative anatomy, in: *R. Coll. Surg. Mus. Cat. Physiol. Ser.* Volume 2, 2nd ed., Taylor & Francis, London.

Ferrington, D. G., and Rowe, M. J., 1980, Differential contributions to the coding of cutaneous vibratory information by cortical somatosensory areas I and II, *J. Neurophysiol.* **43:**310–331.

Fisher, A. M., Harting, J. K., Martin, G. F., and Stuber, M. I., 1969, The origin, course and termination of corticospinal fibers in the armadillo (*Dasypus novemcinctus mexicanus*), *J. Neurol. Sci.* **8:**347–361.

Fisher, G. R., Freeman, B., and Rowe, M. J., 1983, Organization of the parallel projections from Pacinian afferent fibers to somatosensory cortical areas I and II in the cat, *J. Neurophysiol.* **49:**75–97.

Foster, R. E., and Donoghue, J. P., 1979, Ipsilateral corticocortical connections of the SI forepaw area in the parietal cortex of the Virginia opossum, *Anat. Rec.* **193:**540–541.

Foster, R. E., and Ebner, F. F., 1977, Interhemispheric connections between the neocortical forepaw representations in the Virginia opossum, *Soc. Neurosci. Abstr.* **3:**67.

Foster, R. E., Donoghue, J. P., and Ebner, F. F., 1981, Laminar organization of efferent cells in the parietal cortex of the Virginia opossum, *Exp. Brain Res.* **43:**330–336.

Fuster, J. M., 1980, *The Prefrontal Cortex*, Raven Press, New York.

Gates, G. R., and Aitkin, L. M., 1982, Auditory cortex in the marsupial possum *Trichosurus vulpecula*, *Hearing Res.* **7:**1–11.

Gates, G. R., Saunders, J. C., Bock, G. R., Aitkin, L. M., and Elliott, M. A., 1974, Peripheral auditory function in the platypus, *Ornithorhynchus anatinus*, *J. Acoust. Soc. Am.* **56:**152–156.

Gerard, R. W., Marshall, W. H., and Saul, L. J., 1936, Electrical activity of the cat's brain, *Arch. Neurol. Psychiatry* **36:**675–738.

Goldby, F., 1939a, An experimental investigation of the motor cortex and pyramidal tract of *Echidna aculeata*, *J. Anat.* **73:**509–524.

Goldby, F., 1939b, An experimental investigation of the motor cortex and its connexions in the phalanger, *Trichosurus vulpecula*, *J. Anat.* **74:**12–33.

Goldby, F., 1943, An experimental study of the thalamus in the phalanger, *Trichosurus vulpecula*, *J. Anat.* **77:**195–224.

Goldby, F., and Gamble, H. J., 1957, The reptilian cerebral hemispheres, *Biol. Rev.* **32:**383–420.

Gould, H. J., Hall, W. C., and Ebner, F. F., 1978, Connections of the visual cortex in the hedgehog (*Paraechinus hypomelas*), *J. Comp. Neurol.* **177:**445–472.

Grant, T., 1984, *The Platypus*, New South Wales University Press, Sydney.

Gray, P. A., Jr., 1924, The cortical lamination pattern of the opossum, *Didelphys virginiana*, *J. Comp. Neurol.* **37:**221–263.

Gregory, J. E., Iggo, A., McIntyre, A. K., and Proske, U., 1987, Electroreceptors in the platypus, *Nature* **326:**386–387.

Gregory, J. E., Iggo, A., McIntyre, A. K., and Proske, U., 1988, Receptors in the bill of the platypus, *J. Physiol. (London)* **400:**349–366.

Griffiths, M., 1978, *The Biology of the Monotremes*, Academic Press, New York.

Griffiths, M., 1988, The platypus, *Sci. Am.* **256:**84–90.

Haight, J. R., and Murray, P. F., 1981, The cranial endocast of the early Miocene marsupial, *Wynyardia bassiana*: An assessment of taxonomic relationships based upon comparisons with recent forms, *Brain Behav. Evol.* **19:**17–36.

Haight, J. R., and Neylon, L., 1978a, Morphological variation in the brain of the marsupial brush-tailed possum, *Trichosurus vulpecula*, *Brain Behav. Evol.* **15:**415–445.

Haight, J. R., and Neylon, L., 1978b, The organization of neocortical projections from the ventroposterior thalamic complex in the marsupial brush-tailed possum, *Trichosurus vulpecula*: A horseradish peroxidase study, *J. Anat.* **126:**459–485.

Haight, J. R., and Neylon, L., 1979, The organization of neocortical projections from the ventrolateral thalamic nucleus in the brush-tailed possum, *Trichosurus vulpecula*, and the problem of motor and somatic sensory convergence within the mammalian brain, *J. Anat.* **129:**673–694.

Haight, J. R., Sanderson, K. J., Neylon, L., and Patten, G. S., 1980, Relationships of the visual cortex in the marsupial brushtailed possum, *Trichosurus vulpecula:* A horseradish peroxidase and auto-radiographic study, *J. Anat.* **131:**387–413.

Hall, R. D., and Lindholm, E. P., 1974, Organization of motor and somatosensory neocortex in the albino rat, *Brain Res.* **66:**23–38.

Harman, P. J., 1947, Quantitative analysis of the brain–isocortex relationship in Mammalia, *Anat. Rec.* **97:**342.

Hassler, R., and Muhs-Clement, K., 1964, Architektonischer Aufbau des sensomotorischen und Parietalen Cortex der Katze, *J. Hirnforsch.* **6:**377–420.

Hayhow, W. R., 1967, The lateral geniculate nucleus of the marsupial phalanger, *Trichosurus vulpecula.* An experimental study in relation to the intranuclear optic nerve projection fields, *J. Comp. Neurol.* **131:**571–604.

Heath, C. J., and Jones, E. G., 1971, Interhemispheric pathways in the absence of the corpus callosum, *J. Anat.* **109:**253–270.

Herrick, C. L., 1898, The cortical motor centres in lower mammals, *J. Comp. Neurol.* **8:**92–98.

Hines, M., 1929, The brain of *Ornithorhynchus anatinus, Philos. Trans. R. Soc. London Ser. B* **217:**155–259.

Hore, J., Phillips, C. G., and Porter, R., 1973, The effects of pyramidotomy on motor performance in the brush-tailed possum (*Trichosurus vulpecula*), *Brain Res.* **49:**181–184.

Hubel, D. H., and Wiesel, T. N., 1962, Receptive fields, binocular interaction and functional architecture in the cat's visual cortex, *J. Physiol. (London)* **160:**106–154.

Hubel, D. H., and Wiesel, T. N., 1965, Receptive fields and functional architecture in two nonstriate visual areas (18 and 19) of the cat, *J. Neurophysiol.* **28:**229–289.

Hummelsheim, H., and Wiesendanger, M., 1985, Is the hindlimb representation of the rat's cortex a "sensorimotor amalgam"? *Brain Res.* **346:**75–81.

Ivy, G. O., and Killackey, H. P., 1982, Ontogenetic changes in the projections of neocortical neurons, *J. Neurosci.* **2:**735–743.

Jacobson, M., 1978, *Developmental Neurobiology,* Plenum Press, New York.

Jenny, A. B., 1979, Commissural projections of the cortical hand motor areas in monkeys, *J. Comp. Neurol.* **188:**137–146.

Jerison, H. J., 1961, Quantitative analysis of evolution of the brain in mammals, *Science* **133:**1012–1014.

Jerison, H. J., 1973, *Evolution of the Brain and Intelligence,* Academic Press, New York.

Johnson, J. I., 1977, Central nervous system of marsupials, in: *The Biology of Marsupials* (D. Hunsaker, ed.), Academic Press, New York, pp. 157–278.

Johnson, J. I., Haight, J. R., and Megirian, D., 1973, Convolutions related to sensory projections in cerebral neocortex of marsupial wombats, *J. Anat.* **114:**153 (abstr.).

Johnson, J. I., Rubel, E. W., and Hatton, G. I., 1974, Mechanosensory projections to the cerebral cortex of sheep, *J. Comp. Neurol.* **158:**81–108.

Jones, E. G., 1985, *The Thalamus,* Plenum Press, New York.

Jones, E. G., 1986, Connectivity of the primate sensory-motor cortex, in: *Cerebral Cortex,* Volume 5 (E. G. Jones and A. Peters, eds.), Plenum Press, New York, pp. 113–183.

Jones, E. G., and Wise, S. P., 1977, Size, laminar and columnar distribution of efferent cells in the sensory-motor cortex of monkeys, *J. Comp. Neurol.* **75:**391–438.

Joschko, M. A., and Sanderson, K. J., 1987, Cortico-cortical connections of the motor cortex in the brushtailed possum (*Trichosurus vulpecula*), *J. Anat.* **150:**31–42.

Kaas, J. H., 1980, A comparative survey of visual cortex organization in mammals, in: *Comparative Neurology of the Telencephalon* (S. O. E. Ebbesson, ed.), Plenum Press, New York, pp. 483–502.

Kato, H., Bishop, P. O., and Orban, G. A., 1978, Hypercomplex and simple/complex cell classifications in cat striate cortex, *J. Neurophysiol.* **41:**1071–1095.

Killackey, H. P., and Ebner, F. F., 1972, Two different types of thalamocortical projections to a single cortical area in mammals, *Brain Behav. Evol.* **6:**141–169.

Killackey, H., and Ebner, F., 1973, Convergent projection of three separate thalamic nuclei on to a single cortical area, *Science* **179:**283–285.

Kirsch, J. A. W., 1977, The classification of marsupials, in: *The Biology of Marsupials* (D. Hunsaker, ed.), Academic Press, New York, pp. 1–50.

Lende, R. A., 1963a, Sensory representation in the cerebral cortex of the opossum (*Didelphis virginiana*), *J. Comp. Neurol.* **121:**395–403.

Lende, R. A., 1963b, Motor representation in the cerebral cortex of the opossum (*Didelphis virginiana*), *J. Comp. Neurol.* **121:**405–415.

Lende, R. A., 1963c, Cerebral cortex: A sensorimotor amalgam in the Marsupialia, *Science* **141:**730–732.

Lende, R. A., 1964, Representation in the cerebral cortex of a primitive mammal. Sensorimotor, visual, and auditory fields in the echidna (*Tachyglossus aculeatus*), *J. Neurophysiol.* **27**:37–48.

Lende, R. A., 1969, A comparative approach to the neocortex: Localization in monotremes, marsupials and insectivores, *Ann. N.Y. Acad. Sci.* **167**:262–276.

Lende, R. A., and Sadler, K. M., 1967, Sensory and motor areas in neocortex of hedgehog (*Erinaceus*), *Brain Res.* **5**:390–405.

Lende, R. A., and Woolsey, C. N., 1956, Sensory and motor localization in cerebral cortex of porcupine (*Erithizon dorsatum*), *J. Neurophysiol.* **19**:544–563.

Leonard, C. M., 1972, The connections of the dorsomedial nuclei, *Brain Behav. Evol.* **6**:524–541.

LeVay, S., and Sherk, H., 1981, The visual claustrum of the cat. I. Structure and connections, *J. Neurosci.* **1**:956–980.

Lyne, G., 1967, *Marsupials and Monotremes of Australia*, Angus & Robertson, Sydney.

Magalhães-Castro, B., and Saraiva, P. E. S., 1971, Sensory and motor representation in the cerebral cortex of the marsupial *Didelphis azarae azarae*, *Brain Res.* **34**:291–299.

Marshall, W. H., Woolsey, C. N., and Bard, P., 1941, Observations on cortical somatic sensory mechanisms of cat and monkey, *J. Neurophysiol.* **4**:1–24.

Martin, C. J., 1898, Cortical localisation in *Ornithorhynchus*, *J. Physiol. (London)* (Suppl.) **23**:383–385.

Martin, G. F., Megirian, D., and Roebuck, A., 1970, The corticospinal tract of the marsupial phalanger (*Trichosurus vulpecula*), *J. Comp. Neurol.* **139**:245–257.

Martin, G. F., Megirian, D., and Conner, J. B., 1972, The origin, course and termination of the corticospinal tracts of the Tasmanian potoroo (*Potorous apicalis*), *J. Anat.* **111**:263–281.

Martin, G. F., Beals, J. K., Culberson, J. C., Dom, R., and Humbertson, A. O., 1978, Observations on the development of brainstem–spinal systems in the North American opossum, *J. Comp. Neurol.* **181**:271–290.

Merzenich, M. M., and Brugge, J. F., 1973, Representation of the cochlear partition on the superior temporal plane of the macaque monkey, *Brain Res.* **50**:275–296.

Merzenich, M. M., Knight, P. L., and Roth, G. L., 1975, Representation of cochlea within primary auditory cortex in the cat, *J. Neurophysiol.* **38**:231–249.

Merzenich, M. M., Kaas, J. H., and Roth, G. L., 1976, Auditory cortex in the grey squirrel: Tonotopic organization and architectonic fields, *J. Comp. Neurol.* **166**:387–401.

Meyer, J., 1981, A quantitative comparison of the parts of the brains of two Australian marsupials and some eutherian mammals, *Brain Behav. Evol.* **18**:60–71.

Moeller, H., 1973, Zur Evolutions höhe des Marsupialia gehirns, *Zool. Jahrb. Abt. Anat. Ontog. Tiere* **91**:434–448.

Molliver, M. E., Kostovic, I., and Van der Loos, H., 1973, The development of synapses in cerebral cortex of the human fetus, *Brain Res.* **50**:403–407.

Morest, D. K., 1964, The neuronal architecture of the medial geniculate body in the cat, *J. Anat.* **98**:611–630.

Mountcastle, V. B., 1957, Modality and topographic properties of single neurons of cat's somatosensory cortex, *J. Neurophysiol.* **20**:408–434.

Mountcastle, V. B., 1978, An organizing principle for cerebral function: The unit module and the distributed system, in: *The Mindful Brain* (G. M. Edelman and V. B. Mountcastle, eds.), MIT Press, Cambridge, Mass., pp. 7–50.

Mountcastle, V. B., 1986, The neural mechanisms of cognitive function can now be studied directly, *Trends Neurosci.* **9**:505–508.

Murphy, E. H., and Berman, N., 1979, The rabbit and the cat: A comparison of some features of response properties of single cells in the primary visual cortex, *J. Comp. Neurol.* **188**:401–428.

Nelson, J. E., 1987, The early development of the eye of the pouch-young of the marsupial *Dasyurus hallucatus*, *Anat. Embryol.* **175**:387–398.

Nelson, J. E., and Stephan, H., 1982, Encephalization in Australian marsupials, in: *Australian Carnivorous Marsupials* (M. Archer, ed.), Royal Zoological Society of New South Wales, Sydney, pp. 699–706.

Norita, M., 1983, Claustral neurons projecting to the visual cortical areas in the cat: A retrograde double labelling study, *Neurosci. Lett* **36**:33–36.

Ogren, M., and Hendrickson, A., 1976, Pathways between striate cortex and subcortical regions in *Macaca mulatta* and *Saimiri sciureus*: Evidence for a reciprocal pulvinar connection, *Exp. Neurol.* **53**:780–800.

Packer, A. D., 1941, An experimental investigation of the visual system in the phalanger, *Trichosurus vulpecula*, *J. Anat.* **75**:309–329.

Pandya, D. N., and Yeterian, E. H., 1985, Architecture and connections of cortical association areas, in: *Cerebral Cortex*, Volume 4 (A. Peters and E. G. Jones, eds.), Plenum Press, New York, pp. 3–61.

Penfield, N., and Boldrey, E., 1937, Somatic motor and sensory representation in the cerebral cortex of man as studied by electrical stimulation, *Brain* **60**:389–443.

Petras, J. M., 1969, Some efferent connections of the motor and somatosensory cortex of simian primates and felid, canid and procyonid carnivores, *Ann. N.Y. Acad. Sci.* **167**:469–505.

Pirlot, P., and Nelson, J., 1978, Volumetric analyses of monotreme brains, *Aust. Zool.* **20**:171–179.

Porter, R., 1955, Antidromic conduction of volleys in the pyramidal tract, *J. Neurophysiol.* **18**:138–150.

Potter, H., and Nauta, W. J. H., 1979, A note on the problem of olfactory associations of the orbitofrontal cortex in the monkey, *Neuroscience* **4**:361–367.

Poulton, E. B., 1885, On the tactile terminal organ and other structures in the bill of *Ornithorhynchus*, *J. Physiol. (London)* **5**:15–16.

Poulton, E. B., 1894, The structure of the bill and hairs of *Ornithorhynchus paradoxus* with a discussion of the homologies and origin of mammalian hair, *Q. J. Microsc. Sci.* **36**:143–199.

Powell, T. P. S., Cowan, W. M., and Raisman, G., 1965, The central olfactory connections, *J. Anat.* **99**:791.

Pubols, B. H., 1968, Retrograde degeneration study of somatic sensory thalamocortical connections in brain of Virginia opossum, *Brain Res.* **7**:232–251.

Pubols, B. H., 1977, The second somatic sensory area (SmII) of opossum neocortex, *J. Comp. Neurol.* **174**:71–78.

Pubols, B. H., Jr., and Pubols, L. M., 1971, Somatotopic organisation of spider monkey somatic sensory cerebral cortex, *J. Comp. Neurol.* **141**:63–76.

Pubols, B. H., Donovick, P. J., and Pubols, L. M., 1973, Opossum trigeminal afferents associated with vibrissal and rhinarial mechanoreceptors, *Brain Behav. Evol.* **7**:360–381.

Pubols, B. H., Pubols, L. M., Dipette, D. J., and Sheely, J. C., 1976, Opossum somatic sensory cortex: A microelectrode mapping study, *J. Comp. Neurol.* **165**:229–246.

Ravizza, R., Heffner, H., and Masterton, B., 1969, Hearing in primitive mammals. I: Opossum (*Didelphis virginiana*), *J. Aud. Res.* **9**:1–7.

Reale, R. A., and Imig, T. J., 1980, Tonotopic organization in auditory cortex of the cat, *J. Comp. Neurol.* **192**:265–292.

Rees, S., and Hore, J., 1970, The motor cortex of the brush-tailed possum (*Trichosurus vulpecula*): Motor representation, motor function and the pyramidal tract, *Brain Res.* **20**:439–452.

Regidor, J., and Divac, I., 1987, Architectonics of the thalamus in the echidna (*Tachyglossus aculeatus*): Search for the mediodorsal nucleus, *Brain Behav. Evol.* **30**:328–341.

Renfree, M. B., Holt, A. B., Green, S. W., Carr, J. P., and Cheek, D. B., 1982, Ontogeny of the brain in a marsupial (*Macropus eugenii*) throughout pouch life, *Brain Behav. Evol.* **20**:57–71.

Reynolds, M. L., and Saunders, N. R., 1988, Differentiation of the neocortex, in: *The Developing Marsupial* (C. H. Tyndale-Biscoe and P. A. Janssens, eds.), Springer-Verlag, Berlin, pp. 101–116.

Reynolds, M. L., Cavanagh, M. E., Dziegieliewska, K. M., Hinds, L. A., Saunders, N R., and Tyndale-Biscoe, C. H., 1985, Postnatal development of the telencephalon of the tammar wallaby (*Macropus eugenii*). An accessible model of neocortical differentiation, *Anat. Embryol.* **173**:81–94.

Rezak, M., and Benevento, L. A., 1979, A comparison of the organization of the projections of the dorsal lateral geniculate nucleus, the inferior pulvinar and adjacent lateral pulvinar to primary visual cortex (area 17) in the macaque monkey, *Brain Res.* **167**:19–40.

Robinson, C. J., and Burton, H., 1980, Somatotopographic organization in second somatosensory area of *M. fascicularis*, *J. Comp. Neurol.* **192**:43–68.

Rocha-Miranda, C. E., Linden, R., Volchan, E., Lent, R., and Bombardieri, R., 1976, Receptive field properties of single units in the opossum striate cortex, *Brain Res.* **104**:197–219.

Rockel, A. J., Heath, C. J., and Jones, E. G., 1972, Afferent connections to the diencephalon in the marsupial phalanger and the question of sensory convergence in the 'posterior group' of the thalamus, *J. Comp. Neurol.* **145**:105–130.

Rose, J. E., and Woolsey, C. N., 1948, The orbitofrontal cortex and its connections with the mediodorsal nucleus in rabbit, sheep and cat, *Proc. Assoc. Res. Nerv. Ment. Dis.* **27**:210–232.

Rowe, M. J., Ferrington, D. G., Fisher, G. R., and Freeman, B., 1985, Parallel processing and distributed coding for tactile vibratory information within the sensory cortex, in: *Development, Organization and Processing in Somatosensory Pathways* (M. J. Rowe and W. D. Willis, eds.), Liss, New York, pp. 247–258.

Royce, G. J., Ward, J. P., Bade, B. B., and Harting, J. K., 1975, Retinogeniculate pathways in two marsupial opossums, *Didelphis virginiana* and *Marmosa mitis*, *Anat. Rec.* **181**:467–468.

Royce, G. J., Ward, J. P., and Harting, J. K., 1976, Retinofugal pathways in two marsupials, *J. Comp. Neurol.* **170**:391–414.

Sanderson, K. J., Pearson, L. J., and Dixon, P. G., 1978, Altered retinal projections in brush-tailed possum, *Trichosurus vulpecula*, following removal of one eye, *J. Comp. Neurol.* **180**:841–868.

Sanderson, K. J., Haight, J. R., and Pearson, L. J., 1980, Transneuronal transport of tritiated fucose and proline in the visual pathways of the brushtailed possum, *Trichosurus vulpecula*, *Neurosci. Lett.* **20**:243–248.

Sanderson, K. J., Welker, W., and Shambes, G. M., 1984, Reevaluation of motor cortex and of sensorimotor overlap in cerebral cortex of albino rats, *Brain Res.* **292**:251–260.

Sanides, F., 1972, Representation in the cerebral cortex and its areal lamination patterns, in: *Structure and Function of the Nervous System*, Volume 5 (G. H. Bourne, ed.), Academic Press, New York, pp. 329–453.

Saraiva, P., and Magalhães-Castro, B., 1975, Sensory and motor representation in the cerebral cortex of the three-toed sloth (*Bradypus tridactylus*), *Brain Res.* **90**:181–193.

Saunders, N. R., 1985, Plasma proteins and cerebral cortical development, in: *Development, Organization, and Processing in Somatosensory Pathways* (M. J. Rowe and W. D. Willis, eds.), Liss, New York, pp. 79–86.

Scheich, H., Langner, G., Tidemann, C., Coles, R. B., and Guppy, A., 1986, Electroreception and electrolocation in platypus, *Nature* **319**:401–402.

Schuster, E., 1910, Preliminary note upon the cell lamination of the cerebral cortex of the echidna, with an enumeration of the fibres in the cranial nerves, *Proc. R. Soc. Med. Ser. B* **82**:113–123.

Sherk, H., 1986, The claustrum and the cerebral cortex, in: *Cerebral Cortex*, Volume 5 (E. G. Jones and A. Peters, eds.), Plenum Press, New York, pp. 467–499.

Simons, D. J., 1978, Response properties of vibrissa units in rat SI somatosensory neocortex, *J. Neurophysiol.* **41**:798–820.

Snell, O., 1891, Die Abhängigkeit des Hirngewichtes von dem Körpergewicht und den geistigen Fähigkeiten, *Arch. Psychiatr. Nervenkr.* **23**:436–446.

Sousa, R., Aglai, P. B., Gattass, R., and Oswaldo-Cruz, E., 1978, The projection of the opossum's visual field on the cerebral cortex, *J. Comp. Neurol.* **177**:569–588.

Stanfield, B. B., O'Leary, D. D. M., and Fricks, C., 1982, Selective collateral elimination in early postnatal development restricts cortical distribution of rat pyramidal tract neurons, *Nature* **298**:371–373.

Stephan, H., Bauchot, R., and Andy, O. J., 1970, Data on size of the brain and various parts in insectivores and primates, in: *The Primate Brain* (C. R. Noback and W. Montagna, eds.), Appleton, New York, pp. 289–297.

Stone, J., 1983, *Parallel Processing in the Visual System*, Plenum Press, New York.

Suga, N., and Jen, P. H. S., 1976, Disproportionate tonotopic representation for processing CF-FM sonar signals in the moustache bat auditory cortex, *Science* **194**:542–544.

Tyndale-Biscoe, C. H., 1973, *The Life of Marsupials*, Arnold, London.

Tyndale-Biscoe, C. H., and Renfree, M., 1987, *Reproductive Physiology of Marsupials*, Cambridge University Press, London.

Ulinski, P. S., 1984, Thalamic projections to the somatosensory cortex of the echidna, *Tachyglossus aculeatus*, *J. Comp. Neurol.* **229**:153–170.

Van der Loos, H., and Welker, E., 1985, Development and plasticity of somatosensory brain maps, in: *Development, Organization, and Processing in Somatosensory Pathways* (M. J. Rowe and W. D. Willis, eds.), Liss, New York, pp. 53–67.

Van Essen, D. C., 1979, Visual areas of the mammalian cerebral cortex, *Annu. Rev. Neurosci.* **2**:227–263.

Van Essen, D. C., and Maunsell, J. H. R., 1983, Hierarchical organization and functional streams in the visual cortex, *Trends Neurosci.* **6**:370–375.

Vogt, C., and Vogt, O., 1906, Zur Kentniss der elektrisch erregbaren Hirnrindgebiet bei der Säugetieren, *J. Psychol. Neurol.* **8**:277–456.

von Bonin, G., 1937, Brain weight and body weight in mammals, *J. Gen. Psychol.* **16**:379–389.

Ward, L., and Watson, C. R. R., 1973, An experimental study of the ventrolateral nucleus of the brush-tailed possum, *J. Anat.* **116**:472.

Welker, C., 1976, Receptive fields of barrels in the somatosensory neocortex of the rat, *J. Comp. Neurol.* **166**:173–190.

Welker, W., and Lende, R. A., 1980, Thalamocortical relationships in echidna (*Tachyglossus aculeatus*), in: *Comparative Neurology of the Telencephalon* (S. O. E. Ebbesson, ed.), Plenum Press, New York, pp. 449–481.

Welker, W. I., and Seidenstein, S., 1959, Somatic sensory representation in the cerebral cortex of the racoon (*Procyon lotor*), *J. Comp. Neurol.* **111**:469–502.

Weller, W. L., 1972, Barrels in somatic sensory neocortex of the marsupial *Trichosurus vulpecula*, *Brain Res.* **43**:11–24.

Weller, W. L., and Haight, J. R., 1973, Barrels and somatotopy in SI neocortex of the brush-tailed possum, *J. Anat.* **116**:474.

Weller, W. L., Haight, J. R., Neylon, L., and Johnson, J. I., 1977, A re-assessment of the mechanoreceptor projections to cerebral neocortex in marsupial wallabies (*Thylogale*), *J. Anat.* **124**:531–532.

Werner, G., and Whitsel, B. L., 1973, Functional organisation of the somatosensory cortex, in: *Handbook of Sensory Physiology. II. Somatosensory System* (A. Iggo, ed.), Springer-Verlag, Berlin, pp. 621–700.

Whitsel, B. L., Petrucelli, L. M., and Werner, G., 1969, Symmetry and connectivity in the map of the body surface in somatosensory area II of primates, *J. Neurophysiol.* **32**:170–183.

Wilson, J. T., and Martin, C. J., 1893, On the peculiar rod-like tactile organs in the integument and mucous membrane of the muzzle of *Ornithorynchus*, in: *The Macleay Memorial Volume* (J. J. Fisher, ed.), Linn. Soc. N.S W., Sydney, pp. 190–200.

Wilson, J. T., and Martin, C. J., 1894, Further observations upon the anatomy of the integumentary structures in the muzzle of *Ornithorhynchus*, *Proc. Linn. Soc. N.S.W. Ser. 2* **9**:660–681.

Woolsey, C. N., 1952, Patterns of localization in sensory and motor areas of the cerebral cortex, in: *Biology of Mental Health and Disease,* Hoeber, New York, pp. 193–206.

Woolsey, C. N., 1958, Organization of somatic sensory and motor areas of the cerebral cortex, in: *Biological and Biochemical Bases of Behavior* (H. F. Harlow and C. N. Woolsey, eds.), University of Wisconsin Press, Madison, pp. 63–81.

Woolsey, C. N., 1964, Cortical localization as defined by evoked potential and electrical stimulation studies, in: *Cerebral Localization and Organization* (G. Schaltenbrand and C. N. Woolsey, eds.), University of Wisconsin Press, Madison, pp. 17–32.

Woolsey, C. N., and Fairman, D., 1946, Contralateral, ipsilateral and bilateral representation of cutaneous receptors in somatic areas I and II of the cerebral cortex of pig, sheep and other mammals, *Surgery* **19**:684–702.

Woolsey, T. A., and Van der Loos, H., 1970, The structural organization of layer IV in the somatosensory region (SI) of mouse cerebral cortex. The description of a cortical field composed of discrete cytoarchitectural units, *Brain Res.* **17**:205–242.

Zecevic, N. R., and Molliver, M. E., 1978, The origin of the monoaminergic innervation of immature rat neocortex: An ultrastructural analysis following lesions, *Brain Res.* **150**:387–397.

Ziehen, T., 1897, Das Centralnervensystem der Monotremen und Marsupialier. I. Theil: Makroskopische Anatomie, in: *Zoologische Forschungsreisen in Australien und dem Malayischen Archipel* (R. Semon, ed.), Volume 3, Denkschiften der medicinisch-Naturwissenschaftlichen Gesellschaft zu Jena, Fischer, Jena, **6**:677–728.

Comparative Development of Somatic Sensory Cortex

15

JOHN IRWIN JOHNSON

1. Introduction

1.1. Plan of Approach

In the currently popular conception of the development of life forms on earth, mammals have progressively diversified from a single, or small, group of reptilian ancestral forms. Their brains have presumably diversified along with their other components, and these include their somatic sensory cortices. The premise of this chapter is to examine this diversification of somatic sensory cortex, and to do so from an evolutionary point of view rather than an outlook based on the history of neuroscience, or one based on how-does-it-relate-to-humans. To do this, the available data concerning similarities and differences in organization of sensory cortex have been arranged as if on a mammalian family tree, to see if this ordering will reveal evolutionary trends or processes. The hazards of this approach are many: data are spotty and too often not comparable, and the structure of the family tree itself is still discouragingly obscure. Nevertheless the wealth of information that has been accumulated has tempted me into pursuing this plan, however foolhardy it may prove, to see what it may reveal.

For a family tree, the summary tree of Novacek and Wyss (1986) has been adopted. This tree represents a conservative view based on current generally accepted conclusions. Certain branch points have been "spun" (turning branches

JOHN IRWIN JOHNSON • Anatomy Department, and Neuroscience Program, Michigan State University, East Lansing, Michigan 48824.

on the branch point does not alter the relationships depicted) so the tree illustrated in Fig. 1 differs in this respect from that published by Novacek and Wyss. The alterations leave certain data better juxtaposed for some interesting comparisons.

1.2. Somatosensory Projections to Forebrain Pallium in Nonmammalian Vertebrates Compared with the Organization of the Forebrain Somatosensory System in Mammals

Very little is known about somatic sensory input to the telencephalon in anamniotes. Evidence was obtained for telencephalic projections in sharks and rays from combined electrosensory and mechanosensory stimulation (Platt *et al.*,

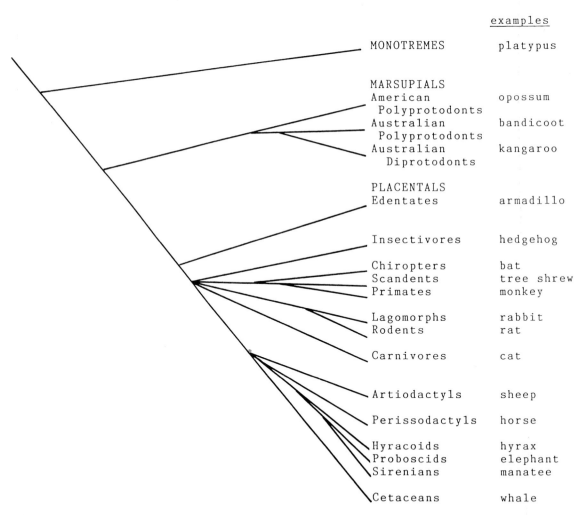

Figure 1. The family tree of the major orders of mammals as proposed by Novacek and Wyss (1986). This tree differs from theirs in that some taxa have been rotated around points of divergence (this does not alter the relationships depicted), marsupials have been divided into three subgroupings with relationships proposed by Kirsch (1977), and a few smaller taxa whose sensory cortices are unexplored have been omitted.

1974); limited attempts at purely mechanosensory stimulation yielded no telencephalic response but these were not systematic enough to constitute negative evidence. In a teleost bony fish (*Sebasticus marmoratus*), a thalamic relay for somatic sensory information, between trigeminal input and one or more telencephalic regions, was hypothesized on the basis of anatomical connections (Ito *et al.*, 1986). There is some evidence for somatosensory projections to the telencephalic pallium in frogs (Kicliter and Ebbesson, 1976).

For the amniotes, a common current hypothesis (Fig. 2) holds that an ancestral amphibian-type simple telencephalic hemisphere has undergone two or three types of evolutionary elaboration (e.g., Karten, 1969; Ebner, 1976; Butler, 1978; Northcutt, 1978; Ulinski, 1986). In this view, a portion of the dorsolateral pallium in most more recent reptiles has expanded into the ventricle forming the dorsal ventricular ridge. A similar process may have yielded the various "hyperstriata" of the avian telecephalon. In mammals, in contrast, the expansion has taken place in more dorsal pallium, leading to a stretched-out and multilaminated "neocortex."

In reptiles and birds, a major telencephalic target for somatosensory pathways is the anterior dorsal ventricular ridge, based on evidence from lizards, crocodilians, and pigeons (Ulinski, 1983, pp. 131–140, 1986; Pritz and Stritzel,

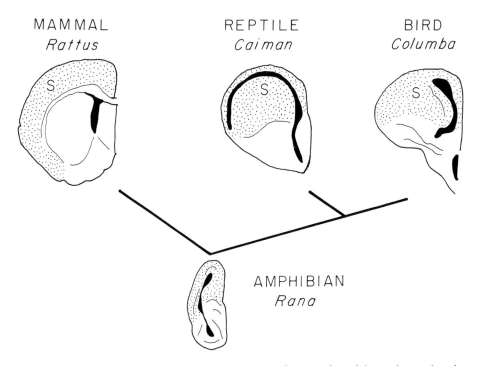

Figure 2. Possible derivation of somatic sensory cortex of mammals and its analogues in other amniote classes, shown in diagrams of coronal sections through right cerebral hemispheres. Lateral ventricles are shown black. The pallium as seen in some adult amphibians (which resemble early developmental stages of all amniote classes) is stippled, as are its apparent derivatives: the cerebral cortex of mammals, and the cortex and dorsal ventricular ridge of reptiles and birds. Regions specialized for somatic sensory input are labeled S, in the mammalian neocortex and in the dorsal ventricular ridge of reptiles and birds (in birds this region is also designated the hyperstriatum). These diagrams are based on figures by Ulinski (1983, Figs. 1.3 and 4.34; 1986, Fig. 5).

1986). These pathways converge upon a thalamic region whose cells project to the ridge rather than to cortex as do somatosensory thalamic regions in mammals. Responses to somatic sensory stimulation are also found in dorsal cortex of turtles and alligators and probably other reptiles; these responses are, however, more variable, have longer latency and large receptive fields, and are less specifically somatic sensory (they also respond to other sensory modalities) (reviewed by Belekhova, 1979). The somatosensory pathways to dorsal cortex have not been elucidated. These data lead to the view that in reptiles, the dorsal ventricular ridge rather than the dorsal cortex is carrying out functions more like those of the somatic sensory cortex of mammals (Ulinski, 1986).

The most distinctive feature of mammalian brains, distinguishing them from those of the other vertebrate classes, is the conversion of the telencephalic pallium into a complex, but consistently, laminated cerebral cortex. While retaining a basic cytoarchitecture common to all cortical regions, specific regions of the cortex are specialized to receive, from thalamic sources, precisely organized arrays of sensory information. One of these specialized regions receives a massive input from the thalamic terminals of the somatic sensory pathways, and it is this specialized somatic sensory cortex that is the topic of this chapter. Somatic sensory cortex is defined here as that region of the cortex whose most prominent characteristic is the presence of somatic sensory projections which dominate all other inputs.

1.3. Survey of Data, in Phylogenetic Order

For each of the taxa in the following account, information about somatic sensory cortex has been arranged in a standard sequence:

- Sensory projections
- Relation to other areas
- Structure
- Thalamic connections
- Corticocortical connections
- Other connections
- Comparison summary

Not all types of data are available for all taxa, and when a subheading is not present it is because there is no information available.

2. Monotremes

The most divergence (hence assumed to be the earliest divergence) is between the egg-laying monotremes (the extant prototherians) and all other surviving mammals (collectively designated as therian mammals). Characters found in both branches of this divergence, monotremes and therians, can most safely be assumed to be those typical of the earliest ancestral mammals and those that will be characteristic of all mammals.

2.1.1. Sensory Projections

In the simplest of the extant monotreme brains, that of the duckbill or platypus *Ornithorhynchus anatinus,* the somatic sensory region occupies a majority of the neocortical surface (Bohringer and Rowe, 1977). There is a single representation of the surface of the contralateral body, and most of this somatotopically organized representation is devoted to projections from the bill (Fig. 3). Projections from the trunk are located dorsomedially to those from the bill, and those from the arm and hand progressively anterior to those from the trunk. Projections from the tail are found around the medial rim of the sensory region. A small region of hindlimb projections is tucked between the anterior parts of the trunk and tail representations. The large extent of the representation of the bill reflects the small size of the peripheral receptive fields projecting to a given cortical locus: more cortical volume is devoted to processing of information from small regions of the bill. These finely detailed projections from the bill are precisely somatotopically organized.

2.1.2. Relation to Other Areas

As shown in Fig. 3, somatic sensory cortex is close to much smaller cortical regions activated by visual and by auditory stimulation; there is very little "sensory-silent" cortex intervening between somatic sensory, auditory, and visual regions.

Electrical stimulation of a large rostral portion of the sensory region produced muscular movements, and the parts of the body which moved were those which sent sensory projections to that particular region being stimulated. A band of cortex anterior to the sensory region also yielded movements of muscles when stimulated. These data were described as indicating largely, but not completely overlapping somatic sensory and "motor" regions of neocortex. Together, the motor and sensory regions occupy almost the entire dorsolateral surface of the hemisphere (Bohringer and Rowe, 1977).

2.2. Spiny Anteater (Echidna)

In the more complex, gyrencephalic cortex of the spiny anteater or echidna *Tachyglossus aculeatus,* representing the other extant family of monotremes, the somatic sensory region occupies a gyrus constituting about a third of a "sensory lobe" at the caudal aspect of the hemisphere (Lende, 1964, 1969; Allison and Goff, 1972) (Fig. 4).

2.2.1. Sensory Projections

Within the somatic sensory gyrus, the pattern of representations reflects the principles seen in the cortex of *Ornithorhynchus:* projections are all from the contralateral body; they are precisely somatotopically organized; the largest representation (with smallest receptive fields) is from the bill; trunk and tail projec-

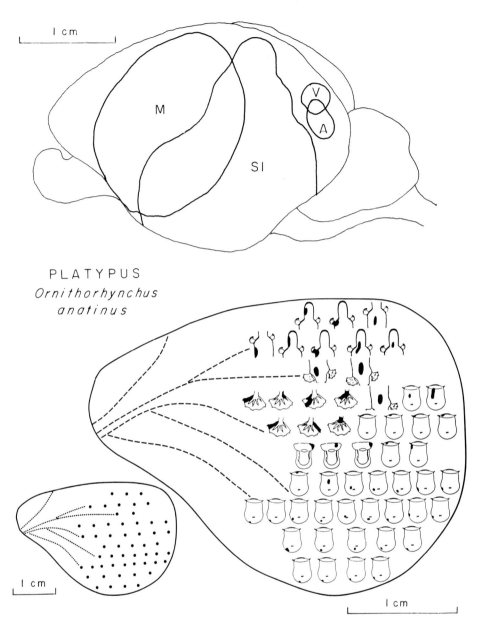

PLATYPUS
*Ornithorhynchus
anatinus*

Figure 3. Organization of projections to somatic sensory cortex of the monotreme (Prototheria) duckbill platypus *Ornithorhynchus anatinus*. *Top:* Outline of a dorsolateral view of the left side of the brain, anterior to the left, showing the relative extents and positions of motor (M), sensory (SI), visual (V), and auditory (A) neocortical regions as determined by extracellular recording or stimulation with microelectrodes (from Bohringer, 1977, with alterations, and permission from R. C. Bohringer). *Bottom left:* Outline of a lateral view of the left cerebral hemisphere, with dots showing the locations of microelectrode penetrations yielding the information about sensory projections shown at lower right. Dotted lines indicate major blood vessels on the cerebral surface. *Lower right:* Receptive fields of cortical units activated by mechanosensory stimulation are indicated by black patches on sketches of body parts, placed at the approximate location on the cerebral surface of microelectrode penetrations yielding evoked unit activity. Most of the somatic sensory region contains cortical units activated by mechanical stimulation of small receptive fields on the bill. Much of the remaining sensory cortex is activated by stimulation of the skin of the hand. Projections are arranged somatotopically: the relative location of projections in cortex mimics the relative locations of receptors in the skin. Body parts with smaller receptive fields project to larger cortical areas. (From Bohringer and Rowe, 1977, with permission from R. C. Bohringer and Alan R. Liss, Inc.)

tions lie medially, and those from the limbs and extremities lie progressively more anteriorly in cortex.

2.2.2. Relation to Other Areas

The other two-thirds of the "sensory lobe" contain separate auditory and visual regions. Incipient or fully developed sulci often intervene between visual, auditory, and somatic sensory regions. As in *Ornithorhynchus*, the somatic sensory cortex qualifies as a motor cortex in that the lowest threshold electrical stimulation induces muscular movements, the motor map replicating the sensory map. In *Tachyglossus* there is an additional motor region of equal size in front of the sensory region, where no sensory projections are found. Lende termed this region MI, and the more posterior sensory–motor region SMI (SMI is designated SI in Fig. 4).

2.2.3. Structure

A sulcus, called sulcus alpha, separates MI and SMI. Two cytoarchitectural fields were identified in SMI and a third in MI (Ulinski, 1984). The MI field has a strongly developed layer 5 and a reduced layer 4. The rostral SMI field, which occupies the rostral, and part of the caudal, bank of sulcus alpha, has a strong layer 4 and a less developed layer 5. The caudal SMI field, occupying most of the gyrus caudal to sulcus alpha, has a most developed layer 4 and a scanty layer 5.

2.2.4. Thalamic Connections

Separate thalamic regions projecting to MI and SMI were identified by retrograde degeneration (W. Welker and Lende, 1980). A more ventral nucleus called the ventrobasal (VB) degenerated following lesions in SMI; just rostral and dorsal to VB a nucleus called the ventrolateral (VL) showed effects following MI lesions.

Retrograde transport of horseradish peroxidase (Ulinski, 1984) again showed SMI receiving projections from VB—now called ventroposterior (VP): the rostral SMI field receives projections from the rostrodorsal part of the thalamic VP nucleus (bordering VL); the caudal SMI field receives projections from the ventral part of VP.

2.2.5. Corticocortical Connections

Electrical stimulation in both MI and SMI evokes responses from the corresponding point in the contralateral hemisphere suggesting detailed interhemispheric communication via the anterior commissure (Allison and Goff, 1972).

2.2.6. Other Connections

Corticospinal fibers extending the length of the spinal cord have been found in *Tachyglossus;* however, the only cortical origin examined in these studies was dorsal to MI on the gyrus in front of sulcus alpha (Goldby, 1939; Griffiths, 1978, pp. 198–200). Thus, the contribution of sensory cortex to the corticospinal tract in monotremes remains to be determined.

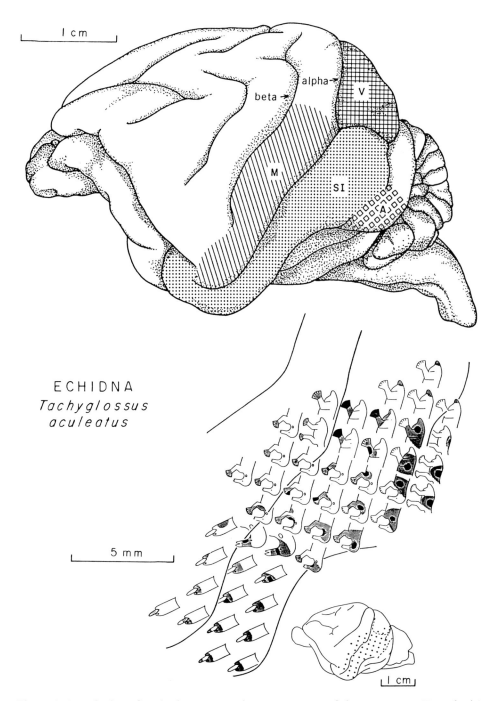

Figure 4. Organization of projections to somatic sensory cortex of the monotreme (Prototheria) echidna *Tachyglossus aculeatus.*

Top: Outline of a lateral view of the left side of the brain, anterior to the left, showing the relative extents and positions of motor (M), sensory (SI), visual (V), and auditory (A) neocortical regions as determined by surface recording or stimulation with macroelectrodes (from W. Welker and Lende, 1980, with alterations, and permission from W. I. Welker and Plenum Press). Lende's sensorimotor region SMI is here designated SI. In this specimen a sulcus intervenes between visual and somatic sensory regions; in other specimens there is a complete sulcus between somatic sensory and auditory regions.

The major difference between the cerebral cortices of the platypus and the echidna is the greatly expanded neocortex of the latter. While platypus cortex is nearly all sensory and motor regions, the corresponding regions in the echidna are relatively small and are displaced to the caudolateral corner of the hemisphere. The functional significance of the additional "silent" cortex of the echidna remains to be determined.

3. Marsupials

The therian subdivision of the mammalian class has in turn diversified into two major radiations, the metatherian marsupials and the eutherian placentals. The surviving marsupials are confined to Australia and the Americas.

3.1. Opossums

The most studied of marsupial brains is that of the North American *Didelphis virginiana*, the Virginia opossum; its somatic sensory cortex is the best known of those of the metatherian subclass.

3.1.1. Sensory Projections

The primary sensory representation (Fig. 5) has many of the characteristics of the somatic sensory cortex seen in the monotremes: projections are from the contralateral body; they are somatotopically organized; the largest and most detailed projections are from the front of the face, in this case the nose and mystacial vibrissae; they are arranged with face to tail represented lateral to medial on the surface of the hemisphere (Bodemer and Towe, 1963; Lende, 1963a,c; Pubols *et al.*, 1976). Similar findings were reported in the South American congener *Didelphis albiventris (azarae)* (Magalhães-Castro and Saraiva, 1971).

Some new features, not present in monotreme cortex, appear in the representation patterns in opossum sensory cortex (and in that of all other therian mammals; Ulinski, 1986). In addition to the primary (SI) representation, there is a smaller additional representation (SII) located caudolaterally adjoining SI. SII projections are also somatotopically arranged, forming a mirror image of the SI representations; receptive fields are larger and many of them are bilateral, representing input from both contralateral and ipsilateral body surfaces (Lende,

Bottom right: Outline of a lateral view of the left side of the brain, with dots showing the surface locations of macroelectrodes yielding the information about sensory projections shown just above and to the left. Receptive fields of cortical potentials activated by mechanosensory stimulation are indicated by shaded patches on sketches of body parts, placed at the approximate location on the cerebral surface of the recording macroelectrodes. Black spots within shaded patches show the body regions from which potentials of greatest amplitude were evoked by minimal mechanical stimulation. Much of the more ventral part of the somatic sensory region is activated by mechanical stimulation of small receptive fields on the bill. (From Lende, 1964, with alterations, and permission from the American Physiological Society.)

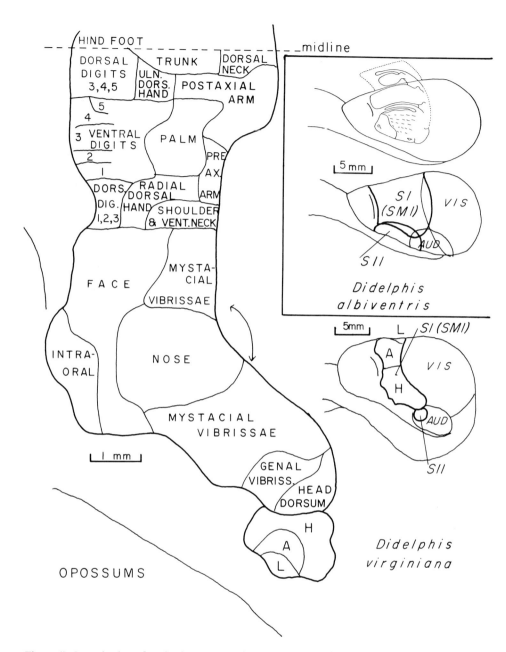

Figure 5. Organization of projections to somatic sensory cortex of American opossums (marsupials, Metatheria). Anterior is to the left in all diagrams.

Lower right: Outline of a lateral view of the neocortex of the North American Virginia opossum Didelphis virginiana, showing the location of auditory (*AUD*), visual (*VIS*), and first (*SI*) and second (*SII*) somatic sensory projection regions. SI is also the motor region, thus SMI. Within SI, H denotes projections from the head, A projections from the arm and hand (forelimb), and L from the leg and foot (hindlimb). This diagram is constructed from data presented by Lende (1963a–c), Pubols *et al.* (1976), and Pubols (1977).

Left: Details of projections in SI and SII (from Pubols *et al.*, 1976, and Pubols, 1977, with alterations, and permission from B. H. Pubols and Alan R. Liss, Inc.). Abbreviations H, A, and L denote one pattern of projections to SII from head, arm and hand (forelimb), and leg and foot (hindlimb). In other specimens the details of SII projections vary somewhat, but the basic relationships among SII projections, and between SI and SII are reasonably constant (Pubols, 1977).

1963a; Magalhães-Castro and Saraiva, 1971; Pubols, 1977; RoBards and Ebner, 1977). When large recording electrodes are used, SII is also an auditory area (Pubols, 1977); with smaller electrodes the auditory input is not recorded (RoBards and Ebner, 1977).

Within the SI representation, there are two additions to the single somatotopic representation of the entire contralateral body surface (Pubols *et al.*, 1976): within the snout representation there are a few neurons activated by receptive fields on the ipsilateral side of the midline; and there is a second representation of the contralateral mystacial vibrissae. The second vibrissal representation forms a mirror image of the first vibrissal representation—and is not to be confused with the SII projections from vibrissae which have the different SII properties of receptive fields (larger, bilateral, and integrated into the SII representation).

3.1.2. Relation to Other Areas

As with the monotremes, SI sensory cortex borders directly upon visual and auditory areas, and SI is also primary motor cortex in that the lowest threshold electrical stimulation evokes muscular movements (Lende, 1963b,c, 1969; Bodemer and Towe, 1963; Magalhães-Castro and Saraiva, 1971). The arrangement of relations with the peripheral body is the same for both sensory and motor functions (stimulation of the sensory forelimb region produces movements of the forelimb). This convergence of sensory and motor regions is "complete" in opossums, there are no regions which show one function without the other; each of the monotremes has some extent of "pure" sensory and motor regions.

3.1.3. Structure

The convergence of sensory and motor functions in the SI (more properly SMI) region of opossums is reflected in the cytoarchitecture of the region: it possesses throughout a well-developed layer 4 typical of sensory regions, along with a well-developed layer 5 characteristic of motor cortex (Walsh and Ebner, 1970). This contrasts with the cytoarchitectonic gradations seen in echidnas as described above (Section 2.2.3). In this cortical region of opossums, Walsh and Ebner also describe small cells oriented tangentially in layer I, and layer II cells with bifurcated or doubled apical dendrites widely branching in layer I; these features were later deemed evidence of resemblance to paleocortical formations (see Section 5.3).

Regions labeled with words are the locations of projections to SMI from the contralateral body surface (along with some projections in nose, face, and intraoral regions from ipsilateral receptive fields) (Pubols *et al.*, 1976). There is a duplicate representation of the mystacial vibrissae (arrows); one representation is a mirror image of the other.

Inset at right: Similar findings in the South American congener *D. albiventris* (= *azarae*) from Magalhães-Castro, and Saraiva (1971, with alterations, and permission from B. Magalhães-Castro, P. E. S. Saraiva, and Elsevier Scientific Publications BV). The upper diagram depicts the pattern of projections as a cartoon of the body surface; the lower diagram shows the relationships among sensory areas *AUD* auditory, *VIS* visual, *SI* (*SMI*) and *SII* first and second somatic sensory.

3.1.4. Thalamic Connections

A similar contrast with echidnas is seen in the projection from thalamus to SMI cortex in opossums, in that there are no separate projection regions from thalamic VL and VP nuclei. The VL nuclei receive input from the cerebellum while the VP nuclei receive projections from the cuneate and gracile nuclei (Walsh and Ebner, 1973). A given locus in opossum SMI cortex receives projections from an anteroposterior row of cells in the somatotopically corresponding part of VP (Pubols, 1968); this VP row is continuous with additional cells of the adjacent VL which project to the same cortical cells, which also receive input from cells of thalamic intralaminar nuclei (Killackey and Ebner, 1972, 1973; RoBards and Ebner, 1977; Donoghue and Ebner, 1981a,b). VL and VP project largely to layer 4, the intralaminar nuclei project mostly to layers 1 and 6 (with substantial projections to the putamen as well).

Cells in layer 6 and a few in layer 5 of SMI project to thalamus; it was not determined just where in the ventral thalamus their fibers terminate (Foster *et al.*, 1981). These corticothalamic cells can be expected to form part of the thalamocortical reciprocal circuitry found in all mammals studied.

Projections from VL were not found in SII; its input is from somatotopically appropriate regions of VP and intralaminar nuclei (Donoghue and Ebner, 1981a). In the absence of a clear demonstration of motor responses from stimulation of SII, this difference in thalamic projections leads to the continuing designation of this region as SII (not SMII), in contrast to SMI which has a motor function by all applicable criteria.

3.1.5. Corticocortical Connections

Both SMI and SII regions receive input from the contralateral hemisphere through the anterior commissure; this commissural input is most concentrated in the region of the face representation (Ebner, 1967). Stimulation of a region within SMI evokes a response in the homotopic region of the contralateral SMI (Nelson and Lende, 1965; Putnam *et al*, 1968); anatomically there are both homotopic and heterotopic commissural projections (Martin, 1967).

In SMI, cells of origin of commissural fibers were found in two patterns (Foster *et al.*, 1981): (1) for example, around the borders of the forepaw representation, cells of origin are seen in all layers 2 through 6, with more in layers 2 and 3 than in deeper layers; and (2) for example, in the center of the forepaw representation, cells of origin are restricted to layers 2 and 3 with very few in deeper layers. Cabana and Martin (1985) found cells of origin in layer 3 (most), 2 (somewhat fewer), 5 and 6 (still fewer) with only occasional cells seen in layer 4; however, some groups of cells are seen in certain locations in layer 4; these locations probably correspond to the first pattern described by Foster *et al.*

The location of commissural terminals has been described variously: in layers 6, 5, 4, sometimes in 3, and infrequently in 2 (Ebner, 1967); in many combinations of layers, commonly in layers 1, 2, 3, 5, and 6 (Ebner, 1969); and as corresponding to the locations of cells of origin, i.e., mostly in layers 2 and 3, fewer in 5 and 6, and occasional patches of terminals at certain locations in 4 (Cabana and Martin, 1985).

In addition to commissural connections, ipsilateral corticocortical connections to other (unspecified) regions of parietal cortex were found to originate in cells whose locations were similar to those giving rise to commissural connections (Foster *et al.*, 1981).

3.1.6. Other Connections

Other connections of sensory cortex that have been determined in opossums include corticofugal pathways to pontine nuclei, dorsal column nuclei, and the spinal gray matter (Bautista and Matzke, 1965; Martin and Fisher, 1968; Foster *et al.*, 1981). Projections to spinal cord, pontine nuclei, and dorsal column nuclei originate mostly in layer 5 with a few in layer 6 (Foster *et al.*, 1981). The corticospinal fibers travel in the medullary pyramids; most but not all of them decussate. Both ipsilateral and contralateral fibers form two descending tracts: the larger travels at the base of the dorsal column, the smaller in the lateral column alongside lamina 5 of the spinal gray. Terminals are confined to cervical spinal segments, most of them in the base of the dorsal horn.

3.1.7. Comparison Summary

Features common to opossums and monotremes are candidates for general or ancestral mammalian characteristics, since they occur in both branches of the earliest great divergence in the mammalian radiation. These include sensory projections from the contralateral body surface, arranged somatotopically, with those from the hindlimb medial and those from the head lateral in the sensory cortex; commissural connections between the sensory cortices of the two hemispheres; and a close approximation of somatic sensory, auditory, and visual regions of the cortex.

The differences seen in opossum as compared with monotreme sensory cortex may represent specializations which have occurred in one or the other taxa, and may in fact represent species-specific peculiarities of opossums; this will be clarified by consideration of more therian species. These differences include an additional complete sensory representation (SII); multiplication of representations of body parts in SMI; and the complete convergence of sensory and motor regions in opossums along with complete convergence of their corresponding thalamic projections.

3.2. Australian Marsupials

3.2.1. Sensory Projections

Scattered findings from a number of Australian marsupials indicate that several features found in *Didelphis* species occur also in marsupials of other families. These common features include the presence of SI (SMI) and SII and the arrangement of projections within SI. While the double representation of mystacial vibrissae seen in *D. virginiana* has not been reported for any other marsupial species, in wallabies and wombats there is a peculiar second representation of hairy maxillary skin, between the upper lip and vibrissae, out of somatotopic order adjoining the chin representation (Fig. 6).

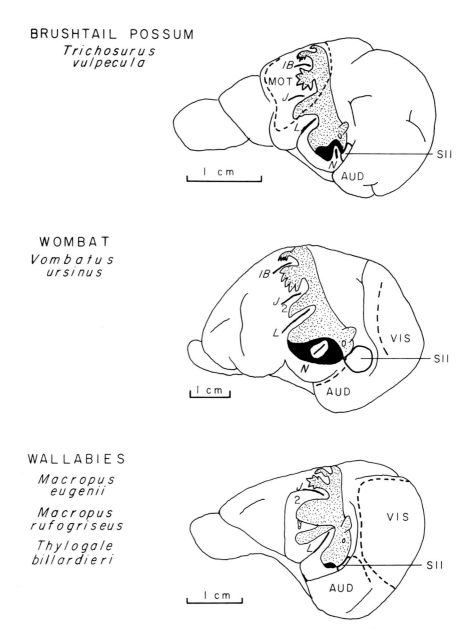

Figure 6. Organization of projections to somatic sensory cortex of three types of Australian diproto-dont marsupials (Metatheria) (from Johnson, 1980, with alterations, and permission from Plenum Press). Anterior is to the left in all diagrams. For each, the pattern of mechanosensory projections to SI is depicted as a cartoon of the contralateral body surface; the solid black area represents projections of the glabrous rhinarium. Consistent sulci demarcating projections within SI are labeled as follows: *IB*, interbrachial sulcus separating projections from fore- and hindlimbs; *J*, jugular sulcus separating forelimb from head projections; *L*, labial sulcus marking junction of upper and lower lip projections; *N*, narial sulcus at the representation of the nostril. A peculiar second representation of maxillary hairy skin, out of somatotopic order, seen in wallabies and wombats, is indicated by the numeral 2. The boundary of SII is indicated by a heavy solid line; heavy dashed lines indicated boundaries of other functional regions: AUD auditory, MOT primary motor, VIS visual.

For *Trichosurus* the motor region is that inferred from the pattern of thalamic projections by Haight and Neylon (1979) and from cortical stimulation by Rees and Hore (1970). SI and SII are as located by Adey and Kerr (1954), Haight and Weller (1973), and W. Weller and Haight (1973).

Also similar to findings in *Didelphis* are the relations to neighboring cortical fields for visual and auditory input (Adey and Kerr, 1954; Lende, 1963c; W. Weller *et al.*, 1976; Johnson, 1980) (Fig. 6). There is evidence that the overlap of sensory and motor regions in SMI, which is complete and precise in opossums, is less so in Australian species including the quoll or native cat *Dasyurus viverrinus* (Haight and Neylon, 1981) which is a polyprotodont as are the American opossums, and the diprotodont brushtail possum *Trichosurus vulpecula* (Rees and Hore, 1970; Haight and Neylon, 1978, 1979). These Australian species are thought to possess a region of purely motor cortex (MI) anterior to SMI; SMI is both sensory and motor as in the American opossums (but see Section 3.2.4). The condition in these Australian marsupial species is reminiscent of the relation between MI and SMI in the monotreme echidnas (Section 2.2.2) Lende (1963c), however, reported complete sensory-motor overlap in Tammar wallabies *Macropus (= Thylogale = Wallabia) eugenii*.

3.2.3. Structure

Two new features, not seen in the monotremes and opossums, are found in some Australian marsupials; they are related to the structure of the somatic sensory cortical region: sulci demarcating projection regions, and cytoarchitectonic specializations in layer 4 in certain projection regions.

1. In addition to sulcal boundaries between somatic sensory, visual, and auditory regions (as seen in monotreme echidnas; see Section 2.2.2), sulci separating projections of particular body parts occur in brains of larger diprotodonts (Fig. 6), including wallabies, wombats, and large possums (Lende, 1963c; Haight and Weller, 1973; Johnson, 1980). An interbrachial sulcus separates the projections from fore- and hindlimbs; a jugular sulcus divides forelimb from face projections; a labial sulcus marks the junction of projections from the upper and lower lips and in some cases a narial sulcus locates the nostril in the representation of the nose.

2. Cellular aggregates described as "barrels" (Fig. 7) occur in layer IV of gyral crowns (or corresponding regions in lissencephalic animals) in the SMI region in several members of the families Phalangeridae and Petauridae, the possums and gliders (W. Weller, 1972; W. Weller and Haight, 1973). In brushtails, limb projection regions in SMI have well-developed layers 4 and 5 as in opossums; while in the more "pure sensory" face region layer 4 is more strongly developed (Martin and Megirian, 1972).

Brushtail possums are remarkable in two related respects. (1) Some specimens are lissencephalic, others gyrencephalic. In the gyrencephalic specimens the sulci appear between sensory representations as described above. (2) In

---

In *Vombatus* SI and SII are from Johnson *et al.* (1973) and Johnson (1980); in these studies the partial boundaries of visual and auditory regions were established but not previously published.

SI for wallabies is from a combination of data from *M. eugenii* (Lende, 1963c), *T. billardieri* (W. Weller *et al.*, 1976), and my unpublished findings in *M. rufogriseus*. In regions sampled by any two or more of these studies, there is agreement in all details of the projection pattern. SII is from W. Weller *et al.* (1976), and the boundaries of the visual and auditory regions are those reported by Lende (1963c).

lissencephalic specimens tangential sections can be prepared, such as that shown in Fig. 7, which reveals not only barrels in layer 4, but around the barrels regions of dense cellular aggregation in layer 4 like those called "granular regions" in rats (see Section 10.1.3) separated by "dysgranular" regions of lesser cell density in layer 4. In modestly gyrencephalic specimens it can be shown that the sulci

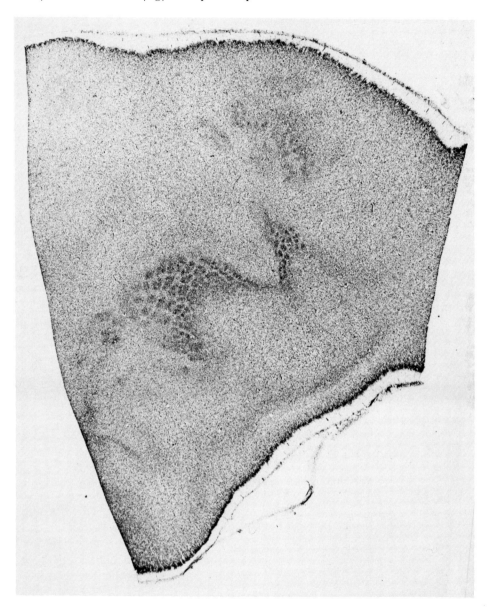

Figure 7. Tangential section through layer 4 of somatic sensory cortex of brushtail possum *Trichosurus vulpecula,* stained with thionin to show groupings of densely packed cell bodies, known as "barrels" because of their three-dimensional shape. (Photo courtesy of Dr. W. L. Weller,, reprinted from Johnson, 1980, with permission from Plenum Press.) The barrels are a portion of a subregion of SI similar to that termed "granular" in rats (see Section 10.1.3); intervening regions of lesser cell density in layer 4 in rats are termed "dysgranular." Brushtail possums are remarkable in that some specimens are gyrencephalic, others lissencephalic (Haight and Weller, 1973), and in the gyrencephalic species sulci appear in SI along the centers of the dysgranular strips (W. L. Weller and J. R. Haight, unpublished observations).

appear in the middle of the dysgranular strips (W. L. Weller and J. R. Haight, unpublished observations).

351

COMPARISONS OF
SOMATIC SENSORY
CORTEX

3.2.4. Thalamic Connections

In quolls and in brushtails as in opossums, a given locus in the limb representation within the somatic sensory SMI cortex receives projections from an anteroposterior column of cells in VP and an extension of this column in the neighboring region of VL (Haight and Neylon, 1978, 1979, 1981); but in these animals, unlike opossums, there are additional projections from more anterior regions of VL to motor cortex anterior to SMI; and in the face representation in SMI there are many regions receiving input from VP but not from VL (this relation is of particular interest in comparing the projections with the greater development of layer 4 and the diminution of layer 5 in the face region; Martin and Megirian, 1972). Equation of VP input with sensory cortex, and VL input with motor cortex, leads to the expression that in these Australian representatives of two major marsupial subgroups, the limb representations are completely overlapped sensory and motor regions, the face representations are incompletely overlapped sensory and motor regions, and the region anterior to these is a purely motor cortex.

In the most recent study of thalamic connections in brushtails (Joschko and Sanderson, 1987), the limb representations were found to have reciprocal connections with the thalamic posterior nucleus (PO) as well as with VP and VL.

3.2.5. Corticocortical Connections

3.2.5a. Ipsilateral. In brushtails the limb representation of sensorimotor cortex has reciprocal connections with the more anterior purely motor cortex, and both regions have reciprocal connections with the purely sensory region in the face representation and with SII (Joschko and Sanderson, 1987). Cells of origin of these corticocortical connections were mostly in layers 2 and 3, with some in layers 4, 5, and 6 (much like cells of origin of commissural connections in opossums). Terminals of these corticocortical connections in brushtails were reported in all layers.

3.2.5b. Commissural. As in opossums, there is commissural input to SMI and SII in brushtails, concentrated in the face regions (Heath and Jones, 1971). Tail and trunk regions also receive heavy commissural input, while in the limb representations the commissural input is present but very sparse. The commissural fibers to and from more basal and lateral portions of the cortex travel in the anterior commissure, those serving more dorsal and medial regions pass through the fasciculus aberrans, a pathway unique to Australian diprotodont marsupials, which travels alongside the internal capsule to near the midline, which the fibers cross just dorsal to the anterior commissure. Commissural fibers were reported to terminate in layers 1 and 2 and in the adjoining parts of layers 3 and 4. It would be of interest to see if these terminals in layer 4 were really in contrast to the situation in *Didelphis* where in at least some descriptions (see Section 3.1.5) terminals avoid layer 4 in some areas of SMI; the illustrations provided in these various papers do not allow meaningful judgments on this matter. Cells of origin of commissural fibers in brushtails were reported to be in layer 5 (Joschko and Sanderson, 1987) without further comment; this does not agree with findings in opossums and most if not all other species where most commissural fibers originate from cells in or near layer 3.

3.2.6. Other Connections

Many corticofugal connections of somatic sensory regions have been determined in brushtails. Reciprocal connections with the claustrum were found, as were projections from the basal forebrain (Joschko and Sanderson, 1987). Projections from SMI terminate in the corpus striatum (Heath and Jones, 1971; Joschko and Sanderson, 1987). Additional output from somatic sensory cortex of brushtails arrives in the red nucleus; deep layers of superior and inferior colliculi; substantia nigra; periaqueductal gray; pontine nuclei; pontine and medullary reticular formations; and cuneate, gracile, commissural, and spinal trigeminal nuclei (Rees and Hore, 1970; Martin *et al.*, 1971; Martin and Megirian, 1972; Joschko and Sanderson, 1987). Corticospinal tracts in brushtails are arranged as they are in opossums, with the differences that in brushtails the pyramids are larger, and terminals are found in thoracic segments (to T8 and T10 from the lateral and dorsal column tracts, respectively) as well as cervical regions (Rees and Hore, 1970; Martin *et al.*, 1970).

Corticospinal projections from SMI (especially the limb projection regions) have also been traced in other diprotodont macropod species: potoroos (Martin *et al.*, 1972), quokka wallabies (Watson, 1971), and red and gray kangaroos (Watson and Freeman, 1977). The corticospinal tracts of these animals vary from those of brushtails only in their caudal extent: the caudalmost fibers are at T6 in the kangaroos, T7 in the quokkas, T8 (lateral column) and T10 (dorsal column) in brushtails, and T8 and T12 in potoroos.

3.2.7. Comparison Summary

The similarity between monotremes and the Australian quolls and brushtail possums in the relations between motor and sensory regions suggests that the complete convergence seen in opossum SMI is a peculiarity of opossums or perhaps of the American family Didelphidae, rather than a general feature of therians or marsupials.

Multiplication of representations within SI, seen in the double projections from mystacial vibrissae in opossums, occurs again in the second representation of maxillary hairy skin in Australian wombats and wallabies. We shall see that this occurs from time to time among placentals, so can be expected among all therians. More extensive investigations of the prototherians (or if more prototherians had survived to be investigated) might reveal this as a general mammalian characteristic.

The fasciculus aberrans, commissurally connecting sensory and other cortical regions, is a distinctive feature peculiar to the Australian diprotodonts (Johnson *et al.*, 1982a,b). Two other new features seen in members of this group— the presence of barrel formations in layer 4, and sulci between representations of body parts—will be seen later to occur in other therian taxa and thus represent some basic feature of therian (or perhaps mammalian) brain organization which becomes apparent only in certain grades of development.

The peculiar coincidence of properties occurring in brushtail possums, where in the same animals it is possible to observe granular and dysgranular regions, barrel formations, and sulci demarcating sensory projections, will be taken up again in discussing the possible general mammalian properties of variations in SI layer 4 and the formation of gyri and sulci (see Sections 10.1.7 and 16.3).

4. Edentates

The majority of extant mammals belong to the eutherian or placental radiation, the largest and most extensively differentiated of the three surviving subclasses (Prototheria, Metatheria, Eutheria). The first bifurcation within the placental radiation separates the edentates from all of the other eutherians. This renders the edentates a most interesting taxon in that they can be expected to be maximally different from other placentals, and characters they have in common with other placentals will most likely represent the ancestral placental condition. Characteristics shared with monotremes and marsupials, and particularly members of this category not shared with other placentals, are possible ancestral characters of early mammals.

4.1. Sensory Projections

Somatic sensory projections to cerebral cortex have been studied in three edentate species: two sloths (two-toed *Choloepus hoffmanni*, 3 specimens, Meulders *et al.*, 1966; three-toed *Bradypus tridactylus*, 32 specimens, Saraiva and Magalhães-Castro, 1975) and one armadillo (*Dasypus novemcinctus*, 12 specimens, Royce *et al.*, 1975). The mediolateral sequence of somatotopically arranged projections in the primary (SI) sensory region is similar to that seen in monotremes and marsupials, with hindquarters represented medially and cranial structures laterally (Fig. 8). A secondary (SII) sensory region was reported in both sloths, but there was no mention of its presence or absence in armadillos. In SI in the sloths there is an enlarged representation of the forelimb, with a relatively small face representation. Armadillos displayed a large face representation relative to those of the limbs and trunk, more similar to the relative sizes seen in montremes and marsupials.

4.2. Relation to Other Areas

In the two-toed sloth, sensory cortex was reported to be posterior to motor cortex as found by Langworthy (1935). Figure 8 shows some overlap between Langworthy's motor regions and the sensory regions mapped by Meulders et al. In the three-toed sloth, sensory and motor areas were reported to be completely and precisely overlapped, as in marsupial opossums (Saraiva and Magalhães-Castro, 1975); Langworthy (1935) had mapped motor cortex in this species and found it to be essentially similar to that of the two-toed species. Discrepancies in methodology and interpretation must be resolved before a claim to interspecies difference in sensory–motor overlap can be made for these sloths. In the armadillo, Royce *et al.* (1975) decided there was partial overlap of sensory cortex with

TWO-TOED SLOTH
*Choloepus
hoffmanni*

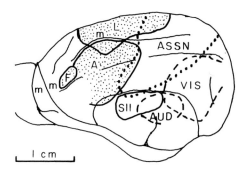

THREE-TOED SLOTH
*Bradypus
tridactylus*

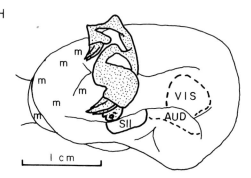

ARMADILLO
*Dasypus
novemcinctus*

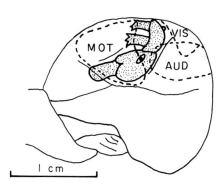

Figure 8. Organization of projections to somatic sensory cortex of three edentates (placentals, Eutheria) as seen in dorsolateral views of the cerebral hemispheres. Anterior is to the left in all diagrams. SI is stippled for each.

Sensory regions for the two-toed sloth represent those reported by Meulders *et al.* (1966): F, A, and L denote respectively projections from face, arm and hand (forelimb), and leg and foot (hindlimb); boundaries of SI and SII, where determined, are marked by a solid line; auditory (AUD) and visual (VIS) regions are enclosed in dashed lines (boundaries were not completely mapped); dotted line encloses what these authors call association cortex (ASSN), wherein they recorded long-latency somatic sensory responses. Regions from which Langworthy (1935) evoked muscular movement by electrical stimulation are designated by m.

For the three-toed sloth, m's again mark the locations from which muscular movements were evoked by Langworthy (1935). In contrast, Saraiva and Magalhães-Castro (1975) found SI (stippled) and motor cortex to be precisely coextensive. The representation of the body surface in SI indicated by the Bradypunculus with an enlarged forelimb, and the locations and extents of SII, auditory

the motor cortex as mapped by Dom *et al.* (1971). Overlap was greatest in the sensory face region, in contrast to the overlaps reported in brushtail possums (Fig. 6) and in rats (see Section 10.1.2), where the overlap is greatest in limb regions and least in face regions.

In armadillos, somatic sensory cortex directly abuts on visual and auditory areas. In both sloths, however, a new phenomenon is seen. While somatic sensory, auditory, and visual areas are all contiguous at certain points, there is a large area intervening among them dorsally. Meulders *et al.* named this association cortex; long-latency responses to somatic sensory (though not visual or auditory) stimulation were found throughout this region (ASSN in Fig. 8).

4.3. Structure

In sloths there may be a sulcal division between forelimb and hindlimb representations in SI, and another between SI medially and SII and auditory cortex laterally; these gyral relationships were not directly addressed in the experimental studies. In armadillos, SI is bounded anteriorly by a sagittal sulcus, posteriorly by a suprasylvian sulcus, and lateroventrally by the rhinal fissure (Fig. 8). There are no sulci within SI.

Gerebtzoff and Goffart (1966) described all of the isocortex of two-toed sloths (*Choloepus hoffmanni*) as "primitive" resembling the mesocortex of other mammals. Layer II is characterized by large cells occurring in clumps; there is no distinct layer IV, layer III merges into layer V, and there are few myelinated intracortical fibers other than a coarse plexus in the superficial layers. All these characteristics are seen in SI cortex. As in the primary visual and auditory areas, SI cortex shows some accumulation of small cells in the deep portion of layer III, suggesting a layer IV without precise limits (Fig. 9). The number of these small cells varies from place to place in SI. There are many large cells in a distinct layer V throughout SI.

The region presumed to be SII has fewer granule cells, and cells of layers II and III are grouped into columns (Fig. 9) capped by clumps of large cells. Similar clumps or knobs in layers II and III are seen throughout the face region of SI in armadillos (Fig. 9). No suggestions have been forthcoming as to the significance of these columns or knobs; modern fine-grain mapping studies might well reveal functional correlates of interest.

In contrast to the reported primitive-undifferentiated laminae of sloth cortex, Royce *et al.* recognized all six layers as well developed in SI of armadillos. They also described peculiar clusters of cells in layer V in that part of the forelimb motor region where they found no sensory responses.

(AUD), and visual (VIS) regions are those reported by Saraiva and Magalhães-Castro (1975); this drawing is in large part a replication of their figures (with permission from P. E. S. Saraiva and Elsevier Science Publishers BV).

The data for armadillo are from Royce *et al.* (1975, with permission from G. J. Royce and Alan R. Liss, Inc.), this drawing is a combination of two of their figures; they made no mention of SII. Three unlabeled sulci bound SI: anterior is the small sagittal sulcus, posterior is the suprasylvian sulcus, and ventrolateral is the rhinal fissure.

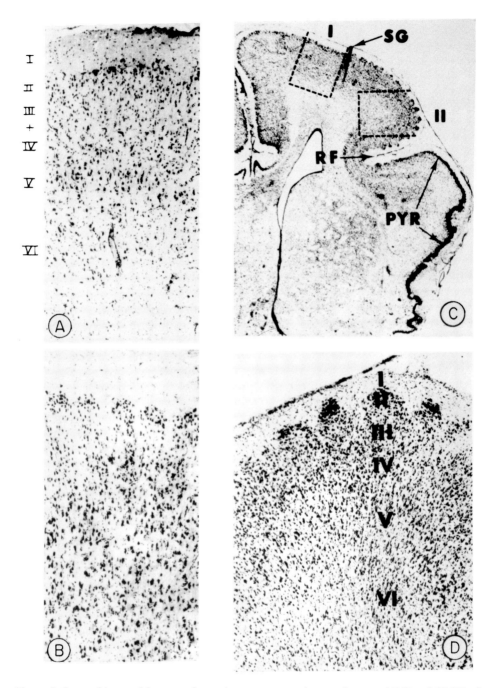

Figure 9. Cytoarchitectural features of somatic sensory cortex in two edentates. (A) SI and (B) SII of the two-toed sloth *Choloepus hoffmanni* (from Gerebtzoff and Goffart, 1966, with permission from M. A. Gerebtzoff and Alan R. Liss, Inc.). Laminar boundaries are obscure, and in SII the upper cell layers form columns capped by knobs or clumps of cell bodies. (C) Low-power photo and (D) enlarged portion outlined by II in C, from armadillo *Dasypus novemcinctus* (from Royce *edt al.*, 1975, with permission from G. J. Royce and Alan R. Liss, Inc.). I and II refer to postorbital areas I and II, II includes all of sensory cortex; PYR: pyriform cortex, RF: rhinal fissure at ventrolateral boundary of SI; SG: sagittal sulcus at anterior boundary of face region of SI. Cell clumps form knobs in lamina II across this face region of SI in armadillo.

4.4. Corticocortical Connections

Edentates possess a corpus callosum, a bundle of fibers passing from the cerebral cortex of one hemisphere to that of the other through the hippocampal formation. All other placentals have this structure; it is not found in marsupials or monotremes (Johnson *et al.*, 1982a,b), and it is the major route of commissural interconnections of somatic sensory cortex in placentals.

4.5. Other Connections

Strominger (1969) studied the corticospinal path by tracing degeneration following large cortical lesions which included the sensorimotor areas in three two-toed sloths and five armadillos. He found degenerating fibers partially decussating in the medulla and extending to thoracic spinal levels. Caudal to the decussation the degeneration was located in the ventral and lateral funiculi, most of them on the side contralateral to the lesion. The major portion were in the outer margin of the lateral funiculi in the sloths, and in the dorsal edge of the ventral funiculi in the armadillos. It cannot be known what portion of these fibers originated from sensory cortex, but it seems safe to conclude that any possible spinal input from sensory cortex lies in the funicular loci mentioned, and does not extend caudal to thoracic regions. A series of related reports of corticofugal paths in armadillos used small lesions, many of them in motor regions which may or may not have impinged on sensory areas, but with none clearly in sensory cortex (A. Fisher *et al.*, 1969; Harting and Martin, 1970a,b; Dom *et al.*, 1971); conclusions, based on these studies, about the output of sensory cortex are difficult to make.

4.6. Comparison Summary

The corpus callosum is the most prominent feature distinguishing edentate (and all placental) cortex from that of monotremes and marsupials. In all other respects the sensory cortex of the edentates is very similar in most general details to that seen in the Prototheria and Metatheria.

In sloths (but not armadillos) the expanded region of "association" cortex intervening between somatic sensory and visual regions may represent something of an evolutionary trend, but (depending on detail of exploration) some intervening cortex was seen in, for example, the prototherian platypus (Fig. 3) and metatherian wombat (Fig. 6).

The relative absence of clear laminae in sloths (but again, not in armadillos) could be some kind of primitive character, but here we would have to assume that prototherians, metatherians, armadillos, and other placentals have then all evolved clear laminae in parallel; the alternative explanation that the cortical homogeneity of sloths is a sloth peculiarity seems equally reasonable.

The enlarged representation of the forelimb seen in sloths is a departure from the pattern seen in all the other species we have so far considered; these others have all had a dominating representation of parts of the face. It does appear that a dominating sensory projection from a nonfacial region is found only among placentals (we shall see it again as we proceed through the eu-

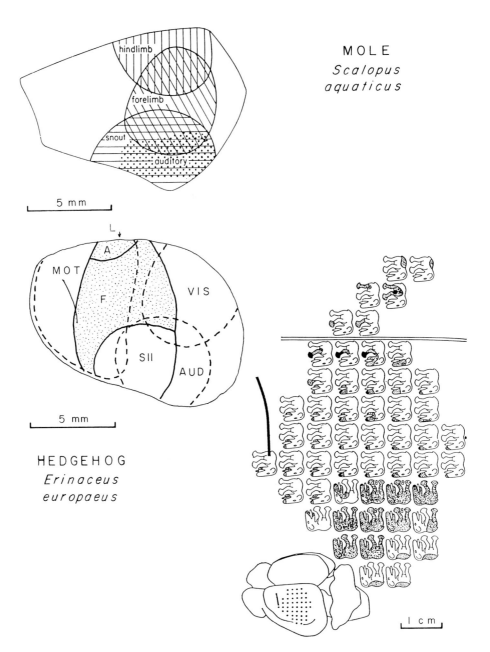

Figure 10. Organization of projections to somatic sensory cortex of two insectivores as seen in dorsolateral views of the cerebral hemispheres. Anterior is to the left in all diagrams.

Data for the mole are reproduced from Allison and Van Twyver (1970, with permission from T. Allison and Alan R. Liss, Inc.). SII was reported to be within the snout representation as indicated for SI but was not further localized. Visual projections were absent.

Data for hedgehogs are those reported by Lende and Sadler (1967, with permission from Elsevier Science Publishers BV). In the diagram at the left, SI representations are stippled, with face (F) regions much larger than those for arm and hand (A = forelimb) and for leg and foot (L = hindlimb; these projections were all on the mesial surface). SI is largely, but not completely, overlapped by motor cortex (MOT), and there is some overlap of auditory (AUD) and visual (VIS) regions with SI and/or SII. The detailed map at lower right is reproduced from their figure, but reversed to keep anterior to the left. As in Fig. 4, at bottom is the outline of a dorsolateral view of the left side of the brain, with dots showing the surface locations of macroelectrodes yielding the information about

therians). This observation can suggest wide-ranging speculations, such as whether a corpus callosum allows more dorsal cortical expansion that would permit greater elaboration of more dorsal (nonfacial) regions of sensory cortex.

359

COMPARISONS OF
SOMATIC SENSORY
CORTEX

5. Insectivores

Turning from the edentate line to the other fork in the path of placental relationships (Fig. 1), we come to a fundamental conundrum in mammalian phylogeny. Rather than an orderly sequence of successive bifurcations, data so far available leave us at the next node with a burst of manifold divergences from a single origin into several separate lines of development. Whether this is due to absence of data or whether there really was a sudden, many-directional spate of differentiation may never be known.

For our account, we are taking each of the branches from this common origin in what is essentially a random order. The insectivores are taken up first, somewhat fearfully, since there are persistent and possibly erroneous suggestions that this group is somehow more primitive or ancestral than the others (overall, it is not). But their brains are tiny and relatively simple and it is convenient to deal with them before taking up other groups which include examples of more complex organization.

With one exception, the few studies on specifically somatic sensory cortex of Insectivora have used the European hedgehog (*Erinaceus europaeus*); this species has come to bear a great burden in speculations about brain evolution due to the popular (and largely unfounded) concept of insectivores as representing a primitive or ancestral form of mammalian brain organization.

5.1. Sensory Projections

The nonhedgehog study was that by Allison and Van Twyver (1970), of sensory representation in the neocortex of the mole, *Scalopus aquaticus*. Recording from large electrodes outside the dura, they found roughly equal-sized hindlimb, forelimb, and snout regions in the usual dorsomedial-to-ventrolateral order within SI, with the snout representation completely overlapping the auditory cortex (Fig. 10); the overlap is presumably due to the size and extradural location of the recording electrode. A secondary (SII) sensory region was noted but not explored. They reported that on the cortical surface SI appeared to be shifted posterolaterally, related to absence of a visual cortex.

In a more detailed study of sensory cortex of *Erinaceus*, Lende and Sadler (1967) used fine-grain recording directly from the cortical surface with 0.25-mm-diameter tungsten macroelectrodes. They found all parts of the contralateral body represented in the primary (SI) sensory region, with no ipsilateral

---

sensory projections shown just above. Receptive fields of cortical potentials activated by mechanosensory stimulation are indicated by shaded patches on sketches of body parts, placed at the approximate location on the cerebral surface of the recording macroelectrodes. Black spots within shaded patches show the body regions from which potentials of greatest amplitude were evoked by minimal mechanical stimulation.

projections. The snout representation was predominant (Fig. 10). SII was present, cortical loci in SII had larger receptive fields than those in SI, these fields were bilateral, but stronger responses were obtained to contralateral compared to ipsilateral stimulation. A later microelectrode study (Kaas *et al.*, 1970) yielded similar results.

5.2. Relation to Other Areas

As mentioned above, the mole showed overlap of sensory and auditory cortex, and it was concluded that *Scalopus* has no visual cortical representation, resulting in the caudalward shift of the somatic sensory region (Allison and Van Twyver, 1970).

Lende and Sadler (1967), using the same methods with both species, found the relations of sensory and primary motor cortices to differ in opossums and hedgehogs: in opossums sensory and motor regions completely overlapped; in hedgehogs a wide region of overlap was bounded by a purely motor region anteriorly and a purely sensory region posteriorly (see Fig. 10). In this respect hedgehogs resembled monotremes, Australian marsupials, and armadillos in contrast to American opossums and possibly sloths (see Sections 2.1.2, 2.2.2, 3.1.2, 3.2.2, and 4.2). As with all species except sloths which we have thus far considered, in hedgehogs there were no substantial cortical regions intervening between the primary sensory regions: the somatic sensory region met and overlapped with auditory and visual regions posteriorly (Kaas *et al.*, 1970) (Fig. 10).

5.3. Structure

Relative difficulty in discriminating laminae was reported in early studies of hedgehog neocortex (Brodmann, 1909; Ebner, 1969). Detailed modern studies (D. Sanides and Sanides, 1974; Valverde and López-Mascaraque, 1981; Valverde and Facal-Valcerde, 1986) resolve this difficulty into the absence of a definite layer 4 anywhere except in visual cortex. These studies showed the most prominent feature of hedgehog neocortex to be layer 2, a conspicuous cell band of densely packed, polymorphic, large neurons, often aggregated into clumps. In the somatic sensory region layer 2 has a predominance of spiny stellate or pyramidal cells with numerous branches in a wide layer 1, which these authors consider the most distinctive feature of this cortex. These layer 2 pyramidal cells have two, three, or more apical dendrites, richly covered by spines, predominating over the smaller basal dendrites. (In this respect they resemble opossum layer 2 cells which have either two, or one apical dendrite which bifurcates near the soma, predominating over basal dendrites; see Section 3.1.3.) A few layer 2 cells have one dendrite a little more prominent, approaching a sort of truly apical condition. These characteristics of layer 2, along with the wide layer 1 containing small horizontally oriented cells, were considered evidence of early stages of evolutionary development. The layer 1 cells resemble fetal cells seen in other species; the layer 2 organization was considered similar to that seen in paleocortical regions. Deeper layers were reported to be more typical of neocortical regions. Spaces between the clumps in layer 2 were shown in Golgi preparations to be occupied by bundles of apical dendrites of deep pyramidal layers.

Moles (*Talpa europaea*) showed layer 2 features similar to those of hedge-hogs, but in contrast to hedgehogs they exhibited a well-defined layer 4 in parietal regions which thereby allowed easy discrimination of all cortical layers (Ferrer, 1986).

5.4. Thalamic Connections

In a directly comparative study of hedgehogs and opossums, Killackey and Ebner (1972) found the sensory cortex of both species to receive thalamic inputs from ventral nuclei of the dorsal thalamus to layers 3 and 4, and from intra-laminar nuclei to layers 1 and 6 (and also to putamen).

5.5. Comparison Summary

Overall, there are no features of the somatic sensory cortex of these insec-tivores that distinguishes its organization from that of edentates or from those of the marsupials and monotremes. Such distinctive features as have been observed are peculiarities of individual species, not of taxonomic groups.

The caudalward displacement of the somatic sensory region in *Scalopus* can be ascribed to the lack of visual projections. The clumps of cells in layer 2 of sensory cortex, separated by bundles of apical dendrites, may have something in common with the similar clumps and knobs seen in edentates (see Fig. 9) whose detailed architecture remains to be determined. The apparent high degree of overlap among the various primary sensory regions seen in these studies of insectivores is to some extent a function of the small size of the brains and the large size of the electrodes used.

The advent of a clear patch of association cortex seen in sloths is revealed as a sloth peculiarity and not a general feature of placental brains. In this respect it is the sloths and not the armadillo that are distinctive: the armadillo is like the insectivores, the sloths are not.

6. Chiroptera

The next branch from the starburst node undergoes a further trifurcation, indicating a closer relationship among the orders Chiroptera, Scandentia, and Primates. The bats are considered next; some bats are considered flying insec-tivores, others have primate affinities as do the tree shrews, thus there is some rationale in considering them after the Insectivora and before the Scandentia and Primates.

6.1. Sensory Projections

Somatosensory cortex has been mapped in two Australian bats: the mega-chiropteran, fruit-eating, tree-climbing, flying fox *Pteropus poliocephalus* (Calford *et al.*, 1985), and the microchiropteran, insectivorous, ghost bat *Macroderma gigas*

(L. Wise *et al.*, 1986). While the general location of, and the mediolateral arrangement of projections in, SI and SII followed the usual mammalian pattern, in these bats there was a striking difference from other mammals in the anteroposterior sequence of representations (Fig. 11). In most mammals the tips of the digits are represented most anteriorly in SI; in bats these representations are the most posterior. The investigators ascribed this difference to the fact that the tips of the digits trail rather than lead during ordinary bat locomotion. Other features of interest include the large representations of the wing (hand) membranes; the enlarged representation of the pinna in the echolocating insectivorous *Macroderma;* and the enlarged representation of the tongue and the hind foot in the frugivorous and tree-climbing *Pteropus.*

6.2. Structure

Two cytoarchitectonic features of neocortex, including somatic sensory regions, described in Section 5.3 for hedgehogs, are also true of the bats (*Myotis locifugus*) studied by Sanides and Sanides (1972, 1974): (1) layer 2 pyramidal cells with several distal dendrites in a wide layer 1 and small basal dendrites, and (2) an indistinct layer 4.

6.3. Comparison Summary

Auditory cortex (of remarkable complexity) has been well studied in a few bat species, but no studies have combined auditory and somatic sensory investigations in the same subjects. Bats are so numerous and varied (one in five of the world's mammalian species are bats) that it would be rash to draw conclusions about cortical relations from such different studies of different species. Expect for the auditory work and the somatic sensory studies cited above, bat brains remain a fertile and unexplored field for future studies of brain evolution.

The same argument can be applied to the isolated studies of cortical architecture. The distinctive arrangement of the forelimb projections in SI, however, was found in representatives of the most widely divergent varieties of bats and has a better claim to being a general property of the whole chiropteran order, distinguishing them from the rest of the mammals. This difference in brain organization may be a cortical consequence of limb use, arising in each individual; L. Wise *et al.* (1986) suggest it will be interesting to see if these relations are also distinctive at subcortical levels less subject to determination by individual experiences.

7. Scandentia

Tree shrews have been considered so closely related to (but yet distinct from) primates that in the history of classification they have frequently been shifted to and from one of two states: (1) as a separate small order as is now the case, or (2) as a peculiar small subdivision of the order Primates. This position as the innermost outgroup leaves them as something of a key to the origins of

FLYING FOX
Pteropus poliocephalus

RAT

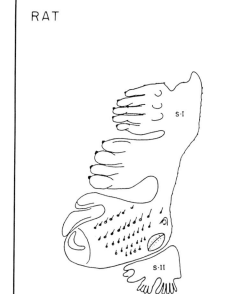

GHOST BAT
Macroderma gigas

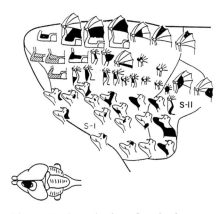

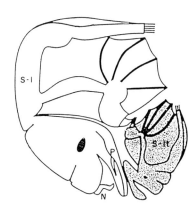

Figure 11. Organization of projections to somatic sensory cortex of two bats as seen in dorsal views of the cerebral hemispheres. Anterior is to the left in all diagrams.

Bottom left: Outline of the dorsal aspect of the brain of the insectivorous microbat *Macroderma gigas*, the Australian ghost bat. SI is blackened and SII is outlined. Above and to the right, figurines indicate details of projections to these regions: receptive fields recorded by extracellular micro-electrodes are indicated by black patches on drawings of body parts, placed relative to electrode locations in sensory cortex as viewed from above. Bottom right, summary of the pattern of projections presented as a cartoon of the body surface. P = pinna, N = nose leaf. Drawings are from L. Wise *et al.* (1986, with permission from J. D. Pettigrew, M. B. Calford, and Alan R. Liss, Inc.).

Top left: The pattern of projections in the frugivorous megabat *Pteropus poliocephalus*, the gray-headed flying fox. *Top right:* The contrasting pattern seen in other mammals, exemplified by the rat. T = tongue. Drawings are from Calford *et al.* [1985, with alterations, and permission from M. B. Calford and from *Nature* Vol. 313, p. 477–479, copyright (c) 1985 Macmillan Magazines Ltd.].

Both bats show extensive representation of the wing (hand) membranes, and the distinctive feature (as contrasted with the rat and other mammals) that the tips of the digits lie caudalmost in both the SI and SII representations. The flying fox has distinctively large representations of the tongue and hindfoot; the ghost bat has large representations of the pinna and the nose leaf probably related to their use in echolocation guidance.

primate specializations, and has induced what would otherwise have been an inordinate amount of research on a small obscure taxon.

7.1. Sensory Projections

Somatic sensory projections to SI and SII of tree shrews have been mapped in detail using microelectrodes (Fig. 12) (Sur *et al.*, 1980b, 1981a,b). In SI, projections follow the general mediolateral sequence seen in the mammals so far considered; particular features of interest include: hand digits represented in the rostral half of SI with tips pointing anteriorly, but with the representation of the volar (palmar) surface of the hand reaching the caudal border of SI; an anterior strip of arm represented laterally to the hand and a posterior strip of leg represented medially to the foot; an extensive representation of the glabrous snout proportionally larger than in any other mammal studied so far (Sur *et al.*, 1980b); and a divided representation of the trunk with the ventral portion represented between the fore- and hindlimbs and the dorsal portion represented medial to the foot and continuous with the representation of the upper hindlimb (Sur *et al.*, 1981b).

In SII, projections from the head adjoin head representations in SI; representations of the distal digits point laterally away from SI; responses are to light tactile stimulation; and all receptive fields were contralateral using the microelectrode mapping from within the cortical cell layers (Sur *et al.*, 1981a). Cells in SII respond to peripheral stimulation in the absence of SI, contrary to what is found in monkeys (see Section 8.2) (Garraghty *et al.*, 1989).

In addition to SI and SII, two additional sensory areas were found in tree shrews (Sur *et al.*, 1980b). Along the rostral border was a thin high-threshold zone, which invaginated between the hand and face representations, wherein responses were restricted to high-amplitude stimulation. A second, wider, high-threshold zone lay immediately caudal to SI and SII [labeled "PSF" (posterior somatic field) in Fig. 12]. Some of the high-threshold responses were to stimulation of deep-lying tissues.

7.2. Relation to Other Areas

Unlike any of the mammals so far surveyed, except the sloths, there is a substantial expanse of parietal cortex intervening between the primary somatic sensory, auditory, and visual areas (Fig. 12) (Cusick *et al.*, 1985). This "association" cortex includes areas 18, TD, and PSF in Fig. 12. The auditory area borders SII, and the dorsomedial extreme of the visual cortex approaches the medial portion of SI.

7.3. Structure

While Sur *et al.* (1981b) decided that sensory koniocortex was not well developed in tree shrews, and that the medial boundary was difficult to discern cytoarchitecturally, Sur *et al.* (1980b) (Fig. 13) showed an anteroposterior coincidence of SI projections with a pronounced increase in density in layers 3 and 4.

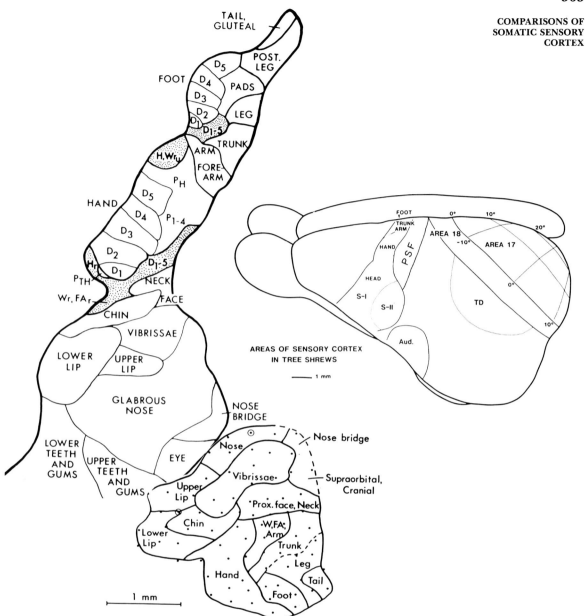

AREAS OF SENSORY CORTEX
IN TREE SHREWS

Figure 12. Organization of projections to somatic sensory cortex of a tree shrew as seen in a dorsolateral view of the left cerebral hemisphere. Anterior is to the left.

Right: Outline of the hemisphere showing the locations of somatic sensory (S-I, S-II), auditory (Aud., and several visual (AREAS 17, 18, TD) areas (from Cusick *et al.,* 1985, with the addition of the posterior somatic field PSF from Sur *et al.,* 1981a, with alterations, and permission from C. G. Gusick, M. Sur, and Alan R. Liss, Inc.).

Left: Examples of details of projections to SI (from Sur

et al., 1980b) and SII (from Sur *et al.,* 1981a) (with alterations, and permission from M. Sur and Alan R. Liss, Inc.). In SI the representations of the dorsal hairy surfaces of the hand and foot, the dorsoradial wrist and forearm, and the dorsoulnar wrist are stippled. Digits of the hand and foot are numbered from the thumb or great toe to the little finger or toe, D_{1-5}. The palmar pads of the hand are interdigital, P1–P4, the hypothenar, P_H, and the thenar, P_{TH}. FA, forearm; H, hand; Prox., proximal; r, radial; u, ulnar; W, Wr, wrist.

Cusick *et al.* (1985) showed in tangential sections that SI and SII, like primary auditory and visual regions, are characterized by increased myelination. Furthermore, within SI the dense myelin is interrupted in SI at the approximate location that SI is invaded by the rostral high-threshold region. In some cases a second such interruption occurred in the general region of the boundary between fore- and hindlimb representations. These interruptions in myelination occur at locations analogous to those of sulci in the SI representations seen in the gyrencephalic Australian marsupials (see Section 3.2.3).

7.4. Corticocortical Connections

SI and SII of tree shrews are commissurally connected reciprocally and homotopically (R. Weller and Sur, 1981). Some regions within the representation of each body part have interhemispheric connections; there are relatively more of these in the face representations than in forepaw regions (Cusick *et al.,* 1985). The only information presented relative to laminar location of commissural connections was that cells of origin in both SI and SII were uniformly distributed in infragranular layers, and unevenly distributed in supragranular layers.

7.5. Comparison Summary

Primate affinities are suggested, as shall be seen, by the rostrocaudal extension of the volar hand representation to the caudal border of SI; by the arrangement of SI into a narrow mediolateral strip of cortex bisected by this volar hand representation; and by the larger amount of cortex intervening among the primary auditory and visual (area 17) regions and SI. The presence of the high-

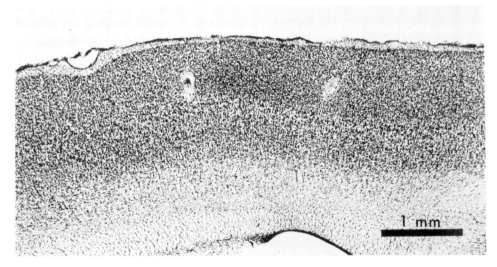

Figure 13. Cytoarchitectural features of somatic sensory cortex in a tree shrew (from Sur *et al.,* 1980b, with permission from M. Sur and Alan R. Liss, Inc.). A parasagittal section is shown. Microlesions mark the rostral (left) and caudal (right) boundaries of SI as determined electrophysiologically. These lesions enclose somatic koniocortex which is characterized by a layer IV densely packed with cells.

characteristic; but there is the possibility that this was found in tree shrews because investigators were searching for primate characteristics. An equally careful search in nonprimate species will be necessary before this can be established as a character distinguishing scandents and primates from other mammals. The peculiar absence of studies of motor cortex and of thalamic projections prevents opportunities for interesting theorizing about trends in sensorimotor segregation between scandents and primates.

8. Primates

Primates include two major subgroups, the mostly small prosimians, and the larger anthropoids (monkeys, apes, and humans) which have more specialized brains. The anthropoids are in two lineages, one from the New World, the other from the Old Word. The Old World line includes the great apes and humans; the New World group has one specialized subgroup, the marmosets.

8.1. Prosimians and Marmosets

Marmosets are considered here with prosimians rather than with the monkeys and apes since their sensory cortex has more features in common with those of prosimians than with those of the other anthropoids (Carlson *et al.,* 1986).

8.1.1. Sensory Projections

8.1.1a. SI. Sensory projections have been mapped in the prosimian lorises *Nycticebus coucang* (Krishnamurti *et al.,* 1976; Carlson and Fitzpatrick, 1982), pottos *Perodicticus potto* (Boisacq-Schepens *et al.,* 1977; FitzPatrick *et al.,* 1982), bushbabies *Galago senegalensis* and *G. crassicaudatus* (Sur *et al.,* 1980a; Carlson and Welt, 1980; Burton and Carlson, 1986), and in marmosets of the genus *Saguinus* (Carlson *et al.,* 1986) (see Fig. 14).

Within the usual sequence of somatotopic projections in SI, lorises have a relatively large representation of glabrous regions of the foot, hand, and face. As is usual with large representations, individual loci within these representations exhibit the smallest receptive fields (Krishnamurti *et al.,* 1976). Two separate representations of the glabrous hand appear in the SI of lorises (Carlson and FitzPatrick, 1982), one rostral to the neighboring representation of the dorsal hairy hand and the other smaller one medial to it (Fig. 14). In the pottos, relatives of the lorises, only a single complete representation was found, otherwise the patterns in both animals were similar (FitzPatrick *et al.,* 1982). In the bushbabies, the main difference from this common pattern of projections was the extension of the representation of the digits of the hand through the entire rostrocaudal extent of SI (Sur *et al.,* 1980a; Carlson and Welt, 1980). The most distinctive feature added to the common pattern in SI of marmosets was the large extent of the representation of the glabrous tips and the claws of the hand digits (Carlson *et al.,* 1986).

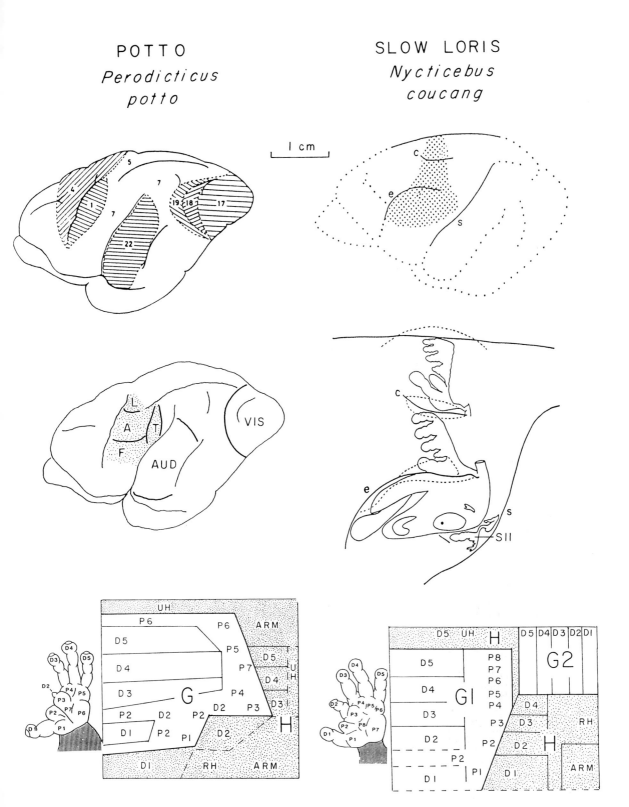

POTTO
*Perodicticus
potto*

SLOW LORIS
*Nycticebus
coucang*

1 cm

Figure 14.

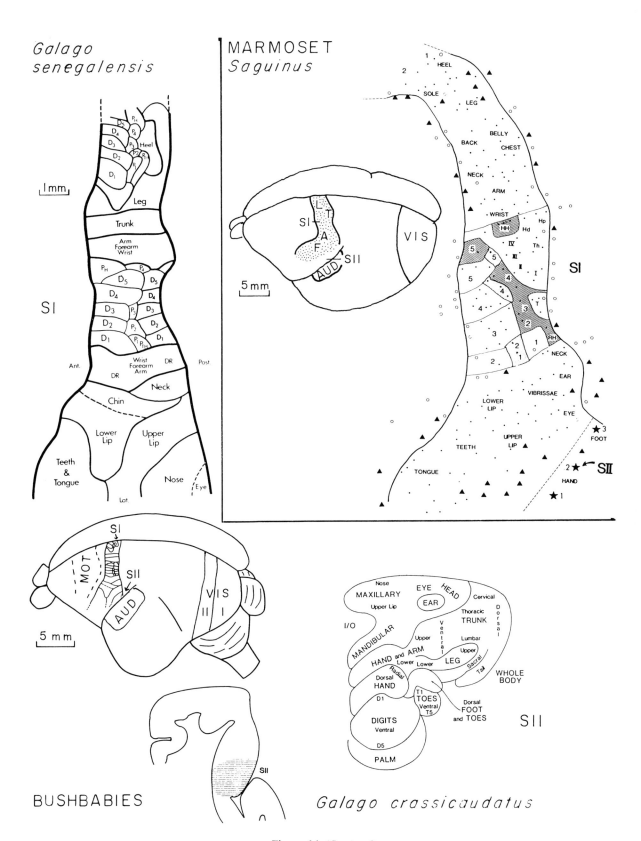

Figure 14. (*Continued*)

In only two respects did SI of marmosets show more similarity to other anthropoids than to prosimians (Carlson *et al.,* 1986): there were representations of neck and occiput both medial and lateral to the hand representation (in prosimians these representations are all lateral to the hand projections); and the forelimb representation was all medial to the hand projections (in the prosimians the forelimb representation is split, portions lying lateral as well as medial to the hand representation).

8.1.1b. Border Zones. In lorises, galagos, and marmosets, as in tree shrews, there were high-threshold zones anterior and posterior to SI that were responsive to strong mechanical stimulation.

8.1.1c. SII. SII was identified in lorises and marmosets, each showing a large representation of the hand and receptive fields larger than their counterparts in SI. SII was thoroughly mapped in *Galago crassicaudatus* (Burton and Carlson, 1986); they found it to lie in the upper or medial bank of the lateral sulcus, with receptive fields of cortical projections primarily contralateral except for a few bilateral fields in the representations of the head and the trunk. The face representation in SII was rostromedial, next to the enlarged hand representation, and caudal and lateral to these were projections from the hindlimb, tail, and sacrum (Fig. 14).

Figure 14 (pages 368–369). Organization of projections to somatic sensory cortex of three prosimians and a marmoset as seen in dorsolateral views of the left cerebral hemispheres. Anterior is to the left, dorsal is to the top for all diagrams.

Top left (page 368): Cytoarchitectural areas corresponding to primary sensory and motor regions of pottos numbered according to the Brodmann system. *Center left:* primary sensory areas as shown by partial mapping studies (from Boisacq-Schepens *et al.,* 1977, with permission from N. Boisacq-Schepens and *Primates,* Japan Monkey Centre): within SI, which is shaded, F denotes projections from the face, A projections from the arm and hand (forelimb), T from the trunk, and L from the leg and foot (hindlimb); AUD = auditory, VIS = visual. *Bottom left:* detailed arrangement of projections from the hand (from FitzPatrick *et al.,* 1982, with alterations, and permission from K. A. FitzPatrick and Alan R. Liss, Inc.); shaded area marked H represents projections from hairy surfaces, area marked G represents glabrous surfaces; D1–5 and P1–8 represent digits and palm pads as in the drawing of the hand to the left; UH = ulnar hand, RH = radial hand.

Top right (page 368): Outline of the hemisphere of a slow loris, showing SI (shaded) and sulci c, e, and s. *Center right:* An enlarged view of SI showing details of projections as a cartoon of the body surface (from Krishnamurti *et al.,* 1976, with alterations, and permission from A. Krishnamurti and S. Karger, AG, Basel); dotted lines enclose projections found in the walls of sulci; the approximate location of SII is also shown. *Bottom right:* Detailed arrangement of projections from the hand (from Carlson and FitzPatrick, 1982, with alterations, and permission from M. Carlson and Alan R. Liss, Inc.); symbols are the same as those for the potto at lower left except that there are two separate representations of the glabrous digits, G1 and G2.

Top left (page 369): Details of projections to SI in the lesser bushbaby, from Sur *et al.* (1980a); DR = dorsoradial, PTH = thenar, and PH = hypothenar palm pads. *Center left:* Location on the cerebral surface of SI and SII, auditory (AUD), visual (VIS), and motor (MOT) regions (from Brugge, 1982, and Kaas, 1982a, with alterations, and permission from J. H. Kaas and *The Lesser Bushbaby (Galago) as an Animal Model: Selected Topics,* pp. 169–181, copyright CRC Press, Inc., Boca Raton). *Bottom left:* Locations of SII in a coronal section through the wall of the lateral sulcus; *bottom right:* details of projections to SII in the greater bushbaby (from Burton and Carlson, 1986, with permission from H. Burton and Alan R. Liss, Inc.); I/O = intraoral.

Top right (page 369): Location on the cerebral surface of marmosets of SI and SII (*Saguinus* sp., Carlson *et al.,* 1986), auditory (AUD, *Callithrix jacchus,* Aitkin *et al.,* 1986), and visual (VIS, *C. jacchus,* Kunz and Spatz, 1985) regions; within SI (shaded) F denotes projections from the face, A projections from the arm and hand (forelimb), T from the trunk, and L from the leg and foot (hindlimb). At far right are details of projections to SI in *Saguinus* (from Carlson *et al.,* 1986, with alterations, and permission from M. Carlson and Alan R. Liss, Inc.); dots indicate locations of electrode penetrations in which cells responded to light cutaneous (low threshold) stimulation, open circles those in which cells responded to more intense somatic (high threshold) stimulation, triangles those in which cells did not respond to somatic stimulation, and stars those in SII; Hd = accessory hypothenar eminence, HH = hairy hand, Hp = hypothenar eminence, RH = radial hand, T was not identified, Th = thenar eminence; arabic numerals indicate digits of the hand or foot; roman numerals indicate digital palm pads; crosshatching indicates dorsal hairy surfaces; fine stipple indicates middle and proximal phalanges.

In pottos, even using surface potentials recorded by macroelectrodes (Boisacq-Schepens *et al.*, 1977), there was a substantial amount of cortex intervening between somatosensory and visual areas, and between visual and auditory regions (Fig. 14). Auditory and somatosensory regions met and overlapped. The ventral portion of the central sulcus separated the anterior edge of somatosensory cortex from the motor cortex as determined physiologically (Zuckerman and Fulton, 1941) and cytoarchitectonically (Boisacq-Schepens *et al.*, 1977).

In galagos (Fig. 14) there is a large parietotemporal region intervening between somatosensory, auditory, and primary visual fields (MT is a nonprimary visual field found within this "association" region; R. Weller and Kaas, 1981). A motor region estimated from cytoarchitectonic characteristics lies immediately anterior to the high-threshold border zone anterior to SI (Kaas, 1982a).

8.1.3. Structure

8.1.3a. Sulci. Sulcal boundaries delimiting SI projections were identified in lorises (Krishnamurti *et al.*, 1976). Their sulcus *c* corresponds to the interbrachial sulcus seen in marsupials (Section 3.2.3) and lies between hindlimb and forelimb projections; the caudomedial end of their sulcus *e* resembles the jugular sulcus of marsupials demarcating forelimb from face projections; the rostrolateral portion of sulcus *e* marks the anterior boundary of SI and was thought to corre-

---

Figure 15 (pages 372–373). Locations and organization of projections to the SI region of somatic sensory cortex of New and Old World monkeys as seen in dorsolateral views of the left cerebral hemispheres. Anterior is to the left, dorsal is to the top for all diagrams. AUD = auditory, MOT = motor, VIS = visual.

Left (page 372): Location of motor, visual, auditory regions, and architectonic fields 3a, 3b, 1, and 2 related to SI in owl monkeys (from Kaas, 1982b, 1983, with alterations, and permission from J. H. Kaas, Academic Press, and the American Physiological Society). Details of the representations of the body surface are shown for fields 3b and 1. A. leg = region devoted to anterior portion of the leg; d = dorsal; D_{1-5} = locations of glabrous digit surfaces of hand and foot; L. lip = region devoted to lower lip; P. leg = region devoted to posterior portion of leg; U. lip = region devoted to upper lip; V. and Vib. = regions devoted to mystacial vibrissae; v = ventral; shaded regions = representations of dorsal hairy surfaces of hand and foot.

Right (page 372): Location of motor (F. Sanides, 1968), visual (Livingstone and Hubel, 1987), auditory (Burton and Jones, 1976) regions and architectonic fields 3b and 1 related to SI (Sur *et al.*, 1982) in squirrel monkeys. Details of the representations of the body surface are shown for fields 3b and 1 (from Sur *et al.*, 1982, with alterations, and permission from M. Sur and Alan R. Liss, Inc.). The middle portion of field 3b is buried in the central sulcus; the dashed line rostral to 3b indicates the inability to establish the precise border since the sulcus limited the spacing of recording sites; the dotted line CS marks the central sulcus. The

dashed line between 3b and 1 indicates the estimated architectonic boundary on the medial wall of the cerebral hemisphere. Ch = chin; D_{1-5} = digits of hand and foot; $Foot_L$ = lateral dorsal foot; F_M = medial dorsal foot; H_{DR} = dorsoradial hand; H_{DU} = dorsoulnar hand; L. face = lateral face; L. Lip = lower lip; Occ. = occiput; Sh. = shoulder; U. Lip = upper lip. Shaded areas correspond to representations of the dorsal hairy surfaces of hand and foot.

Left (p. 373): Organization of the SI representation in spider monkeys (Pubols and Pubols, 1971, with alterations, and permission from B. H. and L. M. Pubols and Alan R. Liss, Inc.). A = arm and hand; F = face and head; IO = intraoral; L = leg and foot; T = trunk; T1 = tail. The dashed line indicates the fundus of the central sulcus. Note the size of the representation of the tail (including the prehensile glabrous tip) compared with the corresponding representations in squirrel and cynomolgus monkeys.

Right (p. 373): Location of auditory (Burton and Jones, 1976; Seltzer and Pandya, 1978), motor, and visual (Brodmann, 1909; C. Woolsey, 1958) regions and architectonic fields 3b and 1 related to SI (from Nelson *et al.*, 1980, with alterations, and permission from R. J. Nelson and Alan R. Liss, Inc.) in macaque monkeys. Most of the auditory and visual fields are buried in sulci and are not visible in this surface view. Details of the representations of the body surface are shown for fields 3b and 1 (Nelson *et al.*, 1980). D_{1-5} = digits of hand and foot; shaded areas = hairy dorsum of digits; dotted line = central sulcus; dashed line = portion of the representation contained in cortex on the medial wall of the hemisphere.

OWL MONKEY
Aotus trivirgatus

SQUIRREL MONKEY
Saimiri sciureus

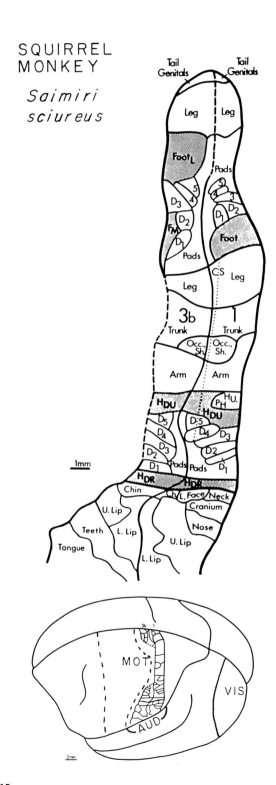
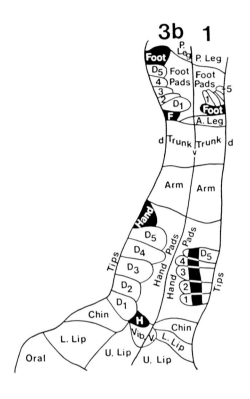
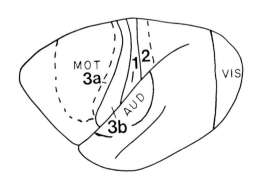

Figure 15.

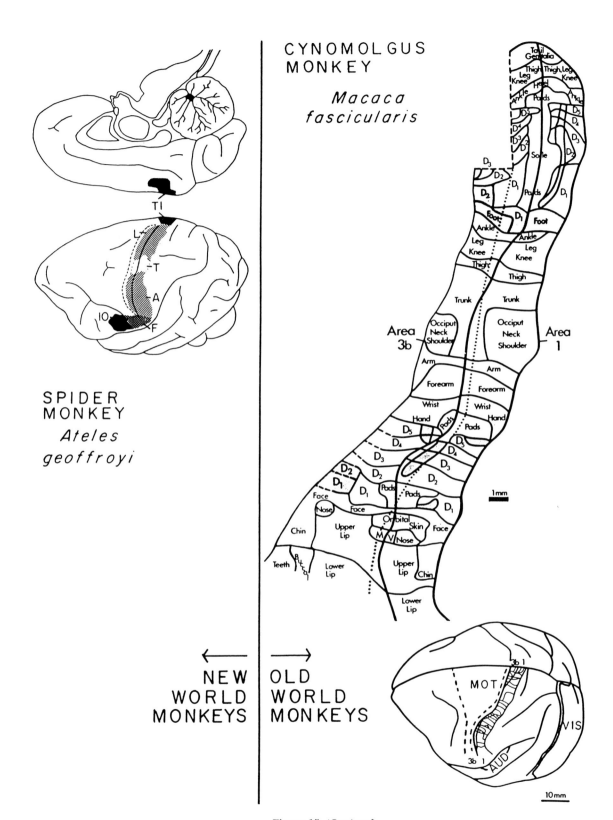

Figure 15. (*Continued*)

spond to the central sulcus of anthropoid primates. A similar central sulcus analogue was described for pottos (Boisacq-Schepens *et al.,* 1977; FitzPatrick *et al.* 1982).

In galagos, the lateral sulcus separates SI and SII (which lies in the medial wall of the sulcus) (Kaas, 1982a; Burton and Carlson, 1986), from the auditory region on the lateral wall and bank of the sulcus (Brugge, 1982).

8.1.3b. Cytoarchitecture. In the hand representation of lorises, Carlson and FitzPatrick identified koniocortex of F. Sanides and Krishnamurti (1967) as coincident with the larger of the two representations of the glabrous surfaces, while dorsal hairy surfaces and the second and smaller glabrous projections were represented in parakoniocortex. Somatic sensory koniocortex in lorises has a dense granular layer clearly separated from a cell-poor layer 5; there is no clear boundary between the granular and the more superficial layers. Within layer 5, variations in the size of the sparse pyramidal cells led to the recognition of three subdivisions separated by sulci; these subdivisions corresponded to the respective representations of (1) hindlimb, with large pyramidal cells; (2) forelimb, with medium-sized pyramidal cells; and (3) face, with small pyramidal cells. Parakoniocortex is characterized by a lesser density of granule cells in layers 3 and 4, and a large number of larger pyramidal cells in layer 3 forming a border distinguishing layer 3 from layer 4.

In pottos, the entire SI representation was described as coincident with similar koniocortex (FitzPatrick *et al.,* 1982), characterized by: fusion of layers 2, 3, and 4 into a dense band of granule cells with some pyramidal cells in layer 3; a sharp border between layers 4 and 5, due to sparsity of cells in 5; and 5 not easily distinguished from 6. This koniocortex extended rostrally only to the bank of the central sulcus; down the bank layer 4 was attenuated, and on the rostral bank the large pyramidal cells appeared in layer 5 characteristic of area 4 and motor cortex.

These gradations in cytoarchitecture parallel those described in monotreme spiny anteaters. Krishnamurti *et al.* (1976) suggest that the rostral high-threshold sensory area occupies the intermediate zone between koniocortex and motor cortex in lorises.

In galagos, the single SI representation was deemed coextensive with koniocortex with dense packing of cells in layers 4 and 6 (Sur *et al.,* 1980a).

SII of lorises (F. Sanides and Krishnamurti, 1967) and galagos (Burton and Carlson, 1986) was located in prokoniocortex, characterized by a layer 4 thickened but less dense and uniform than in the koniocortex of SI, with some pyramidal cells invading from layers 3 and 5; and layer 3 subdivided into 3a with smaller and 3b with large pyramidal cells with 3a not clearly distinct from layer 2.

8.1.4. Thalamic Connections

There is a somatotopic projection from the VP nucleus of the thalamus to SI cortex in *Galago senegalensis:* the cortical face region receives input from the medial part of the nucleus (VPM), successively more lateral parts of the nucleus (VPL) project to forelimb and hindlimb cortical representations (J. Pearson and Haines, 1980; Kaas, 1982a). In *G. crassicaudatus,* Burton and Carlson (1986) found a region of the VPL thalamic nucleus projecting to both SI and SII cortex. SII also received input from ventroposteroinferior (VPI), posterior (PO), and central lateral (CL) thalamic nuclei. Projections from VP and VPI nuclei to SII were observed in a marmoset, *Callithrix jacchus* (Krubitzer and Kaas, 1986, 1987).

With most dorsal thalamic nuclei, there are reciprocal connections with cortex, and SI cortex in *G. senegalensis* does indeed project to the VP thalamic nucleus (Kaas, 1982a).

8.1.5. Comparison Summary

Features of interest in sensory cortex of prosimians and marmosets include high-threshold border zones and expanded association regions resembling those in tree shrews (see Section 7.1) and in the anthropoids (see Section 8.2.1). The lorisoid members of the prosimian group have sulci subdividing representations in SI as previously described in the larger marsupials. The second representation of the glabrous hand seen in lorises is reminiscent of the second representation of the facial vibrissae seen in opossums (Section 3.1.1), and foreshadows the double representation of all cutaneous receptive fields shown by monkeys (Section 8.2.1).

8.2. Other Anthropoids (Monkeys, Apes, and Humans)

(While marmosets are classified as anthropoids, here we will henceforth use the terms *anthropoids* and *monkeys* to describe these groups as excluding marmosets, since the marmoset sensory cortex is more like that of prosimians and has already been described with that of prosimians.) As might be expected, the somatic sensory cortex of anthropoids has been among the most thoroughly investigated of any group of mammals. These studies have been extensively reviewed elsewhere (e.g., Burton and Robinson, 1981; Kaas, 1983; Jones, 1986), so here we will give only the briefest account necessary for making comparisons with findings in other mammals. In most respects the sensory cortex is similar in both New World and Old World monkeys.

8.2.1. Sensory Projections

8.2.1a. SI. In both New and Old World monkeys the striking new feature of the SI region, not seen in prosimians, marmosets, or other mammals, is the presence (observed under appropriate anesthetic conditions; see McKenna *et al.*, 1982) of two complete representations of the cutaneous body surface (in *Aotus, Saimiri, Cebus, Macaca*), one lying anterior to the other (reviewed by Kaas, 1983, who decided that only the anterior representation was SI). Additional projections, largely from deeper-lying tissues, including muscles and joints, are found in two more zones, one anterior and one posterior to the cutaneous representations (Jones and Porter, 1980; Kaas, 1983); these may correspond to the anterior and posterior high-threshold regions described for prosimians. Rather than sharp segregation of cutaneous versus deep projections in these four zones, many studies report a gradation of relative density of deep projections, reaching a peak frequency in the anteriormost and posteriormost regions (e.g., Powell and Mountcastle, 1959; McKenna *et al.*, 1982). Detailed studies of such multiple representations in apes or humans have not been performed, but similar results are expected (Kaas, 1983). Human cortical potentials evoked by median nerve stimulation showed evidence of two foci corresponding in location to the anterior and posterior cutaneous representations of the hand as seen in monkeys (Allison *et al.*, 1989). Within the cutaneous projections there are, as usual, regions of increased cortical area with smaller receptive fields devoted to representations of regions of skin of particular behavioral importance to the respective species; e.g., (Fig. 15) projections from the hands in all monkeys studied, and from the glabrous tip of the tail in spider monkeys *Ateles* (Pubols and Pubols, 1971). While most projections are from contralateral receptive fields, in the face representation there are a few projections from ipsilateral fields; e.g., 8% of neurons in the face representation of *Macaca mulatta* responded to ipsilateral as well as contralateral receptive fields (Dreyer *et al.*, 1975).

An interesting variation in the anterior (Kaas's true SI) body representation was pointed out by Sur *et al.* (1982): the dorsal midline of the trunk is represented at the rostral edge of the representation, and the ventral midline at the posterior edge (the abdomen-rear position), in Old World macaques and in New World owl monkeys, while in New World squirrel monkeys (and cebus monkeys; Felleman *et al.*, 1983a) the sequence is reversed (the abdomen-forward position). In all four species the posterior body representation mirrors the anterior in this respect. In the only map sufficiently detailed that we have considered so far (Fig. 4), the monotreme spiny anteater (echidna) showed the abdomen-forward sequence like the squirrel and cebus monkeys.

8.2.1b. SII. To resolve inconsistencies in earlier studies, Burton and Robinson (1981) adopted a restrictive definition of SII in Old World macaque monkeys, based upon cytoarchitecture and connections. The SII "proper" was located on the parietal operculum of the lateral sulcus and a portion of the adjacent insula, and was characterized by units with small receptive fields just over half of which were contralateral, most of the remainder being bilateral and a small number ipsilateral. Projections from the body surface formed a mostly somatotopic representation, illustrated in Fig. 16. Responsiveness of units in SII was found to be dependent upon an intact SI in the same hemisphere (Pons *et al.*, 1987). Ablation of the SI representation of a particular body part eliminated responses from that body part in the ipsilateral SII. This contrasts with findings in tree shrews (Section 7.1).

A similar SII "proper" was reported in New World owl monkeys (Cusick *et al.*, 1989), but here receptive fields were contralateral and larger than fields in SI.

8.2.1c. Other Somatosensory Areas Near SII. Robustly responsive somatic sensory regions excluded from, but directly adjoining, SII "proper" by Burton and Robinson (1981) included retroinsular, postauditory, granular insular and lateral area 7 regions (Fig. 16). Retroinsular units had receptive fields similar to those in SII but formed a separate somatotopic organization via projections from

Figure 16. Organization of projections to SII (shaded) and neighboring cortical areas in cynomolgus monkeys (*Macaca fascicularis* (from Robinson and Burton, 1980a–c; Burton and Robinson, 1981, with permission from C. J. Robinson, H. Burton, Alan R. Liss, Inc., and Humana Press). Ig = granular insula; MAND = mandibular; MAX = maxillary; Ri = retroinsular field; 7B = cytoarchitectonic area 7B. Diagram at lower right shows schematically the location of the detailed map on an exposed view of the cortical surface that is normally buried within the lateral sulcus.

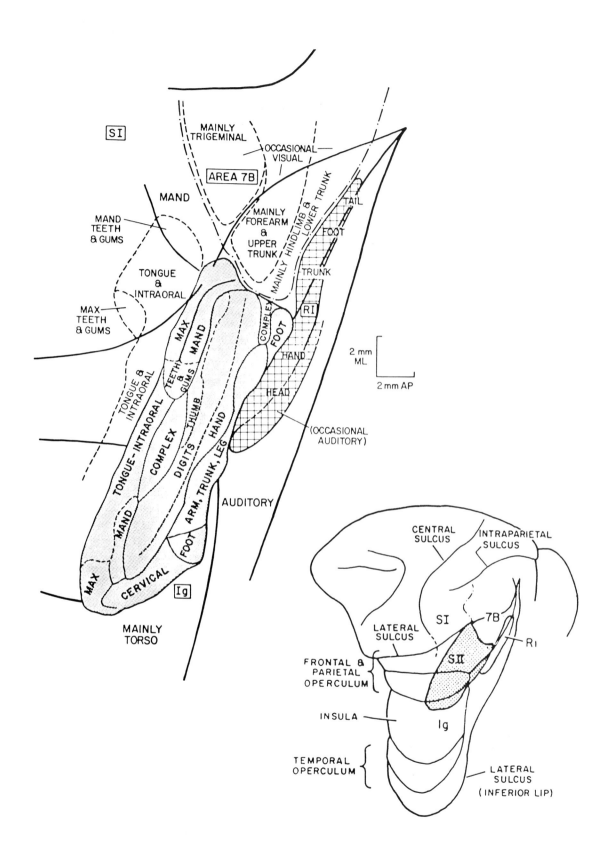

the posterior thalamic nucleus. In the postauditory regions, receptive fields were mostly bilateral and from face, neck, and upper trunk regions, and cells in the region were also responsive to auditory stimuli, some convergently with mechanosensory stimulation which convergence was never seen in SII proper. Neurons in the granular insular cortex had large, poorly defined receptive fields with no topographic organization. In area 7b posterior to SII, units had a large range of receptive field sizes, from largely bilateral fields, and projections were not somatotopically organized.

In owl monkeys (Cusick *et al.*, 1989), there was evidence of regions corresponding to the granular insular and lateral area 7 regions of macaques. Most prominent was a region adjoining, and just lateral to, SII, with receptive fields forming a separate somatotopic organization which resembled a mirror image of the SII projections (but with some bilateral receptive fields). This region was labeled VS (ventral somatic area) and resembled the retroinsular region of macaques in cytoarchitecture, general location, and inclusion of regions responsive to deep stimulation and to stimuli thought to preferentially activate Pacinian receptors.

8.2.1d. Supplementary Sensory Area. Still another sensory representation is found in macaques, in a region designated the supplementary sensory area (Murray and Coulter, 1981), adjoining the posteromedial end of SI on the medial surface of the hemisphere in banks of the cingulate sulcus. Responsive neurons in this region have large receptive fields on the head, neck, or forelimb.

8.2.2. Relation to Other Areas

In all of the anthropoid primates, the separation between primary sensory areas reaches a maximum, denoting a maximal extent of "association" cortex (Fig. 15). In most, gyrencephalic, primate species, motor cortex is clearly separated from SI by a prominent central sulcus, but in general other sulcal demarcations around and within SI and SII are not seen (although in one unusual spider monkey, a sulcus did appear in the postcentral gyrus at the demarcation between forelimb and hindlimb projections; Pubols and Pubols, 1979).

8.2.3. Structure

Four cytoarchitectural regions (Fig. 17) have been related to the four sets of representations seen in the region of SI (Kaas, 1983). The anterior zone of deep projections lies within area 3a of Vogt and Vogt (1919), described as cortex intervening between Brodmann's areas 3 and 4 but lacking the criteria of either 3 or 4, although further specification of consistency of structure, or even coextensivity of projections and area 3a, are not possible (Jones and Porter, 1980). The two complete representations of the cutaneous surface have been related to Brodmann's area 3 (or rather that portion termed 3b by Vogt and Vogt and constituting koniocortex characterized by densely packed small cells in layers 4 and 3) and 1 (with a lesser density in layers 4, 3, and 6), respectively. The posteriormost zone with a higher proportion of projections from deep tissues has been related to Brodmann's area 2 (with cell density in layers 4 and 6 greater than in area 1).

SII is distinguished by greater overall cortical thickness compared with SI and other neighboring fields, a prominent layer 4, and indistinct separation and sublamination of infragranular layers (Burton and Robinson, 1981).

8.2.4. Thalamic Connections

The SI region including areas 3a, 3b, 1, and 2 receives somatotopic projections from the VP thalamic nucleus (including its medial VPM facial and lateral VPL postcranial divisions) (reviewed by Jones, 1986). The deep projections to areas 3a and 2 are from an outer shell of the nucleus; the cutaneous projections to area 3b (and possibly area 1, data are not definitive) are from a central core of the nucleus. In areas 3a and 3b, most thalamic terminals are in layer 4 and the

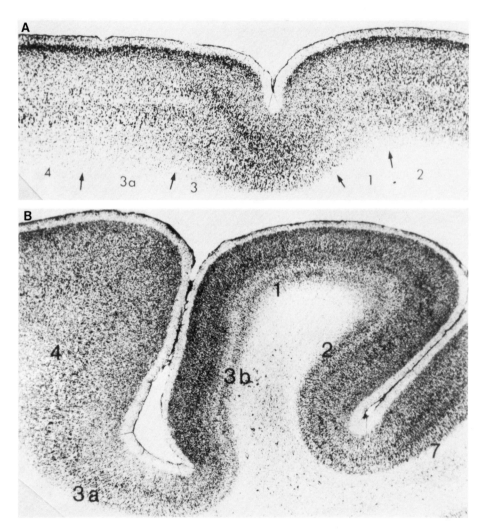

Figure 17. (A) Nissl-stained parasagittal section through cortex of squirrel monkey *Saimiri sciureus* showing cytoarchitectural areas 4, 3a, 3b (here labeled 3), 1, and 2 (reproduced from Jones, 1975, with permission from E. G. Jones and Alan R. Liss, Inc.). (B) Nissl-stained parasagittal section through cortex of rhesus monkey *Macaca mulatta* showing cytoarchitectural areas 4, 3a, 3b, 1, 2, and 7 (reproduced from Jones *et al.*, 1978, with permission from E. G. Jones and Alan R. Liss, Inc.).

overlying layer 3; in areas 1 and 2 they are in layer 3 and not 4. In all regions there are a few thalamic terminals at the border between layers 5 and 6.

SII was defined as a region receiving input, as does SI, from VP thalamic nuclei, but it has also been reported to receive projections from the VPI thalamic nucleus (Friedman *et al.*, 1983; Friedman and Murray, 1986). Thalamic terminals in SII are at the borders between layers 3 and 4 and between layers 5 and 6. Regions neighboring SII are reported to receive thalamic projections as follows (Burton and Robinson, 1981): retroinsular and postauditory areas from posterior and medial geniculate thalamic nuclei; and area 7b from the pulvinar thalamic nucleus.

Intralaminar thalamic nuclei project to SI and SII, probably terminating in layer 1, but Macchi and Bentivoglio (1986) concluded that the somatic sensory regions do not represent preferential targets of intralaminar nuclear projections.

For the corticothalamic portion of the reciprocal circuits, the current supposition is that small pyramidal cells in layer 6 of SI and SII project to the thalamic VP and reticular nuclei, and a smaller number of similar cells in layer 5 project to thalamic intralaminar nuclei (Jones, 1986).

The supplementary sensory region in the cingulate sulcus receives projections from the lateral posterior thalamic nucleus (Murray and Coulter, 1981).

8.2.5. Corticocortical Connections

8.2.5a. Ipsilateral. SII and most of the SI-related regions (areas 3a, 3b, 1, 2) have reciprocal and somatotopic connections with one another as well as with motor cortex (MI, area 4) on the same side (Jones, 1986). Exceptions to this rule include lack of projections from 3a or 3b to area 4, and from 3a to 3b. Terminals of these connections are distributed mainly in layers 1 through 4, but a few are also found in layers 5 and 6. The vast majority of cells of origin are in layer 3 (DeFelipe *et al.*, 1986).

In addition to the reciprocal ipsilateral connections among sensory and motor regions in monkeys, there are ipsilateral projections from areas 1 and 2 to supplementary motor cortex, and from area 3b to 3a. These connections originate in patches of large pyramidal cells deep in layer 2 and in layer 3 (Jones, 1986). Then there are generally somatotopic projections from SI (largely from area 2) to area 5 posterior to SI; rostral parts of SI project to caudal parts of area 5 and caudal parts of SI project to rostral parts of area 5; terminals are in layers 4 and 3 of area 5 (R. Pearson and Powell, 1985).

8.2.5b. Commissural. Each of the SI-related areas (3a, 3b, 1, 2) and SII has reciprocal and somatotopic commissural connections with its counterpart in the other hemisphere, with a striking general exception: in each of these fields, regions that make up the representations of the hands and feet neither send nor receive commissural connections (Jones, 1986). In addition, each of the SI-related areas projects to the contralateral SII.

From a given locus in one hemisphere, fibers project to one or more columnar patches in the contralateral cortex, wherein the commissural terminals are found mainly in layers 1–4 with a few in deeper layers. The pattern is much like that seen for ipsilateral corticocortical terminals.

Most of the commissural projections from sensory regions originate from mostly large pyramidal cells deep in layer 3, but some smaller cells, and some of these in layer 6, also appear to give rise to commissural fibers (Jones, 1986).

8.2.6. Other Connections

As do most regions of neocortex, SI and SII regions send projections to claustrum, and to corpus striatum, midbrain tectum, pons, medulla, and spinal cord (reviewed by Jones, 1986). Projections from SI (probably originating in layer 6) terminate in the dorsal part of the dorsal claustrum, which in turn projects back to SI (reviewed by Sherk, 1986). Corticostriatal projections originate from small pyramidal cells in the upper part of layer 5 and terminate in islands or patches in the putamen separated by terminal-free regions. Cortico-tectal, -pontine, and -bulbar axons originate in medium-to-large sized pyramidal cells in the middle and deep portions of layer 5. Those few that project to the midbrain tectum appear to end in the deep gray layer of the superior colliculus, near tectal cells with somatosensory receptive fields. More numerous corticopontine fibers have multiple, columnlike terminals in the dorsomedial portion of the pontine nuclei. The dorsal column nuclei are the principal targets of corticobulbar axons from somatic sensory cortex. Corticospinal fibers originate in medium- and large-sized pyramidal cells in the deep part of layer 5 of all of the SI and SII regions (fewer originate in area 3a than in areas 3b, 1, or 2); they terminate in the spinal dorsal horn in Rexed's laminae 3, 4, and 5 (those from area 2 tend to end deeper than those from area 1 and 3b).

8.2.7. Comparison Summary

At this point in our survey, the large question at hand is whether the wealth of differentiation newly observed in monkey sensory cortex is due to brain evolution, or rather to the number and intensity of the studies of monkeys. The few studies that are believably comparable using species we have so far considered, mainly those of the prosimians, indicate that evolutionary processes are responsible for at least some of the observed increase in complexity. Subdivision of the SI region into subfields of contrasting cytoarchitecture and multiplication of sensory representations, when deliberately searched for, occurs in all monkeys (excluding marmosets) and in no prosimians or marmosets that have been adequately studied. Kaas (1983) suggests that the SI of prosimians corresponds to only area 3b of monkeys, that the anterior and posterior high-threshold zones are seen in monkeys as areas 3a and 2, and that area 1 has no counterpart in species outside the anthropoidea.

A further peculiarity of monkeys is that responsiveness of SII depends upon SI, which is not the case with tree shrews, rabbits, and cats (see Sections 7.1, 9.1, and 11.1.1). It has been expressed as serial processing of tactile information in monkeys contrasted with parallel processing in other mammals, or that thalamic input is sufficient to drive SII in tree shrews, rabbits, and cats but connections from SI are needed to drive SII in monkeys (Pons *et al.*, 1987; Garraghty *et al.*, 1989).

In another set of comparable studies, those of opossums and of monkeys with regard to patterns of thalamic terminals in sensory cortex, a clear contrast is seen. Opossum sensory cortex has terminals in layer 1 from intralaminar nuclei, and in layer 4 from VL and VP nuclei; in monkeys sensory cortex has only the

VP terminals in any quantity, the VL and IL terminals being segregated into motor cortex.

In another instance of anthropoid peculiarity in thalamocortical relations, Krubitzer and Kaas (1987) concluded that the VPL–VPM projection to SII seen in most mammals has, in monkeys (but also in raccoons, see Section 11.2.4), been reduced and replaced to a large extent by a strong projection from an extraordinarily well developed VPI nucleus.

9. Lagomorphs

Returning to the first of the two starburst nodes on the trunk of the placental family tree (Fig. 1), the next groups considered are the lagomorphs and rodents. Evidence is inconclusive as to their relationships to one another and to other placentals. Recently, lagomorphs had been considered an early divergent line much like the edentates forming another inner-outgroup (e.g., McKenna, 1975), but Novacek and Wyss (1986) decided that evidence now favors a common origin with the rodents. In either case, lagomorphs constitute an interesting, possibly "baseline" group for the analyses of divergent characteristics among the placentals. Among the lagomorphs the only detailed studies of sensory cortex have used domestic rabbits *Oryctolagus cuniculus*.

9.1. Sensory Projections

The somatic sensory cortex of rabbits has been the subject of early, general (Adrian, 1941; C. Woolsey and Wang, 1945; C. Woolsey and Fairman, 1946) and recent, comprehensive and detailed (Gould, 1986) studies.

SI of rabbits contains a single representation of the body surface, in the usual mammalian arrangement. The largest proportion (0.864; Gould, 1986) of projections are from perioral structures: lips, philtrum, nose, and vibrissae (Fig. 18). Unusual features of the projection pattern include a sizeable "displaced" representation of the pinna at the caudolateralmost corner of SI; a small representation of the dorsal midline of the trunk at the mediocaudal corner of SI (rabbits thus join spiny anteaters and squirrel and cebus monkeys with the abdomen-forward position in contrast to owl and macaque monkeys; see Section 8.2.1a); the hindlimb representation is not split around that of the foot (as in rats but unlike monkeys, squirrels, and galagos); and in the forepaw representation

Figure 18. Organization of projections to somatic sensory cortex of rabbits as seen in a dorsolateral view of the left cerebral hemisphere. Anterior is to the left.

Lower left: The location of SI and SII relative to auditory and visual regions (redrawn from C. Woolsey and Fairman, 1946, with permission from C. N. Woolsey and C. V. Mosby (Co.). aud: auditory; f: face, a: arm (forelimb), l: leg (hindlimb) representations in SI and SII; vis: visual.

Right: Details of projection to SI and SII, reproduced from Gould (1986, with permission from H. J. Gould and Alan R. Liss, Inc.). Individual vibrissae are indicated by rows A–F (A most dorsal on the face) and columns 1–5 (1 most caudal on the face); Ar: arm; d: dorsal; D1–5: forepaw digits; FA: forearm; LIO: lower intraoral area; M: medial; Occ: occipital area; PhIO: intraoral portion of philtrum; R: rostral; r: radial; Sh: shoulder; T & G: tail and genitalia; UIO: upper intraoral area; UZ: "unresponsive" zones; u: ulnar; v: ventral.

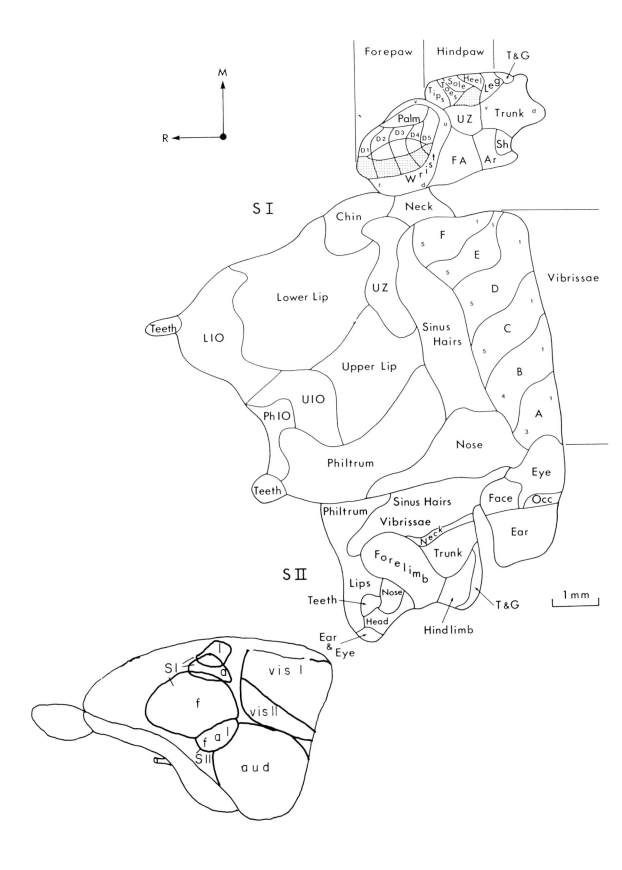

projections from digit 1 are rostralmost and those from digit 5 are caudalmost (other mammals usually have the digits arranged mediolaterally with digit 1 caudolateral).

Within SI are two distinct unresponsive zones that occur at the respective locations, between fore- and hindlimb representations and between forelimb and head representations, where the interbrachial and jugular sulci occur in the gyrencephalic marsupials (Section 3.2.3) and prosimian lorises (Section 8.1.3).

Gould (1986) noted high-threshold zones rostral and caudal to SI as seen in tree shrews and prosimians, but these were not investigated in detail.

SII borders on SI (Fig. 18), and the SI and SII representations of the midline of the head abut one another. The SII representations of the limbs and tail extend caudolaterally. Receptive fields activating SII are contralateral, and form a single uncomplicated representation without the complexities seen in monkeys and cats (Gould, 1986). Responses in SII are evoked via a pathway separate from that activating SI (C. Woolsey and Fairman, 1946), thus revealing rabbits to be like tree shrews as "parallel processors" in contrast with the "serial processing" seen in monkeys (Section 8.2.1).

9.2. Relation to Other Areas

C. Woolsey and Fairman (1946), referring to C. Woolsey and Wang (1945) and unpublished data, illustrated somatic sensory, auditory, and visual regions of rabbit cortex closely approximating one another, with no substantial intervening regions of association neocortex (Fig. 18), unless visual II is classified as an association region.

9.3. Structure

Gould (1986) found SI to occupy a single koniocortical region, with cytoarchitectural subdivisions proposed by earlier students (M. Rose, 1931; Fleischauer et al., 1980) possibly related to projections from different body parts. In the region of projections from mystacial vibrissae, distinctive barrel-like structures are found (Rice, 1983; T. Woolsey et al., 1975), resembling those seen in some marsupials (Section 3.2.3).

While unresponsive zones occurred at loci corresponding to those of sulci in marsupials and lorises, and those of unmyelinated regions in tree shrews (Section 7.3), Gould (1986) could find no structural correlate in rabbits of these electrophysiologically determined zones.

While SII was in a sensory type of cortex, Gould (1986) reported it to be less distinctly laminated than that in SI.

9.4. Thalamic Connections

Direct studies of thalamocortical connections in rabbits seem not to have been done; it can be expected that the sensory projections mapped in ventrobasal thalamus (J. Rose and Mountcastle, 1952) give rise to projections to SI as in other mammals.

Origins and terminals of commissural projections in rabbits were found to be dense in the SI and SII representations of the whole postcranial body and of the midline regions of the head, and sparse or absent in representations of the lateral head (including sinus hairs, lateral lips, and vibrissae) (Ledoux *et al.*, 1987). Cells of origin of commissural fibers are located in layers 2, 3, and 5, with only a few in layers 4 and 6. Terminals are found from inner layer 1 to outer layer 6, are densest in layers 1–3 and sparsest in layer 4 of commissurally connected regions.

9.6. Other Connections

As with all neocortex so studied (Section 8.2.6), sensory regions in rabbits have corticostriate and corticoclaustral projections (Carman *et al.*, 1963, 1964).

9.7. Comparison Summary

The presence of high-threshold zones rostral and caudal to SI indicates that these are not primate–scandent specializations. The possibilities thus are (1) that they are general mammalian features, seen in any mammal that is carefully studied, or (2) that lagomorphs have a closer relationship in this respect to primates and tree shrews than to the other groups considered thus far. The shifts in the direction of the order of projections of the digits can be merely evidence of a relative rotation in the projection of the whole extremity, of no great functional or phylogenetic significance. The large representations of facial structures indicate the importance of facial sensation for a grazing mammal. Barrels represent the main divergence from the "simple-cortical" unspecialized condition that we have seen previously in sensory regions of monotremes, opossums, armadillos, and insectivores; and barrels would now seem to be a specialization that appears convergently in several lines, correlated with dependence on sensory input from vibrissae. As with the case with tree shrews, studies of motor cortex, or, better, comparisons of cerebellar with lemniscal projections to neocortex, in rabbits would provide critical evidence for the "primitivity" or unspecialized nature of cortical "sensory–motor overlap."

The sparseness of commissural terminals in layer 4 parallels that in some reports of opossums (Section 3.1.5); in this respect, rabbits and opossums stand in contrast to primates where layer 4 has strong commissural input (Section 8.2.5).

The "parallel processing" in SI and SII of rabbits and tree shrews suggests that this is the common mode, and that the "serial processing," SI to SII, of monkeys (Section 8.2.1) is an anthropoid specialization.

10. Rodents

We come now to the most biologically successful of all mammalian groups. In numbers and in variety, rodents surpass all other mammalian taxa: almost half of all extant mammalian species are rodents. For reasons not unrelated to this predominance, rodents have become (but only recently) the model research mammals for brain research as well as for other fields. While their brains may be small and simple, they are certainly biologically adequate; knowledge of their brain organization is vital as a basis of comparative study as well as for understanding of biological success. In this regard, what is true of brains is true of sensory cortex.

The large order of rodents has been classified into three or more suborders. Two are generally unquestioned, the ratlike Myomorpha with 70% of rodent species and the squirrel-like Sciuromorpha with 20%. The remaining 10% of rodent species have been lumped into the porcupinelike Hystricomorpha, although some classifiers subdivide out of these the guinea pig-like Caviomorpha (which include the American porcupines).

The most thoroughly studied rodent cortices are those of the myomorph rats *Rattus norvegicus* and mice *Mus musculus* that have become the standard laboratory animals. In addition, there is a recent and extremely informative literature on the sensory cortex of sciuromorph gray squirrels *Sciurus carolinensis*.

10.1. Rats and Mice

10.1.1. Sensory Projections

10.1.1a. SI. In rats and mice SI contains a single representation of the body surface (Figs. 19, 20), with small representations of the limbs rostromedially and a large face representation laterally. There is a particularly large representation of the facial vibrissae (C. Welker, 1971; Hall and Lindholm, 1974; Chapin and Lin, 1984; T. Woolsey, 1967).

In rats the core of SI is activated primarily by light tactile stimuli, responses to stimulation of deep tissues are more frequent along the anterior edge of SI, with some seen posterior to SI in waking preparations (W. Welker *et al.,* 1984; Sievert and Neafsey, 1986). A distinct zone of projections from muscles was identified along the anterior edge of the limb representations (Chapin and Lin, 1984); such projections extended into the region between the limb representations (W. Welker *et al.,* 1984). Within the single representation of the body there is a double representation of the palmar surface of the forepaw; the second representation lies anterior to the first which is in somatotopic register with the rest of the forelimb representation; the two forepaw representations meet at the tips of their digits (as in gray squirrels and unlike monkeys; see Fig. 21) (Chapin and Lin, 1984).

10.1.1b. SII. In mice, the prominent projections from the face, especially the vibrissae, with subordinate concentrations from the paws, are seen again in SII (Carvell and Simons, 1986). The rostrum of the face and the digits of the paws are represented laterally. Receptive fields are larger than in SI, but as in SI the smallest receptive fields are in the face representation. Some receptive fields are bilateral and cover the whole face or body.

10.1.2. Relation to Other Areas

The limb representations in rat SI overlap the motor cortex (Hall and Lindholm, 1974; Sanderson *et al.,* 1984). This appears to be true also in mice, as judged from thalamic projections (Carvell and Simons, 1987).

In mice, SI abuts SII, auditory, and visual cortices (T. Woolsey, 1967) and auditory responses were found in the body representation in mouse SII (see Fig. 19) (T. Woolsey, 1967; Carvell and Simons, 1986, 1987). No association cortex intervenes between these sensory regions. Similar relations seem to occur in rats, based on separate studies of sensory projections and the juxtapositions of the related cytoarchitectonic regions (Fig. 19).

10.1.3. Structure

SI cortex in rats shows all six layers, with 2 and 3 lacking a clear boundary (Wise and Jones, 1978).

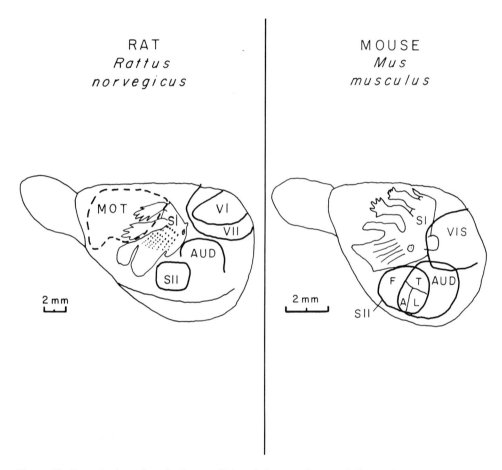

Figure 19. Organization of projections to SI in relation to other cortical areas in rats and mice as seen in dorsolateral views of the left hemisphere; anterior is to the left in both diagrams.

Data for rat SI are from C. Welker (1971, 1976, with permission from C. Welt, Alan R. Liss, Inc., and Elsevier Science Publishers BV) and are shown in relation to other areas determined electrophysiologically (SII, C. Welker and Sinha, 1972; motor = MOT, Hall and Lindholm, 1974; Sanderson *et al.*, 1984; auditory = AUD, Sally and Kelly, 1988; primary and secondary visual, VI and VII, Montero *et al.*, 1973; Espinoza and Thomas, 1983) and cytoarchitectonically (Zilles and Wree, 1985).

Data for mice are from T. Woolsey (1967, with alterations, and permission from T. A. Woolsey and The Johns Hopkins University Press) except for details of projections to SII (from Carvell and Simons, 1986, 1987) from face = F, arm (forelimb) = A, leg (hindlimb) = L, and trunk = T. Auditory projections overlap postcranial projections in SII.

C. Welker (1971, 1976) showed cutaneous projections in rat SI to be coterminous with concentrations of small cells in layer 4, by sectioning flattened cortex through the layer (Fig. 20). Also prominent in this figure are barrel formations marking the representations of the mystacial vibrissae (C. Welker and Woolsey, 1974); the first such barrels were discovered in mice (T. Woolsey, 1967; T. Woolsey and Van der Loos, 1970). We have already noted similar barrels in marsupials and rabbits (Sections 3.2.3 and 9.3). Anterior to, and between, patches of concentrated cells ("granular cortex") in layer 4 are regions of "dysgranular" cortex; projections in granular regions are largely cutaneous, while dysgranular regions contain projections from deep tissues and from large receptive fields (W. Welker *et al.*, 1984; Sievert and Neafsey, 1986). Dysgranular regions invading SI are at locations corresponding to sulci in marsupials, lorises, and other mammals (Sections 3.2.3, 8.1.3, 11.2.3, and others below).

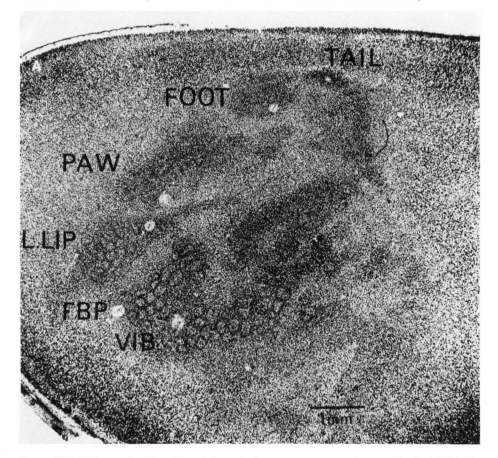

Figure 20. (A) Flattened section through layer 4 of sensory neocortex of a rat, stained with thionin. White circular patches are microlesions marking the sites of projections, determined electrophysiologically, from TAIL, hindFOOT, forePAW, Lower LIP, Furry Buccal Pad, and small anterior mystacial VIBrissae. (B) Cellular condensations (granular cortex) form morphological counterparts of the body regions projecting to them as seen in the superimposed sketch. Black dots represent the large posterior mystacial vibrissae which project to barrels. Regions of "dysgranular" cortex between granular projection regions can be labeled: interbrachial (IB) between the condensations representing hindFOOT and forePAW, jugular (J) between forePAW and Lower LIP, and labial (L) between Lower LIP and Furry Buccal Pad. Reproduced, with alterations, from C. Welker (1976, with permission from C. Welt and Alan R. Liss, Inc.).

SII cortex in rats is cytoarchitecturally similar to SI except that the pronounced condensations of granule cells of layer 4 characteristic of SI are not seen in SII (C. Welker and Sinha, 1972; Wise and Jones, 1978).

10.1.4. Thalamic Connections

In rats, thalamic projections to SI cortex arise from the ventrobasal complex (VB) and the central lateral (CL) nucleus of the intralaminar group (Jones and Leavitt, 1974). Those from VB terminate in somatotopic order (Saporta and Kruger, 1977) in layers 4 and (to a lesser degree) 6 of SI cortex (Chmielowska *et al.*, 1989); those from CL may be those seen ending in layer 1 (Wise and Jones, 1978). Similar projections from VB were found in SII (Wise and Jones, 1978).

In the hindlimb representations of rats, where sensory and motor regions overlap, there are projections from both VB (which receives lemniscal input) and the ventrolateral nucleus (VL; which receives cerebellar input). In the face representations the separate motor cortex receives VL but not VB projections, and the sensory cortex receives input from VB but not VL (Donoghue *et al.*, 1979).

Projections from the medial division of the posterior thalamic nucleus (POm) of rats are located in dysgranular regions and in septa separating barrels

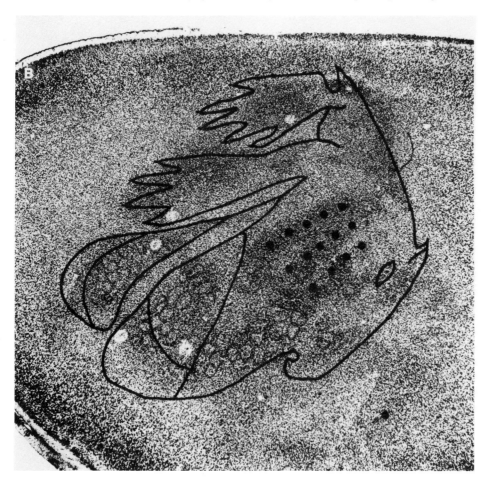

Figure 20. (*Continued*)

(Koralek *et al.*, 1988; Chmielowska *et al.*, 1989). The pattern of the POm terminals is complementary to that of input from VB: input from VB arrives in the granular regions of cellular concentration in layer 4, including the barrels.

As is usual, there are corticothalamic respondents to the thalamocortical projections. In SI and SII of rats, cells in layer 6 project to the ventrobasal thalamus in somatotopic order (Wise and Jones, 1977). In the SI vibrissal representation, thalamocortical cells projecting to VB in layer 6 (and some in lower layer 5) are congregated deep to the barrels and are sparse deep to the septa in layer 4 (Chmielowska *et al.*, 1989).

In mice (Carvell and Simons, 1987), SI face regions receive input from VB, while limb regions receive input from both VB and VL as in the sensorimotor overlap regions of rats. There are some projections from posterior nuclei as well as from VB in the SI vibrissal representation (White and DeAmicis, 1977); they may be patterned in septa as is the case in rats but this was not determined. In mouse SII, there are projections from VB and thalamic posterior nuclei, and in the trunk and limb representations there are also projections from the auditory medial geniculate nucleus.

At least the vibrissal representation in mouse SI sends reciprocating projections to the VB, posterior, and reticular nuclei of the thalamus (White and DeAmicis, 1977).

10.1.5. Corticocortical Connections

In considering connections of SI in rats, a distinction must be made between granular and dysgranular regions (Wise and Jones, 1976; Akers and Killackey, 1978; Olavarria *et al.*, 1984; Koralek *et al.*, 1988): each has a distinct pattern of connections.

10.1.5a. Ipsilateral Corticocortical Connections in Rats. Granular regions in SI of rats have no input from ipsilateral somatosensory cortex (reviewed by Koralek *et al.*, 1988), while dysgranular regions receive some axons from neighboring granular regions and more from other nearby dysgranular regions (Chapin *et al.*, 1987). The cells of origin of these connections are pyramidal cells, mostly in layers 3 and 2, with a few in layer 5 and fewer still in layer 4 (Chapin *et al.*, 1987). Terminals were reported in dysgranular cortex in layers 1, 2, and 3 (Akers and Killackey, 1978) and in all layers except layer 4 (Chapin *et al.*, 1987). Dendrites of the cells of origin, whose cell bodies lie in dysgranular zones, often reach well into granular regions, forming possible avenues of conduct of information from granular to dysgranular regions, and also directly from axons from VB thalamus to dysgranular regions (Chapin *et al.*, 1987). An output from granular SI to ipsilateral motor cortex has been noted (Akers and Killackey, 1978).

There are projections from primary visual striate cortex to the head representations in SI (Olavarria and Montero, 1984); it was not determined if the terminals are present in granular or dysgranular regions. Reciprocal connections were found between dysgranular regions of somatosensory cortex and frontal cortex (Isseroff *et al.*, 1984); cells of origin lay in bands in layer 5 and clumps in layers 2 and 3; terminals were in layers 1–3 and 5, avoiding layer 4.

In rat SII there is input from granular regions of SI (Akers and Killackey, 1978); it was not determined if dysgranular SI regions also project to SII. In SII this ipsilateral corticocortical input terminates in layer 4 as does the thalamic input from VB.

10.1.5b. Commissural Connections in Rats. Granular regions of SI in rats do not receive commissural input (Wise and Jones, 1976; Akers and Killackey, 1978). These granular regions include representations of facial structures as well as of the limb extremities. We see here something of a combination of the arrangements seen in primates, where representations of the extremities are acallosal in their connectivity, and in rabbits, where lateral facial regions are acallosal. However, it was reported that rats are different from rabbits in that axial as well as lateral facial representations are included in acallosal granular regions (Akers and Killackey, 1978).

Dysgranular regions of rat SI receive commissural input from contralateral dysgranular regions. Thus, terminals of both contralateral and ipsilateral corticocortical connections are confined to dysgranular cortex (including septa between barrels) in the same pattern as seen for projections from the thalamic POm nucleus (reviewed by Koralek *et al.*, 1988). Cells of origin of commissural fibers are found in all layers, but mostly in layers 3 and 5; terminals are arranged in columns, mostly in layers 1–3, with some also in 5 and 6 and few if any in layer 4 (Wise and Jones, 1976). Similar findings (Akers and Killackey, 1978) were contrasted with the situation in primates, where corresponding terminals are found in all cortical layers with most in layers 1, 2, 3, *and 4* (see Section 8.2.5).

In rats SII there are heterotopic connections from the contralateral SI; terminals are densest in layer 4 (as is the case with ipsilateral corticocortical and thalamocortical input) and sparsest in layer 2 (Wise and Jones, 1976). Commissural input from the contralateral SII might also be expected but apparently has not been investigated in rats.

10.1.5c. Ipsilateral Corticocortical Connections in Mice. In looking for similarity of connections between rats and mice, a major conclusion is that, despite the relative wealth of data, those available are as yet still inadequate for making many generalizations about connectivity in these two murid species.

The analysis of connections, or lack of them, between granular and dysgranular regions of SI has not been carried out in mice, and may not be possible due to the small size of mouse brains.

The visual projections to SI seen in rats have not been investigated in mice. Reciprocal connections to frontal cortex shown in rats may have something of a counterpart in reciprocal and homotopic connections between vibrissal representations in SI and in MI (primary motor cortex) shown in mice (White and DeAmicis, 1977); cells of origin of these connections in mice were in layers 5 (more) and 3 (fewer) (in rats the cells of origin were reported in layers 5, 2, and 3); terminals in mice were in layers 1–3 (in rats they were reported in layers 1–3 and 5).

Projections were shown from SI to SII in rats; in mice SI and SII were shown to be reciprocally connected (White and DeAmicis, 1977; Carvell and Simons, 1987) and this may well be the case in rats given further investigation. Terminals in SII are in layer 4 in both species; cells of origin are in layer 3 and upper layer 6 in mice (not determined in rats). The postcranial representations in SII of mice have reciprocal connections with auditory cortex (Carvell and Simons, 1987) (not investigated in rats).

In mice, in addition to the reciprocal corticocortical connections just described, projections were found to contralateral motor cortex from SI, and to the ipsilateral motor cortex from SII postcranial representations (Carvell and Simons, 1987). These projections originated from cells in layer 3. (Their counterparts have not been studied in rats.)

10.1.5d. Commissural Connections in Mice. In mice there are regions free of commissural input (and output) corresponding to the major granular regions of rats, including the representations of the facial vibrissae and the limb extremities (Yorke and Caviness, 1975). Otherwise SI regions, as in the dysgranular areas of rats, are commissurally and somatotopically connected (Carvell and Simons, 1987); cells of origin are found in layers 3 and 5 in mice, as in rats; terminals in both species lie in layers 1–3, and 5 but not 4 (and upper 5 in mice). In mice SI and SII were reported to be reciprocally commissurally connected, with projections from SII to SI weaker than those from SI to SII (Carvell and Simons, 1987); more detailed study may reveal corresponding connections in rats, as only the SI to SII connections have been reported thus far. In mice, as in other species investigated, SII is strongly connected with the contralateral SII; it is peculiar that these connections have not been studied in rats.

10.1.6. Other Connections

10.1.6.a. Rats. In SI and SII of rats, cells of the upper part of layer 5 project to the corpus striatum, cells in the lower part of layer 5 project to the midbrain, pons, dorsal column nuclei, and spinal cord; all of these projections maintain some somatotopic order (Wise and Jones, 1977; McGeorge and Faull, 1989).

From an intensively studied region of rostral SI in rats, projections were described to the tectum in the anterior colliculus, to the principal sensory trigeminal and the interpolar spinal trigeminal nuclei, and to the spinal cord as sampled at the pyramidal decussation of the corticospinal tracts (Killackey *et al.*, 1989). Cells projecting to the tectum were small and restricted to the superficial part of layer 5b, but were distributed throughout both granular and dysgranular regions of the area studied; between 5 and 10% of these cells had branches projecting to the trigeminal nuclei or spinal cord. Cells projecting to the trigeminal nuclei were seen throughout the width of layer 5b but only in a lateral dysgranular region; those projecting to spinal cord were also situated from top to bottom of layer 5b but were all located in medial granular regions of the area studied. Between 10 and 15% of cells projecting to the principal trigeminal nucleus had branches to the interpolar spinal trigeminal nucleus and vice versa; cells projecting exclusively to one or the other of these trigeminal nuclei were not segregated in the cortex. Between 5 and 10% of cells projecting to interpolar spinal trigeminal nuclei had spinally projecting branches in the pyramidal decussation. Corticospinal cells, in contrast, showed no branches to trigeminal or tectal targets.

10.1.6b. Mice. At least the vibrissal representation in mouse SI sends projections to the caudate nucleus and to the ventral pontine nuclei (White and DeAmicis, 1977.) Those to the caudate correspond to those seen in rats.

Granular regions of rat cortex have much in common with area 3b of monkeys. The anterior dysgranular regions in rats may correspond to some degree with area 3a of primates. It has been suggested (Chapin *et al.*, 1987) that areas 1 and 2 in monkeys may represent coalescences of dysgranular zones arranged to better facilate somatotopic granular-to-dysgranular connections (3b to 1 to 2). Cytoarchitectural correspondences (1 and 2 are dysgranular compared with 3b) as well as connectivity patterns offer some support for this suggestion.

Some of those dysgranular regions intervening between granular patches in rats have, in their position at least, parallels with the sulci in the corresponding locations in SI seen in diprotodont marsupials and lorises (see Sections 3.2.3 and 8.1.3) and carnivores (Sections 11.1.3 and 11.2.3); sulci and dysgranularity may be two manifestations of a structural property common to all mammals (Johnson, 1980); in the one species (brushtail possums) where both sulci and the granular–dysgranular distinction can be observed the sulci and the dysgranular interruptions are·perfectly congruent (see Section 3.2.3).

Similar input patterns to sensorimotor overlap regions in rats and opossums led to the prediction that all such regions would show converging projections from thalamic VB and VL nuclei (Donoghue *et al.*, 1979). The partial overlap of sensory and motor regions seen in rats and mice recalls that seen in monotremes and some marsupials, in particular that in quolls and brushtail possums. In the quolls and possums, there is overlap in the limb regions, as in rats and mice, while at least part of the face region is "pure" sensory as is all of the face region in rats and mice. (Other instances of reported partial overlap among edentates and hedgehogs are not sufficiently documented to allow detailed comparison.) All of the species just mentioned contrast with the primates (and carnivores, as shall be seen) where there is complete segregation of cortical sensory and motor regions, and of thalamic VB (VP) and VL projections.

Sensory–motor overlaps, and laminar segregation of corticocortical (to layers 2 and 3) and thalamocortical (to layer 4) inputs to sensory cortex, have been suggested as somehow conjoint properties of small brain size (Akers and Killackey, 1978). In this view, in small brains such as those of opossums and rats, sensory and motor cortex have to share the same region, while in large brains like those of monkeys and cats each can have its own space. Then in small brains it may be necessary to keep inputs segregated by laminae, while in large brains laminar segregation is functionally not so critical. Thus, small-brained rats, mice, opossums, rabbits, and possibly hedgehogs have corticocortical inputs avoiding layer 4 in SI where thalamic terminals are concentrated; while larger-brained primates and carnivores have corticocortical terminals in all layers, including layer 4. Brushtail possums, with overlap *and* corticocortical terminals in layer 4, can feed extended speculation on this point; before making too much of it, data on contrasting species using the same procedures and investigators would be helpful, to ensure that common definitions of laminar boundaries and other criteria and methods are truly comparable across species.

Thalamic input in rats and mice, from CL to layer 1 and from VB (VP) to layer 4, is similar to that seen in the other mammals thus far considered. Thalamic projections from POm to SI have been noted thus far in our survey only in brushtail possums; they will be seen in carnivores. Posterior thalamic projections in SII seen in mice parallel those noted in *Galago crassicaudatus* (Section 8.1.4), and with further investigation may prove to be a common mammalian condition.

The convergence of mechanosensory and auditory (via cortical and medial geniculate projections) in SII of mice is the first well-documented overlap of auditory and somatic sensory cortical regions that we have seen thus far in our survey. Studies of small brains using large electrodes and slow-wave evoked potentials have reported overlap of SII with auditory regions in opossums (Section 3.1.1, but this was not seen with microelectrodes), moles and hedgehogs (Fig. 10), and prosimian pottos (Section 8.1.2). No overlap was seen in tree shrews (Section 7.2); and in macaque monkeys there were no auditory responses in "SII proper," but neighboring cortex had convergent auditory and mechanosensory input (Section 8.2.1).

The connections of SI and visual cortex seen in rats have not been noted in any of the other mammals we have considered thus far. A specific search for them may be in order.

In animals considered thus far, outputs to extracortical targets from specifically somatosensory cortex have been investigated, to the detailed degree they have in rats, only in monkeys (Section 8.2.6), and, interestingly, in the marsupial brushtail possums (Section 3.2.6). No striking differences are evident among these species; specifically comparative studies may yet reveal species-distinctive features of interest. The spinal levels at which fibers from somatosensory cortex terminate may differ; in brushtail possums they are restricted, as are corticospinal terminals in general, to cervical and thoracic levels.

10.2. Gray Squirrels

Many, but by no means all, members of the second great suborder of rodents, the Sciuromorpha, are diurnal and arboreal (as are most of the anthropoid primates). Among these is the species whose somatosensory cortex has received detailed attention, the American gray squirrel *Sciurus carolinensis*.

10.2.1. Sensory Projections

The SI representation of the body surface in gray squirrels features a double representation of the forepaw in the rostral part of the forelimb representation, large lip and intraoral representations of the lips and intraoral surfaces, and a sizable "unresponsive zone" (UZ) between the face and forepaw representations where no activity is elicited by tactile stimulation (Sur *et al.*, 1978; Krubitzer *et al.*, 1986). In the trunk representation the dorsal midline is represented rostrally and the ventral midline caudally.

The SII representation in squirrels includes units with receptive fields larger than SI, and is organized as illustrated in Fig. 21, and is similar to that of mice, rabbits, and most other mammals studied recently (Nelson *et al.*, 1979; Krubitzer *et al.*, 1986).

In gray squirrels, a third area, adjoining SI and SII and called the parietal ventral (PV), contains another complete representation of the body (Krubitzer *et al.*, 1986). Receptive fields in PV are contralateral and otherwise similar to those in SII. Many cells in PV are also responsive to auditory stimulation. Krubitzer *et al.* (1986) suggest that detailed study may reveal a PV in other mammals; its close juxtaposition to SII may have resulted in both PV and SII being identified as a single area SII in other studies.

395

COMPARISONS OF
SOMATIC SENSORY
CORTEX

10.2.2. Relation to Other Areas

In some contrast to rats and mice, the primary auditory and visual areas of squirrels are separated from the three somatosensory regions by substantial strips of neocortex (Fig. 21).

10.2.3. Structure

In squirrels, SI is coterminous with a field of koniocortex with densely packed granule cells in layer 4; the UZ forms a prominent island within this koniocortex where cell packing in layer 4 and in layer 6 is much less pronounced (Sur *et al.*, 1978). Barrels can be seen (although with some difficulty) in the small representation of the mystacial vibrissae (T. Woolsey *et al.*, 1975).

SI is also coextensive with a heavily myelinated region including all cortical layers (Krubitzer *et al.*, 1986); the unresponsive zone is evident as a patch of lesser myelination, and representations of body parts can be recognized as related to gradients within the dense myelination. SII and PV can be recognized by moderate myelination in the middle, and poor myelination in the other, cortical layers.

10.2.4. Thalamic Connections

Projections from thalamus to the somatosensory regions in gray squirrels were analyzed in detail by Krubitzer and Kaas (1987). They found that the major thalamic input to SI, SII, and PV is from the VP nucleus (which corresponds more or less to VB of rats and mice). They recognize three separate subnuclei around VP which also contribute some input to possibly restricted regions of SI as well as to SII and to PV. These additional subnuclei were tentatively identified as the ventroposteroinferior nucleus (VPI), and the lateral and medial regions of a posterior complex (POl and POm). The internal magnocellular division of the medial geniculate was also found to project to PV, and may be responsible for the auditory input found in PV (Krubitzer *et al.*, 1986). All these thalamic regions receive reciprocal corticothalamic connections.

10.2.5. Corticocortical Connections

10.2.5a. Ipsilateral Corticocortical Connections. In squirrels, there are major connections from granular SI to UZ, recalling the granular-to-dysgranular projections in rats. Granular SI also has reciprocal connections with ipsilateral SII, PV, motor cortex, a parietal medial area posterior to SI, and a parietal rhinal area lateral to PV (Krubitzer *et al.*, 1986). These connections appeared to be somatotopically organized, except for those with the parietal rhinal area.

The squirrel SII has ipsilateral reciprocal somatotopic connections with, besides SI, PV and the parietal medial area. Other connections were found (not determined to be somatotopic) with the ipsilateral parietal rhinal area, the cortex

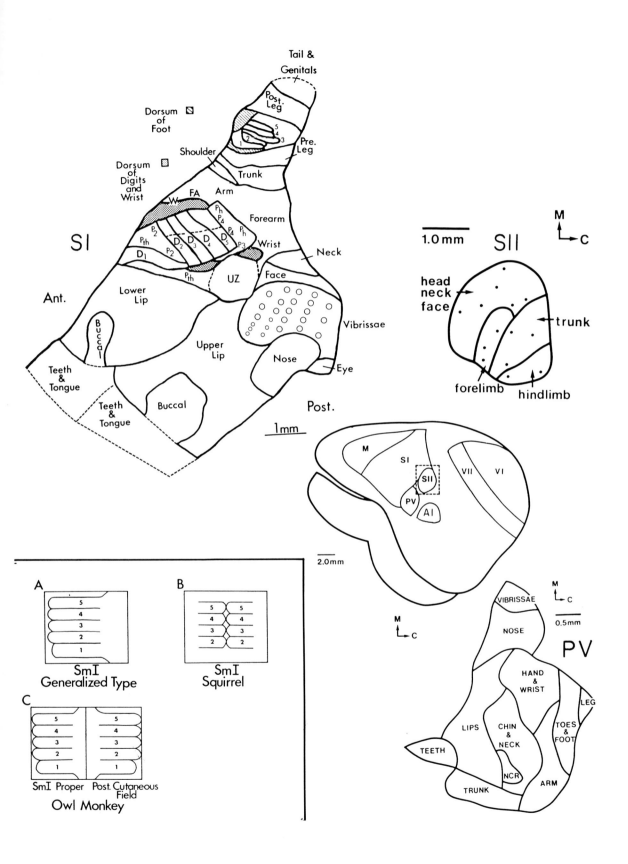

SI

Tail &
Genitals

Dorsum
of
Foot

Post.
Leg

Pre.
Leg

Shoulder

Dorsum
of
Digits
and
Wrist

Trunk

Arm

FA

W

Forearm

P_h
P_4

P_2

P_4

P_h

P_{th}

D_2 D_3 D_4 D_5

P_3

Wrist

Neck

D_1

P_2

P_{th}

UZ

Face

Ant.

Lower
Lip

Vibrissae

Buccal

Upper
Lip

Nose

Eye

Teeth
&
Tongue

Teeth
&
Tongue

Buccal

Post.

1mm

1.0 mm   SII

M
C

head
neck
face

trunk

forelimb   hindlimb

M

SI

SII

VII   VI

PV

AI

2.0mm

M
C

A

5
4
3
2
1

SmI
Generalized Type

B

5   5
4   4
3   3
2   2

SmI
Squirrel

C

5   5
4   4
3   3
2   2
1   1

SmI Proper   Post. Cutaneous
Field

Owl Monkey

M
C

VIBRISSAE

NOSE

0.5mm

PV

HAND
&
WRIST

LEG

LIPS

CHIN
&
NECK

TOES
&
FOOT

TEETH

NCR

ARM

TRUNK

neighboring SII caudolaterally, and cortex medial to the motor area. Unexpectedly, no connections with the motor area itself were seen.

PV has reciprocal connections with ipsilateral SI (mainly) and SII as just mentioned, and also with motor cortex, the parietal medial and the parietal rhinal areas, other cortex just dorsal to the rhinal fissure, entorhinal cortex, and possibly subdivisions of auditory cortex. Since connections were found between PV and motor cortex, and not between SII and motor cortex as reported in other animals, it was suggested that these purported SII-to-motor cortex connections may in fact be from a hitherto undetected analogue of PV in other species (Krubitzer *et al.*, 1986).

10.2.5b. Commissural Connections. In the SI region of squirrels, the UZ is a major zone of callosal terminals (Gould and Kaas, 1981), which arrive from the contralateral UZ, SII, PV, motor cortex, parietal medial and parietal rhinal areas (Krubitzer *et al.*, 1986). Other areas in the SI region that may correspond to the dysgranular regions of rats have substantial amounts of callosal terminals, but so do "granular" representations of midline face and body structures (unlike rats) (Gould and Kaas, 1981). Callosal terminals were, in contrast, sparse in representations of the lateral lips and vibrissae (like rabbits) and of the glabrous surfaces of the fore- and hindpaws (like primates). The callosal regions are somatotopically connected.

In squirrels, SII is reciprocally and somatotopically connected with the contralateral SII, and there were commissural connections with contralateral cortex encircling SII (Krubitzer *et al.*, 1986).

PV has more extensive callosal connections than does SI or SII; these are with the contralateral PV, with the parietal rhinal area, and (less dense) with the parietal medial area, and with SII and cortex caudal to SII (Krubitzer *et al.*, 1986).

Figure 21. Location and organization of somatic sensory projections to cortex of gray squirrels (from Sur *et al.*, 1978, and Krubitzer *et al.*, 1986, with permission from M. Sur, L. A. Krubitzer, and Alan R. Liss, Inc.). Anterior is to the left in all diagrams.

Center: Location of SI, SII, and parietal ventral (PV) somatic sensory regions in relation to motor (M), primary auditory (AI), and primary (VI) and secondary (VII) visual regions as seen on flattened cortex.

Upper left: Organization of projections in SI. The digits and palm pads P_{2-4}, P_h (hypothenar), and P_{th} (thenar) of the forepaw are represented twice; the dashed line separates the two representations of the digits. Digits of the foot are numbered 1–5, Pre. and Post. Leg denote preaxial and postaxial leg; FA = forearm; W = wrist; UZ = unresponsive zone.

Lower left: A schematic illustration of the ways the glabrous digits are represented in somatosensory cortex of different mammals.

(A) The orientation of the digits and palm in SmI of most mammals, the "generalized type." The digit tips are along the rostral border of SmI.

(B) SmI of gray squirrels has two representations of the digits, which meet at the tips of the digits. The caudal representation is like the generalized type.

(C) In owl monkeys and other monkeys, the orientation of the digits in the rostral representation, SmI proper (architectonic field 3b), is like that of the generalized type; digits in the posterior cutaneous field (architectonic field 1) point in the opposite direction.

Lower right: Example of the organization of projections in PV.

Upper right: Example of the organization of projections in SII.

10.2.6. Comparison Summary

The UZ has parallels with a distinct portion of dysgranular cortex in rats (Krubitzer *et al.*, 1986) and also with the jugular sulcus, the most universal sulcus appearing within SI in all types of mammals (Johnson, 1980). It may be the squirrel manifestation of a feature of SI common to all mammals.

A deliberate search for a PV region in mice similar to that seen in squirrels showed only a single, SII, representation lateral to SI (Carvell and Simons, 1986, 1987). Thus, the auditory role of PV (auditory responses and connections with the medial geniculate and auditory cortex) appears to be a real difference between squirrels and mice (in mice these auditory functions are in SII), rather than due to failure to distinguish SII and PV in mice. Further specifically comparative study is needed to establish any parallels that may exist between PV and the various neighbors of SII that have been documented in monkeys (Section 8.2.1) and cats (Section 11.1.1).

The difference between callosal (reported in squirrels and rabbits) and acallosal (reported in rats) representations of axial facial regions needs further study. The difference as it now exists could be a difference between investigators (one group has studied squirrels and rabbits; a different group reported the rat distinctiveness). A directly comparative study in the same laboratory would establish if the difference is truly between species.

Squirrels join owl and macaque monkeys with the abdomen-rear arrangement in the SI trunk representations; they are unlike spiny anteaters, cebus and squirrel monkeys, and rabbits, which have the abdomen-forward arrangement.

10.3. Other Rodents

Several other rodents have been the subjects of mapping studies of SI. One of these was the largest of Sciuromorpha, the North American beaver (sometimes split into a separate suborder Castorimorpha); the others were all caviomorphs (or hystricomorphs if that classification is preferred); the capybara (the largest of all rodents), its closer relatives the agouti and the guinea pig, and the more distantly related North American porcupine. The results of these mapping studies are presented in Fig. 22.

Features of interest include the dominance of perioral structures in the SI representations of all these animals; agoutis, porcupines, and beavers have a relatively larger representation of the forelimb than do capybaras. Motor, SI, SII, auditory, and visual cortices meet one another in all of these species where each has been investigated. The question of overlap of sensory and motor regions has not been seriously investigated in any of these animals, and the orientation of the SII representation in capybaras and porcupines would probably be represented differently using modern methods.

The three largest brains show interesting sulci related to SI. In capybaras, sulci mark the representation of the lips (a *labial sulcus* in the terminology of Johnson, 1980), the boundary between forelimb and face representations (a *jugular sulcus* in the position of the squirrel UZ), and part of the border between sensory and motor cortex (a possible *central sulcus* analogue). The sulci in agouti and beaver SI separate the fore- and hindlimb representations (thus are *in-*

terbrachial sulci which are commonly seen in forepaw-using mammals of sufficient brain size).

Cytoarchitecturally, barrels have been seen in SI of guinea pigs, and chinchillas, other small caviomorphs, but could not be located in capybaras, agoutis, American porcupines or in large sciuromorph beavers, mountain beavers *Aplodontia rufescens*, and woodchucks *Marmota monax* (T. Woolsey et al., 1975; Johnson *et al.*, 1982b), raising the speculation that they may be present, or visible only in smaller brains. The largest rodent brain with visible barrels was the true hystricomorph African porcupine *Hystrix cristata*; rodents surveyed with smaller brains showed barrels: myomorph mice, rats, gerbils *Gerbillus gerbillus* and *Meriones unguiculata*, hamsters *Cricetus cricetus*, muskrats *Ondatra zibethica*; dormice *Glis glis*, two species of kangaroo rat *Dipodomys*, and five species of deer mice *Peromyscus*; sciuromorph flying squirrels *Glaucomys volans* and *Pteromys* sp., chipmunk *Tamias striatus*, ground squirrel *Spermophilus tridecemlineatus*, praire dog *Cynomys ludovicianus*, and gray squirrel (T. Woolsey *et al.*, 1975; Johnson *et al.*, 1982b).

11. Carnivores

Returning for the penultimate time to the starburst node on the phylogenetic tree of Fig. 1, we come to the order Carnivora. The carnivores are a moderately diversified group, of middling size among mammalian orders; they retain many primitive characters along with their specializations for predation. For our purposes they are of great importance since they include domestic cats, which until recently were by far the most frequent subjects of studies of sensory cortex (Fig. 23). The other remarkable carnivore for such studies is the North American raccoon, which represents an extreme in the sheer extent of neocortex devoted to mechanosensory input.

11.1. Cats

11.1.1. Sensory Projections

Doubtless due to the great number of investigations rather than to specializations of the species, no less than five distinct somatic sensory areas have been identified and formally numbered in cat neocortex.

11.1.1a. SI. The primary sensory area (SI) of cats contains a single representation of the body surface, with substantial representations of the paws and face (Dykes *et al.*, 1980; Felleman *et al.*, 1983b; McKenna *et al.*, 1981; Rubel, 1971) (see Fig. 24). Projections are from the contralateral body surface, and also from a substantial portion of ipsilateral oral and perioral regions (Taira, 1987). The dorsal midline of the trunk is represented rostrally and the ventral caudally. These representations of the midline include projections from receptive fields that extend to include ipsilateral as well as contralateral tissues (Barbaresi *et al.*, 1984).

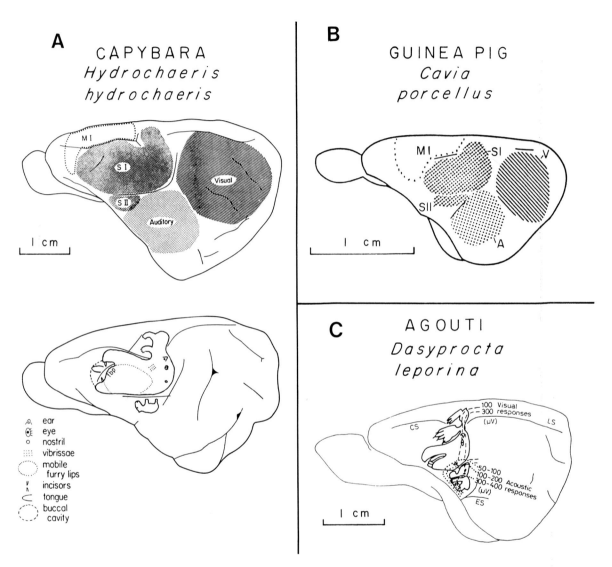

Figure 22. Location and organization of somatic sensory projections in four hystricomorph rodents and myomorph beavers seen in dorsolateral or lateral views of left cerebral hemispheres. Anterior is to the left in all diagrams.

(A) *Top.*: Relative locations of SI, SII, primary motor (MI), auditory, and visual regions. *bottom:* Organization of projections within SI in capybaras *Hydrochaeris hydrochaeris* (= *H. hydrochoerus*) (from Campos and Welker, 1976, with permission from G. B. Campos and S. Karger AG, Basel). The orientation of projections illustrated for SII was suggested on presumption but was not verified. fbp = furry buccal pad.

(B) Relative locations of SI, SII, primary motor (MI), auditory (A), and visual (V) regions in guinea pigs *Cavia porcellus* (from Zeigler, 1964, and Campos and Welker, 1976, with permission from G. B. Campos and S. Karger, AG, Basel).

(C) Organization of projections within SI (large figurine) and SII (small figurine) of agoutis *Dasyprocta leporina* (= *D. aguti*) (from Pimentel-Souza *et al.*, 1980, with permission from F. Pimentel de Souza and S. Karger AG, Basel). Boundaries of auditory and visual regions near and overlapping SI and SII are indicated by dotted and dashed "isopotential" lines representing the loci of mean amplitudes in

D

PORCUPINE
Erethizon dorsatum

MII CC

MI SI VIS

SII

SI VIS

MI SII AUD

└─┘ I cm

E

BEAVER
Castor canadensis

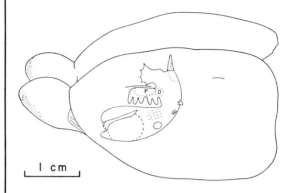

└─┘ I cm

⌂	ear
𝄞	eye
o	nostril
⋮⋮⋮	vibrissae
⌒	mobile furry lip
K	incisors
P	palm
Ð	hand dorsum
⌒	scaly tail
⬭	furry tail

microvolts of unit (microelectrode) or slow wave (macroelectrode) responses evoked by visual or auditory stimuli. Similar amplitudes and boundaries were obtained using micro- or macroelectrodes. CS = coronal sulcus; ES = ectosylvian sulcus; LS = lateral sulcus.

(D) Organization of projections in cerebral cortex of porcupines *Erethizon dorsatum* (from Lende and Woolsey, 1956, with alterations, and permission from C. N. Woolsey and the American Physiological Society). In addition to the

left lateral view (bottom), dorsal (middle) and medial (top) views are shown. AUD = auditory; CC = corpus callosum; MI, MII = primary and secondary motor; VIS = visual.

(E) Organization of projections in SI of North American beavers; SII was not located (from Carlson and Welker, 1976, with alterations, and permission from M. Carlson and S. Karger AG, Basel).

Reports of gradations of modality representation, with rostral and caudal regions showing more projections from deep receptors (e.g., Mountcastle, 1957; McKenna *et al.*, 1981) were questioned by the suggestion (Felleman *et al.*, 1983b) that these subcutaneous projections are actually from rostral and caudal regions bordering an "SI proper" whose representations are all cutaneous. The rostral bordering region has been well characterized as receiving projections from muscle afferents and possibly receptors from joints and other deep-lying tissues involved in kinesthetic perception (see Feldman and Johnson, 1988, for review);

	1966–1971	1972–1982	1983–1989
A – All titles	8.8	16.6	41.0
C – with Cats	2.7	5.0	9.8
R – with Rats	1.2	3.3	11.0
M – with Monkeys	.8	2.3	4.3
m – with mice	.2	.4	2.5

PROPORTION:

	1966–1971	1972–1982	1983–1989
C – with Cats	.302	.302	.240
R – with Rats	.132	.201	.268
M – with Monkeys	.094	.136	.114
m – with mice	.019	.025	.065

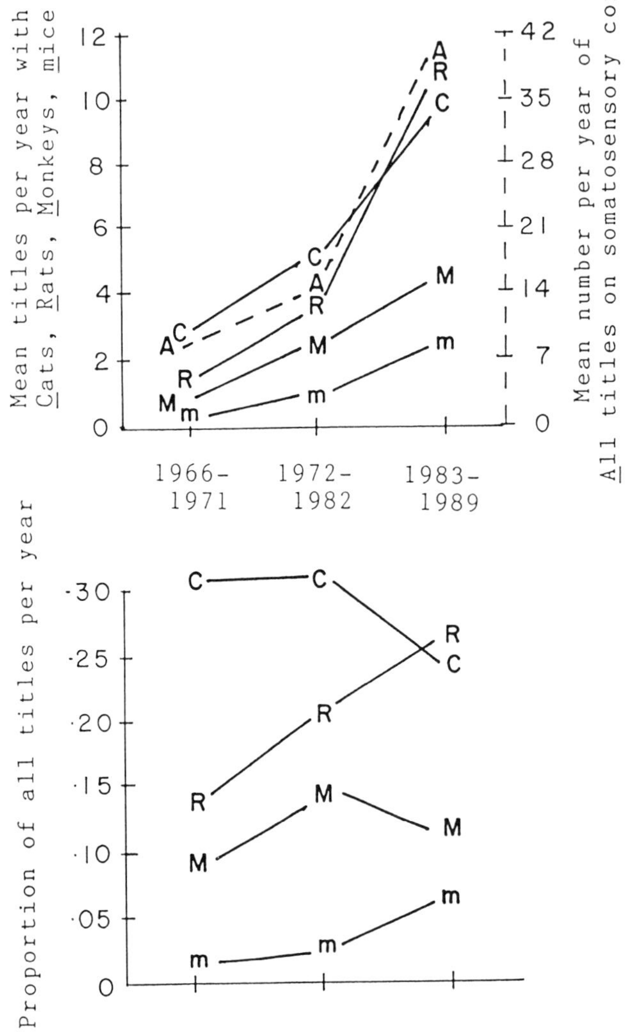

Figure 23. Trends in relative popularity as experimental subjects. As indicated by titles of articles compiled in the Medline database for the years 1966–1989, rats have recently overtaken cats in both absolute numbers and proportions of publications about somatic sensory cortex. Shown in the tables and graphs are means per year of: A, the total number of all titles including somatic sensory (or somatosensory) cortex, and of these the number which also include C, cat(s); R, rat(s); M, monkey(s); or m, mouse (or mice). Absolute numbers of articles per year have steadily increased for all groups, but most rapidly for rats.

its counterparts have been described above in monkeys (Section 8.2.1) and rats (Section 10.1.1).

A region of units with distinctive large and disjoint cutaneous receptive fields (e.g., including separate areas on each of several digits) has been described along the anterolateral periphery of the small-receptive-field SI forepaw representation in cats (Welt *et al.,* 1967; Iwamura and Tanaka, 1978; McKenna *et al.,* 1981).

Within the area of small-receptive-field cutaneous projections, two separate regions have been described, one containing rapidly adapting, the other slowly adapting responsive cells; these regions form irregular and interdigitating bands across SI (Sretavan and Dykes, 1983). Such proposals of distinct subareas, segregating intermingled categories, will be more convincing when the proposed subareas are mathematically tested for coherence against subareas plotted from randomly generated bicategorical data.

11.1.1b. SII. Figure 24 shows the arrangement of projections in SII of cats: there is a large representation of the forelimb digits, and a second smaller representation of the distal limbs along the medial edge of SII (Burton *et al.,* 1982; Clemo and Stein, 1983). This additional representation was considered part of SII (and called medial SII) rather than a separate sensory area because of similarities of response properties, cytoarchitecture and connectivity. The face region in cat SII has not been mapped in the degree of detail as have the postcranial regions. Most receptive fields in SII are, like those in SI, cutaneous and contralateral; but there are a few bilateral fields, disjunctive fields, and fields with stockinglike extent around the distal limbs such as are not seen in SI (Haight, 1972). A posteriormost region of SII contains neural units with large receptive fields, some including the whole body; some cells in this region responded to auditory stimulation, some to nociceptive stimulation, and some multimodal cells responded to auditory or mechanical, some to nociceptive or mechanical, and some to auditory or nociceptive stimulation (Carreras and Andersson, 1962; Burton *et al.,* 1982). A focus of projections in or near SII (the region was localized within a cytoarchitectural field rather than within projection maps) has been identified as carrying input from Pacinian corpuscles (Dykes and Herron, 1986).

In cats, SII responsiveness to peripheral stimulation survives ablation of the ipsilateral SI (J. I. Johnson, E. W Rubel, and R. L. Raisler, unpublished observations); cats thus join tree shrews and rabbits as parallel processors in SII in contrast to the serial processing seen in monkeys (Section 8.2.1b).

11.1.1c. SIII. SIII, formally identified thus far only in cats, lies caudal to, and adjacent to SI (Fig. 24) and has been reported to contain a complete representation of the body surface (Garraghty *et al.,* 1987); receptive fields and discharge characteristics of cells in SIII are very like those in SI (Tanji *et al.,* 1978; Garraghty *et al.,* 1987) except for a striking absence of receptive fields on the glabrous surfaces of the fore- and hindpaws (Garraghty *et al.,* 1987).

11.1.1d. SIV. Just lateral to, and adjoining, SII of cats is another, smaller, sensory representation of the complete body surface (Fig. 24). Its cytoarchitecture and connections differ from those of SII and this region has therefore been designated SIV (Burton *et al.,* 1982; Clemo and Stein, 1983; Stein *et al.,* 1983).

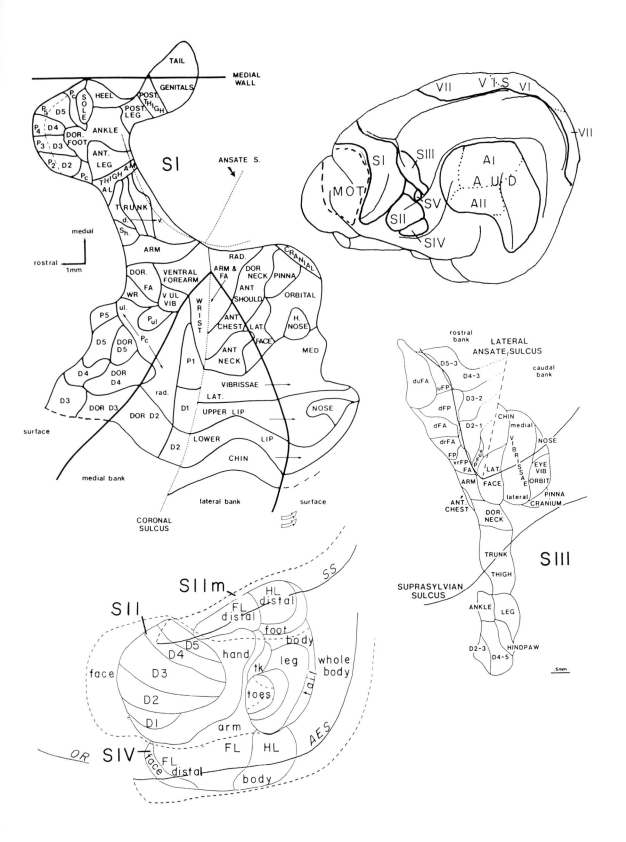

Units in SIV, like those in SII, respond to gentle cutaneous stimulation and have discrete, stable, and topographically organized contralateral receptive fields (Clemo and Stein, 1983).

11.1.1e. SV. Another representation of the body in cat neocortex has been termed SV (Mori *et al.*, 1985); it consists of what seems to be the hindlimb representation of SIII (Avendaño *et al.*, 1988) with nearby projections from forelimb and face, all in the medial bank of the anterior suprasylvian sulcus.

11.1.2. Relation to Other Areas

The question of overlap of SI with primary motor cortex has not been directly addressed experimentally in cats using modern methods. Motor and sensory maps (e.g., most recently, Felleman *et al.*, 1983b; Nieoullon and Rispal-Padel, 1976) show a boundary of some ambiguity in the motor and sensory representations of the forepaw in the coronal gyrus; trunk and hindlimb representations, in contrast, are clearly and consistently separated (in part by the postcruciate dimple), as are the associated cytoarchitectural regions (Fig. 25). Studies of thalamic projections do not suggest significant overlap of VL with VP projections (e.g., Jones and Powell, 1969; Jones and Burton, 1974; Asuncion-Moran and Reinoso-Suarez, 1988).

What was described in the previous section as the posteriormost region of SII can be considered a multimodal area rather than a strictly somatic sensory region; it has a distinctive cytoarchitecture which has been designated the suprasylvian field; its thalamic projections are from the lateral PO (POl) and the medial geniculate nuclear complex; it adjoins and receives input from auditory

---

Figure 24. Location and organization of somatic sensory projections to cortex of cats. Anterior is to the left in all diagrams.

Upper right: Location of SI, SII, SIII, SIV, and SV somatic sensory regions in relation to motor cortex (MOT) (Nieoullon and Rispal-Padel, 1976), to auditory cortex (AUD) including primary (AI) and secondary (AII) regions (Imig *et al.*, 1982), and to visual cortex (VIS) including primary (VI) and secondary (VII) regions (Tusa *et al.*, 1981). These references also describe numerous additional visual and auditory areas which occupy much of the intervening association regions between the somatic sensory, auditory, and visual regions as depicted here; such designations at far remove from the sensory input render rather meaningless the distinction between sensory and association areas. The boundaries as shown here indicate only the positions of regions relative to one another: many boundaries and much of the actual areas lie in sulcal walls not visible in this surface view.

Upper left: Organization of projections to SI of cats (from Felleman *et al.*, 1983b, with alterations, and permission from D. J. Felleman and the *Journal of Neuroscience*). Dotted lines indicate the ansate sulcus and the fundus of the coronal sulcus; dashed lines indicate undetermined borders. ANT., anterior; A-L, anterolateral; A-M, anteromedial; D, digit; d., DOR., dorsal; FA, forearm; H., hairy; LAT., lateral; MED., medial; P, glabrous digit pad; Pc, large central pad and adjoining surface of forepaw and hindpaw; POST., posterior; P$_{ul}$, ulnar pad at wrist; RAD., rad., radial; S., sulcus; Sh., SHOULD, shoulder; UL, ul., ulnar; V, v., ventral; VIB, vibrissa; WR, wrist.

Lower left: Organization of projections to SII, medial SII (SIIM), and SIV of cats; the approximate borders of these regions are indicated by dashed lines (from Burton *et al.*, 1982, with alterations, and permission from H. Burton and Alan R. Liss, Inc.). AES, anterior ectosylvian sulcus; D1–5, hand digits 1–5; FL, forelimb; HL, hindlimb; OR, orbital sulcus; SS, suprasylvian sulcus; tk, trunk.

Lower right: Organization of projections to SIII of cats (from Garraghty *et al.*, 1987, with permission from P. E. Garraghty and Guilford Press). The lateral wing of the ansate sulcus has been opened; the dashed line represents the fundus and the solid line the rostral and caudal lips. ANT., anterior; d, dorsal; D, digit; FA, forearm; FP, forepaw; r, radial; u, ulnar; v, ventral; VIB, vibrissa.

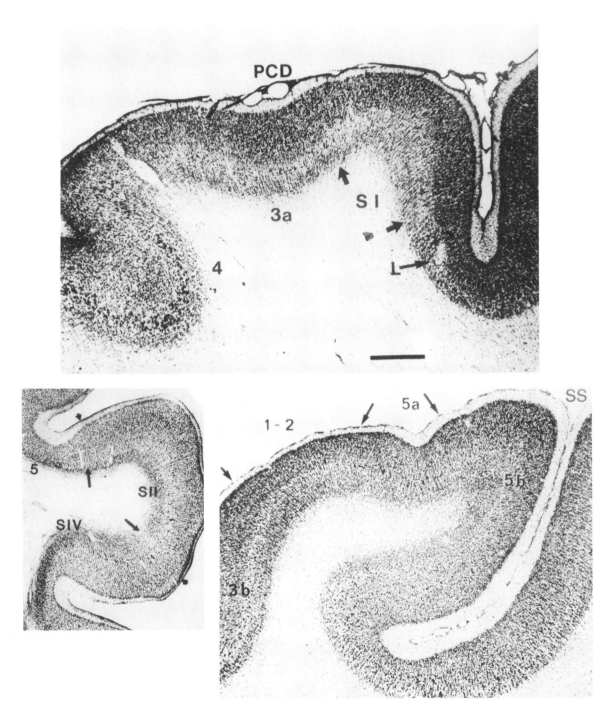

as well as somatic sensory cortex (reviewed by Burton *et al.*, 1982). Several other *n*th-order auditory and visual regions (so designated because auditory or visual stimuli influence activity in these regions under certain conditions) overlap the somatosensory areas (Imig *et al.*, 1982; Tusa *et al.*, 1981). Using the more parsimonious understanding of a sensory region as one wherein a particular modality or class of stimuli reliably, consistently, and exclusively evoke activity in an anesthetized preparation, the somatosensory regions of cat neocortex are clearly separated from other sensory regions by substantial bands of intervening cortex ("association" regions in our terminology) (Fig. 24).

11.1.3. Structure

11.1.3a. Sulci. In cats, the ansate sulcus forms a posterior boundary for much of SI, and the coronal sulcus functions as a jugular sulcus demarcating forelimb and face projections. The postcruciate dimple, when present, serves double duty, first as an analogue of the central sulcus between sensory and motor regions, and second as an interbrachial sulcus between the representations of the fore- and hindlimbs (Johnson, 1980).

11.1.3b. Cytoarchitecture of SI. Hassler and Muhs-Clement (1964) described areas 3a, 3b, 1, and 2 in cat SI cortex, mimicking the parcellation established in primates. Area 3a, distinguished from the more caudal SI by large cells in layer 5 (Fig. 25), has some relationship with the anterior zone of kinesthetic projections (reviewed by Dykes *et al.*, 1986). A well-researched absence of physiological correlations with the distinctions among areas 3b, 1, and 2 led Felleman *et al.* (1983b) to propose that these subdivisions in fact do not exist in cats, and that instead a single koniocortical region comprises all of SI in cats and is similar to area 3b of primates. Connectional data (Jones and Powell, 1968a–c; McKenna *et al.*, 1981; Burton and Kopf, 1984b; Jones, 1985, p. 363; Barbaresi *et al.*, 1987) support this proposition.

Figure 25. Cytoarchitectural features of somatic sensory cortex in cats as seen in Nissl-stained sections.

Top: A parasagittal section through the region of SI representing the forearm (from Felleman *et al.*, 1983b, with permission from D. J. Felleman and the Society for Neuroscience). Rostral is to the left. The rostral border of SI (leftmost arrow) corresponds to a transition in responses from those driven by deep receptors [to the left of this arrow, in area 3a, at the postcruciate dimple (PCD)] to those driven by cutaneous receptors (to the right of this arrow). The caudal border of SI (next arrow to the right) corresponds to the start of a cutaneous projection thought to be part of SIII. The arrow from L points to an electrolytic lesion made at the end of an electrode penetration in the bank of the ansate sulcus. Area 4 (motor cortex) lies in the banks of the cruciate sulcus in this section. Bar = 1 mm.

Below, left: A coronal section through SII (part of the distal forelimb zone) and SIV in the rostral half of the anterior ectosylvian gyrus between the suprasylvian and ectosylvian gyri; cytoarchitectonic borders are marked by arrows (from Burton *et al.*, 1982, with permission from H. Burton and Alan R. Liss, Inc.).

Below, right: A parasagittal section through the lateral end of the ansate sulcus showing cytoarchitectonic areas 3b, 1–2, 5a, and 5b (from Tanji *et al.*, 1978, with permission of D. G. Tanji and the American Physiological Society). Arrows mark cytoarchitectonic boundaries. Rostral is to the right. SIII is located in area 5a on the floor of the ansate sulcus. SS, suparasylvian sulcus.

11.1.3c. Cytoarchitecture of SII. Burton *et al.* (1982) described the cytoarchitecture of SII in detail, contrasting it with neighboring regions of SI (which they call area 2 after Hassler and Muhs-Clement) and SIV. The distinctive features of SII are a widening of layer 4, and a blurring of the boundaries between layers 2 and 3, 3 and 4, and between layer 6 and the underlying white matter. Within SII, the lateral region (SII proper) has broader layers 5 and 6 than does medial SII (Fig. 25).

11.1.3d. Cytoarchitecture of SIII. SIII lies within, but is not coextensive with, area 5a of Hassler and Muhs-Clement (1964) (Tanji *et al.*, 1978; Avendaño *et al.*, 1988). It is distinguished from the neighboring area 2 by several large pyramidal cells in layer 5 (Fig. 25).

11.1.3e. Cytoarchitecture of SIV. Unlike the neighboring SII, SIV has clear boundaries between layers 2, 3, 4, 5, 6 and the underlying white matter; and layers 4, 5, and 6 are narrower (Burton *et al.*, 1982) (Fig. 25).

11.1.4. Thalamic Connections

11.1.4a. SI. Representation of particular body regions in SI of cats have reciprocal connections with corresponding regions of the ventroposterolateral (VPL) and ventroposteromedial (VPM) thalamic nuclei. For example, the SI forepaw representation is connected with an architecturally distinct medial sector of VPL (designated VPLm) and the trunk representation with a dorsal sector of VPL (Hand and Morrison, 1970, 1972; Jones and Leavitt, 1973; Spreafico *et al.*, 1983; Barbaresi *et al.*, 1984, 1987; Burton and Kopf, 1984a). Projections from VPM are found in the face representation (Jones and Powell, 1969; Hand and Morrison, 1970, 1972). The anterior region of kinesthetic projections from the limbs (related to area 3a) has its connections with a rostrodorsal cap of VPL (Dykes *et al.*, 1986), corresponding to the outer shell region of monkeys (see Section 8.2.4).

Terminals of thalamocortical fibers are most dense in layer 4, with some spread into neighboring layers 3 and 5; a number of fine fibers ascend to terminate in layer 1 (Jones and Powell, 1969; Hand and Morrison, 1970). Cells of origin of corticothalamic fibers are located throughout layer 6 with some in layer 5 (Rustioni *et al.*, 1983). The corticothalamic portion of reciprocal connections includes connections to the thalamic reticular nucleus (Jones and Powell, 1968c) as is believed to be the case with most thalamocortical circuits (Jones, 1985, p. 218).

A region of the thalamic ventrolateral nucleus which receives input from the spinal cord was reported to have reciprocal connections with SI (Jones and Powell, 1968c; Jones and Leavitt, 1973); this may have something in common with the region just described as the rostrodorsal cap of VPL.

There are also sparse projections to SI from the intralaminar CL (central lateral) and centre médian nuclei (Jones and Leavitt, 1974; Bentivoglio *et al.*, 1983; Barbaresi *et al.*, 1987). Some of the CL projections may be branches of CL projections to the caudate nucleus (Macchi *et al.*, 1984). Projections to CL from SI (but not to céntre median) were observed (Jones and Burton, 1974).

The question arises as to whether in cats there are projections from thalamic

POm to SI like those interesting ones seen in rats (Section 10.1.4). SI input from POm in cats was reported by Spreafico *et al.* (1981) but denied in earlier and later studies (Jones and Leavitt, 1973; Barbaresi *et al.*, 1987). Confusion with POm projections known to arrive in neighboring regions of SIII was denied (Spreafico *et al.*, 1981) but both anatomical and physiological boundaries between SI and SIII are very ambiguous (Avendaño *et al.*, 1988). SI does project to POm (Jones and Powell, 1968c; Jones and Burton, 1974) in what seems thus far to be a case of a "nonreciprocal" corticothalamic connection. [Jones (1975, p. 206) has pointed out that such cases usually turn out to be reciprocal after all with sufficient further study.]

11.1.4b. SII. The main thalamic connections of cat SII are with VP (Jones and Powell, 1968c; Hand and Morrison, 1970, 1972; Jones and Leavitt, 1973; Spreafico *et al.*, 1981; Bentivoglio *et al.*, 1983; Fisher *et al.*, 1983; Burton and Kopf, 1984a; Barbaresi *et al.*, 1987). Cells projecting to a particular part of the body representation of SII are found in that portion of VPL–VPM that projects to the homotopic representation in SI (Guillery *et al.*, 1966; Jones and Powell, 1969; Burton and Kopf, 1984a). A few, but very few, cells have branched projections to both SI and SII (Spreafico *et al.*, 1981, 1983; Fisher *et al.*, 1983). Multiple and varied reports of distinctive VPL regions projecting to SII as opposed to SI have not been confirmed with careful control of cortical sites and comparability of homotopic regions (Burton and Kopf, 1984a; Jones, 1985, p. 368). The pattern of terminals in SII from VP is similar to that in SI, except that the total density of fibers is less in SII than in SI (Jones and Powell, 1969; Hand and Morrison, 1970). SII also has reciprocal connections with the medial portion (POm) of the posterior group of thalamic nuclei (Jones and Powell, 1968c; Hand and Morrison, 1972; Bentivoglio *et al.*, 1983; Burton and Kopf, 1984a; Barbaresi *et al.*, 1987). Corticothalamic projections to the thalamic reticular nucleus form part of the reciprocal circuits for SII as for SI (Jones and Powell, 1968c). The region of Pacinian projections, localized in SII of cats by cytoarchitectural criteria, was reported to have reciprocal connections with a newly redefined VPI thalamic nucleus, as well as with the POl (Dykes and Herron, 1986).

SII receives sparse projections from the thalamic intralaminar CL and central medial (not to be confused with the more posterior centre médian) nuclei (Bentivoglio *et al.*, 1983; Spreafico *et al.*, 1983; Burton and Kopf, 1984a; Barbaresi *et al.*, 1987).

11.1.4c. SIII. Projections to the face representation in SIII are from the medial portion (POm) of the posterior group of thalamic nuclei, a region which receives direct input from the spinal cord and from SIII (Tanji *et al.*, 1978; Bentivoglio *et al.*, 1983; Jones, 1985, p. 592; Garraghty *et al.*, 1987). Projections to the hindlimb region of SIII were from a region of POm just dorsal to VPL; those to the face region were from a more medial location in POm (Garraghty *et al.*, 1987).

SIII projects to a larger region within POm including the suprageniculate nucleus, and to a portion of the LP thalamic nucleus (not to be confused with POl) (Jones and Powell, 1968c; Garraghty *et al.*, 1987) and to CL and the thalamic reticular nucleus (Tanji *et al.*, 1978). At least a portion of the projection to POm reciprocates the thalamocortical projection to SIII.

11.1.4d. SIV. SIV also has reciprocal connections with POm. While there appears to be some distinction in the various regions of POm that project, respectively, to SII. SIII. and SIV, there is also overlap among these regions (Burton and Kopf, 1984a).

11.1.5. Corticocortical Connections

11.1.5a. Ipsilateral Reciprocal. In cats there are reciprocal and homotopic connections between SI and ipsilateral SII (Jones and Powell, 1968b; Manzoni *et al.,* 1979; Graziosi *et al.,* 1982; Burton and Kopf, 1984b; Alloway and Burton, 1985; reviewed in Barbaresi *et al.,* 1987). Cells of origin of SI-to-SII fibers are mostly pyramidal cells in layer 3 (Burton and Kopf, 1984b; 90%, Barbaresi *et al.,* 1987), most in the outer part of the layer, with a few cells in layers 2, 5, and 6 and least in 4 and upper 5 (Manzoni *et al.,* 1979; Graziosi *et al.,* 1982). In SII cells of origin of SII-to-SI fibers were reported variously as equally dense in layers 3 and 5, with a few in layer 6 and none in 1, 2, or 4 (Alloway and Burton, 1985), or as numerous in all layers, with a peak in layer 6 and fewest in 2 and 4 (Barbaresi *et al.* 1987). Terminals of these and all other ipsilateral corticocortical fibers were reported concentrated in layers 6, 5, 4, and the neighboring edge of 3 (Jones and Powell, 1968b); terminals in SII of projections from SI were later reported concentrated in layer 3b with some in neighboring 3a and 4 as well as 6 (Alloway and Burton, 1985). SI also has reciprocal and homotopic connections with motor cortex (Jones and Powell, 1968b), and receives input from insular cortex (Guldin *et al.,* 1986).

SII has homotopic and reciprocal connections with motor cortex as well as with SI (Jones and Powell, 1968b; Burton and Kopf, 1984b). Additional reciprocal connections were reported between SII and area 5 including at least some parts of SIII, and between SII and insular, perirhinal, and ventrolateral orbital cortex (Burton and Kopf, 1984b).

SIII has homotopic reciprocal connections with SI (Jones and Powell, 1968b; Tanji *et al.,* 1978; Garraghty *et al.,* 1987; Avendaño *et al.,* 1988) and some evidence suggests homotopic connections with SII and SIV (Garraghty *et al.,* 1987). SIII is part of a wider cortical region receiving projections from motor cortex, prefrontal cortex, and granular insular cortex (Garraghty *et al.,* 1987; Avendaño *et al.,* 1988).

SIV showed strong reciprocal connections with area 5 including SIII, and less dense with the "suprasylvian fringe" anterior to auditory cortex and with insular cortex (Burton and Kopf, 1984b).

11.1.5b. Ipsilateral One-Way. Besides the reciprocal connections with SII, SIII, and motor cortex, SI projects to supplementary motor cortex (Jones and Powell, 1968b).

SII also projects to supplementary motor cortex, and to the region caudal to SII where there are convergent somatic sensory and auditory inputs (Jones and Powell, 1968b).

SIII projects to all of area 6, including the supplementary motor cortex (Jones and Powell, 1968b).

SIV has, in addition to its reciprocal connections, projections to area 6 in the region of supplementary motor cortex and to dorsolateral orbital cortex (Burton and Kopf, 1984b).

11.1.5c. Commissural. SI receives callosal fibers homotopically from the representations of the axial body in the contralateral SI; the representations of the limb extremities are not callosally connected (Ebner and Myers, 1965; Jones and Powell, 1968a; Caminiti *et al.*, 1979; Manzoni *et al.*, 1980; Graziosi *et al.*, 1982; McKenna *et al.*, 1981; Barbaresi *et al.*, 1987). The SI forepaw representations were reported to receive fibers from the contralateral SII (Barbaresi *et al.*, 1985, 1987) although earlier studies showed no projections from SII to any of SI (Caminiti *et al.*, 1979) or only a small projection to the bilateral representation of the face in SI (Jones and Powell, 1968a). Cells of origin of SI callosal fibers to the contralateral SI, in the axial body representation, are nearly all in layers 3 and 6 (Caminiti *et al.*, 1979; Manzoni *et al.*, 1980; Graziosi *et al.*, 1982; McKenna *et al.*, 1981; Barbaresi *et al.*, 1987). Cells in SII projecting to contralateral SI were mainly layer 3 pyramidal cells (Barbaresi *et al.*, 1985). Terminals of SI-to-SI callosal fibers are concentrated in layer 4 and deep layer 3 with possible lesser amounts in all other layers (Jones and Powell, 1968a).

SII in cats receives callosal input from the contralateral SII and from the axial body representations in the contralateral SI (Jones and Powell, 1968a; Caminiti *et al.*, 1979; Barbaresi *et al.*, 1985, 1987). The cells of origin in SII and in SI are mostly in layer 3 with a few in layer 6. Callosal terminals in SII, as in SI, are densest in layers 4 and deep 3 with possible terminals in all other layers (Jones and Powell, 1968a).

In addition to the callosal connections to SII from the SI representations of axial body regions, Caminiti *et al.* (1979) reported a peculiar region in the coronal sulcus in SI which sends callosal projections to the contralateral SII. The cells of origin were judged, based on different experiments, to be in the SI representation of the radial forepaw digits. Why the radial digit region, and no other portions of the representations of the extremities, would have such callosal connections, is not easily explained. An alternative hypothesis would be that these cells are not in the SI representation, but rather adjoining it, between the SI representations of forepaw and face. The coronal sulcus, on whose banks these cells are found, is in location analogous to that of the unresponsive zone (UZ) of squirrels, which is a major zone of callosal connections (see Section 10.2.5b) and also lies between the SI representations of forepaw and face. (In squirrels, however, the many callosal projections from UZ do not include fibers to the contralateral SII or PV; Krubitzer *et al.*, 1986). This hypothetical cat UZ analogue might also account for the conflict about the existence of callosal fibers from SII to SI (see two paragraphs above; the projections might be to the UZ analogue rather than to forepaw SI).

No commissural projections from SI or SII of cats were found to contralateral regions other than SI and SII (Jones and Powell, 1968a).

11.1.6. Other Connections

11.1.6a. Claustrum. As with most, if not all, neocortex, the somatic sensory areas of cats receive topographically organized input from both the ipsilateral and contralateral claustrum, more from the ipsilateral than from the contralateral (Narkiewicz, 1964; Norita, 1977; Macchi *et al.*, 1981, 1983; Druga, 1982, Guldin *et al.*, 1986); and at least the hindlimb representation in SI has a reciprocal homotopic corticoclaustral projection (Olson and Graybiel, 1980).

11.1.6b. Corpus Striatum. Corticostriate projections arise from somatic sensory regions, as from all neocortical regions, in cats (Webster, 1965) as in monkeys, rabbits, rats, and mice (Sections 8.2.6, 9.6, 10.1.6).

11.1.6c. Brain Stem and Spinal Cord. Regions within or near SI or SII project to the zona incerta, substantia nigra, red nucleus, and superior colliculus (Jones and Powell, 1968c). Corticopontine fibers, and many corticospinal fibers of the pyramidal tract originate from layer 5 pyramidal cells in SI (Yamamoto *et al.*, 1987).

Fibers originating in SIV project to deep layers of the superior colliculus and the ventrolateral periaqueductal gray (Burton and Kopf, 1984a); in this regard SIV is unlike SII, which sends no projections to these locations.

SI and SII are significant sources of corticospinal projections; the face representations project to the sensory trigeminal nuclei; and the limb representations send substantial projections to the cuneate and gracile nuclei (reviewed by Brodal, 1981, pp. 188 ff., 81 ff., 512 ff.).

11.1.7 Comparison Summary

SI of cats appears to be a simple basic mammalian SI with few if any distinctive features. In this respect, cats have indeed been good experimental examples for generalizations to mammals (though not for generalizations to humans since the anthropoid SI is so unusual in its organization). Cats exhibit no multiple representations in SI. There are no connections from visual cortex to any of the somatic sensory regions (Jones and Powell, 1968b) in contrast to rats where visual cortex projections to SI were seen. The usual jugular and interbrachial–central sulci appear in cat SI. There is no evidence of special features in the architecture of layer 4 of SI of cats. There are no unusual thalamic projections.

Somewhat distinctive features of SI of cats include an ipsilateral representation of mouth parts, more than in monkeys, and far more than in the other mammals so far considered. SI in cats has the abdomen-rear position, placing cats in what was a minority but which now becomes a more equal cohort (cats, owl and macaque monkeys, and squirrels versus spiny anteaters, squirrel and cebus monkeys, and rabbits).

In its proximity to SII, and its mirroring of the somatotopy of SII, SIV shows parallels with areas Ri of macaques and VS of owl monkeys (Section 8.2.1c). Careful localization of the focus of Pacinian-activated responses in SII or SIV might establish a better functional parallel with owl monkey area VS.

SIII, located in area 5a of cats, invites comparison with area 5a of monkeys due to their similar cytoarchitecture, location, and the fact that both receive substantial topographic projections from SI (Sections 8.2.5a, 11.1.5a). They have in many respects similar thalamic connections as well (Garraghty *et al.*, 1987; Hyvärinen, 1982). They are different in that SIII in cats is responsive to mechanical stimulation under anesthesia, area 5a in monkeys is not; and in the unanesthetized state responses in monkey 5a are mostly to movements of joints (reviewed by Hyvärinen, 1982) while in cats SIII responses are mostly from cutaneous projections. It would be very interesting to learn if these mechanosensory responses in either species are dependent upon input from SI (implying "serial processing") or whether input from thalamic projections alone is sufficient for cortical activation by peripheral stimulation.

A cat counterpart of the supplementary sensory area of monkeys (Section 8.2.1d) has been suggested (Avendaño *et al.*, 1988) based upon a focus of projections from SI to the corresponding region on the mesial surface of the hemisphere in cats.

11.2. Raccoons

11.2.1. Sensory Projections

11.2.1a. SI. The SI region in raccoons contains a single representation of the body surface (Fig. 26). What had initially appeared to be a possible second representation of the trunk (Johnson, 1985), upon further study was determined to be a pleated single representation folded into a small cortical space (Johnson, unpublished studies). The SI representation is dominated by an imposing enlarged representation of the glabrous volar surface of the hand (Papez and Hunter, 1929; W. Welker and Seidenstein, 1959). This glabrous cutaneous hand representation contains responsive cells with very small receptive fields arranged in somatotopic order.

Along the anterior border and extending caudally along the medial and lateral borders of the glabrous volar hand representation, and invaginating between the representations of the volar skin of the individual digits, there is a zone containing a somatotopic representation of the claws and dorsal hairy skin of the hand. More anteriorly, around this claw and hairy skin representation, and possibly intermingled with it, is a zone containing cells with larger and more complex receptive fields and less somatotopic ordering, called the heterogeneous zone (Johnson *et al.*, 1982c; Kelahan and Doetsch, 1984). Examples of complex receptive fields of cells in the heterogeneous zone include several or all claws, large areas on the dorsal and volar surfaces of the hand and forearm, and/or deep subcutaneous tissues.

A distinct zone of kinesthetic projections is found bordering the heterogeneous zone still more anteriorly, and also extending caudally along the medial border of the hand representation (between hand and hindfoot regions, actually between the heterogeneous zones bordering these representations of the extremities). In this kinesthetic zone most cells respond to displacements of joints and muscles; the majority respond to muscle stretch (Feldman and Johnson, 1988).

11.2.1b. SII. In raccoons, projections in SII are as usual arranged somatotopically, the representations of the extremities pointing away from SI (Herron, 1978). Receptive fields are larger than in SI, but as in SI the largest receptive fields are on the trunk and the smallest on the volar glabrous hand. Correspondingly, the largest representation is that of the volar hand; it accounts for three-fourths of the total area of representation of the postcranial body surface, clearly reflecting the proportions of projections from different body regions seen in SI. A very few projections (9 of 190) from postcranial surfaces were from bilateral receptive fields, the rest being contralateral. All hand projections were from contralateral receptive fields. Only one auditory response was encountered, and that was on the posterior border of the SII postcranial representation.

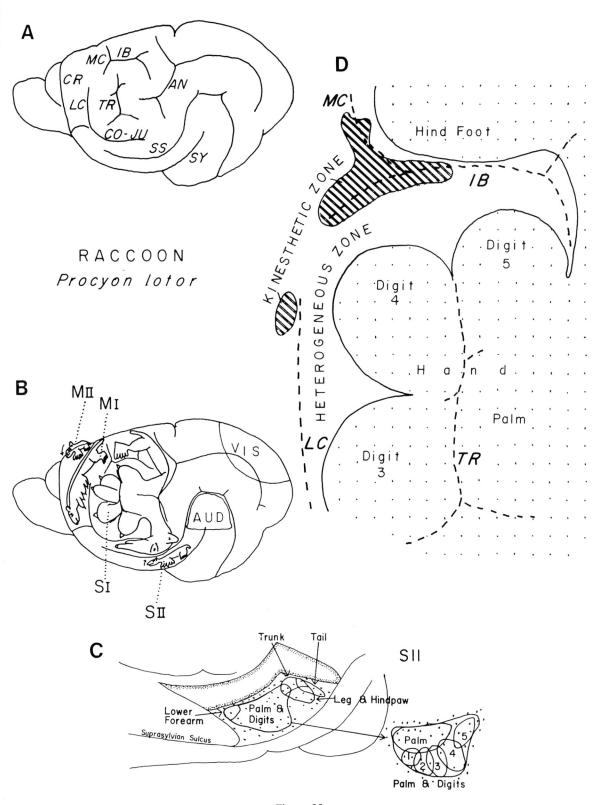

A

MC IB

CR

AN

LC TR

CO-JU

SS

SY

RACCOON

Procyon lotor

B

MII MI

VIS

AUD

SI

SII

C

Trunk Tail

SII

Lower
Forearm

Palm &
Digits

Leg & Hindpaw

Suprasylvian Sulcus

Palm

5

1
2 3

4

Palm & Digits

D

MC

Hind Foot

IB

KINESTHETIC ZONE

Digit
5

HETEROGENEOUS ZONE

Digit
4

Hand

Palm

LC

Digit
3

TR

Figure 26.

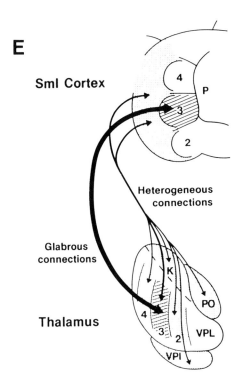

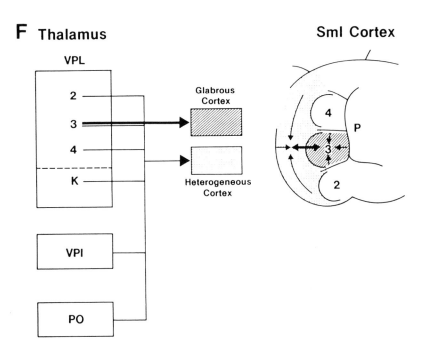

Figure 26. (*Continued*)

11.2.2. Relation to Other Areas

Primary (MI) and secondary or supplemental (MII) motor cortical regions lie anterior to SI (Hardin *et al.*, 1968; Jameson *et al.*, 1968) (Fig. 26). Detailed studies of other functional regions in raccoon cortex remain to be done. The approximate locations of auditory and visual regions were roughly determined (W. Welker and Seidenstein, 1959) and are presented in Fig. 26.

11.2.3. Structure

Raccoons were the introductory examples of the functional significance of sulci in somatosensory cortex (W. Welker and Seidenstein, 1959; W. Welker and Campos, 1963). As in primates, there is a central sulcus demarcating sensory from motor cortex. As in marsupials, prosimian lorises, and some large rodents, there is a jugular sulcus between fore- and hindlimb projections. The forelimb representation in raccoons occupies the large and distinct "elliptical hand gyrus" (W. Welker and Seidenstein, 1959), which surrounds a triradiate sulcus. The triradiate sulcus with its spurs marks the separations of the representations of the five individual digits of the hand and that of the palm.

The kinesthetic zone lies in the depths of the central and interbrachial sulci; the heterogeneous zone lies on the walls of those sulci and in their spurs that project into the hand representation (Johnson *et al.*, 1982c; Feldman and Johnson, 1988). These spurs of the central and interbrachial sulci approach and sometimes meet the corresponding spurs of the triradiate sulcus (thus forming boundaries between representations of individual digits). The heterogeneous zone is confined to the central and interbrachial spurs: the triradiate sulcus and its spurs include only the zone of precise somatotopic projections from the glabrous surface of the hand.

Figure 26 (pages 414–415). Features of somatic sensory cortex in raccoons.

(A) Outline of the left cerebral hemisphere from a dorsolateral viewpoint. Sulci in the somatic sensory region are labeled: *AN*, ansate; *CO-JU*, coronal (jugular); *CR*, cruciate; *IB*, interbrachial; *LC*, lateral central; *MC*, medial central; *SS*, suprasylvian; *SY*, sylvian; *TR*, triradiate.

(B) Relative locations of primary somatic sensory SI, second somatic sensory SII, primary motor MI, and second motor MII regions (from Johnson, 1985, with permission from Springer-Verlag). The general locations of auditory (AUD) and visual (VIS) regions were determined but not mapped in detail (W. Welker and Seidenstein, 1959). The lateral and medial central sulci separate sensory from motor regions. The jugular and interbrachial sulci demarcate SI representations of the limbs. The triradiate sulcus and its spurs outline the representations of the digits of the hand in SI. SII lies in the banks of the suprasylvian sulcus.

(C) Details of projections in SII (from Herron, 1978, with permission from P. Herron and Alan R. Liss, Inc.). The upper bank of the suprasylvian sulcus has been cut away to reveal the positions of representations of postcranial body regions on the lower bank. Dots indicate sites of microelectrode penetrations.

(D) Details of projections in SI (from Feldman and Johnson, 1988, with alterations, and permission from S. H. Feldman and Alan R. Liss, Inc.), depicted as if on flattened cortex; dashed lines indicate the fundi of sulci. Dotted region indicates the glabrous or gyral zones with projections in precise somatotopic order from small receptive fields. Shaded regions along the *LC*, *MC*, and *IB* sulci indicate the kinesthetic zone with projections from subcutaneous tissue of muscles and joints. Between these zones is the heterogeneous zone with projections from variegated, including many complex, receptive fields.

(E) Contrasting thalamic connections of gyral (glabrous) and sulcal (heterogeneous) zones of SI (from Doetsch *et al.*, 1988a, with permission from G. S. Doetsch and the *Journal of Neuroscience*). P, 2, 3, 4, SI representations of palm and digits 2, 3, and 4 of the hand in the gyral zone of SI and the ventroposterolateral thalamic nucleus VPL; K, kinesthetic region of VPL; PO, posterior thalamic nucleus; VPI, ventroposteroinferior thalamic nucleus.

(F) Summary of thalamocortical and corticocortical connections to gyral (glabrous) and sulcal (heterogeneous) zones of raccoon SI (from Doetsch *et al.*, 1988b, with permission from G. S. Doetsch and the *Journal of Neuroscience*).

In at least the limb representations in SI of raccoons, the kinesthetic and heterogeneous zones have been classed together as a zone of "sulcal cortex" (Herron and Johnson, 1987), which in position, connections, and possibly function, has much in common with the dysgranular regions of rat SI. The complementary "gyral cortex" (= the "glabrous area" of Doetsch *et al.*, 1988a,b) on the crowns of neighboring gyri (but which also includes the walls of the triradiate sulcus) is similar to the granular regions of rat SI (and area 3b of monkeys) in that it receives projections from highly innervated surfaces, with correspondingly small receptive fields represented in precise somatotopic order. There are a number of correspondences in the connectivity of rat granular and raccoon "gyral" regions (see Section 11.2.5). The "gyral" regions of raccoons are thickly myelinated as are the granular regions in squirrels (Section 10.2.3). However, unlike granular regions in rats and area 3b of monkeys, there is not a pronounced and distinct accumulation of granule cells in layer 4 in "gyral" regions of raccoons: while additional granule cells are present they are intermingled with the larger cells of deep layer 3. The distinctive cytoarchitectural feature of this area in raccoons is, rather, a prominent cell-free outer stripe of Baillarger between layers 4 and 5. This stripe is greatly attenuated in the depths of the central and interbrachial (but not the triradiate) sulci, much as is the granulous layer 4 in the corresponding regions in rats and monkeys; but unlike the abrupt attenuation of the granular layer in these animals, in raccoons the attenuation of the stripe is gradual. Thus, in raccoons sharp boundaries between "gyral" (3b- and granular-like) and "sulcal" (dysgranular-like) zones cannot be drawn cytoarchitectonically although they are apparent electrophysiologically (Johnson *et al.*, 1982c; Kelahan and Doetsch, 1984).

In raccoons SII lies on the banks of the anterior suprasylvian sulcus (W. Welker and Seidenstein, 1959; Herron, 1978).

11.2.4. Thalamic Connections

There is input to both "gyral" and "sulcal" regions of raccoon SI from the ventrobasal [(VB) = ventroposterior (VP) = ventroposterolateral (VPL) + ventroposteromedial (VPM)] nucleus of the thalamus. Separate subdivisions (lobules, lamellae), readily visible in sections stained for cells, fibers, or cytochrome oxidase activity, project to corresponding separate gyral formations representing discrete body parts: tail, hindlimb, and parts of the hand (each of the five digits and the palm) (W. Welker and Johnson, 1965; Herron, 1983; Warren and Pubols, 1984; Wiener *et al.*, 1987a,b; Doetsch *et al.*, 1988a). A rostrodorsal cap subdivision of VB projects to the rostral kinesthetic subdivision of "sulcal" SI cortex.

As would be expected, there is a precise reciprocal projection from raccoon SI to the appropriate lamellae or lobules of the ventrobasal thalamus (Petras, 1969).

While projections to "gyral" ("glabrous") regions are strictly somatotopic (a gyral crown receives projections only from its "own" lamella or lobule in VB) (Fig. 26), "sulcal" heterogeneous zone regions receive thalamic projections not only from the homotopic lamella, but also from neighboring lamellae, the kinesthetic rostrodorsal cap, the VPI nucleus, and portions of the PO nucleus (Doetsch *et al.*, 1988a). These PO projections to sulcal regions recall similar projections to dysgranular regions of rat SI. In addition, sparse projections from PO to gyral regions have been reported (Warren and Pubols, 1984).

Projections from the VL thalamic nucleus are confined to primary motor cortex (Sakai, 1982; no input from VL is found in SI (Herron, 1983).

The major input to SII is from the VPI; no projections to SII from VB were found (Herron, 1983). Some cells in thalamic intralaminar nuclei (central lateral, centromedian, and parafascicular nuclei) project to SII.

11.2.5. Corticocortical Connections

11.2.5a. Ipsilateral Corticocortical. In the forepaw representation of raccoon SI, in gyral (glabrous) regions there are reciprocal corticocortical connections between areas (both gyral and sulcal) within the representation of a single digit, but only sparse input from other cortical regions (Herron and Johnson, 1987; Doetsch *et al.*, 1988b). Contrastingly, in sulcal regions (heterogeneous and possibly kinesthetic cortex) there are such connections not only within a digit representation, but with other digit representations, with SII, with motor cortex, and with kinesthetic regions; there are no connections from the face or hindlimb representations. The cells of origin of all these connections are primarily in layer 3, with some in layers 2 and 4 on either side of layer 3, and some in layer 6 with a very few in layer 5.

Raccoon SII has reciprocal connections, both homotopic and heterotopic with sulcal regions of SI. In addition, a few projections from SII to gyral regions have been reported (Standage and Doetsch, 1988). The cells of origin within SI are distributed as were the projections to other SI regions (most in layer 3, fewer in 2, 4, and 6, fewest in 5); the cells of origin in SII were reported in layers 3 and 5 (Herron and Johnson, 1987), and in layers 5 and 6 (Standage and Doetsch, 1988).

11.2.5b. Commissural. In SI of raccoons, the hand representation, both gyral and sulcal regions, is free of commissural connections; face and hindlimb representations have substantial commissural input (Ebner and Myers, 1965; Herron and Johnson, 1987). Raccoon SII, as SI, has a hand representation free of commissural input, but a well-connected representation of the trunk and proximal hindlimb. Commissural connections in both SI and SII are homotopic, and cells of origin of commissural fibers are found in layers 3 and 5 (Herron and Johnson, 1987).

Terminal fields of corticocortical connections have not been analyzed in raccoons.

11.2.6. Other Connections

Projections from claustrum to SI have been observed (Standage and Doetsch, 1988).

11.2.7. Comparison Study

The contrasting feature of raccoon somatic sensory cortex is its vast extent. Among the features revealed by this expansion is the heterogeneous region in the anterior SI area, adjoining the kinesthetic ("3a") cortex, which may be a feature of many or all other mammals. Traces of a heterogeneous zone were seen in cats, and together with the kinesthetic zone they may correspond to the dysgranular region of rats. Common features of rat dysgranular cortex and raccoon heterogeneous cortex include feedforward from granular (gyral) regions, as a first stage in hierarchical processing; a relative abundance of commissural connections, and extension back into SI receiving regions between the limb representations. Following the suggestion of Chapin *et al.* (see Section 10.1.7), raccoons and rats (and possibly cats and most other mammals) would contrast with anthropoid primates by locating the first stage of higher-order processing anterior to SI input in the heterogeneous–dysgranular zone, where anthropoids locate it posterior to SI input in cytoarchitectonic areas 1 and 2. This alliance of raccoons with cats and rodents in opposition to primates contrasts with the relations seen in several other aspects of the somatic sensory pathway where raccoons are like monkeys and unlike cats and other mammals (Johnson, 1985). The correspondences of raccoon and monkey brains appear to be due to convergence associated with similar evolved behavior patterns; the contrasts between raccoons and monkeys may reflect phylogeny.

Consistent with the massive extent of SI, the usual demarcating sulci (interbrachial, jugular, and central) are supplemented by additional grooves demarcating projection regions. Cytoarchitectionically, the large raccoon SI does not present distinguishing features, the only peculiarity being difficulty of separating layers 3 and 4 because of intermingling of cell types in these layers (Johnson *et al.*, 1982c).

The thalamocortical connections of readily identifiable subdivisions in SI and VPL make raccoons subjects of choice in analyzing relationships between these regions. The limited observations of PO projections place raccoons for the moment in support of the idea of PO projecting to SI in all mammals.

11.3. Other Carnivores

Other carnivores have been subjects of occasional studies of somatic sensory cortex. These include some other available members of the raccoons' family Procyonidae, and dogs, fur seals, and ferrets.

11.3.1. Procyonids

To examine possible phylogenetic factors in the genesis of the expansion and elaboration of somatic sensory cortex in raccoons, SI was mapped in several members of the family Procyonidae, to which raccoons belong (W. Welker and Campos, 1963) (Fig. 27). Lesser pandas (*Ailurus fulgens*), ringtailed cats (*Bassariscus astutus*), and kinkajous (*Potos flavus*) all showed a more conservative SI organized similar to that in cats, with jugular and interbrachial sulci between representations of head and forelimb, and fore- and hindlimbs, respectively; in ringtailed cats the interbrachial sulcus also bounded a portion of SI anteriorly and probably is a central sulcus analogue like the postcruciate dimple or sulcus seen in some cats (*Felix catus*). Coati mundis (*Nasua nasua*) show all of these features, but in addition there is a greatly expanded representation of the glabrous surface of the nose, including a narial sulcus marking the representation of the nostril, like that of wombats (Section 3.2) and pigs (Section 12.1).

Coati mundis use the nose as an exploring and manipulating organ, much as raccoons use the hand. In each species the somatic sensory cortex has expanded and gyrated in correspondence with this behavioral use of the tactile surface.

11.3.2. Dogs

In view of their long use as experimental subjects, the sparsity of studies of dog sensory cortex is surprising. An early mapping study (Pinto Hamuy *et al.*, 1956) found SI and SII in the usual locations (Fig. 28) in the carnivores previously considered. SI showed no specialized features, organized very similarly to that of cats and the conservative procyonids (all but raccoon and coati mundi, Fig. 27) with a jugular sulcus between head and forelimb representations, and a postcruciate dimple or sulcus in the position of interbrachial and partial central sulci. Projections from bilateral and ipsilateral receptive fields inside the mouth were found at the anteriormost edge of the face representation in SI, just anterior to contralateral projections from the mouth.

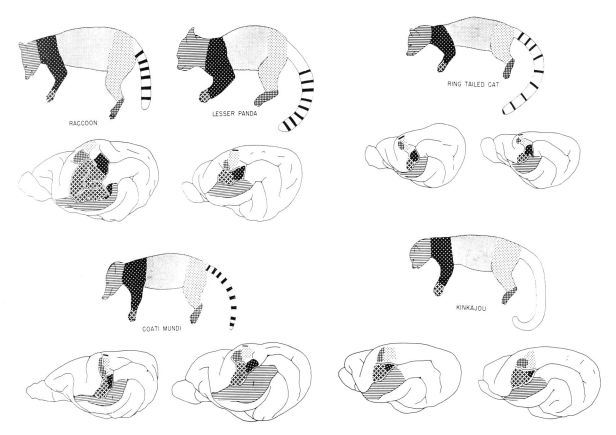

Figure 27. Projections from body parts to SI cortex in five members of the family Procyonidae (from W. Welker and Campos, 1963, with alterations, and permission from W. Welker and Alan R. Liss, Inc.). The "standard" pattern common to most carnivores (and seen here in ringtailed cat, kinkajou, and lesser panda) has been markedly altered by expanded and gyrated representations of the hand in raccoons and of the nose in coati mundis. The sulcus (a narial sulcus) in the center of the face region in coati mundi cortex denotes the position of the nostril in the representation of the glabrous nose. All species show sulci separating representations: hand from face (jugular) and forelimb from hindlimb (interbrachial).

In the most recent and detailed study in a long history of investigations of the motor cortex of dogs (beginning with the discovery of motor cortex itself, reviewed by Breazile and Thompson, 1967), Gorska (1974) reported that primary motor (MI, Fig. 28) directly adjoined but did not overlap SI, at least in the postcranial representations of SI and MI. Gorska did not study face motor regions. A face motor region was described in the face representation of SI (Breazile and Thompson, 1967), but this study did not discriminate between the low-threshold motor responses of MI and the higher-threshold motor responses characteristic of all SI (Gorska, 1974).

Retrograde degeneration studies of thalamocortical projections to SI, SII and motor cortex of dogs showed not only expected projections from VL to motor cortex and VPL to SI and SII, but also some projections from VL to SI and from VPL to motor cortex (Sych, 1976, 1977). Conclusions about sensory–motor overlap in dogs must therefore await further study directed specifically at this problem.

A second auditory region (AII), which receives projections from the medial geniculate of the thalamus, is near and may adjoin SII (Tunturi, 1944, 1970). SII itself was reported as a third auditory area, but without projections from the medial geniculate (Tunturi, 1945, 1970).

As in cats a band of association cortex separates somatic sensory (and auditory) regions from visual cortex (Fig. 28).

11.3.3. Northern Fur Seals

Sensory cortex has been mapped in the Northern fur seal *Callorhinus ursinus* (Ladygina *et al.*, 1985). The most remarkable feature is the large specialized representation of facial vibrissae (Fig. 28). The medial limb of the coronal sulcus forms a substantial jugular sulcus, with much of the forelimb representation in its anteromedial wall. Another sulcus between the postcruciate and the coronal may represent an interbrachial sulcus medially and portion of a central sulcus laterally. As in other carnivores the ansate sulcus marks a posterior boundary of the SI representation of the postcranial body.

11.3.4. Ferrets

In one of his early mapping studies (notable in their accuracy as judged from findings of later experiments), Adrian (1943) located somatic sensory cortex in a ferret (Fig. 28). Projections are organized as in cats and dogs, with the ansate and coronal (jugular) sulci in the usual boundary locations and a postcruciate dimple located so as to serve as a central and interbrachial sulcus analogue. (Adrian designated the species *Putorius foetidus*, a little-used name now discarded in favor of *Mustela putorius*.)

12. Artiodactyls

The last branch from the starburst node on the tree of Fig. 1 leads to another point of multiple branches, indicating a group of orders thought to have some closer relation to one another than to the other orders just reviewed. These

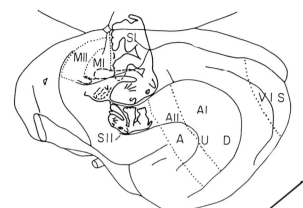

DOG
Canis familiaris

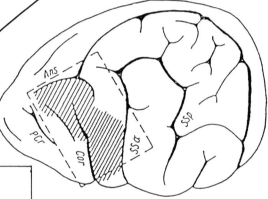

NORTHERN FUR SEAL
Callorhinus ursinus

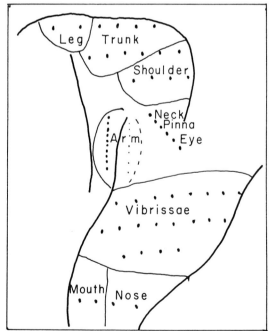

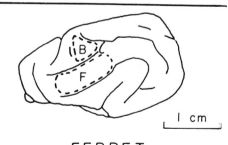

FERRET
Mustela putorius

include the hoofed artiodactyls and perissodactyls; three still more closely related orders grouped under the name *paenungulates:* Hyracoidea, Sirenia, and Proboscidea; and finally the aquatic Cetacea. Studies of sensory cortex in all of these groups are rare; most is known of these regions in the Artiodactyla.

Like bats, cetaceans, and sirenians, artiodactyls (the even-toed hoofed mammals) represent something of an extreme in bodily specialization. Members of the order can be arranged into a series showing ever-increasing specialization for (1) cursorial digitigrade locomotion, and (2) utilization of plant structural carbohydrate as an energy source with consequent alterations in dentition and chambering of the stomach (Eisenberg, 1981, p. 194). Three major suborders have been recognized which show increasing degrees of these specializations, reflected in some interesting increasing specializations in sensory cortex. Somatic sensory cortex has been mapped in detail in representatives of each of the suborders: pigs (the most conservative suborder, Suiformes), llamas (suborder Tylopoda), and sheep (the most specialized suborder, Ruminantia). Some partial maps of goats confirm findings in sheep; goats and sheep are in the same family and subfamily within Ruminantia.

12.1. Pigs

Early sensory maps of pig cortex were published by Adrian (1943) and C. Woolsey and Fairman (1946) who used 5- to 8-month-old pigs. A recent detailed study used neonatal pigs (Craner, 1988; Ray and Craner, 1988). Considering

---

Figure 28. *Top:* The general arrangement of SI and SII representations in the dog (from Pinto Hamuy *et al.*, 1956, with permission from T. Pinto Hamuy and the American Physiological Society), showing also the relative positions of motor (MI and MII; Gorska, 1974), visual (Popova, 1968), and auditory (Tunturi, 1944, 1945) regions. An additional auditory region was found within SII (Tunturi, 1945; Pinto Hamuy *et al.*, 1956) but did not have direct projections from the medial geniculate as did the auditory regions shown here (Tunturi, 1970). In SI the dashed outlines of mandible, tongue, and radial forepaw represent projections to the banks of the coronal sulcus (which here forms a jugular sulcus); they do not extend into limb and trunk regions of MI and MII. The projections on the anteriormost part of the SI face representation were from bilateral and ipsilateral receptive fields on the palate and upper teeth. A jugular (the coronal) sulcus lies between face and forelimb representations in SI; and a small postcruciate sulcus does double duty as a small central sulcus between SI and MI and as an interbrachial sulcus between hand and foot representations in SI.

Center: Organization of somatic sensory projections recorded in the northern fur seal (from Ladygina *et al.*, 1985, with permission from Plenum Press and Naukova Dumka, Publishers of Akademiya Nauk Ukrainskoi S.S.R.). Again an arm of the coronal sulcus serves as a jugular sulcus; much of the representation of the arm lies on the medial bank of the sulcus, indicated here by small dots within the dashed line representing the obscured surface of the medial bank. The dominant representation is that of the facial (mystacial) vibrissae. Sulci: Ans, ansate; Cor, coronal; PCr, postcruciate; SSa, anterior suprasylvian; SSp, posterior suprasylvian. As in cats and raccoons, the ansate sulcus forms a posterior boundary for SI. The unlabeled sulcus between PCr and Cor may represent the interbrachial medially and portion of a central sulcus laterally, corresponding to the postcruciate dimple or sulcus of cats and dogs and the medial central and interbrachial sulci of raccoons.

Lower right: Results from an early and brief mapping study of ferret (from Adrian, 1943, with alterations, and permission from Oxford University Press) showing representations of face (F) and postcranial body (B) located similarly to those in cats, dogs, and conservative procyonids. Again the coronal sulcus serves as a jugular sulcus between face and limb projections, the ansate sulcus lies posterior to the postcranial projections, and a postcruciate dimple is appropriately situated for a central sulcus analogue.

differences in methodology over almost 5 decades, the findings of all these studies are in remarkable agreement.

Sensory Projections

SI. Pigs (Fig. 29) show the most extreme case of domination of SI by projections from nose, complete with a large narial sulcus (see Sections 3.2.3 and 11.3.1 on wombats and coatis) (Adrian, 1943; C. Woolsey and Fairman, 1946; Craner, 1988). This large expanse of nose-related cortex has regions, easily identified by casual observation, that contain abundant known projections from specific peripheral receptive fields, like that of the hand representation in raccoon SI. This nose region in pigs should afford an excellent opportunity for detailed study of cortical sensory organization, particularly since the receptive fields themselves are on a large flat surface. (Miniature pig varieties have been developed for

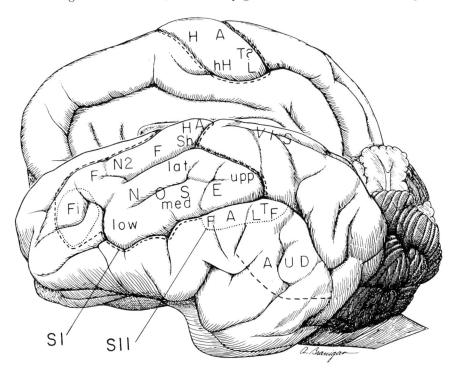

Figure 29. Locations of somatic sensory projections to SI and SII of young (Craner, 1988; Ray and Craner, 1988) and adult (Adrian, 1943; C. Woolsey and Fairman, 1946) pigs (*Sus scrofa*). The left hemisphere is depicted, revealing both the lateral surface and the mesial surface as it would be reflected in a mirror. Anterior is to the left. (Reproduced from Craner, 1988, with alterations and permission of Dr. S. L. Craner and the East Carolina University School of Medicine). The general locations of auditory (AUD) and visual (VIS) regions were determined but not mapped in detail (Adrian, 1943; C. Woolsey and Fairman, 1946). Representations in SI and SII are depicted according to Craner (1988), whose findings are in full agreement with, but more extensive than, those of Adrian and Woolsey and Fairman. A, arm (foreleg); F, face; Fi, ipsilateral face; H, fore hoof; hH, hind hoof; L, hind leg; lat (lateral), low (lower), med (median), upp (upper) aspects of the large representation of the flat rostrum of the rhinarium (NOSE), which occupies a large elliptical gyrus around a sulcus that occurs where the nostril is located in the cortical representation (a giant narial sulcus); N2, a second complete representation of the nose in SI; Sh, shoulder; T?, site of occasional few and inconsistent responses to stimulation of the trunk. The face (F) is represented twice in SII, at its anterior and posterior poles.

research: size of subject animals should not be a deterrent to prospective investigators.)

A second representation of the nose within the face representation was described (Craner, 1988; Ray and Craner, 1988).

The early studies did not explore the mesial surface of the hemisphere (Adrian, 1943; C. Woolsey and Fairman, 1946) and so did not find the projections from the trunk and hindlimb, although Woolsey and Fairman predicted they would be found where in fact Craner did find them. They were found with difficulty, however, and Craner (1988) reported special difficulty in locating any projections from the trunk; they were encountered, inconsistently, in relatively few animals. This marks the beginning of a trend (trends have been rare in our survey) to be evident as we further consider artiodactyls, toward elimination of SI representation of postcranial body parts.

Another possible trend also starts in pigs with a substantial representation of the ipsilateral face in SI, although in pigs considered alone the ipsilateral region is not much larger than those seen in carnivores (Section 11.1.1a, Fig. 28) and hyraxes (Section 14, Fig. 33).

SII. Two representations of facial regions were also found in SII (Craner, 1988), one on either side of projections from the trunk and limbs which were in the usual locations for mammalian SII (Fig. 29).

An auditory region was located near and caudolateral to SII (Adrian, 1943; C. Woolsey and Fairman, 1946).

12.2. Llamas

Llamas are representatives of the suborder Tylopoda, more specialized than the conservative pigs (suborder Suiformes) and less specialized than the sheep and goats (of the suborder Ruminantia) to be considered next. Detailed mapping study of SI and SII (W. Welker *et al.*, 1976) showed two features (Fig. 30) reflecting brain specialization which parallels general anatomical and behavioral specializations. The most striking of these is the complete absence of projections from the trunk and limbs in SI. SI consists entirely of a large representation of the face, and most of this is devoted to projections from the mobile grasping lips. The upper lip of llamas is split at the midline, providing them with three fingerlike manipulatory organs (two upper and one lower independently mobile lips).

The dominance of lip projections, and the absence of postcranial projections to llama SI brings to mind the "disappearing" trunk and hindlimb projections of pigs along with an expanded representation of an exploring nose; in llamas trunk and both limb representations have completely "disappeared" in favor of an expanded representation of exploring and manipulating lips.

Llama SI shows an intermediate stage in expansion of the ipsilateral face representation in SI; it is larger than that seen in pigs, though much smaller than that of sheep and goats.

In contrast to SI, a complete representation of the body was found in llama SII. This representation was judged to be SII because of its position in relation to SI and auditory cortex and the orientation of the projections with the limbs pointing caudolaterally.

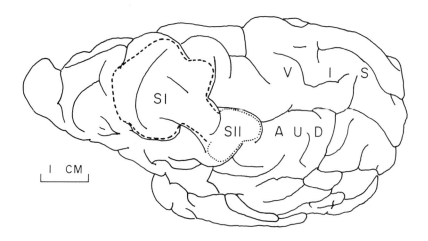

LLAMA
Lama glama

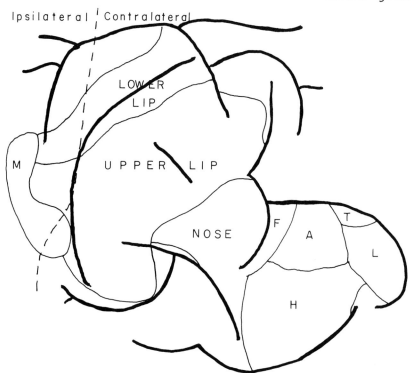

Figure 30. Location and organization of somatic sensory projections to cerebral cortex of llama (from W. Welker *et al.*, 1976, with alterations, and permission from W. I. Welker and S. Karger AG, Basel).

Above: Dorsolateral view of left hemisphere showing locations of SI and SII, and the general location of auditory (AUD) and visual (VIS) regions which were not mapped in detail.

Below: Organization of projections in SI and SII. A, arm (foreleg); F, face; H, forehoof; L, hindlimb; M, mouth (intraoral teeth, palate, and tongue). All projections to SI were from the mouth and the front of the face; the dominant representation is that of the mobile, grasping lips. All body surfaces were represented in SII.

Sheep show a culmination of both trends seen among artiodactyls in the organization of projections to SI (Fig. 31). First, as in llamas, there are no projections from the postcranial body evident in SI (projections from the trunk and hindlimbs were difficult to find in pigs). Second, the proportion of ipsilateral projections in SI has grown (they were substantial in pigs and llamas) to dominate SI: most projections are from ipsilateral receptive fields. These receptive fields are of course all on the face, largely on the lips and nose, used presumably for exploration and selection of foods for grazing.

SII in contrast has a complete representation of the body, mostly from contralateral surfaces, as in llamas.

Adrian's early maps of sensory projections in goats show all the features later reported in sheep (Adrian, 1943; C. Woolsey and Fairman, 1946; Johnson *et al.*, 1974).

SI and SII are located in sensory-type cytoarchitectonic cortex (see Dinopoulos *et al.*, 1985, for review). Both receive projections from the VP thalamic nucleus, with an interesting difference. SI is connected only with VPM, as might be expected since only face is represented in SI. SII does have connections with the small VPL (Dinopoulos *et al.*, 1985); connectivity with VPM was not analyzed. VPM and VPL show the same proportions of ipsilateral and contralateral representations as do SI and SII (Cabral and Johnson, 1971).

Just medial to SI is motor cortex (Fig. 31) as determined electrophysiologically (Simpson and King, 1911) and cytoarchitectonically (King, 1911). Motor cortex is connected with VL and not VPM; SI does not receive projections from VPM or VPL (Dinopoulos *et al.*, 1985). Sensory–motor overlap is not evident in sheep.

Judged by incomplete recording studies (Adrian, 1943; C. Woolsey and Fairman, 1946) and projections from visual, auditory, somatic sensory, and VL thalamic nuclei (Dinopoulos *et al.*, 1985), the primary sensory and motor regions in sheep and goats appear to be closely juxtaposed much as they are in animals with much smaller brains (e.g., spiny anteaters, hedgehogs, rabbits, rats). Lacking are the belts of association cortex seen in large-brained primates and carnivores (and smaller-brained sloths and tree shrews).

13. Perissodactyls

The perissodactyls are another group of specialized grazing animals, less numerous and less specialized than the artiodactyls. Among the perissodactyls the horse family became cursorial specialists, developing hooves with odd numbers of toes in contrast to the even-numbered toes of the hooves of the artiodactyls.

The domestic horse *Equus caballus* (or more precisely, the Shetland pony) is the only perissodactyl whose somatic sensory cortex has been investigated, and this was again by Adrian (1943). He found an elaborate representation of the skin around the nostril, and a representation of the limbs, both being projections from contralateral receptive fields (Fig. 32). A motor cortex was located medial to these sensory representations (Breazile *et al.*, 1966).

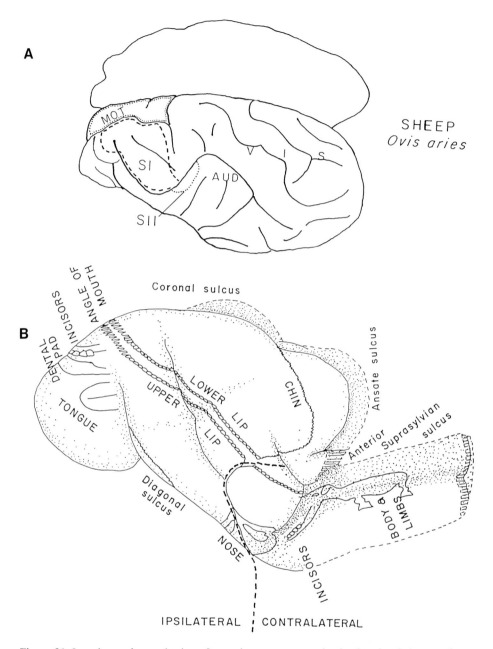

Figure 31. Location and organization of somatic sensory cortex in closely related sheep and goats.

Sheep. (A) Dorsolateral view of the left hemisphere of a sheep, anterior to the left, showing the location of SI and SII, and the general (but unmapped) locations of auditory (AUD) and visual (VIS) regions (Adrian, 1943; C. Woolsey and Fairman, 1946; Johnson *et al.*, 1974) and their relation to motor cortex (MOT) (Simpson and King, 1911; King, 1911).

(B) Details of projections to SI and SII of sheep (from Johnson *et al.*, 1974, with alterations, and permission from Alan R. Liss, Inc.). The sensory region is shown as if dissected free from the rest of the hemisphere, with the anterior suprasylvian sulcus spread open to reveal SII on its lateral bank. As in the llama, all projections to SI are from the front of the face, but in sheep the greater proportion of these are from ipsilateral receptive fields. All body parts are represented in SII, and projections to SII are almost all contralateral.

The next line leading from the secondary manifold node on the tree of Fig. 1 is that leading to the three related orders of paenungulates: the Hyracoidea (hyraxes), the Proboscidea (elephants), and the aquatic Sirenia (manatees and dugongs). Understandably but regrettably, considering their flamboyant bodily and behavioral specializations, the sensory cortices of elephants and sirenians remain unstudied.

The most conservative of these orders is that of the hyraxes, and one hyrax species, *Procavia capensis*, was the subject of a sensory cortical mapping study (W. Welker and Carlson, 1976). They found a conservative mammalian organization of SI (Fig. 33), with two features of interest: a substantial representation of

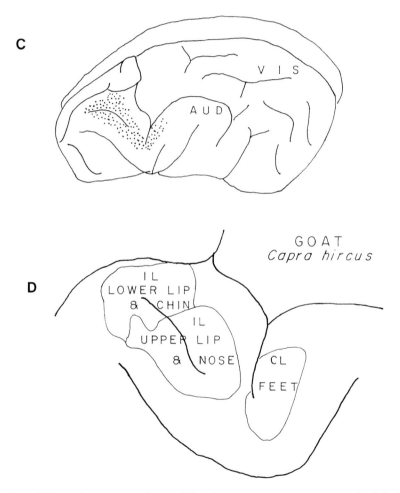

Goat. (C) Dorsolateral view of the left hemisphere of a goat, anterior to the left, showing the location of somatic sensory (stippled), auditory (AUD), and visual (VIS) projections found in the early mapping study of Adrian (1943).

(D) Details of the somatic sensory projections in goats. As in sheep, most projections were from the ipsilateral lips, chin, and nose; those from the limbs were contralateral and probably correspond to SII of sheep and llamas (from Adrian, 1943, with alterations, and permission from Oxford University Press).

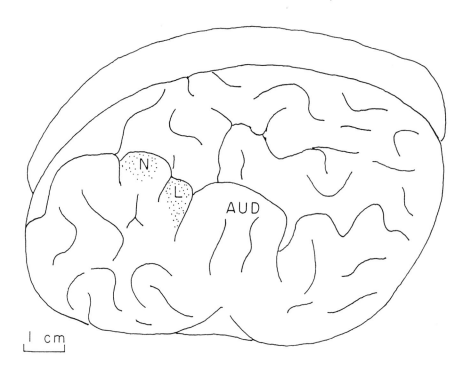

1 cm

HORSE
Equus caballus

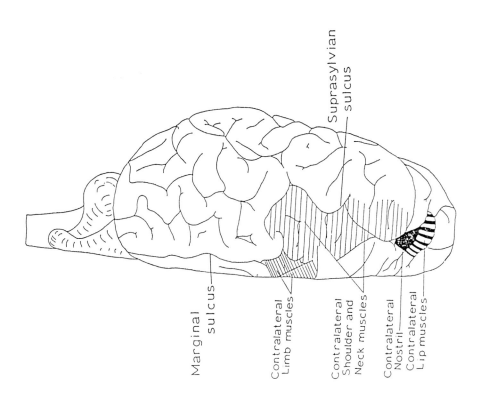

Marginal sulcus

Contralateral Limb muscles

Suprasylvian sulcus

Contralateral Shoulder and Neck muscles

Contralateral Nostril

Contralateral Lip muscles

ipsilateral mouth parts (as have many of their neighbors on the tree of Fig. 1); and an abdomen-forward representation of the trunk in SI, lending support to this arrangement as the basic or primitive sequence if indeed the variation in trunk representations is at all phylogenetic in origin. (Our final lineup, for now, is thus: abdomen-forward in spiny anteaters, squirrel and cebus monkeys, rabbits, and hyraxes; abdomen-rear in owl and macaque monkeys, cats, and gray squirrels.)

15. Cetaceans

Cetaceans, the whales and dolphins, are completely adapted for aquatic existence, and are an extreme of mammalian specialization, at the farthest branch of the tree of Fig. 1.

Partial mapping studies of the bottlenose dolphin *Tursiops truncatus* revealed a somatosensory area at the rostral aspect of the brain (Fig. 34) (Lende and Welker, 1972; Ladygina *et al.*, 1978). Responses were to delicate mechanical stimulation of bilateral fields on the face and head. Lende and Welker believed these might be auditory, but Ladygina *et al.* reported a separate auditory area caudal to this somatosensory area, which lies adjacent to a motor region (Lende and Akdikmen, 1968). According to the summary figures from these studies (Fig. 34), visual, auditory, somatosensory, and motor areas lie adjacent to one another with no intervening association cortex. There is, however, abundant cortex lying outside this primary sensory–motor region. On the basis of these preliminary studies, these dolphins (and by extension in the absence of data from other species, all cetaceans) may be regarded as having a cortex organized like the artiodactyls and many smaller-brained mammals in that primary sensory and motor areas are directly adjacent to one another.

16. Discussion: Constancies, Variations, and Trends in the Organization of Somatic Sensory Cortex

A first general finding, from the survey of mammalian somatic sensory cortices just completed, is that a great many features are constant across all mammals, from platypus to monkey, rat, cat, and sheep. Variations from the standard pattern occur here and there, but are usually peculiarities (of adaptation or accident) that are restricted to a single species. General trends seen across large groups of animals are extremely rare, as are serial progressive changes.

Figure 32. Sensory and motor regions reported for horses, shown in left hemispheres, anterior to the left.

Above: As seen in a dorsolateral view, the locations of somatic sensory projections from contralateral nostril (N) and limbs (L), and of the auditory region (AUD) (from Adrian, 1943, with alterations, and permission from Oxford University Press).

Below: As seen in a dorsal view, motor cortex in horse (reproduced from Breazile *et al.*, 1966, with permission from J. E. Breazile and the *American Journal of Veterinary Research*). The motor regions were reported to be all medial to Adrian's sensory regions. The differences in the published sketches of the horse brain preclude precise rendition of the relations between the sensory and motor regions.

16.1. Sensory Projections

16.1.1. SI

16.1.1a. Constancies. As a first constancy of sensory projections to cortex, all mammals have a somatotopically organized set of projections from at least those parts of the body surface used in exploratory and manipulative behaviors. These projections, mostly from cutaneous receptors, form a representation of the sensory surface in the cortex. In the representation, a larger volume is represented by peripheral regions with dense innervation; and in these regions the receptive fields of activated units are smaller.

Second, there is a common general ordering of the representation of the body formed by the projections to the primary sensory cortex (SI): hindlimb projections are medial and cranial projections arrive more laterally in the cortical mantle.

Third, at the anterior edge of the largely cutaneous representation of the body, there is a specialized cortical sensory region receiving input from deeper-lying subcutaneous tissue, largely from muscle stretch receptors.

16.1.1b. Variations. Variant features include multiplication of representations of certain body parts in the SI cortical region: we have seen double representations of vibrissae in opossums; upper lips in diprotodont marsupials; hands in lorises, rats, and squirrels; and the nose in pigs. Other variations include the pointing backwards of the digits in the cortical representation in bats, and the oscillating position of the representation of the ventral midline along the abdomen (at the front of the representation in spiny anteaters, cebus and squirrel

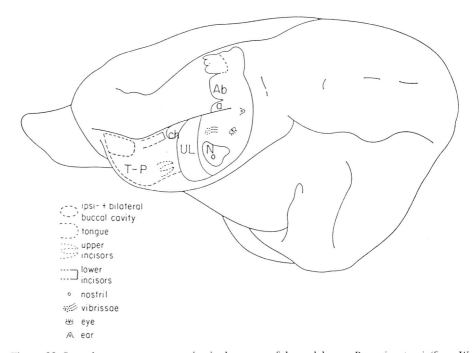

Figure 33. Somatic sensory representation in the cortex of the rock hyrax, *Procavia capensis* (from W. Welker and Carlson, 1976, with alterations, and permission from W. I. Welker and S. Karger (AG, Basel). a, arm (forelimb); Ab, abdomen; ch, chin; N, nose (glabrous surface of the rhinarium); T-P, teeth and palate; UL, upper lip.

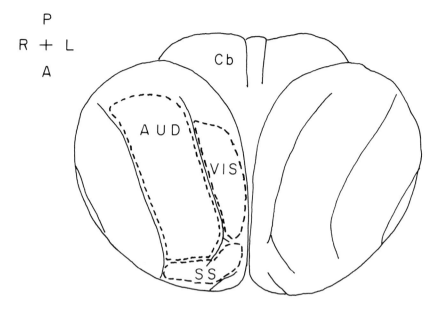

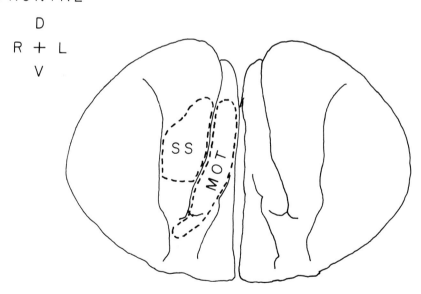

Figure 34. Sketches of sensory and motor regions in the brain of bottlenose dolphin *Tursiops truncatus*. A, anterior; Cb, cerebellum; D, dorsal; L, left; R, right; P, posterior; V, ventral.

Above: Dorsal view of cerebrum, caudal toward the top, showing somatosensory (SS), auditory (AUD), and visual (VIS) regions (redrawn from data presented in Ladygina *et al.*, 1978).

Below: Frontal view of cerebrum showing somatosensory (SS) and motor (MOT) regions (from Lende and Welker, 1972, with alterations, and permission from W. I. Welker and Elsevier Science Publishers BV).

monkeys, rabbits, and hyraxes; at the rear in owl and macaque monkeys, squirrels, and cats). The function of these individual and species-specific variations has remained entirely speculative.

16.1.1c. Trends. One trend observed in the organization of SI is the progressive loss of postcranial projections in the cortex of progressively more specialized artiodactyls. As species became more cursorial, we can speculate that the exploratory–manipulative function of the trunk and limbs was downgraded, relegated to SII or transferred to facial receptors projecting to SI, the limbs becoming specialized as more strictly locomotor organs. A second trend in the artiodactyls, toward increased ipsilateral components of SI projections, defies functional explanation.

Another group-variant phenomenon is the multiplication of the representation of the whole body surface in the anthropoid primates (all monkeys studied except marmosets). This may be related to another general feature, the relay of information from a central thalamo-recipient core of SI to surrounding regions for processing. As suggested by Chapin *et al.* (Section 10.1.7), this may be a common feature of mammals, but is organized differently in the granular-to-dysgranular progression of rats, mice, and squirrels; the gyral-to-sulcal progression of raccoons; and the area 3b-to-area 1 and 2 progression involving, and perhaps creating, the multiple representations seen in monkeys.

16.1.2. Additional Somatic Sensory Regions

A major variation is the absence of SII in the prototherian monotremes, contrasting with its constant presence in all the therian mammals both marsupial and placental. In these animals, SII is remarkably consistent, adjacent to SI with a distorted mirror image of the SI projections, with the images meeting at the representations of the top of the head. Even when most of the body is missing in the SI projection in artiodactyls, the SII representation is complete and in its standard location and orientation.

A possible trend is the recently described "dependence" of SII upon SI in monkeys (a "serial" processing order) in contrast to the independence of SII seen in tree shrews, rabbits, and cats ("parallel" processing) (Sections 7.1, 8.2.1b, 8.2.7, 9.1.1, 11.1.1). The effect of anesthetics upon this dependence needs to be determined, as do other factors which would prevent the response of monkey SII to stimulation despite the presence of connections from the periphery.

Numbers of additional somatic sensory cortical representations beyond SI and SII that have been reported range from 0 in mice and 1 in squirrels to 3 or more in cats and monkeys. Some of these may turn out to be counterparts of one another, perhaps cat SIV with macaque Ri and owl monkey VS, and cat SIII with monkey area 5 as has been discussed above (Section 11.1.7). The VP of squirrels has so far defied comparison with additional regions seen in other species.

16.2. Relation to Other Areas

As a constancy, SI (and SII adjoining it in the therians) has two consistent neighbors: a motor region next to SI anteriorly, and an auditory region close to SI or SII posteriorly.

As a first variation, there is a variable amount of "association" cortex intervening between the visual cortex and the somatic-sensory-and-auditory array.

There is little or none in monotremes, marsupials, edentate armadillos, insectivores, rabbits, rodent mice and rats and hystricomorphs, in dolphins nor apparently in the artiodactyls. A substantial band of association cortex is seen here in edentate sloths, and in tree shrews, in primates, in rodent squirrels, and in carnivores. This perhaps surprising array precludes thinking of parietal association cortex as a standard consequence of increasing brain size. It seems, rather, to have something to do with the use of limbs as information-gathering and manipulating organs. This somewhat unexpected (to me, anyway) conclusion is forced by the recognition that this feature is all that connects the diverse species showing the association region and divides them from the even more diverse species lacking it.

There are even more problems explaining the next relational variation: the variable amount of overlap between SI and motor cortex. Well-documented sensory–motor overlap, judged by cortical stimulation and recording, and more securely by overlapping thalamic projections from VP and VL thalamic nuclei, is complete in opossums, and occurs in limb representations in brushtail possums and rats and mice. Overlap does not occur in monkeys, cats, or sheep. More detailed investigation directed to this specific question is needed to securely determine the presence or absence of overlap in other species. As speculative explanation, none better has appeared, however unsatisfactory it may seem at first glance, than that of Akers and Killackey (Section 10.1.7), that overlap occurs in small crowded brains. Study of this problem in small prosimians and tree shrews would be a good first test of this proposition.

16.3. Structure

A chief commonality is in the architecture of the thalamic-input portion of SI (SI proper, or true SI). This region is marked by a greater packing density of small cells in layer 4 (making it "koniocortex"), and along with this there is a greater density of myelinated fibers leading into layer 4 from subjacent layers, and a greater concentration of activity-related enzymes in layer 4 (see for example and review Cusick *et al.*, 1989). These features are distributed in SI cortex according to the somatotopic pattern of incoming projections, such that images of the body surface can be seen with appropriate stains (Fig. 20). The gaps in cytoarchitectural continuity (cell packing, myelin density, enzyme concentration) occasioned by space between representations of body parts (e.g., head, limbs, tail) are also the site of sulci in gyrencephalic species. It is not yet clear whether just another case of koniocortex with interruptions is represented by the barrels seen in a diverse array of species: mice, rats, and many other small rodents, some diprotodont marsupials, rabbits, and the mysterious colugo (Johnson *et al.*, 1982b) or flying lemur (placed by itself in the order Dermoptera which we have not mentioned heretofore). The barreled species all use vibrissae as an important information-gathering system, but many other animals with such use do not show barrels, e.g., cats, seals, some large rodents, and opossums.

16.4. Thalamic Connectivity

The chief constancy here is orderly connectivity of SI with the VP (VPL and VPM) thalamic nuclei. Related regions of the thalamic reticular nucleus and sparse projections from the intralaminar CL nucleus also appear to be a common feature. Projections of some sort from thalamic PO, more pronounced in the dysgranular–sulcal–surround regions in or near SI, may turn out to be another.

Projections to SII from thalamus are still not well enough known in a sufficient number of species to draw broad conclusions. Projections to SII from VP are common, as are those from PO. The primate and raccoon feature of VPI projections to SII may be another convergent characteristic related to hand use. Projections from some part of PO to the additional sensory regions beyond SI and SII are frequent. Mice show medial geniculate projections to the part of SII that responds to auditory stimuli; this variant may be more widespread.

16.5. Corticocortical Connections

16.5.1. Ipsilateral

The constant feature is that SI, SII, and motor cortex of one hemisphere all have reciprocal and somatotopic connections with one another. When additional somatic sensory areas are present, they generally participate in similar reciprocal and homotopic interarea connectivity.

Variations are seen in the detailed routes of connectivity, particularly from the thalamic-recipient core (TRC) zone of SI.

In monkeys this TRC zone is area 3b, which communicates with motor cortex only indirectly, via connections through areas 1 and 2. In raccoons, the TRC zone is gyral cortex, which also communicates with motor cortex mainly indirectly, through connections in sulcal cortex. In rats, the TRC zone is granular cortex, which is reported to project directly to motor cortex, although careful study of the relative contributions of granular and dysgranular cortex to the projection to motor cortex may reveal a closer parallel to the case in monkeys and raccoons.

The TRC granular cortex in rats projects directly to SII, but the projections back to SI from SII go to dysgranular cortex. In raccoons, communications between the TRC granular cortex and SII are indirect, via sulcal cortex, in both directions. In monkeys projections are directly from TRC area 3b to and from SII.

A distinct TRC subarea has not been described in cats, and projections to and from motor cortex and SII seem to be direct.

These apparent interspecies variations in connectivity are derived from a large number of very different experiments of questionable comparability. Directly comparable studies, in the same laboratory using the same methods, will contribute greatly to securely establishing the fact of variations, and some explanation of why and how they occur. Meaningful speculations about general trends and functional significance may then be possible.

Another constancy in ipsilateral corticocortical connectivity is the general concentration of cells of origin of these connections in or near layer 3. Terminals are found in all layers, but a possible consistent variation is seen in the degree to which they avoid layer 4 in SI. Such avoidance was reported in rats and mice, in contrast to cats, monkeys, and brushtail possums. Akers and Killackey (1978) suggested this may be another feature of small crowded brains.

16.5.2. Commissural

Commissural connections also originate largely from cells of layer 3 and sometimes neighboring layer 2, with a lesser concentration of cells of origin in layers 5 and 6; this seems to be a constant mammalian feature. Terminals of commissural connections again avoid layer 4 in rats and mice, and in opossums and rabbits as well; but they do not, again, in cats, monkeys, and brushtail possums.

Pronounced variations are seen in regions of SI and SII that have greater and lesser amounts of commissural connections, which are reciprocal and somatotopic whatever their relative density, with their counterparts in the contralateral hemisphere. Representations of the limb extremities have few or no commissural connections in opossums, brushtail possums, tree shrews, monkeys, rats, mice, squirrels, cats, and raccoons. But in rabbits these regions are well-connected commissurally: rabbits may have minimal use of extremities as lateralized sources of information. (They are grazing animals, as are the artiodactyls which seem to have given up extremities completely as sources of information for SI.) Rabbits instead have as noncommissurally connected regions the representations of the lateral vibrissae; also commissure-free are the vibrissae regions of squirrels, rats, and mice, probably because they all use vibrissae as lateralized information sources.

One major trend is seen in the route of commissural connections. In the monotremes and polyprotodont (all American and some Australian) marsupials, all commissural connections are via the anterior commissure. In Australian diprotodont marsupials, commissural fibers from more dorsal regions, including mediodorsal portions of SI, travel instead in the fasciculus aberrans. And in placentals most commissural fibers are in the corpus callosum, only a few from ventrolateral cortex remain in the anterior commissure, and these last include few if any fibers from somatic sensory regions.

16.6. Other Connections

Many of the connections, of somatic sensory cortical regions with extracortical structures, that have been seen are probably not only constant features across mammals, but also are probably general features of all neocortex. These include reciprocal connections with the claustrum, and projections to the corpus striatum, and will probably be found to include projections received from the basal forebrain, locus coeruleus, dorsal raphe nuclei of the brain stem although these last three have not commonly been reported in studies of somatic sensory cortex. No consistent interspecies differences have been documented for projections from sensory cortex to superior colliculi, pontine nuclei, and other brainstem structures. Projections from limb representation regions to cuneate and gracile nuclei, and from face representations to trigeminal nuclei also seem to be constant features across species. Somatic sensory cortex is an important source of corticospinal fibers, and these vary among species in the rostral-to-caudal spinal levels in which they terminate. In some species they are restricted to cervical or to cervical and thoracic levels; in other species they are found at all levels. This variation is a feature, however, of the whole corticospinal tract, not just that part arising from somatic sensory cortex. In summary, no consistent variations among different groups of mammals have as yet been demonstrated in the extracortical connections of specifically the somatic sensory cortex.

ACKNOWLEDGMENT. Supported by NSF Grant BSR 85-03687.

17. References

Adey, W. R., and Kerr, D. I. B., 1954, The cerebral representation of deep somatic sensibility in the marsupial phalanger and the rabbit: An evoked potential and histological study, *J. Comp. Neurol.* **100:**597–625.

Adrian, E. D., 1941, Afferent discharges to the cerebral cortex from peripheral sense organs, *J. Physiol. (London)* **100:**159–191.

Adrian, E. D., 1943, Afferent areas in the brain of ungulates, *Brain* **66:**89–103.

Aitkin, L. M., Merzenich, M. M., Irvine, D. R. F., Clarey, J. F., and Nelson, J. E., 1986, Frequency representation in auditory cortex of the common marmoset (*Callithrix jacchus jacchus*), *J. Comp. Neurol.* **252:**175–185.

Akers, R. M., and Killackey, H. P., 1978, Organization of corticocortical connections in the parietal cortex of the rat, *J. Comp. Neurol.* **181:**513–538.

Allison, T., and Goff, W. R., 1972, Electrophysiological studies of the echidna, *Tachyglossus aculeatus.* III. Sensory and interhemispheric evoked responses, *Arch. Ital. Biol.* **110:**195–216.

Allison, T. A., and Van Twyver, H., 1970, Sensory representation in the neocortex of the mole, *Scalopus aquaticus, Exp. Neurol.* **27:**554–563.

Allison, T., McCarthy, G., Wood, C.C., Darcey, T. M., Spencer, D. D., and Williamson, P. D., 1989, Human cortical potentials evoked by stimulation of the median nerve. I. Cytoarchitectonic areas generating short-latency activity, *J. Neurophysiol.* **62:**694–710.

Alloway, K. D., and Burton, H., 1985, Homotypical ipsilateral cortical projections between somatosensory areas I and II in the cat, *Neuroscience* **14:**15–35.

Asuncion-Moran, M., and Reinoso-Suarez, F., 1988, Topographical organization of the thalamic afferent connections to the motor cortex in the cat, *J. Comp. Neurol.* **270:**64–85.

Avendaño, C., Rausell, E., Perez-Aguilar, D., and Isorna, S., 1988, Organization of the association cortical afferent connections of area 5: A retrograde tracer study in the cat, *J. Comp. Neurol.* **278:**1–33.

Barbaresi, P., Conti, F., and Manzoni, T., 1984, Topography and receptive field organization of the body midline representation in the ventrobasal complex of the cat, *Exp. Brain Res.* **54:** 327–336.

Barbaresi, P., Ugolini, G., and Manzoni, T., 1985, Reciprocal callosal connections between the first (SI) and the second (SII) somatosensory areas in the cat, *Neurosci. Lett.* **22**(Suppl.):S464.

Barbaresi, P., Fabri, M., Conti, F., and Manzoni, T., 1987, D-[³H]Aspartate retrograde labelling of callosal and association neurones of somatosensory areas I and II of cats, *J. Comp. Neurol.* **263:**159–178.

Bautista, N. S., and Matzke, H. A., 1965, A degeneration study of the course and extent of the pyramidal tract of the opossum, *J. Comp. Neurol.* **124:**367–376.

Belekhova, M. G., 1979, Neurophysiology of the forebrain, in: *Biology of the Reptilia,* Volume 10, *Neurology B* (R. G. Northcutt, P. Ulinski, and C. Gans, eds.), Academic Press, New York, pp. 287–359.

Bentivoglio, M., Molinari, M., Minciacchi, D., and Macchi, G., 1983, Organization of the cortical projections of the posterior complex and intralaminar nuclei of the thalamus as studied by means of retrograde tracers, in: *Somatosensory Integration in the Thalamus* (G. Macchi, A. Rustioni, and R. Spreafico, eds.), Elsevier, Amsterdam, pp. 338–363.

Bodemer, C. W., and Towe, A. L., 1963, Cortical localization patterns in the somatic sensory cortex of the opossum, *Exp. Neurol.* **8:**380–394.

Bohringer, R. C., 1977, The Somatosensory System of the Platypus (*Ornithorhynchus anatinus*), Ph.D. thesis, University of New South Wales (Anatomy), Kensington.

Bohringer, R. C., and Rowe, M. J., 1977, The organization of sensory and motor areas of cerebral cortex in the platypus (*Ornithorhynchus anatinus*), *J. Comp. Neurol.* **174:**1–14.

Boisacq-Schepens, N., Gerebtzoff, M. A., and Goffart, M., 1977, Sensory projections to the cerebral cortex in *Perodicticus potto edwarsi* (Bouvier), *Primates* **18:**401–416.

Breazile, J. E., and Thompson, W. D., 1967, Motor cortex of the dog, *Am. J. Vet. Res.* **28:**1483–1486.

Breazile, J. E., Swafford, B. C., and Biles, D. R., 1966, Motor cortex of the horse, *Am. J. Vet. Res.* **27:**1605–1609.

Brodal, A., 1981, *Neurological Anatomy in Relation to Clinical Medicine,* 3rd ed., Oxford University Press, London.

Brodmann, K., 1909, *Vergleichende Lokalisationlehre der Grosshirnrinde in ihren Prinzipien dargestellt auf Grund des Zellenbaues,* Barth, Leipzig.

Brugge, J. F., 1982, Auditory cortical areas in primates, in: *Cortical Sensory Organization*, Volume 3 (C. N. Woolsey, ed.), Humana Press, Clifton, N.J., pp. 59–70.

Burton, H., and Carlson, M., 1986, Second somatic sensory cortical area (SII) in a prosimian primate, *Galago crassicaudatus, J. Comp. Neurol.* **247:**200–220.

Burton, H., and Jones, E. G., 1976, The posterior thalamic region and its cortical projection in new world and old world monkeys, *J. Comp. Neurol.* **168:**249–302.

Burton, H., and Kopf, E. M., 1984a, Connections between the thalamus and the somatosensory areas of the anterior ectosylvian gyrus in the cat, *J. Comp. Neurol.* **224:**173–205.

Burton, H., and Kopf, E. M., 1984b, Ipsilateral cortical connections from the second and the fourth somatic sensory areas in the cat, *J. Comp. Neurol.* **225:**527–553.

Burton, H., and Robinson, C. J., 1981, Organization of the SII parietal cortex: Multiple somatic sensory representations within and near the second somatic sensory area of cynomolgus monkeys, in: *Cortical Sensory Organization*, Volume 1 (C. N. Woolsey, ed.), Humana Press, Clifton, N.J., pp. 67–120.

Burton, H., Mitchell, G., and Brent, D., 1982, Second somatic sensory area in the cerebral cortex of cats: Somatotopic organization and cytoarchitecture, *J. Comp. Neurol.* **210:**109–135.

Butler, A. B., 1978, Forebrain connections in lizards and the evolution of sensory systems, in: *Behavior and Neurology of Lizards* (N. Greenberg and P. D. MacLean, eds.), National Institute of Mental Health, Rockville, Md., pp. 65–78.

Cabana, T., and Martin, G. F., 1985, The development of commissural connections of somatic motor–sensory areas of neocortex in the North American opossum, *Anat. Embryol.* **171:**121–128.

Cabral, R. J., and Johnson, J. I., 1971, The organization of mechanoreceptive projections in the ventrobasal thalamus of sheep, *J. Comp. Neurol.* **141:**17–35.

Calford, M. B., Graydon, M. L., Huerta, M. F., Kaas, J. H., and Pettigrew, J. D., 1985, A variant of a mammalian somatotopic map in a bat, *Nature* **313:**477–479.

Caminiti, R., Innocenti, G. M., and Manzoni, T., 1979, Anatomical substrate of the callosal messages from SI and SII in the cat, *Exp. Brain Res.* **35:**295–314.

Campos, G. B., and Welker, W. I., 1976, Comparisons between brains of a large and a small hystricomorph rodent: capybara, *Hydrochoerus* and guinea pig *Cavia;* neocortical projection regions and measurements of brain subdivisions, *Brain Behav. Evol.* **13:**243–266.

Carlson, M., and FitzPatrick, K. A., 1982, Organization of the hand area in the primary somatic sensory cortex (SmI) of the prosimian primate, *Nycticebus coucang, J. Comp. Neurol.* **204:**280–295.

Carlson, M., and Welker, W. I., 1976, Some morphological, physiological and behavioral specializations in North American beavers *(Castor canadensis), Brain Behav. Evol.* **13:**302–326.

Carlson, M., and Welt, C., 1980, Somatic sensory cortex (SmI) of the prosimian primate *Galago crassicaudatus:* Organization of mechanoreceptive input from the hand in relation to cytoarchitecture, *J. Comp. Neurol.* **189:**249–271.

Carlson, M., Huerta, M. F., Cusick, C. G., and Kaas, J. H., 1986, Studies on the evolution of multiple somatosensory representations in primates: The organization of anterior parietal cortex in the new world callitrichid, *Saguinus, J. Comp. Neurol.* **246:**409–426.

Carman, J. B., Cowan, W. M., and Powell, T. P. S., 1963, The organization of cortico-striate connexions in the rabbit, *Brain* **86:**525–562.

Carman, J. B., Cowan, W. M., and Powell, T. P. S., 1964, The cortical projection upon the claustrum, *J. Neurol. Neurosurg. Psychiatry* **27:**46–51.

Carreras, M., and Andersson, S. A., 1962, Functional properties of neurons of the anterior ectosylvian gyrus of the cat, *J. Neurophysiol.* **26:**100–126.

Carvell, G. E., and Simons, D. J., 1986, Somatotopic organization of the second somatosensory area (SII) in the cerebral cortex of the mouse, *Somatosensory Res.* **3:**213–239.

Carvell, G. E., and Simons, D. J., 1987, Thalamic and corticocortical connections of the second somatic sensory area of the mouse, *J. Comp. Neurol.* **265:**409–427.

Chapin, J. K., and Lin, C.-S., 1984, Mapping the body representation in the SI cortex of anesthetized and awake rats, *J. Comp. Neurol.* **229:**199–213.

Chapin, J. K., Sadeq, M., and Guise, J. L. U., 1987, Corticocortical connections within the primary somatosensory cortex of the rat, *J. Comp. Neurol.* **263:**326–346.

Chmielowska, J., Carvell, G. E., and Simons, D. J., 1989, Spatial organization of thalamocortical and corticothalamic projection systems in the rat SmI barrel cortex, *J. Comp. Neurol.* **285:**325–338.

Clemo, H. R., and Stein, B. E., 1983, Organization of a fourth somatosensory area of cortex in cat, *J. Neurophysiol.* **50:**910–925.

Craner, S. L., 1988, A Developmental Analysis of the Organization of the Somatosensory Cortices of the Domestic Pig, Ph.D. Dissertation, Department of Physiology, East Carolina University, Greenville, N.C.

Cusick, C. G., MacAvoy, M. G., and Kaas, J. H., 1985, Interhemispheric connections of cortical sensory areas in tree shrews, *J. Comp. Neurol.* **235:**111–128.

Cusick, C. G., Wall, J. T., Felleman, D. J., and Kaas, J. H., 1989, Somatotopic organization of the lateral sulcus of owl monkeys: Area 3b, S-II, and a ventral somatosensory area, *J. Comp. Neurol.* **282:**169–190.

DeFelipe, J., Conley, M., and Jones, E. G., 1986, Long-range focal collateralization of axons arising from corticocortical cells in monkey sensory-motor cortex, *J. Neurosci.* **6:**3749–3766.

Dinopoulos, A., Karamanlidis, A. N., Papadopoulos, G., Antonopoulos, J., and Michaloudi, H., 1985, Thalamic projections to motor, prefrontal, and somatosensory cortex in the sheep studied by means of the horseradish peroxidase retrograde transport method, *J. Comp. Neurol.* **241:**63–81.

Doetsch, G. S., Standage, G. P., Johnston, K. W., and Lin, C.-S., 1988a, Thalamic connections of two functional subdivisions of the somatosensory forepaw cerebral cortex of the raccoon, *J. Neurosci.* **8:**1873–1886.

Doetsch, G. S., Standage, G. P., Johnston, K. W., and Lin, C.-S., 1988b, Intracortical connections of two functional subdivisions of the somatosensory forepaw cerebral cortex of the raccoon, *J. Neurosci.* **8:**1887–1900.

Dom, R., Martin, G. F., Fisher, B. L., Fisher, A. M., and Harting, J. K., 1971, The motor cortex and corticospinal tract of the armadillo (*Dasypus novemcinctus*), *J. Neurol. Sci.* **14:**225–236.

Donoghue, J. P., and Ebner, F. F., 1981a, The organization of thalamic projections to the parietal cortex of the Virginia opossum, *J. Comp. Neurol.* **198:**365–388.

Donoghue, J. P., and Ebner, F. F., 1981b, The laminar distribution and ultrastructure of fibers projecting from three thalamic nuclei to the somatic sensory-motor cortex of the opossum, *J. Comp. Neurol.* **198:**389–420.

Donoghue, J. P., Kerman, K. L., and Ebner, F. F., 1979, Evidence for two organizational plans within the somatic sensory-motor cortex of the rat, *J. Comp. Neurol.* **183:**647–664.

Dreyer, D. A., Loe, P. R., Metz, C. B., and Whitsel, B. L., 1975, Representation of head and face in postcentral gyrus of macaque, *J. Neurophysiol.* **38:**714–734.

Druga, R., 1982, Claustro-neocortical connections in the cat and rat demonstrated by HRP tracing techniques, *J. Hirnforsch.* **23:**191–202.

Dykes, R. W., and Herron, P., 1986, The ventroposterior inferior nucleus in the thalamus of cats: A relay nucleus in the Pacinian pathway to somatosensory cortex, *J. Neurophysiol.* **56:**1475–1497.

Dykes, R. W., Rasmusson, D. D., and Hoeltzell, P. B., 1980, Organization of primary somatosensory cortex in the cat, *J. Neurophysiol.* **43:**1527–1546.

Dykes, R. W., Herron, P., and Lin, C.-S., 1986, Ventroposterior thalamic regions projecting to cytoarchitectonic areas 3a and 3b in the cat, *J. Neurophysiol.* **56:**1521–1542.

Ebner, F. F., 1967, Afferent connections to neocortex in the opossum, (*Didelphis virginiana*), *J. Comp. Neurol.* **129:**241–268.

Ebner, F. F., 1969, A comparison of primitive forebrain organization in metatherian and eutherian mammals, *Ann. N.Y. Acad. Sci.* **167:**241–257.

Ebner, F. F., 1976, The forebrain of reptiles and mammals, in: *Evolution of Brain and Behavior in Vertebrates* (R. B. Masterton, M. E. Bitterman, C. B. G. Campbell, and N. Hotton, eds.), Erlbaum, Hillsdale, N.J., pp. 147–168.

Ebner, F. F., and Myers, R. E., 1965, Distribution of corpus callosum and anterior commissure in cat and raccoon, *J. Comp. Neurol.* **124:**353–365.

Eisenberg, J. F., 1981, *The Mammalian Radiations,* University of Chicago Press, Chicago.

Espinoza, S. G., and Thomas, H. C., 1983, Retinotopic organization of striate and extrastriate visual cortex in the hooded rat, *Brain Res.* **272:**137–144.

Feldman, S. H., and Johnson, J. I., 1988, Kinesthetic cortical area anterior to primary somatic sensory cortex in the raccoon (*Procyon lotor*), *J. Comp. Neurol.* **277:**80–95.

Felleman, D. J., Nelson, R. J., Sur, M., and Kaas, J. H., 1983a, Representations of the body surface in areas 3b and 1 of postcentral parietal cortex of cebus monkeys, *Brain Res.* **268:**15–26.

Felleman, D. J., Wall, J. T., Cusick, C. G., and Kaas, J. H., 1983b, The representation of the body surface in S-I of cats, *J. Neurosci.* **3:**1648–1669.

Ferrer, I., 1986, Golgi study of the isocortex in an insectivore: The common European mole (*Talpa europaea*), *Brain Behav. Evol.* **29:**105–114.

Fisher, A. M., Harting, J. K., Martin, G. F., and Stuber, M. I., 1969, The origin, course and termination of corticospinal fibers in the armadillo (*Dasypus novemcinctus mexicanus*), *J. Neurol. Sci.* **8:**347–361.

Fisher, G. R., Freeman, B., and Rowe, M. J., 1983, Organization of parallel projections from Pacinian afferent fibers to somatosensory cortical areas I and II in the cat, *J. Neurophysiol.* **49:**75–97.

FitzPatrick, K. A., Carlson, M., and Charlton, J., 1982, Topography, cytoarchitecture, and sulcal patterns in primary somatic sensory cortex (SmI) of the prosimian primate, *Perodicticus potto, J. Comp. Neurol.* **204:**296–310.

Fleischauer, K., Zilles, K., and Schleicher, A., 1980, A revised cytoarchitectonic map of the neocortex of the rabbit (*Oryctolagus cuniculus*), *Anat. Embryol.* **161:**121–143.

Foster, R. E., Donoghue, J. P., and Ebner, F. F., 1981, Laminar organization of efferent cells in the parietal cortex of the Virginia opossum, *Exp. Brain Res.* **43:**330–336.

Friedman, D. P., and Murray, E. A., 1986, Thalamic connectivity of the second somatosensory area and neighboring somatosensory fields of the lateral sulcus of the macaque, *J. Comp. Neurol.* **252:**348–373.

Friedman, D. P., Murray, E. A., and O'Neill, J. B., 1983, Thalamic connectivity of the somatosensory cortical fields of the lateral sulcus of the monkey, *Soc. Neurosci. Abstr.* **9:**921.

Garraghty, P. E., Pons, T. P., Huerta, M. F., and Kaas, J. H., 1987, Somatotopic organization of the third somatosensory area (SIII) in cats, *Somatosensory Res.* **4:**333–357.

Garraghty, P. E., Florence, S. L., Tenhula, W. N., and Kaas, J. H., 1989, Parallel processing in the first and second somatosensory areas in tree shrews, *Soc. Neurosci. Abstr.* **15:**1052.

Gerebtzoff, M. A., and Goffart, M., 1966, Cytoarchitectonic study of the isocortex in the sloth (*Choloepus hoffmanni* Peters), *J. Comp. Neurol.* **126:**523–534.

Goldby, F., 1939, An experimental investigation of the motor cortex and pyramidal tract of *Echidna aculeata, J. Anat.* **73:**509–524.

Gorska, T., 1974, Functional organization of cortical motor areas in adult dogs and puppies, *Acta Neurobiol. Exp.* **34:**171–203.

Gould, H. J., 1986, Body surface maps in the somatosensory cortex of rabbit, *J. Comp. Neurol.* **243:**207–234.

Gould, H. J., and Kaas, J. H., 1981, The distribution of commissural terminations in somatosensory areas I and II of the grey squirrel, *J. Comp. Neurol.* **196:**489–504.

Graziosi, M. E., Tucci, E., Barbaresi, P., Ugolini, G., and Manzoni, T., 1982, Cortico-cortical neurones of somesthetic area II as studied in the cat with fluorescent retrograde double-labelling, *Neurosci. Lett.* **31:**105–110.

Griffiths, M., 1978, *The Biology of Monotremes*, Academic Press, New York.

Guillery, R. W., Adrian, H. O., Woolsey, C. N., and Rose, J. E., 1966, Activation of somatosensory area I and II of the cat's cerebral cortex by focal stimulation of the ventrobasal complex, in: *The Thalamus* (D. P. Purpura and M. D. Yahr, eds.), Columbia University Press, New York, pp. 197–206.

Guldin, W. O., Markowitsch, H. J., Lampe, R., and Irle, E., 1986, Cortical projections originating from the cat's insular area and remarks on claustrocortical connections, *J. Comp. Neurol.* **243:**468–488.

Haight, J. R., 1972, The general organization of somatotopic projections to SII cerebral neocortex in the cat, *Brain Res.* **44:**483–502.

Haight, J. R., and Neylon, L., 1978, The organization of neocortical projections from the ventroposterior thalamic complex in the marsupial brush-tailed possum, *Trichosurus vulpecula:* A horseradish peroxidase study, *J. Anat.* **126:**459–485.

Haight, J. R., and Neylon, L., 1979, The organization of neocortical projections from the ventrolateral thalamic nucleus in the brush-tailed possum, *Trichosurus vulpecula,* and the problem of motor and somatic sensory convergence within the mammalian brain, *J. Anat.* **129:**673–694.

Haight, J. R., and Neylon, L., 1981, An analysis of some thalamic projections to parietofrontal neocortex in the marsupial native cat, *Dasyurus viverrinus* (Dasyuridae), *Brain Behav. Evol.* **19:**193–204.

Haight, J. R., and Weller, W. L., 1973, Neocortical topography in the brush-tailed possum: Variability and functional significance of sulci, *J. Anat.* **116:**473–474.

Hall, R. D., and Lindholm, E. P., 1974, Organization of motor and somatosensory neocortex in the albino rat, *Brain Res.* **66:**23–38.

Hand, P. J., and Morrison, A. R., 1970, Thalamocortical projections from the ventrobasal complex to somatic sensory areas I and II, *Exp. Neurol.* **26:**291–308.

Hand, P. J., and Morrison, A. R., 1972, Thalamocortical relationships in the somatic sensory system as revealed by silver impregnation techniques, *Brain Behav. Evol.* **5:**273–302.

Hardin, W. B., Arumugasamy, N., and Jameson, H. D., 1968, Pattern of localization in 'precentral' motor cortex of raccoon, *Brain Res.* **11:**611–627.

Harting, J. K., and Martin, G. F., 1970a, Neocortical projections to the mesencephalon of the armadillo *Dasypus novemcinctus, Brain Res.* **17:**447–462.

Harting, J. K., and Martin, G. F., 1970b, Neocortical projections to the pons and medulla of the nine-banded armadillo *Dasypus novemcinctus, J. Comp. Neurol.* **138:**483–500.

Hassler, R., and Muhs-Clement, K., 1964, Architektonischer aufbau des sensorimotorischen und parietalen cortex der Katze, *J. Hirnforsch.* **6:**377–420.

Heath, C. J., and Jones, E. G., 1971, Interhemispheric pathways in the absence of a corpus callosum, *J. Anat.* **109:**253–270.

Herron, P., 1978, Somatotopic organization of mechanosensory projections to SII cerebral neocortex in the raccoon (*Procyon lotor*), *J. Comp. Neurol.* **181:**717–728.

Herron, P., 1983, The connections of cortical somatosensory areas I and II with separate nuclei in the ventroposterior thalamus in the raccoon, *Neuroscience* **8:**243–257.

Herron, P., and Johnson, J. I., 1987, Organization of intracortical and commissural connections in somatosensory cortical areas I and II in the raccoon, *J. Comp. Neurol.* **257:**359–371.

Hyvärinen, J., 1982, Posterior parietal lobe of the primate brain, *Physiol. Rev.* **62:**1060–1129.

Imig, T. J., Reale, R. A., and Brugge, J. F., 1982, The auditory cortex: Patterns of corticocortical projections related to physiological maps in the cat, in: *Cortical Sensory Organization,* Volume 3 (C. N. Woolsey, ed.), Humana Press, Clifton, N.J., pp. 1–42.

Isseroff, A., Schwartz, M. L., Dekker, J. J., and Goldman-Rakic, P. S., 1984, Columnar organization of callosal and associational projections from rat frontal cortex, *Brain Res.* **293:**213–223.

Ito, H., Murakami, T., Fukuoka, T., and Kishida, R., 1986, Thalamic fiber connections in a teleost (*Sebasticus marmoratus*): Visual, somatosensory, octavolateral, and cerebellar relay region to the telencephalon, *J. Comp. Neurol.* **250:**215–228.

Iwamura, Y., and Tanaka, M., 1978, Functional organization of receptive fields in the cat somatosensory cortex. I: Integration within the coronal region, *Brain Res.* **151:**49–60.

Jameson, H. D., Arumugasamy, N., and Hardin, W. B., 1968, The supplementary motor cortex of the raccoon, *Brain Res.* **11:**628–637.

Johnson, J. I., 1980, Morphological correlates of specialized elaborations in somatic sensory neocortex, in: *Comparative Neurology of the Telencephalon* (S. O. E. Ebbesson, ed.), Plenum Press, New York, pp. 423–447.

Johnson, J. I., 1985, Thalamocortical organization in the raccoon: Comparison with the primate, *Brain Res. Suppl.* **10:**294–312.

Johnson, J. I., Haight, J. R., and Megirian, D., 1973, Convolutions related to sensory projections in cerebral neocortex of marsupial wombats, *J. Anat.* **114:**153.

Johnson, J. I., Rubel, E. W., and Hatton, G. I., 1974, Mechanosensory projections to cerebral cortex of sheep, *J. Comp. Neurol.* **158:**81–108.

Johnson, J. I., Kirsch, J. A. W., and Switzer, R. C., 1982a, Phylogeny through brain traits: Fifteen characters which adumbrate mammalian genealogy, *Brain Behav. Evol.* **20:**72–83.

Johnson, J. I., Switzer, R. C., and Kirsch, J. A. W., 1982b, Phylogeny through brain traits: The distribution of categorizing characters in contemporary mammals, *Brain Behav. Evol.* **20:**97–117.

Johnson, J. I., Ostapoff, E.-M., and Warach, S., 1982c, The anterior border zones of primary somatic sensory (S_I) neocortex and their relations to cerebral convolutions, shown by micromapping of peripheral projections to the region of the fourth forepaw digit representation in raccoons, *Neuroscience* **7:**915–936.

Jones, E. G., 1975, Lamination and differential distribution of thalamic afferents within the sensory-motor cortex of the squirrel monkey, *J. Comp. Neurol.* **160:**167–204.

Jones, E. G., 1985, *The Thalamus,* Plenum Press, New York.

Jones, E. G., 1986, Connectivity of the primate sensory-motor cortex, in: *Cerebral Cortex,* Volume 5 (E. G. Jones and A. Peters, eds.), Plenum Press, New York, pp. 113–184.

Jones, E. G., and Burton, H., 1974, Cytoarchitecture and somatic sensory connectivity of thalamic nuclei other than the ventrobasal complex in the cat, *J. Comp. Neurol.* **154:**395–432.

Jones, E. G., and Leavitt, R. Y., 1973, Demonstration of thalamo-cortical connectivity in the cat somato-sensory system by retrograde axonal transport of horseradish peroxidase, *Brain Res.* **63:**414–418.

Jones, E. G., and Leavitt, R. Y., 1974, Retrograde axonal transport and the demonstration of non-specific projections to the cerebral cortex and striatum from thalamic intralaminar nuclei in the rat, cat and monkey, *J. Comp. Neurol.* **154:**349–378.

Jones, E. G., and Porter, R., 1980, What is area 3a? *Brain Res. Rev.* **2:**1–43.

Jones, E. G., and Powell, T. P. S., 1968a, The commissural connexions of the somatic sensory cortex in the cat, *J. Anat.* **103:**433–455.

Jones, E. G., and Powell, T. P. S., 1968b, The ipsilateral cortical connexions of the somatic sensory areas in the cat, *Brain Res.* **9:**71–94.

Jones, E. G., and Powell, T. P. S., 1968c, The projection of the somatic sensory cortex upon the thalamus in the cat, *Brain Res.* **10:**369–391.

Jones, E. G., and Powell, T. P. S., 1969, The cortical projection of the ventroposterior nucleus of the thalamus in the cat, *Brain Res.* **13:**298–318.

Jones, E. G., Coulter, J. D., and Hendry, S. H. C., 1978, Intracortical connectivity of architectonic fields in the somatic sensory, motor and parietal cortex of monkeys, *J. Comp. Neurol.* **181:**291–348.

Joschko, M. A., and Sanderson, K. J., 1987, Cortico-cortical connections of the motor cortex in the brushtailed possum (*Trichosurus vulpecula*), *J. Anat.* **150:**31–42.

Kaas, J. H., 1982a, The somatosensory cortex and thalamus in *Galago*, in: *The Lesser Bushbaby (Galago) as an Animal Model: Selected Topics* (D. E. Haines, ed.), CRC Press, Boca Raton, pp. 169–181.

Kaas, J. H., 1982b, The segregation of function in the nervous system: Why do sensory systems have so many subdivisions?, in: *Contributions to Sensory Physiology*, Volume 7 (W. D. Neff, ed.), Academic Press, New York, pp. 201–240.

Kaas, J. H., 1983, What, if anything, is SI? Organization of first somatosensory area of cortex, *Physiol. Rev.* **63:**206–231.

Kaas, J., Hall, W. C., and Diamond, I. T., 1970, Cortical visual areas I and II in the hedgehog: Relation between evoked potential maps and architectonic subdivisions, *J. Neurophysiol.* **33:**595–614.

Karten, H. J., 1969, The organization of the avian telencephalon and some speculations on the phylogeny of the amniote telencephalon, *Ann. N.Y. Acad. Sci.* **167:**164–179.

Kelahan, A. M., and Doetsch, G. S., 1984, Time-dependent changes in the functional organization of somatosensory cerebral cortex following digit amputation in adult raccoons, *Somatosensory Res.* **2:**49–82.

Kicliter, E., and Ebbesson, S. O. E., 1976, Organization of the "nonolfactory" telencephalon, in: *Frog Neurobiology* (R. Llinas and W. Precht, eds.), Springer-Verlag, Berlin, pp. 946–972.

Killackey, H. P., and Ebner, F. F., 1972, Two different types of thalamocortical projections to a single cortical area in mammals, *Brain Behav. Evol.* **6:**141–169.

Killackey, H. P., and Ebner, F. F., 1973, Convergent projection of three separate thalamic nuclei on to a single cortical area, *Science* **179:**283–285.

Killackey, H. P., Koralek, K.-A., Chiaia, N. L., and Rhaodes, R. W., 1989, Laminar and areal differences in the origin of the subcortical projection neurons of the rat somatosensory cortex, *J. Comp. Neurol.* **282:**428–445.

King, J. L., 1911, Localisation of the motor area in the sheep's brain by the histological method, *J. Comp. Neurol.* **21:**311–321.

Kirsch, J. A. W., 1977, The classification of marsupials, in: *The Biology of Marsupials* (D. Hunsaker, ed.), Academic Press, New York, pp. 1–51.

Koralek, K.-A., Jensen, K. F., and Killackey, H. P., 1988, Evidence for two complementary patterns of thalamic input to the rat somatosensory cortex, *Brain Res.* **463:**346–351.

Krishnamurti, A., Sanides, F., and Welker, W. I., 1976, Microelectrode mapping of modality-specific somatic sensory cerebral neocortex in slow loris, *Brain Behav. Evol.* **13:**267–283.

Krubitzer, L. A., and Kaas, J. H., 1986, The second somatosensory area in primates: Somatotopic organization, architecture, and connections in marmosets (*Callithrix jacchus*), *Soc. Neurosci. Abstr.* **12:**798.

Krubitzer, L. A., and Kaas, J. H., 1987, Thalamic connections of three representations of the body surface in somatosensory cortex of gray squirrels, *J. Comp. Neurol.* **265:**549–580.

Krubitzer, L. A., Sesma, M. A., and Kaas, J. H., 1986, Microelectrode maps, myeloarchitecture, and cortical connections of three somatotopically organized representations of the body surface in the parietal cortex of squirrels, *J. Comp. Neurol.* **250:**403–430.

Kunz, B., and Spatz, W. B., 1985, A callosal projection of area 17 upon the border region of area MT in the marmoset monkey, *Callithrix jacchus*, *J. Comp. Neurol.* **239:**413–419.

Ladygina, T. F., Mass, A. M., and Supin, A. Y., 1978, Multiple sensory projections in the dolphin cerebral cortex, *Zh. Vyssh. Nervn. Deyat. im. I. P. Pavlova* **28:**1047–1054.

Ladygina, T. F., Popov, V. V., and Supin, A. I., 1985, Topicheskaia organizatsiia somaticheskikh proektsii v koru golovnogo mozga morskogo kotika, [Topical organization of somatic projections to the cerebral cortex of the seal Callorhinus ursinus], *Neirofiziologiya* **17:**344–351.

Langworthy, O. R., 1935, A physiological study of the cerebral motor cortex and the control of posture in the sloth, *J. Comp. Neurol.* **62:**333–348.

Ledoux, M. S., Whitworth, R. H., and Gould, H. J., 1987, Interhemispheric connections of the somatosensory cortex in the rabbit, *J. Comp. Neurol.* **258:**145–157.

Lende, R. A., 1963a, Sensory representation in the cerebral cortex of the opossum (*Didelphis virginiana*), *J. Comp. Neurol.* **121:**395–403.

Lende, R. A., 1963b, Motor representation in the cerebral cortex of the opossum (*Didelphis virginiana*), *J. Comp. Neurol.* **121:**405–415.

Lende, R. A., 1963c, Cerebral cortex: A sensorimotor amalgam in the Marsupialia, *Science* **141:**730–732.

Lende, R. A., 1964, Representation in the cerebral cortex of a primitive mammal. Sensorimotor, visual and auditory fields in the echidna (*Tachyglossus aculeatus*), *J. Neurophysiol.* **27:**37–48.

Lende, R. A., 1969, A comparative approach to neocortex: Localization in monotremes, marsupials and insectivores, *Ann. N.Y. Acad. Sci.* **167:**262–275.

Lende, R. A., and Akdikmen, S., 1968, Motor field in cerebral cortex of the bottlenose dolphin, *J. Neurosurg.* **29:**495–499.

Lende, R. A., and Sadler, K. M., 1967, Sensory and motor areas in neocortex of hedgehog (*Erinaceus*), *Brain Res.* **5:**390–405.

Lende, R. A., and Welker, W. I., 1972, An unusual sensory area in the cerebral neocortex of the bottlenose dolphin, *Tursiops truncatus*, *Brain Res.* **45:**555–560.

Lende, R. A., and Woolsey, C. N., 1956, Sensory and motor localization in cerebral cortex of porcupine (*Erethizon dorsatum*), *J. Neurophysiol.* **19:**544–563.

Livingstone, M. S., and Hubel, D. H., 1987, Connections between layer 4B of area 17 and the thick cytochrome oxidase stripes of area 18 in the squirrel monkey, *J. Neurosci.* **7:**3371–3377.

Macchi, G., and Bentivoglio, M., 1986, The thalamic intralaminar nuclei and the cerebral cortex, in: *Cerebral Cortex*, Volume 5 (E. G. Jones and A. Peters, eds.), Plenum Press, New York, pp. 355–402.

Macchi, G., Bentivoglio, M., Minciacchi, D., and Molinari, M., 1981, The organization of the claustroneocortical projections in the cat studied by means of the HRP retrograde axonal transport, *J. Comp. Neurol.* **195:**681–696.

Macchi, G., Bentivoglio, M., Minciacchi, D., and Molinari, M., 1983, Claustroneocortical projections studied in the cat by means of multiple retrograde fluorescent tracing, *J. Comp. Neurol.* **215:**121–134.

Macchi, G., Bentivoglio, M., Molinari, M., and Minciacchi, D., 1984, The thalamo-caudate versus thalamo-cortical projections as studied in the cat with fluorescent retrograde double labeling, *Exp. Brain Res.* **54:**225–239.

McGeorge, A. J., and Faull, R. L. M., 1989, The organization of the projection from the cerebral cortex to the striatum in the rat, *Neuroscience* **29:**503–537.

McKenna, M. C., 1975, Toward a phylogenetic classification of the mammals, in: *Phylogeny of the Primates* (W. P. Luckett and F. S. Szalay, eds.), Plenum Press, New York, pp. 31–46.

McKenna, T. M., Whitsel, B. L., Dreyer, D. A., and Metz, C. B., 1981, Organization of cat anterior parietal cortex: Relations among cytoarchitecture, single neuron functional properties, and interhemispheric connectivity, *J. Neurophysiol.* **45:**667–697.

McKenna, T. M., Whitsel, B. L., and Dreyer, D. A., 1982, Anterior parietal cortical topographic organization in macaque monkey: A re-evaluation, *J. Neurophysiol.* **48:**289–311.

Magalhães-Castro, B., and Saraiva, P. E. S., 1971, Sensory and motor representation in the cerebral cortex of the marsupial *Didelphis azarae azarae*, *Brain Res.* **34:**291–299.

Manzoni, T., Caminiti, R., Spidalieri, G., and Morelli, E., 1979, Anatomical and functional aspects of the associative projection from the somatic area SI to SII, *Exp. Brain Res.* **34:**453–470.

Manzoni, T., Barbaresi, P., Bellardinelli, E., and Caminiti, R., 1980, Callosal projections from the two body midlines, *Exp. Brain Res.* **39:**1–9.

Martin, G. F., 1967, Interhemispheric connections in the opossum, *Didelphis virginiana*, *Anat. Rec.* **157:**607–615.

Martin, G. F., and Fisher, A. M., 1968, A further evaluation of the origin, the course and the termination of the opossum corticospinal tract, *J. Neurol. Sci.* **7:**177–188.

Martin, G. F., and Megirian, D., 1972, Corticobulbar projections of the marsupial phalanger (Trichosurus vulpecula), *J. Comp. Neurol.* **144:**165–192.

Martin, G. F., Megirian, D., and Roebuck, A., 1970, The corticospinal tract of the marsupial phalanger (*Trichosurus vulpecula*), *J. Comp. Neurol.* **139:**245–258.

Martin, G. F., Megirian, D., and Roebuck, A., 1971, Corticobulbar projections of the marsupial phalanger (*Trichosurus vulpecula*), *J. Comp. Neurol.* **142:**275–296.

Martin, G. F., Megirian, D., and Conner, J. B., 1972, The origin, course and termination of the corticospinal tracts of the Tasmanian potoroo (*Potorous apicalis*), *J. Anat.* **111**:263–281.

Meulders, M., Gybels, J., Bergmans, J., Gerebtzoff, M. A., and Goffart, M., 1966, Sensory projections of somatic, auditory, and visual origin to the cerebral cortex of the sloth (*Choloepus hoffmanni* Peters), *J. Comp. Neurol.* **126**:535–546.

Montero, V. M., Rojas, A., and Torrealba, F., 1973, Retinotopic organization of striate and peristriate visual cortex in the albino rat, *Brain Res.* **53**:197–201.

Mori, A., Matsuura, N., Kagaya, K., Seki, T., Hiraba, H., and Sumino, R., 1985, Organization of the fifth somatic sensory cortex (SV) in the cat, *Soc. Neurosci. Abstr.* **11**:288.

Mountcastle, V. B., 1957, Modality and topographic properties of single neurons in cats somatic sensory cortex, *J. Neurophysiol.* **20**:408–434.

Murray, E. A., and Coulter, J. D., 1981, Supplementary sensory area: The medial parietal cortex in the monkey, in: *Cortical Sensory Organization*, Volume 1 (C. N. Woolsey, ed.), Humana Press, Clifton, N.J., pp. 167–196.

Narkiewicz, O., 1964, Frontoclaustral interrelations in cats and dogs, *J. Comp. Neurol.* **123**:335–356.

Nelson, L. R., and Lende, R. A., 1965, Interhemispheric responses in the opossum, *J. Neurophysiol.* **28**:189–199.

Nelson, R. J., Sur, M., and Kaas, J. H., 1979, The organization of the second somatosensory area (SmII) of the grey squirrel, *J. Comp. Neurol.* **184**:473–490.

Nelson, R. J., Sur, M., Felleman, D. J., and Kaas, J. H., 1980, Representation of the body surface in postcentral parietal cortex of *Macaca fascicularis*, *J. Comp. Neurol.* **192**:611–644.

Nieoullon, A., and Rispal-Padel, L., 1976, Somatotopic localization in cat motor cortex, *Brain Res.* **105**:405–422.

Norita, M., 1977, Demonstration of bilateral claustro-cortical connections in the cat with the method of retrograde axonal transport of horseradish peroxidase, *Arch. Histol. Jpn.* **40**:1–10.

Northcutt, R. G., 1978, Forebrain and midbrain organization in lizards and its phylogenetic significance, in: *Behavior and Neurology of Lizards* (N. Greenberg and P. D. MacLean, eds.), National Institute of Mental Health, Rockville, Md., pp. 11–64.

Novacek, M. J., and Wyss, A. R., 1986, Higher-level relationships of the recent eutherian orders. Morphological evidence, *Cladistics* **2**:257–287.

Olavarria, J., and Montero, V. M., 1984, Relation of callosal and striate–extrastriate cortical connections in the rat: Morphological definition of extrastriate visual areas, *Exp. Brain Res.* **54**:240–252.

Olavarria, J., Van Sluyters, R. C., and Killackey, H. P., 1984, Evidence for the complementary organization of callosal and thalamic connections within rat somatosensory cortex, *Brain Res.* **291**:364–368.

Olson, C. R., and Graybiel, A. M., 1980, Sensory maps in the claustrum of the cat, *Nature* **288**:479–481.

Papez, J. W., and Hunter, R. P., 1929, Formation of a central sulcus in the brain of the raccoon, *Anat. Rec.* **42**:60.

Pearson, J. C., and Haines, D. E., 1980, Somatosensory thalamus of a prosimian primate (*Galago senegalensis*). II. An HRP and Golgi study of the ventral posterolateral nucleus (VPL), *J. Comp. Neurol.* **190**:559–580.

Pearson, R. C. A., and Powell, T. P. S., 1985, The projection of the primary somatic sensory cortex upon area 5 in the monkey, *Brain Res. Rev.* **9**:89–107.

Petras, J. M., 1969, Some efferent connections of the motor and somatosensory cortex of simian primates and felid, canid and procyonid carnivores, *Ann. N.Y. Acad. Sci.* **167**:469–505.

Pimentel-Souza, F., Cosenza, R. M., Campos, G. B., and Johnson, J. I., 1980, Somatic sensory cortical regions of the agouti, *Dasyprocta aguti*, *Brain Behav. Evol.* **17**:218–240.

Pinto Hamuy, T., Bromiley, R. G., and Woolsey, C. N., 1956, Somatic afferent areas I and II of dog's cerebral cortex, *J. Neurophysiol.* **19**:485–499.

Platt, C. J., Bullock, T. H., Czóh, G., Kovačević, N., Konjević, D., and Gojković, M., 1974, Comparison of electroreceptor, mechanoreceptor, and optic evoked potentials in the brain of some rays and sharks, *J. Comp. Physiol.* **95**:323–355.

Pons, T. P., Garraghty, P. E., Friedman, D. P., and Mishkin, M., 1987, Physiological evidence for serial processing in somatosensory cortex, *Science* **237**:417–470.

Popova, N. S., 1968, [Dynamics of evoked potential parameters in different regions of the visual cortex and surrounding cortical fields in dogs during defensive conditioning], *Zh. Vyssh. Nervn. Deyat. im. I. P. Pavlova* **18**:940–950.

Powell, T. P. S., and Mountcastle, V. B., 1959, Some aspects of the functional organization of the cortex of the postcentral gyrus of the monkey: A correlation of findings obtained in a single unit analysis with cytoarchitecture, *Bull. Johns Hopkins Hosp.* **105**:133–162.

Pritz, M. B., and Stritzel, M. E., 1986, Reptilian somatosensory midbrain, *Soc. Neurosci. Abstr.* **12**:106.

Pubols, B. H., 1968, Retrograde degeneration study of somatic sensory thalamocortical connections in the brain of Virginia opossum, *Brain Res.* **7**:232–251.

Pubols, B. H., 1977, The second somatic sensory area (SMII) of opossum neocortex, *J. Comp. Neurol.* **174**:71–79.

Pubols, B. H., and Pubols, L. M., 1971, Somatotopic organization of spider monkey somatic sensory cerebral cortex, *J. Comp. Neurol.* **141**:63–76.

Pubols, B. H., and Pubols, L. M., 1979, Variations in the fissural pattern of the cerebral neocortex of the spider monkey (Ateles), *Brain Behav. Evol.* **16**:241–252.

Pubols, B. H., Pubols, L. M., DePette, D. J., and Sheely, J. C., 1976, Opossum somatic sensory cortex: A microelectrode mapping study, *J. Comp. Neurol.* **165**:229–246.

Putnam, S. J., Megirian, D., and Manning, J. W., 1968, Marsupial interhemispheric relation, *J. Comp. Neurol.* **132**:227–234.

Ray, R. H., and Craner, S. L., 1988, The development and topographic organization of the somatosensory cortices of the neonatal pig, *Soc. Neurosci. Abstr.* **14**:224.

Rees, S., and Hore, J., 1970, The motor cortex of the brush-tailed possum (*Trichosurus vulpecula*): Motor representation, motor function and the pyramidal tract, *Brain Res.* **20**:439–451.

Rice, F. L., 1983, A comparative analysis of barrel and lamina formation in SI cortex of small animals, *Anat. Rec.* **205**:161A–162A.

RoBards, M. J., and Ebner, F. F., 1977, Thalamic neurons projecting to the second somesthetic area (SII) of the cortex of the Virginia opossum, *Soc. Neurosci. Abstr.* **3**:490.

Robinson, C. J., and Burton, H., 1980a, Somatotopic organization in the second somatosensory area of *M. fascicularis*, *J. Comp. Neurol.* **192**:43–67.

Robinson, C. J., and Burton, H., 1980b, The organization of somatosensory receptive fields in cortical areas 7b, retroinsular, postauditory, and granular insula of *M. fascicularis*, *J. Comp. Neurol.* **192**:69–92.

Robinson, C. J., and Burton, H., 1980c, Somatic submodality distribution within the second somatosensory (SII), 7b, retroinsular, postauditory and granular insular cortical areas of *M. fascicularis*, *J. Comp. Neurol.* **192**:93–108.

Rose, J. E., and Mountcastle, V. B., 1952, The thalamic tactile region in rabbit and cat, *J. Comp. Neurol.* **97**:441–490.

Rose, M., 1931, Cytoarkitektonischer Atlas der Grosshirnrinde des Kaninchens, *J. Psychol. Neurol.* **43**:353–440.

Royce, G. J., Martin, G. F., and Dom, R. M., 1975, Functional localization and cortical architecture in the nine-banded armadillo (*Dasypus novemcinctus mexicanus*), *J. Comp. Neurol.* **164**:495–522.

Rubel, E. W., 1971, A comparison of somatotopic organization in sensory neocortex of newborn kittens and adult cats, *J. Comp. Neurol.* **143**:447–480.

Rustioni, A., Schmechel, D. E., Spreafico, R., Cheema, S., and Cuénod, M., 1983, Excitatory and inhibitory amino acid putative neurotransmitters in the ventralis posterior complex: An autoradiographic and immunocytochemical study in rats and cats, in: *Somatosensory Integration in the Thalamus* (G. Macchi, A. Rustioni, and R. Spreafico, eds.), Elsevier, Amsterdam, pp. 365–383.

Sakai, S. T., 1982, The thalamic connectivity of the primary motor cortex (MI) in the raccoon, *J. Comp. Neurol.* **204**:238–252.

Sally, S. L., and Kelly, J. B., 1988, Organization of auditory cortex in the albino rat: Sound frequency, *J. Neurophysiol.* **59**:1627–1638.

Sanderson, K. J., Welker, W., and Shambes, G. M., 1984, Reevaluation of motor cortex and of sensorimotor overlap in cerebral cortex of albino rats, *Brain Res.* **292**:251–260.

Sanides, D., and Sanides, F., 1974, A comparative Golgi study of the neocortex in insectivores and rodents, *Z. Mikrosk. Anat. Forsch.* **88**:957–977.

Sanides, F., 1968, The architecture of the cortical taste nerve areas in squirrel monkey (*Saimiri sciureus*) and their relationships to insular, sensorimotor and prefrontal regions, *Brain Res.* **8**:97–124.

Sanides, F., and Krishnamurti, A., 1967, Cytoarchitectonic subdivisions of sensorimotor and prefrontal regions and of bordering insular and limbic fields in slow loris (*Nycticebus coucang coucang*), *J. Hirnforsch.* **9**:225–252.

Sanides, F., and Sanides, D., 1972, The "extraverted neurons" of the mammalian cerebral cortex, *Z. Anat. Entwicklungsgesch.* **136**:272–293.

Saporta, S., and Kruger, L., 1977, The organization of thalamocortical relay neurons in the rat ventrobasal complex studied by the retrograde transport of horseradish peroxidase, *J. Comp. Neurol.* **174**:187–208.

Saraiva, P. E. S., and Magalhães-Castro, B., 1975, Sensory and motor representation in the cerebral cortex of the three-toed sloth (*Bradypus tridactylus*), *Brain Res.* **90**:181–193.

Seltzer, B., and Pandya, D. N., 1978, Afferent cortical connections and architectonics of the superior temporal sulcus and surrounding cortex in the rhesus monkey, *Brain Res.* **149**:1–24.

Sherk, H., 1986, The claustrum and the cerebral cortex, in: *Cerebral Cortex*, Volume 5 (E. G. Jones and A. Peters, eds.), Plenum Press, New York, pp. 467–500.

Sievert, C. F., and Neafsey, E. J., 1986, A chronic unit study of the sensory properties of neurons in the forelimb areas of rat sensorimotor cortex, *Brain Res.* **381**:15–23.

Simpson, S., and King, J. L., 1911, Localisation of the motor area in the sheep, *Q. J. Exp. Physiol.* **4**:53–65.

Spreafico, R., Hayes, N. L., and Rustioni, A., 1981, Thalamic projections to the primary and secondary somatosensory cortices in cat: Single and double retrograde tracer studies, *J. Comp. Neurol.* **203**:67–90.

Spreafico, R., Whitsel, B. L., Rustioni, A., and McKenna, T. M., 1983, The organization of nucleus ventralis postero-lateralis (VPL) of the cat and its relationship to the forelimb representation in cerebral cortical area SI, in: *Somatosensory Integration in the Thalamus* (G. Macchi, A. Rustioni, and R. Spreafico, eds.), Elsevier, Amsterdam, pp. 287–307.

Sretavan, D., and Dykes, R. W., 1983, The organization of two cutaneous submodalities in the forearm region of area 3b of cat somatosensory cortex, *J. Comp. Neurol.* **213**:381–399.

Standage, G. P., and Doetsch, G. S., 1988, Projections from cortical area SmII and claustrum to two functional subdivisions of SmI forepaw digit cortex of the raccoon, *Brain Res. Bull.* **21**:207–213.

Stein, B. E., Spencer, R. F., and Edwards, S. B., 1983, Corticotectal and corticothalamic efferent projections of SIV somatosensory cortex in cat, *J. Neurophysiol.* **50**:896–909.

Strominger, N. L., 1969, A comparison of the pyramidal tracts in two species of edentate, *Brain Res.* **15**:259–262.

Sur, M., Nelson, R. J., and Kaas, J. H., 1978, The representation of the body surface in somatosensory area I of the grey squirrel, *J. Comp. Neurol.* **179**:425–450.

Sur, M., Nelson, R. J., and Kaas, J. H., 1980a, Representation of the body surface in somatic koniocortex in the prosimian *Galago*, *J. Comp. Neurol.* **189**:381–402.

Sur, M., Weller, R. E., and Kaas, J. H., 1980b, Representation of the body surface in somatosensory area I of tree shrews, *Tupaia glis*, *J. Comp. Neurol.* **194**:71–96.

Sur, M., Weller, R. E., and Kaas, J. H., 1981a, The organization of somatosensory area II in tree shrews, *J. Comp. Neurol.* **201**:121–134.

Sur, M., Weller, R. E., and Kaas, J. H., 1981b, Physiological and anatomical evidence for a discontinuous representation of the trunk in S-I of tree shrews, *J. Comp. Neurol.* **201**:135–148.

Sur, M., Nelson, R. J., and Kaas, J. H., 1982, Representation of the body surface in cortical area 3b and 1 of squirrel monkeys: Comparison with other primates, *J. Comp. Neurol.* **211**:177–192.

Sych, B., 1976, Retrograde degeneration in the thalamus following the removal of cerebral cortex in somatosensory areas I and II in the dog, *Folia Biol. (Krakow)* **24**:349–365.

Sych, B., 1977, Retrograde degeneration in the thalamus following the removal of premotor and motor cortex in the dog, *Folia Biol. (Krakow)* **25**:367–379.

Taira, K., 1987, The representation of the oral structures in the first somatosensory cortex of the cat, *Brain Res.* **409**:41–51.

Tanji, D. G., Wise, S. P., Dykes, R. W., and Jones, E. G., 1978, Cytoarchitecture and thalamic connectivity of the third somatosensory area of the cat cerebral cortex, *J. Neurophysiol.* **41**:268–284.

Tunturi, A. R., 1944, Audio frequency localization in the acoustic cortex of the dog, *Am. J. Physiol.* **141**:397–402.

Tunturi, A. R., 1945, Further afferent connections to the acoustic cortex of the dog, *Am. J. Physiol.* **144**:389–394.

Tunturi, A. R., 1970, The pathway from the medial geniculate body to the ectosylvian auditory cortex in the dog, *J. Comp. Neurol.* **138**:131–136.

Tusa, R. J., Palmer, L. A., and Rosenquist, A. C., 1981, Multiple cortical visual areas: Visual field topography in the cat, in: *Cortical Sensory Organization*, Volume 2 (C. N. Woolsey, ed.), Humana Press, Clifton, N.J., pp. 1–32.

Ulinski, P. S., 1983, *Dorsal Ventricular Ridge*, Wiley–Interscience, New York.

Ulinski, P. S., 1984, Thalamic projections to the somatosensory cortex of the echidna, *Tachyglossus aculeatus*, *J. Comp. Neurol.* **229**:153–170.

Ulinski, P. S., 1986, Neurobiology of the therapsid–mammal transition, in: *The Ecology and Biology of Mammal-like Reptiles* (N. Hotton, P. D. MacLean, J. J. Roth, and E. C. Roth, eds.), Smithsonian Institution Press, New York, pp. 149–172.

Valverde, F., and Facal-Valverde, M. V., 1986, Neocortical layers I and II of the hedgehog (*Erinaceus europaeus*), *Anat. Embryol.* **173**:413–430.

Valverde, F., and López-Mascaraque, L., 1981, Neocortical endeavor: Basic neuronal organization in the cortex of hedgehog, in: *Eleventh International Congress of Anatomy: Glial and Neuronal Cell Biology*, Liss, New York, pp. 281–290.

Vogt, C., and Vogt, O., 1919, Allgemeinere Ergebnisse unserer Hirnforschung, *J. Psychol. Neurol.* **25**:279–462.

Walsh, T. M., and Ebner, F. F., 1970, The cytoarchitecture of somatic sensory-motor cortex in the opossum (*Didelphis marsupialis virginiana*): A Golgi study, *J. Anat.* **107**:1–18.

Walsh, T. M., and Ebner, F. F., 1973, Distribution of cerebellar and somatic lemniscal projections in the ventral nuclear complex of the Virginia opossum, *J. Comp. Neurol.* **147**:427–446.

Warren, S., and Pubols, B. H., 1984, Somatosensory cortical connections in the raccoon: An HRP study, *J. Comp. Neurol.* **227**:597–606.

Watson, C. R. R., 1971, The corticospinal tract of the quokka wallaby (*Setonix brachyurus*), *J. Anat.* **109**:127–133.

Watson, C. R. R., and Freeman, B. W., 1977, The corticospinal tract in the kangaroo, *Brain Behav. Evol.* **14**:341–351.

Webster, K. E., 1965, The cortico-striatal projection in the cat, *J. Anat.* **99**:329–337.

Welker, C., 1971, Microelectrode delineation of fine grain somatotopic organization of SmI cerebral neocortex in albino rat, *Brain Res.* **26**:259–275.

Welker, C., 1976, Receptive fields of barrels in the somatosensory neocortex of the rat, *J. Comp. Neurol.* **166**:173–190.

Welker, C., and Sinha, M. M., 1972, Somatotopic organization of SmII cerebral neocortex in albino rat, *Brain Res.* **37**:132–136.

Welker, C., and Woolsey, T. A., 1974, Structure of layer IV in the somatosensory neocortex of the rat: Description and comparison with the mouse, *J. Comp. Neurol.* **158**:437–454.

Welker, W. I., and Campos, G. B., 1963, Physiological significance of sulci in somatic sensory cortex of mammals of the family Procyonidae, *J. Comp. Neurol.* **120**:19–36.

Welker, W. I., and Carlson, M., 1976, Somatic sensory cortex of hyrax (*Procavia*), *Brain Behav. Evol.* **13**:294–301.

Welker, W. I., and Johnson, J. I., 1965, Correlation between nuclear morphology and somatotopic organization in ventrobasal complex of the raccoon's thalamus, *J. Anat.* **99**:761–790.

Welker, W., and Lende, R. A., 1980, Thalamocortical relationships in echidna (*Tachyglossus aculeatus*), in: *Comparative Neurology of the Telencephalon* (S. O. E. Ebbesson, ed.), Plenum Press, New York, pp. 449–481.

Welker, W. I., and Seidenstein, S., 1959, Somatic sensory representation in the cerebral cortex of raccoon (*Procyon lotor*), *J. Comp. Neurol.* **111**:469–501.

Welker, W. I., Adrian, H. O., Lifschitz, W., Kaulen, R., Caviedes, E., and Gutman, W., 1976, Somatic sensory cortex of llama (*Lama glama*), *Brain Behav. Evol.* **13**:284–293.

Welker, W., Sanderson, K. J., and Shambes, G. M., 1984, Patterns of afferent projections to transitional zones in the somatic sensorimotor cerebral cortex of albino rats, *Brain Res.* **292**:261–267.

Weller, R. E., and Kaas, J. H., 1981, Cortical and subcortical connections of visual cortex in primates, in: *Cortical Sensory Organization*, Volume 2 (C. N. Woolsey, ed.), Humana Press, Clifton, N.J., pp. 121–156.

Weller, R. E., and Sur, M., 1981, Some connections of S-I and S-II in the tree shrew, *Tupaia glis*, *Anat. Rec.* **199**:271A.

Weller, W. L., 1972, Barrels in somatic sensory neocortex of the marsupial *Trichosurus vulpecula* (brush-tailed possum), *Brain Res.* **43**:11–24.

Weller, W. L., and Haight, J. R., 1973, Barrels and somatotopy in S I neocortex of the brush-tailed possum, *J. Anat.* **116**:474.

Weller, W. L., Haight, J. R., Neylon, L., and Johnson, J. I., 1976, Single representation of mystacial vibrissae in SI neocortex of rufous wallaby *Thylogale billardierii*, *Soc. Neurosci. Abstr.* **2**:926.

Welt, C., Aschoff, J. C., Kameda, K., and Brooks, V. B., 1967, Intracortical organization of cat's motorsensory neurons, in: *Neurophysiological Basis of Normal and Abnormal Motor Activities* (M. D. Yahr and D. P. Purpura, eds.), Raven Press, New York, pp. 255–293.

White, E. L., and DeAmicis, R. A., 1977, Afferent and efferent projections of the region in mouse SmI cortex which contains the posteromedial barrel subfield, *J. Comp. Neurol.* **175**:455–481.

Wiener, S. I., Johnson, J. I., and Ostapoff, E.-M., 1987a, Organization of postcranial kinesthetic projections to the ventrobasal thalamus in raccoons, *J. Comp. Neurol.* **258**:496–508.

Wiener, S. I., Johnson, J. I., and Ostapoff, E.-M., 1987b, Demarcations of the mechanosensory projection zones in the raccoon thalamus, shown by cytochrome oxidase, acetylcholinesterase, and Nissl stains, *J. Comp. Neurol.* **258**:509–526.

Wise, L. Z., Pettigrew, J. D., and Calford, M. B., 1986, Somatosensory cortical representation in the Australian ghost bat, *Macroderma gigas, J. Comp. Neurol.* **248**:257–262.

Wise, S. P., and Jones, E. G., 1976, Organization and postnatal development of the commissural projection of the rat somatic sensory cortex, *J. Comp. Neurol.* **168**:313–343.

Wise, S. P., and Jones, E. G., 1977, Cells of origin and terminal distribution of descending projections of the rat somatic sensory cortex, *J. Comp. Neurol.* **175**:129–158.

Wise, S. P., and Jones, E. G., 1978, Developmental studies of thalamocortical and commissural connections in the rat somatic sensory cortex, *J. Comp. Neurol.* **178**:187–208.

Woolsey, C. N., 1958, Organization of somatic sensory and motor areas of the cerebral cortex, in: *Biological and Biochemical Bases of Behavior* (H. F. Harlow and C. N. Woolsey, eds.), University of Wisconsin Press, Madison.

Woolsey, C. N., and Fairman, D., 1946, Contralateral, ipsilateral, and bilateral representation of cutaneous receptors in somatic areas I and II of the cerebral cortex of pig, sheep, and other mammals, *Surgery* **19**:684–702.

Woolsey, C. N., and Wang, G.-H., 1945, Somatic sensory areas I and II of the cerebral cortex of the rabbit, *Fed. Proc.* **4**:79.

Woolsey, T. A., 1967, Somatosensory, auditory and visual cortical areas of the mouse, *Johns Hopkins Med. J.* **121**:91–112.

Woolsey, T. A., and Van der Loos, H., 1970, The structural organization of layer IV in the somatosensory region (SI) of mouse cerebral cortex, *Brain Res.* **17**:205–242.

Woolsey, T. A., Welker, C., and Schwartz, R. H., 1975, Comparative anatomical studies of the SmI face cortex with special references to the occurrence of "barrels" in layer IV, *J. Comp. Neurol.* **164**:79–94.

Yamamoto, T., Samejima, A., and Oka, H., 1987, Morphology of layer V pyramidal neurons in the cat somatosensory cortex: An intracellular HRP study, *Brain Res.* **437**:396–374.

Yorke, C. H., and Caviness, V. S., 1975, Interhemispheric neocortical connections of the corpus callosum in the normal mouse: A study based on anterograde and retrograde methods, *J. Comp. Neurol.* **164**:233–246.

Zeigler, H. P., 1964, Cortical sensory and motor areas of the guinea pig, *Arch. Ital. Biol.* **102**:587–598.

Zilles, K., and Wree, A., 1985, Cortex: Areal and laminar structure, in: *The Rat Nervous System*, Volume 1 (G. Paxinos, ed.), Academic Press, New York, pp. 375–416.

Zuckerman, S., and Fulton, J. F., 1941, The motor cortex in *Galago* and *Perodicticus, J. Anat.* **75**:447–456.

16

The Role of Somatic Sensory Cortex in Tactile Discrimination in Primates

MARY CARLSON

> The nature of the sensory changes produced by lesions of the cerebral cortex and other parts of the brain has been the theme of innumerable works by the acutest intellects in medicine of the last fifty years.
>
> Henry Head and Gordon Holmes (1911)

1. Introduction

Research on cerebral cortex function during the 50-year period referred to in the above quote was conducted by clinicians before the development of the neuroanatomical and electrophysiological methods that have dominated research on cortical sensory areas over the last 75 years. As these new experimental techniques gained in prominence in research on nonhuman species (and perhaps occupied the "acutest intellects in medicine"), interest in sensory phenomena and skills associated with sensory areas declined. Many of the same theoretical issues raised in the early clinical studies of tactile function following disease, injury, or surgical removal of parietal cortex remain the topic of contemporary research in the somatic sensory system. Review of the earlier experimental studies of tactile deficits following surgical lesions in nonhuman primates points to several important methodological issues, such as the significance of the age and species of experimental subject, of types of tasks used to assess tactile skills, and the basis for specification of the specific cortical area(s) involved in a

MARY CARLSON • Department of Neurobiology, Harvard Medical School, Boston, Massachusetts 02115.

particular skill, which may account for some of the differences in findings between past and current studies. Recent and ongoing studies from my laboratory on a variety of Old and New World primates are summarized to present both a comparative and a developmental perspective on the role of somatic sensory cortex in tactile discrimination capacity. In these studies, physiological mapping and selective cortical lesions were done, in conjunction with tactile discrimination testing, to determine how normal cortical organization and/or surgical intervention in cortical areas related to tactile capacity. Finally, theories that address the relationship between ontogenetic and phylogenetic changes in brain and behavior will be discussed to bring together the findings on development and evolution of the somatic sensory system and tactile capacities in primates.

1.1. Localization of Tactile Areas in Cerebral Cortex in Primates

A starting basis for the examination of the role of a cortical structure in a particular behavior is the assumption that sensory functions can be localized to distinctive pathways, subcortical nuclei, or cortical projection areas. Confronted with the vast complexity of surface morphology, histological detail, and connectional patterns in the cerebral cortex of primates, early attempts to localize sensory, motor, and cognitive functions in the central nervous system of humans and other primates appeared daunting. Smith (1902, 1910), Campbell (1905), Brodmann (1909, 1925), and Vogt and Vogt (1919) were among the pioneers in establishing the association between sulcal patterns and cytoarchitectonic areas in a variety of simple and complex primate brains. The pattern of cortical projection of specific thalamic nuclei provided another criterion by which functional subdivisions could be established in conjunction with, or in the absence of, architectonic criteria. Monakow (1882), Clark and Boggon (1935), and Walker (1937) were among the first to determine the relationship between thalamic input patterns and SI architectonic areas. The correlation between sulci and granular sensory areas (primary visual, auditory, and somatic sensory regions) and pyramidal (primary motor region) areas served to identify functional subdivisions prior to electrophysiological methods coming into common usage.

The first application of electrical stimulation methods to circumscribe functional areas was by Fritsch and Hitzig (1870) in examination of motor cortex. Barenne (1916) later used strychnine activation of the cortical surface to map projection sites for different skin surfaces by determination of sites causing disturbances in sensation. A momentous achievement in the effort to localize sensory function came with Penfield and Boldrey's (1937) publication of the motor and sensory "homunculi" in humans by means of electrical simulation of pre- and postcentral gyrus in alert patients undergoing surgical treatment of epilepsy. Adrian (1941) and Woolsey *et al.* (1942) were among the first to record evoked potentials on the cortical surface to construct topographic maps of cutaneous sensation in primary (SI), and later secondary (SII) (Woolsey, 1943) somatic sensory receiving areas. These anatomical and physiological studies provided the basis for early efforts to localize tactile functions in SI and SII. More recent studies using microelectrode techniques have refined the details of the correspondence between sulci, topographic maps, architectonic fields, and thalamic and intracortical projections, but the approximate location and organization of tactile receiving area that formed the basis for early clinical and experimental lesion studies still apply today (see Dykes, Volume 5 of this series).

1.2. Clinical Studies of Tactile Deficits in Human Patients

The early studies of tactile localization in cortex conducted by leading neurologists of the time, referred to above by (and including) Head and Holmes (1911), were concerned with many of the same issues that are the current themes of behavioral, physiological, and anatomical investigation today. Conclusions from these early works (Head, 1920) stressed the importance of contralateral parietal cortex in responding to different categories of somatic sensation (e.g., size, shape, roughness) and in relating these submodalities for the appreciation of complex tactile stimuli. A thoughtful text on the function of parietal cortex by Critchley (1953) summarized both earlier work along with more recent studies, characterizing a variety of perceptual and intellectual disturbances, such as finger agnosia, body image, and spatial location, as well as the classical measures of two-point thresholds and punctate thresholds. An important point to be made by this review is that the lesion-deficit approach, whether following injury or disease in humans or experimental lesions in nonhuman primates, remains an important method for demonstration of brain–behavior relations.

A major study appearing in the following decade, by Semmes *et al.* (1960), examined a wide range of sensory and perceptual capacities in veterans suffering missile wounds to the head. In contrast to prior studies, their conclusions stressed the importance of ipsilateral parietal cortex and extraparietal areas in both hemispheres, rather than the contralateral postcentral gyrus, in performance of tactile detection and discrimination tasks. These differences with previous studies may relate to the nature of the patients examined. It is difficult to assess the location and extent of cortical/subcortical damage following a closed head injury and based on site of missile entry only. More precise localization of cortical damage was obtained by Corkin *et al.* (1970) in their study of patients receiving unilateral parietal excisions for relief of focal epilepsy. Results from that study demonstrated that tactile sensitivity and acuity depend primarily on the postcentral gyrus in the contralateral hemisphere as seen by the severe deficits following surgical lesions. The consequences of precentral motor or posterior parietal damage were negligible compared to postcentral damage, and in agreement with most previous studies.

A more recent study of human patients by Roland (1976) also examined subjects with unilateral surgical lesions (mainly for treatment of meningiomas, intracerebral metastasis, arteriovenous malformation) and developed a very sophisticated set of stimuli to quantify size and shape discrimination. Patients with lesions sparing the middle third of the postcentral gyrus performed as normal subjects on these tasks but those involving the middle third had severe deficits on these tasks. In a companion study, performance on these same tasks was found to result in increased cerebral blood flow in the contralateral pre- and postcentral gyrus relative to other cortical areas (Roland and Larsen, 1976). This increase was greatest in the postcentral area when discriminations were made with the hand, consistent with the findings of deficits when damage included this same area.

2. Experimental Lesions and Tactile Testing in Nonhuman Primates

Some investigators approached the study of parietal cortex function by producing surgical lesions in nonhuman primates and examining the pattern of sensory deficits following damage to selective areas. Often these experimental studies were prompted by findings from electrophysiological and cytoarchitectural studies in primates. Among the first studies were those by Minkowski (1917) in which pre- and postcentral gyrus were separately ablated. The general findings were that lesions of postcentral parietal areas affected cutaneous and muscle sense, whereas lesions of motor cortex did not. This study, along with those by Ruch and colleagues, were done prior to evoked potential mapping studies, but the combination of neurological, anatomical, and stimulation studies had done much to suggest the critical role of the contralateral postcentral gyrus in tactile capacity. The important studies of Ruch and Fulton (1935) were the first to use discrimination tasks, in this case weight discrimination as opposed to simple tactile stimulation, to evaluate the significance of cortical areas for tactile sensibility. They sought to remove specific cytoarchitectonic areas estimated by the relationship of these areas to surface features of cortex. The subjects were five immature monkeys—four Old World monkeys (*Cercocebus*) and one mature New World monkey (*Ateles*)—given an assortment of unilateral or bilateral posterior parietal area, motor area, or unilateral postcentral lesions. In most cases, some initial deficit was seen, yet after repeated testing all subjects recovered normal levels of tactile function. Given the emphasis on the role of the postcentral gyrus in tactile abilities from preceding investigations, the finding of minimal and transient impairment was unexpected. Histological examination of the brains of these subjects revealed incomplete removal of the anterior bank of the postcentral gyrus in most cases and is a major factor that distinguishes this early work from more recent studies. Also, as will emerge from these more recent studies, the use of immature animals or New World species may have contributed to the modest sensory consequences observed.

In another study by Ruch *et al.* (1938), chimpanzees and humans were trained to perform discriminations of weights, roughness, and shapes. One chimpanzee with a partial removal of the postcentral gyrus showed complete recovery of weight, texture, and shape discrimination capacity. A second chimpanzee with a complete postcentral removal showed continued texture deficits which were associated with some involvement of motor cortex as well. Subsequent removal of the posterior parietal cortex produced a lasting deficit on both the shape and weight discrimination tasks. By testing of humans with postcentral or posterior parietal lesions on the same tasks, they found more lasting deficits on weight discrimination tasks than were found with chimpanzees or monkeys suffering similar damage. These findings led to the suggestion that humans may depend on cortex for such functions to a greater degree than monkeys and chimpanzees. They also proposed that posterior parietal areas (therefore secondary, rather than primary areas) may have a more important role in mediating sensory function in humans than in nonhuman species. Theories about the "encephalization of function" in primate evolution are a topic of interest that has arisen in our own recent studies of SI and SII in prosimians and Old and New World monkeys.

The next significant series of studies came after the evoked potential maps of SI by Woolsey *et al.* (1942) were published. Cole and Glees (1954) used electrical stimulation of the pre- and postcentral gyrus in adult and immature Old World macaques to localize the hand area. Following removal of the anterior two-thirds of the postcentral gyrus, animals were trained on tasks developed to test motor function, dexterity, and form discrimination. The most obvious disability was on the latter test, but considerable recovery occurred after continued training. They concluded that remaining postcentral gyrus areas and motor cortex may have mediated recovery and maintained the notion that sensorimotor cortex was one functional unit.

Since the previous study did not include SII in the removals, Kruger and Porter (1958) hypothesized that recovery may be mediated by that second region defined by evoked potential studies (Woolsey, 1943). Following unilateral or bilateral SI–SII, unilateral or bilateral MI, and unilateral pre- and postcentral lesions, macaques were trained to discriminate an inverted from an upright L-shaped object or to manipulate a box closed by a hasp, without visual cues. They found that the removal of SI and SII together did not result in permanent deficits unless MI was also removed. They concluded that although there were functional differences between sensory and motor cortical areas, MI could mediate sensory capacities following sensory cortex damage. This same approach was taken by Orbach and Chow (1959) in examination of SI, SII, and SI–SII lesions on a greater variety (i.e., size, form, texture) of sensory tasks than the previous study. The SI lesions were followed by severe, lasting deficits in form and roughness whereas an SII lesion alone caused little to no impairment. The combined SI–SII lesion caused no more impairment than SI alone.

The relative significance of MI and SI, and more recently of SII, in subserving tactile abilities was still uncertain after decades of new details on the location and organization of tactile input to cerebral cortex in primates. A major experimental feature given little attention in these previous studies is the nature of the tactile tasks. Attention to the specific sensory characteristics and level of difficulty of tasks, along with the importance of the age or species of the subjects, will be emphasized as new experimental findings are presented.

3. Comparative Studies of Somatic Sensory Cortex and Tactile Discrimination Capacity in Primates

3.1. Contribution of Multiple SI Hand Areas to Tactile Capacity

Those somatotopic mapping studies of SI and SII discussed in the previous section were obtained using macroelectrodes (with recording tips on the order of 1 mm in diameter) and evoked potential activity recorded on the surface of cortex. Such procedures made it impossible to explore the pattern of input to regions of cortex buried in sulci, without surgical removal of adjacent gyri. Fine detail of input adjacent to, or directly below, the surface location of the electrode could not be resolved. When mapping strategies turned to the use of microelectrodes (with recording tips of $1-5$ μ), activity from cell clusters near the site of thalamic terminations could be obtained. These micromapping techniques, first used by W. Welker and colleagues in the primate *Nycticebus* (Krishnamurti *et al.,* 1976), and in the rat (C. Welker, 1971), provided considerably more detail than earlier evoked-potential maps and led to a more precise understanding of the location, size, and complexity of detail in somatic sensory projections to cortex. It was the application of these micromapping studies by Paul and colleagues (Paul *et al.,* 1972) that first illustrated that the pattern of cutaneous input projecting to postcentral gyrus in the macaque was distributed in the same radial–ulnar pattern from lateral-to-medial across the gyrus but that the proximal–distal axis of the hand did not project in a single pattern from caudal area 1 to anterior area 3 in the depths of the central sulcus (CS). Rather, based on the pattern of receptive fields on the palm, proximal and distal digits, they described two maps of the hand distributed in a serial pattern, one in area 1 and the second in area 3 (see Fig. 1). These findings suggesting two separate projection patterns for cutaneous input from the hand prompted our first experimental lesion study of the role of cortex in sensory discrimination (Randolph and Semmes, 1974).

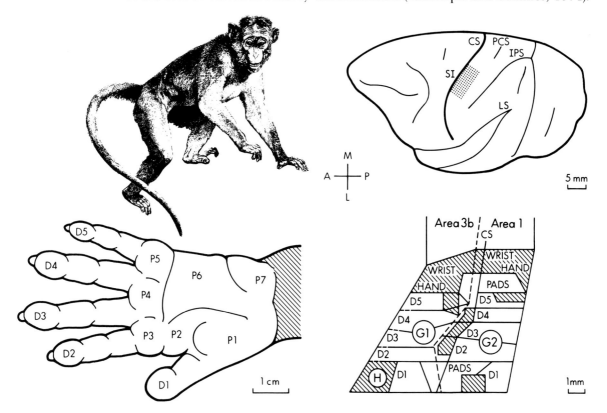

Figure 1. Illustration of the Old World anthropoid, *Macaca,* commonly known as the macaque. The body drawing illustrates the quadrupedal posture assumed during locomotion in this species. The brain drawing of the left cortical hemisphere indicates the location of the cutaneous input from the hand to the SI area (dotted) located posterior to the central sulcus (CS). Area 2 extends from the posterior margin of the cutaneous hand area into the lateral third of the anterior bank of the intraparietal sulcus (IPS), at the location lateral to the postcentral sulcus (PCS). SII is located in the anterior bank of the lateral sulcus (LS), posterior to the tip of the IPS. The drawing of the hand identifies the five gla-brous digits (D1–D5) and the palmar pads (P1–P7) as adapted from Biegert (1961). The map of the hand in areas 3b and 1 of SI displays the general topographic features of the cutaneous projection from the glabrous digits and palm (white) and the hairy digits, hand, and wrist (striped), with the two cutaneous projection patterns (G1 and G2) in areas 3b and 1, respectively, and the single, distributed hairy projection pattern (H) across the two cytoarchitectonic areas (Paul *et al.,* 1972; Nelson *et al.,* 1980). The division between cytoarchitectonic areas 3b and 1 is indicated by a dashed line, while the curve from the crown to the bank of the CS is noted by a solid line.

Cortical lesion studies in macaques by Semmes and Mishkin (1965) had previously examined the role of sensorimotor cortex on the ipsilateral hand and of nonsensorimotor cortex on the contralateral hand in tactile discrimination capacity based on findings from clinical studies referred to in an earlier section (Semmes *et al.*, 1960). Using the broad battery of tactile tasks developed in the earlier study, Semmes and Porter (1972) removed either the anterior or posterior *half* of the precentral or postcentral gyri in search of regional differences in the pattern of tactile deficits. Their findings were of severe impairment following both postcentral lesions but no deficits following either precentral lesion. Based on these significant deficits and the new SI maps by Paul *et al.*, I proposed a study with Semmes in which we evaluated the patterns of deficits following selective lesions of *three* separate cytoarchitectonic subdivisions of SI containing the *two* cutaneous hand areas in areas 3b and 1. From this study (Randolph and Semmes, 1974), evidence for the general importance of area 3b, and the selective contributions of areas 1 and 2, to a tactile discrimination capacity was obtained. Removal of area 3b alone produced severe deficits on all tasks. Whereas only texture-type tasks were impaired following an area 1, but not area 2, lesion. An analogous finding was that size and shape tasks were impaired following an area 2, but not area 1, lesion. A second study of area 1 and 2 lesions verified these selective deficits on size and texture tasks, even after extensive preoperative training on the same tasks (Carlson, 1981). Such a pattern of impairment is regarded as "double dissociation of function" and is considered as strong evidence for localization of function in specific areas (Ruch *et al.*, 1938).

The differential consequences of these subtotal SI removals were consistent with the findings of Powell and Mountcastle (1959b) that cutaneous and noncutaneous input project primarily to areas 3b–1 and areas 3a–2, respectively (see Fig. 2). These results also fit with more recent findings on the pattern of thalamic input of cutaneous and deep input to SI areas (Jones, 1985). As both behavioral and physiological studies of SI in *Macaca* indicate that cutaneous and noncutaneous (kinesthetic) information are important in tactile function, "tactile" in this chapter should be understood as referring to both the tactile and kinesthetic sensations discussed by Rose and Mountcastle (1959). The localization of specific tactile capacities to different SI subdivisions in these behavioral studies led to a renewed interest in the evolution of multiple cortical areas and tactile function in primates (Carlson, 1985).

3.2. Organization of Somatic Sensory Areas (SI and SII) in Prosimian Primates

Based on findings in *Macaca mulatta* of multiple projection patterns in SI (Paul *et al.*, 1972), and our findings of selective behavioral roles of SI cytoarchitectural divisions (Randolph and Semmes, 1974), an important issue emerged as to whether all primates have more complex SI projection patterns than nonprimates or whether the single pattern reported for *Nycticebus* (Krishnamurti *et al.*, 1976) was typical of all prosimians. We decided to study the prosimian *Galago* as its locomotion style of an upright clinger and leaper (Napier and Walker, 1967) was more like that of extinct ancestral prosimians, as suggested by skeletal features, and the external surface of its brain, compared to endocasts of fossil prosimian skulls (Radinsky, 1970; Carlson and Welt, 1981). The sagittal sulcal pattern in sensorimotor cortex, seen in fossil prosimian and most extant prosimians, contrasts with the coronal patterns typical of both extinct and extant Old and New World anthropoid species. *Galago* seemed to be the most generalized of the prosimians and therefore the best subject to use as a model for study of the pattern of SI organization that may have existed in the ancestral prosimians that gave rise to both Old and New World anthropoids. Such a comparative strategy would allow us to make judgments about whether cortical areas in different species are homologous, i.e., inherited from a common ancestor (Campbell and Hodos, 1970), or merely analogous.

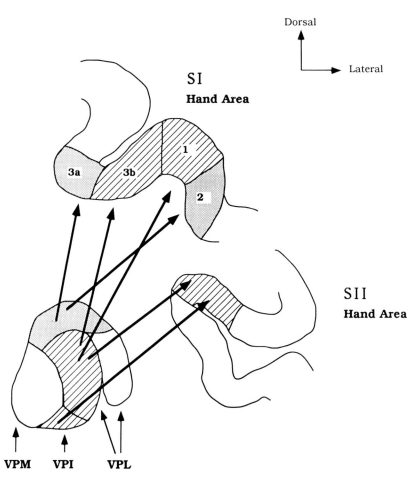

Figure 2. Illustration of a frontal view of the left hemisphere of *Macaca* showing the thalamocortical projection pattern from the ventroposterior nucleus (VP) to cytoarchitectonic areas 3a, 3b, 1, and 2 of the SI hand area. The medial division, VPM, projects to the face area not shown in this section. The medial portion of the lateral division, VPL, projects to the hand areas in SI and SII. The central cutaneous core (striped) portion projects primarily to areas 3b and 1, and the shell of deeply responding input (shaded) projects to areas 3a and 2 (Jones, 1985; Powell and Mountcastle, 1959b). In addition, the inferior portion, VPI, projects to SII and is indicated as a source of tactile input although the source of cutaneous and noncutaneous input to SII remains controversial (Robinson and Burton, 1980; Jones, 1985; Friedman and Murray, 1986; Pons *et al.*, 1986).

3.2.1. SI Map in *Galago*

Using micromapping methods, Welt and I determined the somatotopic organization of the hand area in *Galago crassicaudatus* and, by placing microlesions at anterior and posterior boundaries of cortex that responded to cutaneous stimulation in anesthetized animals, found a single SI projection pattern for the contralateral hand (see Fig. 3). In this pattern the glabrous surface projected to the anterior half, and the hairy hand and digits projected to the posterior half, of the granular area of cortex lying between the two sagittally oriented sulci (Carlson and Welt, 1980). Recordings in awake animals with chronically attached recording chambers allowed us to isolate single neurons driven by passive manipulation or active movement of muscles and joints. Neurons driven by active hand movements were found in the region posterior to the hairy hand and digit

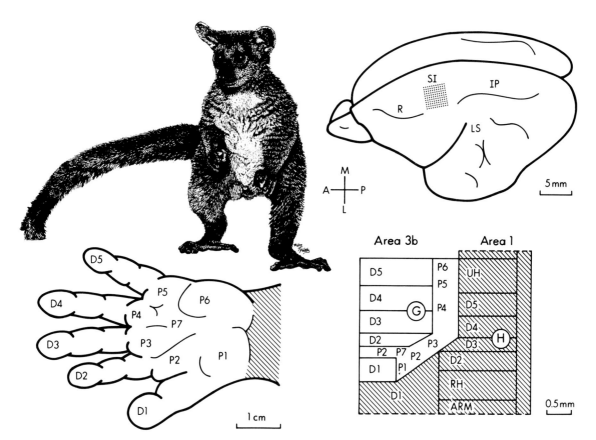

Figure 3. Illustration of the African prosimian, *Galago*, commonly known as the bushbaby. The body drawing illustrates the bipedal posture assumed during locomotion in this species. The brain drawing of the left cortical hemisphere indicates the location of the cutaneous input to the SI hand area (dotted), posterior to the rectus (R) and anterior to the intraparietal (IP) sulcus. SII is located in the anterior bank of the lateral sulcus (LS), just lateral to the anterior tip of the IP (from Burton and Carlson, 1986). The drawing of the hand identifies the five glabrous digits (D1–D5) and the palmar pads (P1–P7) as adapted from Biegert (1961). The map of the hand in areas 3b and 1, of SI (from Carlson and Welt, 1980; Sur *et al.*, 1980), displays the general topographic features of the input from the glabrous digits and palm (G, white) and hairy digits and ulnar (UH) and radial (RH) hand (H, striped). The division between areas 3b and 1 is roughly equivalent to the division between the glabrous and hairy hand and digit projection areas.

region and many forms of noncutaneous stimulation evoked activity in the area anterior to the glabrous hand area. We suggested these to be the homologues of areas 2–5 and areas 3a, respectively. The total glabrous–hairy hand area appeared to be homologous to areas 3b–1 in *Macaca*. Studies of the smaller species *G. senegalenis* by Kaas and colleagues found the same general single pattern of the glabrous–hairy division, with some minor differences in the details of proximal–distal axis of the hairy hand and digits (Sur *et al.*, 1980).

3.2.2. SI Maps in *Perodicticus* and *Nycticebus*

Given the simple and singular pattern of cutaneous input to SI in *Galago*, our next effort was to examine the organization of cutaneous input to SI in two additional prosimian species. Each species, one African (*Perodicticus*) and the other Asian (*Nycticebus*), shows the same unusual behavioral adaptation of slow, cryptic quadrupedal locomotion, yet we found each to have a different projection pattern of cutaneous input from the hand to SI (see Fig. 4 and 5). The pattern in *Perodicticus* is similar to that in *Galago*, with the exception of the attenuated digit 2 area (related to a modified digit) and the glabrous hand and remaining digits project to nearly 75% of an expanded hand area as opposed to a 50–50% split between glabrous and hairy hand in SI of *Galago* (FitzPatrick *et al.*, 1982). In *Nycticebus*, the SI hand area is also relatively enlarged compared to that in *Galago*, and although the projection areas for the glabrous and hairy hand and digits are roughly 50–50%, as in *Galago*), a second projection area for the glabrous hand was found within the hairy hand region in posterior SI (Carlson and Fitzpatrick, 1982).

In these rare animals we could examine only two individuals of each species yet we felt confident that these fine-grained maps were representative as the topographic details were practically identical within, and vastly different between, species. The uniqueness of these maps is especially impressive, in that one clearly represents an expanded map and the other a more differentiated map, yet each has independently acquired the same novel behavioral style. The minimal intraspecies variation compared to the maximal interspecies variation contrasts with the high intraspecies variation seen in the New World species, *Saimiri* and *Aotus* (Merzenich, 1985; Merzenich *et al.*, 1987). The mapping procedures employed in all three prosimian species used sampling densities equal, or exceeding, those used in the New World species, yet all three species show minimal variability in the details of SI organization. The increased complexity and variability seen in the maps of these New World species may be specific to some or all of the members of this primate family and may contribute to the limited tactile capacity found in these species.

Compared to the multiple cutaneous areas in Old and New World anthropoids, we interpret the small second glabrous projection in *Nycticebus* as an independent acquisition of a second cutaneous projection area, rather than as a homologue to the multiple areas in anthropoids. This pattern is an exception from the general prosimian pattern observed and it occurs in a highly specialized species, rather than generalized species like *Galago*. Expansion, duplication and differentiation of cortical areas are seen in the major sensory systems of many mammals, and may be independent mechanisms, or evolutionary strategies, occurring repeatedly in mammalian evolution and associated with advances in the power or complexity of cortical processing.

3.2.3. Sulcal Patterns, Topography, and Cytoarchitectonic Subdivisions in SI of Prosimians

Just as in our studies of *Galago*, we found the cutaneous projection area for the hand to coincide with the granular region in sensorimotor cortex of *Perodicticus* and *Nycticebus*. The cortical sulci in these two species also showed distinctive configurations compared to *Galago* and fossil prosimians. *Perodicticus* has a coronally oriented sulcus in the sensorimotor region, which qualifies as a limiting sulcus as it divides two functionally distinct areas, SI and MI. The cutaneous projection region areas of the glabrous and hairy hand correspond roughly to areas 3b and 1, as in Old World primates (Powell and Mountcastle, 1959a). Such a sulcal pattern is typical of anthropoids, and exceedingly rare in prosimians, another apparent example of convergent evolution. In *Nycticebus* the sagittal sulcal pattern typical of prosimians was seen but, rather than these sulci lying anterior and posterior to SI, sulci were found within SI, separating the face from

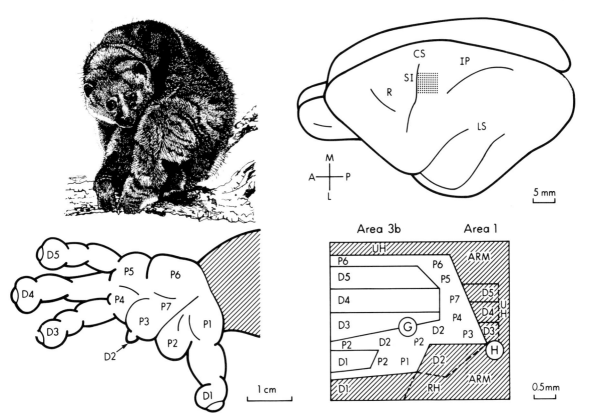

Figure 4. Illustration of the African prosimian, *Perodicticus*, commonly known as the potto. The body drawing illustrates the crouched, quadrupedal posture assumed at rest in the branches by this species and *Nycticebus*. The brain drawing of the left cortical hemisphere indicates the location of the cutaneous input to the SI hand area (dotted), between the rectus (R) and the intraparietal (IP) sulcus as in *Galago*, but adjacent to the unusual central sulcus (CS) in this prosimian species (FitzPatrick *et al.*, 1982; Radinsky, 1970). The drawing of the hand identifies the four glabrous digits (D1, D3, D4, D5 and the vestige of D2) and the palmar pads (P1–P7) as adapted from Biegert (1961). The map of the hand in areas 3b and 1 of SI displays the general topographic features of a single pattern of input from the glabrous digits and palm (G, white) and hairy digits and hand (H, striped). The border between areas 3b and 1 is not indicated in the drawing, but it lies along the line between the radial palm and posterior hairy fields and between the ulnar digits and palm, through the middle of the total SI hand area (FitzPatrick *et al.*, 1982).

the hand and the hand from the foot areas, from lateral to medial across the cortical surface. In both of these species, we found that the distinction between the glabrous and hairy hand and digit projection patterns corresponded to the two distinctive granular cytoarchitectural fields, anterior area 3b and posterior area 1, respectively. The posterior topographic region in *Nycticebus* includes both the hairy and second glabrous region and corresponds to that cytoarchitectural region suggested by Welker and colleagues as the homologue to area 1 in *Macaca* (Krishnamurti *et al.*, 1976; Sanides and Krishnamurti, 1967). The significance of these studies of SI somatotopy, submodality, and cytoarchitecture in these three prosimians is to suggest that elaboration and/or differentiation of cortical projection areas may be selected as neural mechanisms by which greater sensory capacity is achieved in evolution of new species. Whether the simple SI patterns of

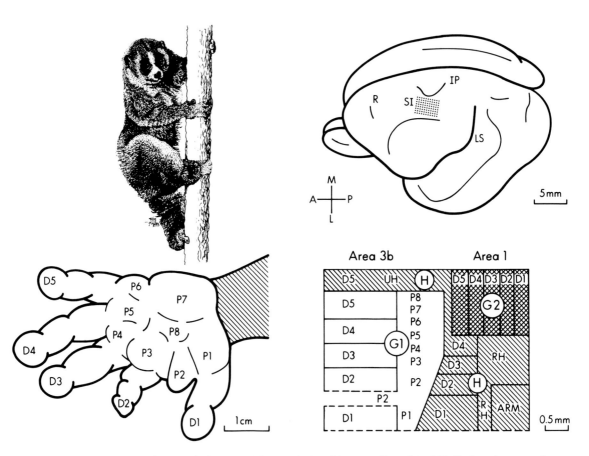

Figure 5. Illustration of the Asian prosimian, *Nycticebus*, commonly known as the slow loris. The body drawing illustrates the quadrupedal, clinging posture assumed during the slothlike locomotion typical of this species and *Perodicticus*. The brain drawing of the left cortical hemisphere indicates the location of the cutaneous input to the SI hand area (dotted), posterior to the rectus sulcus (R), but lateral to the medial segment of the intraparietal sulcus (IP) and medial to a second sagittally oriented sulcus. The drawing of the hand identifies the five glabrous digits (D1–D5) and the palmar pads (P1–P8) as adapted from Biegert (1961). The map of the hand in areas 3b and 1 of SI displays the general topographic features of the input from the glabrous digits and palm (G1, white) and hairy digits and hand (H, striped), similar to that in SI of *Galago* and *Perodicticus*. A second projection pattern from the glabrous digits (G2, cross-hatched) is shown in the posteromedial corner of the D5 and hairy hand projection pattern in this species. The division between areas 3b and 1 lies on the border of the G1 and H projection patterns (Carlson and FitzPatrick, 1982; Sanides and Krishnamurti, 1967).

prosimians imply less tactile capacity compared to species with an expanded and/or more differentiated SI is the topic of the comparative studies of normal and SI-lesioned prosimians and monkeys discussed in the next section.

3.2.4. Organization of SII in *Galago* and the Role of SII in Tactile Capacity

To demonstrate the neural basis for a specific sensory skill, one can begin by searching for neural structures that respond to the specific class of input on which a skill is assumed to be based. From the earliest of evoked potential studies, it has been known that a second somatic sensory projection area exists in the anterior bank of the lateral sulcus in all mammals examined and responds to mechanical stimulation (Woolsey and Fairman, 1946). However, early studies of the behavioral consequences of SII lesion in primates failed to produce the severity of impairment that was expected on the basis of known anatomical or physiological input to this area. Our first behavioral studies of tactile discrimination focused exclusively on the role of SI until it appeared that the input to SII, and its potential role in tactile function, may not be that different from SI. Physiological studies of tactile input to SII and behavioral studies from other laboratories in the past decade heightened the interest in the role of SII. Studies from several laboratories have shown that complete unilateral or bilateral removal of SI does result in tactile defects on size, texture, and form tasks with a severity and permanence similar to those following SI lesions (Ridley and Ettlinger, 1976, 1978; Murray and Mishkin, 1984).

With an interest in the evolution of SII and tactile capacity in primates, we examined tactile input, thalamocortical and corticocortical connections in SII in *Galago* and compared these to the structural and functional properties of SII in *Macaca*. Recent studies by Burton and colleagues (Robinson and Burton, 1980; see Burton, Volume 5 of this series) described the topography and submodal distribution of input to SII and surrounding areas in *Macaca*, showing that the receptive field characteristics of the cutaneous input to SII were not as different from SI as previous studies had implied (Whitsel *et al.*, 1969). For this reason, Burton and I (1986) mapped SII in *Galago* and described the location, size, somatotopy, and submodal composition of tactile input to the anterior bank of the lateral sulcus. We found receptive fields in the SII hand area to be slightly larger than in SI but commonly restricted to localized regions of single digits or the palm or hairy hand. More than 85% of the input was from the contralateral body, as opposed to the greater contribution of ipsilateral input reported by other investigators in SII of *Macaca*. SII in *Galago* was responsive to both low-threshold cutaneous and to noncutaneous input, suggesting to us that it might play a role in both texture and size discrimination behavior. Our anatomical studies showed that SII receives its major thalamic projection from the ventral portion of the ventroposterior lateralis nucleus (VPL), in contrast to SI, which receives input from more dorsal regions (see Fig. 6). Other nuclei, including the ventroposterior inferior (VPI) as recently reported for *Macaca* (Friedman and Murray, 1986), also project to SII. It is interesting to find a greater similarity between SII in *Galago* and *Macaca* than between SI areas in these two species. To determine the relative contribution of these two areas to tactile capacity in these species, behavioral studies of the effects of selective removal of these areas in *Galago* were initiated.

3.3. Behavioral Significance of SI–SII in *Macaca* and *Galago*

In previous studies of tactile discrimination capacity of *Macaca mulatta*, we obtained data on acquisition and performance for both normal and lesioned animals. Interested in the level of tactile capacity in *Galago* (with a less complex SI but comparable SII hand area), we tested normal *Galago* on the same discrimination apparatus and tasks developed for infant *Macaca* (Carlson, 1984a) species. Summary of our findings on normal, SI- and SII-lesioned *Galago* is given in Table 1. Not surprisingly, these prosimians are slower and make more errors in acquiring the easiest-, moderate-, and difficult-level size and texture comparisons. By using two types of tasks and three levels of difficulty, on both acquisition and performance tasks, it becomes possible to distinguish the relative importance of learning from specific discrimination capacities. Although on average *Galago* made more than 10 times as many errors (and required about twice that number of trials) to learn the easiest-level size discrimination, some animals learned the most difficult level with the same efficiency as *Macaca* (Carlson, in preparation). Acquisition of the moderate-level size tasks by *Galago* was also less efficient than in *Macaca* but size threshold task performance was only

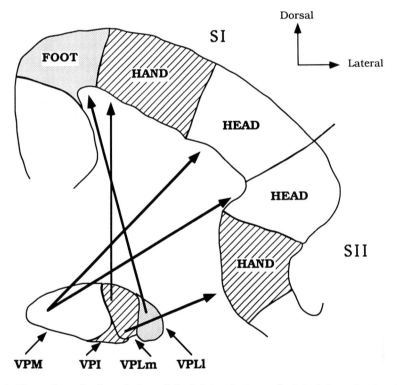

Figure 6. Illustration of a frontal view of the left hemisphere of adult *Galago*, showing the thalamocortical projection pattern from the ventroposterior nucleus (VP) to the foot, hand, and head projection areas of SI and head and hand areas of SII (Burton and Carlson, 1986). The medial division, VPM, projects to the face area, both shown in white. The medial portion of the lateral division, VPLm, projects to the hand areas in SI and SII. In addition to the ventral portion of VPLm, the inferior portion, VPI, projects to SII. Both thalamic (VPLm and VPI) and cortical (SI and SII) hand areas are shown as striped. The lateral division, VPL1, projects to the foot area in SI (shaded) and to SII (which is contained in a more posterior section than illustrated; Burton and Carlson, 1986).

noticeably different on the difficult-level task. By contrast, on texture acquisition *Galago* made 3 times the number of errors prior to criterion as *Macaca* but 10 times the number of errors on difficult texture comparisons with two animals failing to reach criterion after making 20 times the number of errors (and receiving 20 times the number of trials) as required by *Macaca* to achieve 80% correct criterion.

Referring to the acquisition curves illustrated in Fig. 7 for *Macaca* and *Galago*, it can be seen that an average *Galago* required about five sessions to learn the difficult size comparison compared to one session for *Macaca*. On the texture threshold tasks listed in Table 1, *Galago* performance for both the moderate- and most-difficult-level tasks can be seen as significantly lower than for *Macaca*. Our earlier studies of *Macaca* with subtotal SI lesions showed that size capacity was affected by area 2 lesions (a projection area for joint and muscle related input) and texture discrimination by area 1 (receiving cutaneous input) (Randolph and Semmes, 1974; Carlson, 1981). Although some joint-related input was found in areas 3b–1 in *Galago*, posterior areas 2–5 seemed most responsive to passive and active hand movements. Poor size acquisition seemed to be reflecting poor learning capacity initially, as *Galago* was able to perform as well as *Macaca* over all comparisons on size thresholds, the ALLS task. On texture tasks, *Galago* did worse on difficult than easy texture comparisons during acquisition and worse overall than *Macaca* on texture thresholds. These results suggest that input

Table 1. Average Efficiency of Acquisition and Performance on ALLS Threshold Tests

Species[a] (N)[b]	Size acquisition (errors to criterion)				Size ALLS (% correct)			
	7–18 mm	7–12 mm	7–9 mm	Total	7–18 mm	7–12 mm	7–9 mm	Total
Mm-N (9)	7.8	5.2	54.0	115.1	98.4	95.4	76.7	92.3
Gc-N (8)	87.4	77.1	130.4	371.1	98.6	93.5	57.1	87.7
Gc-SI (8)	70.3	190.8	691.1	1046.1	99	90.9	65.1	86.5
GC-SII (8)	235.4	218.5	585.9	1005	99.1	89.2	60.7	85.1
Ss-N (5)	98	108.8	155.6	430	97.3	87.6	64.1	86.3
Ca-N (2)	31.5	10	127.5	205	100	92.1	65.4	88.7
Ca-les (3)	13	19.7	6	113.3	99.3	94.9	66.3	89.4

Species (N)	Texture acquisition (errors to criterion)				Texture ALLS[c] (% correct)			
	320–40[e]	320–80[e]	320–120[e]	Total	320–40[e]	320–80[e]	320–120[e]	Total
Mm-N (10)	77.2	26.5	92.2	249.5	97.8	94.8	63.7	89.2
Gc-N (8)	227	65.8	1061[d]	1583.1	93.8	83.1	54.7	80.4
Gc-SI (8)	263.3	354.8	1115[d]	2193	92.9	75	59.8	76
Gc-SII (8)	450.6[d]	300[d]	1022[d]	1538	97.1	82.9	56.0	81.7
Ss-N (4)	348.8	180.8	1307[d]	2266.5	94.2	80	47.6	76.2
Ca-N (2)	482	248.5	971[d]	2491	88.5	84	60.7	77.8
Ca-les (3)	9	17	231.7	474.7	96	85.3	65.6	83.5

[a]Mm, *Macaca mulatta*; Gc, *Galago crassicaudatus*; Ss, *Saimiri sciureus*; Ca, *Cebus apella*; N, normal; SI, SI lesion; SII, SII lesion; les, area 1 lesion.
[b]N, number of animals included in average score.
[c]Average only includes animals that reached criterion on all levels in acquisition.
[d]Some animals included in average never reached criterion in 20 or more sessions.
[e]Grains/linear inch.

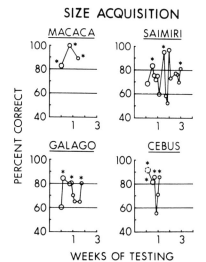

SIZE ACQUISITION

TEXTURE ACQUISITION

Figure 7. Acquisition curves for size and texture discrimination tasks for individual animals representing four primate species. These behavioral data were obtained on an apparatus in which pairs of small handles, differing in size (cross-sectional diameter) or texture (covered with different grades of sandpaper), were presented to determine tactile discrimination capacity (see Carlson, 1984a, and Fig. 11). Animals were trained on easy level discriminations (represented by large circles) followed by moderate and difficult comparisons (represented by middle- and small-sized circles) until an 80% correct criterion was obtained on each level in a single daily session of 50–120 trials. The actual size or texture comparisons presented are described and illustrated in Fig. 11. These curves show the average percent correct on each comparison level for each session, beginning with week 1 until the 80% criterion was obtained on the three levels. The asterisks near data points indicate when the 80% criterion was first achieved on each level. Animals were first trained using only the correct handle (7–0 mm or 320–0 grains/inch; represented by a dashed circle), which was alternated from the upper to the lower position in the apparatus, as is the position of the correct handle when two handles are presented together in regular acquisition. If an animal failed to make 60% correct on a specific comparison (over two consecutive sessions), it would be tested on the next easier level of difficulty until 80% criterion was reached again. Examples of this correction procedure are shown in the size acquisition for *Saimiri* and in the texture acquisition for the three other species. From these repeated sessions on easy- and difficult-level comparisons, it is clear that the poor performance on the difficult-

related to digit movement and position (required for judging size) are not as different as are the differences in cutaneous input to area SI, and the lack of a separate area 1 cutaneous area, found in *Macaca* but not *Galago*. The prosimian *Galago* with a "genetic lesion" of area 1 has the limited capacity of those *Macaca* in which area 1 was surgically removed (Randolph and Semmes, 1974; Carlson, 1981). Evidence that SI and SII both contribute to tactile discrimination in *Galago* is provided by the indication of severe impairment seen on both size and texture tasks following SI or SII lesion as in *Macaca* (see Table 1). The average error scores and threshold performance on the ALLS task indicate that both SI and SII lesions affect both types of tasks, which is consistent with earlier studies in *Macaca*. These behavioral studies were just completed and the brains are being prepared for histological examination of lesions (Carlson, in preparation). A number of animals in each lesion condition failed to master the moderate- or difficult-level tasks in acquisition and the histological studies should show if the size or location of the most devastating lesions differ from those more mildly affected. Speculation about the relative role of these two projection areas in tactile capacity in *Galago* and *Macaca* will be discussed in the review of developmental studies below.

4. Single or Multiple SI Areas and Tactile Capacity in New World Anthropoids

4.1. SI Maps in *Cebus* and *Saimiri*

Earlier evoked potential studies of SI projection areas in *Saimiri* (Benjamin and Welker, 1957) and *Cebus* (Hirsch and Coxe, 1958) described a single topographic pattern situated behind the coronally oriented central sulci in the parietal lobe in these two New World species. More recent studies using microelectrode mapping techniques in these species have shown complex topographic patterns in SI in which the ulnar–radial axis of the hand area is oriented in the medial–lateral direction, as in other primate species, and in which the proximal–distal axis of the hand and digits is oriented in a posterior–anterior direction in area 3b, similar to that in Old World prosimians and anthropoids. However, in area 1, a mirror-image reversal of the proximal–distal axis of the hand in the anterior–posterior direction has been described for both *Saimiri* (Sur *et al.*, 1982) and *Cebus* (Felleman *et al.*, 1983) in studies from the Kaas laboratory (see Figs. 8 and 9). These studies followed micromapping studies by Merzenich, Kaas, and colleagues of the New World anthropoid, *Aotus*, in which this mirror-image double pattern was first proposed (Merzenich *et al.*, 1978). The multiple cutaneous areas in the Old World *Macaca* have been variously described as serial or mirror-image duplication by different groups (Paul *et al.*, 1972; Nelson *et al.*,

---

level texture task is related to task difficulty, not some nonsensory aspect of task performance. Table 1 gives the total number of errors made on each level for size and texture tasks, averaged across all animals of a particular species tested. Errors to criterion are used as an estimate of the efficiency with which animals acquire different levels of size and texture tasks (Carlson, 1984a; Carlson and Burton, 1988).

1980; McKenna *et al.*, 1982). These studies of *Saimiri* and *Cebus* provide the background for behavioral studies to be discussed in a later section and for our mapping study of SI in *Saguinus*.

4.2. SI Map in *Saguinus*

When multiple hand areas were described in these New World anthropoids, our interest was stimulated in the complexity of SI topography in *Saguinus*, as this New World species is a member of the Callithricidae family, believed to be among the earliest evolved of the New World primates. These small primates have a relatively simple, lissencephalic cortex, possessing only a lateral sulcus on the lateral surface. As the prosimian *Galago* provides a good approximation to an

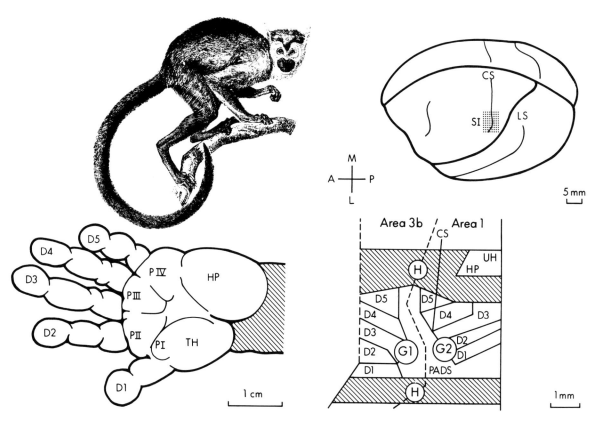

Figure 8. Illustration of the New World anthropoid, *Saimiri*, commonly known as the squirrel monkey. The body drawing illustrates the quadrupedal posture assumed during arboreal locomotion in this species. The brain drawing of the left cortical hemisphere indicates the location of the cutaneous input to the SI hand area (dotted), overlapping the central sulcus (CS) which is not a limiting sulcus between SI and MI in this species (Sur *et al.*, 1982). The drawing of the hand identifies the five glabrous digits (D1–D5) and the palmar pads [PI–PIV, thenar (TH), hypothenar (HP), and accessory hypothenar (HD) pads], with terminology according to Biegert (1961). The map of the hand in areas 3b and 1 of SI displays the general topographic features of the input from the glabrous digits and palm (white) and hairy digits and hand (striped). Two topographic patterns are suggested for the input from glabrous surfaces, G1 and G2, with the palm projecting to both margins of the 3B–1 border and digits projecting to anterior area 3b and posterior area 1. Only one area of input from the hairy surfaces (H), including the hand and digits, is seen on the margins of the G1 and G2 patterns. The division between areas 3b and 1 is indicated by the dashed line, while the CS is noted by the solid line in the medial half of area 1.

ancestral prosimian common to Old and New World anthropoids, *Saguinus* provides an approximation of the level of cortical development in the most primitive anthropoid in the New World lineage. Considerable controversy exists as to whether the major primate groups in the Old and New World diverged at the level of prosimian organization, migrating from Asia through North America to Central and South America, or whether an anthropoid ancestor crossed from Africa or Asia to South America, by rafting when the continents were not as separated as today (Ciochon and Chiarelli, 1980). Comparative studies of brain and behavior of contemporary species, along with evidence from the fossil record, can provide information about the level of cortical organization of the last common ancestor to Old and New World species (Carlson *et al.*, 1986) which may have implications for the debate on primate distribution and diversification.

In collaboration with Kaas and colleagues, we mapped sensorimotor area in *Saguinus* to determine if SI contained a single cutaneous area, as in prosimians, or a double cutaneous area, as in anthropoids (Carlson *et al.*, 1986). Our micro-

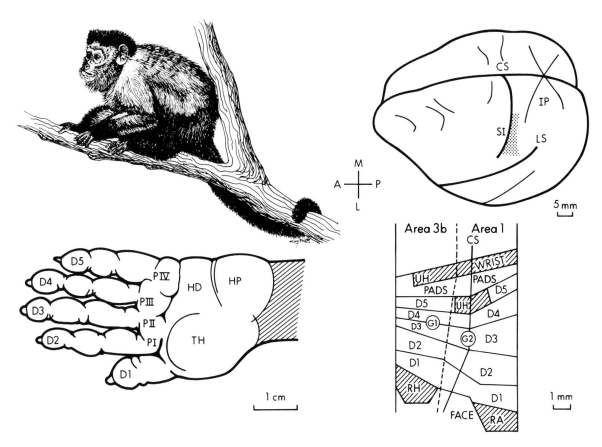

Figure 9. Illustration of the New World anthropoid, *Cebus*, commonly known as the cebus monkey. The body drawing illustrates the quadrupedal posture assumed during rest in the branches in this species. The brain drawing of the left cortical hemisphere indicates the location of the cutaneous input to the SI hand area (dotted), posterior to the central sulcus (CS). The drawing of the hand identifies the digits and the palmar pads with the same nomenclature as in *Saimiri* in Fig. 8. The map of the hand in areas 3b and 1 of SI shows two projection patterns for the glabrous digits (G1 and G2) across the full extent of areas 3b and 1, with the palm and hairy digit, hand (H), and radial arm (RA) projection pattern compressed in the areas medial and lateral to the G1 and G2 patterns (Felleman *et al.*, 1983). The division between areas 3b and 1 is indicated by the dashed line, while the curve of the CS is noted by the solid line.

mapping studies revealed a single SI topographic pattern in which the glabrous digits and "claws" projected to the anterior half and the palm and hairy digits and hand to the posterior half (see Fig. 10). The organization of the digit area was similar to that in prosimian SI but differed in the palm area, which was posterior to the hairy digit and hand fields. The simple pattern found in *Saguinus* suggests, along with the prosimian studies, that multiple SI areas in Old and New World species were independently acquired in these two groups, a product of convergent evolution. The importance of making such distinctions in the present context is to emphasize that if cortical features, such as topographic patterns or cytoarchitectonic fields, appear similar in different species, that does not justify the attribution of "homologous" to cortical areas. Unless comparative studies can provide evidence for similar features in species considered representative of ancestral forms, from which the similar features may have been inher-

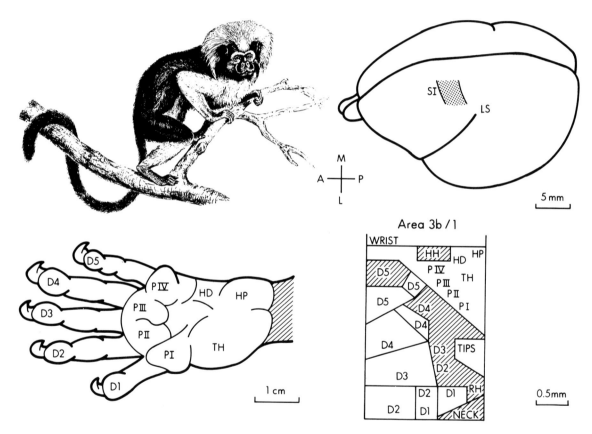

Figure 10. Illustration of the New World anthropoid, *Saguinus*, commonly known as the tamarin. The body drawing illustrates the crouched posture assumed by this species in arboreal locomotion and rest. The brain drawing of the left cortical hemisphere indicates the location of the cutaneous input to the SI hand area (dotted), and the lack of any sulci in the parietal cortex. SII is located in the anterior bank of the lateral sulcus (LS; Carlson *et al.*, 1986). The drawing of the hand identifies the digit and the palmar pads as described for the previous New World species (Biegert, 1961). However, notice the specialized claws on each digit of the hand in this species. The map of the hand in areas 3b and 1 of SI displays the general topographic features of the input from the glabrous digits and palm (white) and hairy digits and hand (HH, striped), each organized in a single topographic pattern. In contrast to other single SI patterns in prosimian species, the palm area is separated from the digit area by the projection of the hairy digits and radial hand (RH). The architectonic division between areas 3b and 1 is not marked within the cutaneous hand area but may occur in the posterior margin of the SI hand area (see Carlson *et al.*, 1986).

ited, species that share topographic or cytoarchitectonic features in SI need not have obtained them through the same lineage or for the same sensory function. As a direct test of functional equivalence is as important as morphological similarity, we examined the tactile capacity in several New World monkeys for comparison to the Old World prosimians and anthropoids.

4.3. Behavioral Significance of Different SI Maps for Tactile Discrimination Capacities in New World Primates

Using the same tactile discrimination apparatus for comparative studies of normal *Galago* and *Macaca*, one can examine the possible behavioral significance of multiple cutaneous areas in SI of normal *Cebus* and *Saimiri*. We trained animals of both species on size and texture tasks to determine if there were any major differences in the capacity to master or perform these tactile discriminations compared to *Macaca* or *Galago*, or to each other, that might be related to known details of SI organization (Carlson and Nystrom, 1986). The contribution of differences in learning capacity (or other nonsensory aspects of task acquisition) is reflected most clearly on the first, easy-level size tasks, as the first exposure to the testing procedure and a level of difficulty for which the sensory demands are minimal (see Carlson and Burton, 1988, for discussion). *Macaca* and *Cebus* made few errors on the initial tasks compared to *Saimiri* and *Galago* (with smaller brain/body ratio than the two other species; Jerison, 1967). On the most-difficult-level tasks, the average errors to criterion (see Table 1) suggest that differences in ability to discriminate small size differences between the four species are minimal compared to the larger differences on initial and easier tasks, more influenced by species-specific difference in nonsensory task demands of the task. The similarity in the performance on the threshold tasks is consistent with this view that sensory differences in size (mediated by noncutaneous input) are minimal compared to the differences in nonsensory aspects of the initial task acquisition.

Texture acquisition, given following the size acquisition and threshold tasks, involved the exact same procedures as size tasks, yet there remains a large species difference, more apparent on the most difficult task. In fact, two of the eight *Galago*, two of the four *Saimiri*, and one of the two *Cebus* trained on texture failed to reach 80% criterion after considerable training. Examination of the acquisition profiles in Fig. 7 shows the number of weeks required to reach criterion by the four species. Although *Macaca* was slightly faster on size tasks than the other three species, on texture acquisition the difference between *Macaca* and the other species is profound. Over all levels of texture acquisition, *Cebus* and *Saimiri* showed error scores more like *Galago* than like *Macaca*, suggesting that the ability of the New World species to perform texture discrimination and the nature of their cutaneous input to SI, and SII, are less developed than in the Old World *Macaca*. Based on details of the SI maps, it would appear that *Cebus* might be as good on texture as *Macaca*, as both have multiple cutaneous areas in SI and, in both species, the digit tip areas are vastly expanded across the full anterior–posterior extent of SI as compared to *Galago* and *Saguinus*. In *Saimiri* the palm is a more prominent part of the two projection patterns than the digit tips. So even though *Cebus* has expanded and complex topographic organization for the digit tips, it does not approach the ability of *Macaca* on texture tasks shown in our earlier work to be dependent on areas 3b and 1 (Randolph and Semmes, 1974; Carlson, 1981).

In order to assess what the area 1 projection in *Cebus* might be doing for texture discrimination capacity, we tested *Cebus* again, this time following removal of area 1. During reacquisition, the error scores on size tasks were identical to those for *Macaca* for original learning and size threshold scores were similar to preoperative *Cebus* and *Macaca* scores. On the texture tasks, postoperative acquisition scores and threshold scores were considerably *better* than preoperative scores for these same animals. Removal of area 1 *improved* the acquisition of the texture tasks and thresholds for one animal, and for the second animal, resulted in obtaining criterion on the difficult-level texture not achieved in preoperative training. These studies of normal and area 1-lesioned *Cebus* suggest that, unlike in *Macaca*, area 1 does not contribute to texture discrimination capacity but that the cutaneous input to that area may actually compete or interfere with texture discrimination capacity and has evolved for a different analysis of cutaneous input. These behavioral results are consistent with the conclusions of our earlier study of the New World species *Saguinus*, that the multiple cutaneous areas found in other New World species must have evolved independent of the multiple areas in Old World species, after diverging from a common ancestor that did not have multiple SI areas. The New and Old World species are known to have a vast number of convergent (therefore analogous but not homologous) features, in part related to their common adaptation to an arboreal environment. These studies clearly point to the importance of examination of actual sensory capacities of normal and SI lesioned animals as a means of attributing functional significance to specific anatomically and topographically described areas in different species.

5. Developmental Studies of Somatic Sensory Cortex and Tactile Discrimination Capacity in *Macaca* and *Galago*

Our comparative approach is to examine the correlation between SI and SII organization and tactile capacity in different species, to determine the correspondence between specific cortical features and behavioral capacity. Surgical lesions allow us to modify cortical structure in different species and compare consequences as another approach to the relationship between structure and function. Developmental studies in my laboratory have been carried out over the same period as the comparative and experimental lesion studies discussed above. To determine the level of morphological, physiological, and behavioral maturity of the somatic sensory system, we have examined the postnatal development of tactile discrimination capacity in normal infant and juvenile macaques and the recovery of tactile function so prominent after damage to the infant cortex. Ongoing studies of thalamocortical projections in *Galago* are intended to address the possible morphological basis for this recovery. Preliminary studies of tactile capacity after nerve crush in the infant are designed to look for critical periods and the role of activity in the maturation of the somatic sensory system. The developmental consequences of cortical lesions have provided important insights into normal developmental events, such as changing patterns of thalamocortical projections, which may form the basis for the level of recovered function possible in the immature macaque.

473

SOMATIC SENSORY
CORTEX AND
TACTILE
DISCRIMINATION

5.1. Tactile Discrimination Capacity in Infant *Macaca*

In order to test the development of tactile discrimination in a newborn macaque, it was necessary to develop an automated apparatus tailored to the motor and intellectual capacities of a young animal (Carlson, 1984a). Primate neonates appear unique among mammals in that they show precocial sensory maturation combined with altricial motor development (Gottlieb, 1972). This same apparatus proved useful for discrimination testing of prosimians, New and Old World monkeys, infants and adults alike. Training of infants began at 2–3 weeks of age, first to drink milk from the apparatus and next to palpate and discriminate the tactile surfaces to obtain their daily milk requirements. Most infants were tested on size discriminations first, as early as 8 weeks of age, and were found to make slightly more errors during acquisition than older animals. By contrast, the youngest animals learned texture tasks more quickly and efficiently than older infants and juveniles. This difference between rate and efficiency of learning for the two tasks indicates that it is not some nonsensory skill, but rather some subtle modality-specific capacity related to cutaneous and noncutaneous modalities, that are changing in the first year of life and that account for developmental differences in normal abilities. In order to assess the possible role of postnatal sensory experience in the tactile discrimination ability, we raised an infant with a gloved hand from birth to 4 months of age. To determine the role that maturation of manual motor skill might play in the ability to perform these tasks, we lesioned the hand area of motor cortex (MI) in another infant. Both animals showed normal acquisition of size and texture tasks, suggesting these two factors do not play a determinant role in early postnatal development of tactile skills (Carlson, 1984a).

5.2. Tactile Capacity following SI or SII Lesions in Infant *Macaca*

Following the finding that infants were capable of adult-level discrimination in the first 2 months of life, the next series of experiments was designed to see if the level or pattern of sensory deficits was the same regardless of the age of lesioning or of testing. If the consequences of lesions are different (although the level of normal function are the same), this would suggest that some of the structures and mechanisms mediating tactile sensory processing must differ as a function of age. At the age that normal capacity and the consequences of lesions are the same, one would suspect that underlying processes must also be the same. With the expectation that normal tactile function may be mediated by remaining SI areas, a partial SI lesion was made in infants at 5 weeks of age. Areas 3b, 1, and 2 are all necessary for normal size and texture discrimination in the adult, yet no one area is sufficient to mediate function (Randolph and Semmes, 1974; Carlson, 1981). Unilateral removal of area 3b or areas 1–2 combined in infants did result in more errors to criterion, particularly on difficult texture tasks, but all lesioned infants obtained 80% correct criterion on all levels of size and texture tasks (see Fig. 11). Thresholds for size were as in normal infants whereas texture thresholds remained slightly raised compared to normal infants (Carlson, 1984b; see Table 2). In contrast to adults with partial SI lesions, animals lesioned as infants could recover function to normal, or near normal, levels.

If remaining SI areas in the damaged hemisphere were to mediate tactile recovery after partial SI lesions in infants, it would be expected that recovery would not be found following a total SI lesion. When the entire SI hand area were removed unilaterally in infants, complete recovery (or perhaps, sparing) of tactile function was obtained. During size acquisition, SI-lesioned infants made fewer errors than SI-lesioned juveniles and performed better on some threshold tasks than lesioned juveniles and normal infants. On texture tasks, SI-lesioned infants made fewer errors than infants with partial SI lesions and SI-lesioned juveniles. Thresholds for SI-lesioned infants were superior to those for normal and partial SI-lesioned infants on the difficult-level texture task (Carlson, 1984c). Though it is clear that infants with total SI removals do not suffer tactile impairments, it is not clear whether it is the remaining areas in the damaged SI area that are responsible for recovered function, or whether as with the total SI lesion in infants, an area outside the contralateral SI mediates recovered tactile function.

This finding of less impairment after a complete rather than partial SI lesion is similar to a fascinating report by Rasmussen and Milner (1977) in young human patients with damage to left hemisphere language areas. Following incomplete lesions of the language areas, impaired language was mediated in the damaged hemisphere, whereas following more complete lesions, normal language was mediated by the right hemisphere. The slower and less complete recovery of tactile function found after partial lesions, contrasted with complete

Table 2. Average Efficiency of Acquisition and Performance on ALLS Threshold Tests

Group[a] (N)[b]	Size acquisition (errors to criterion)				Size ALLS (% correct)			
	7–18 mm	7–12 mm	7–9 mm	Total	7–18 mm	7–12 mm	7–9 mm	Total
Mm-N (9)	7.8	5.2	54.0	115.1	98.4	95.4	76.7	92.0
Mm-SIp (4)	21.5	6.8	153.3	228.5	97.4	89.4	74.2	90.6
Mm-SIt (4)	37.3	14.8	72	146.7	100	93.8	65.8	92.5
Mm-SII (7)	16.6	3	6.9	34.1	99	98.1	79.2	94.6
Mm-SI–SII (6)	30	12.8[d]	176.7[d]	266	99.4	93.2	66.1	90.2

Group (N)	Texture acquisition				Texture ALLS[c]			
	320–40[e]	320–80[e]	320–120[e]	Total	320–40[e]	320–80[e]	320–120[e]	Total
Mm-N (10)	77.2	26.5	92.2	249.5	97.8	94.8	63.7	89.2
Mm-SIp (4)	339.8	112.8	1283.5	1803.2	97.2	84.4	60.6	83.9
Mm-SIt (4)	196.8	79.8	270	781	94.3	82.2	74.8	84.5
Mm-SII (7)	116.1	18	776.9	932.7	99.6	94.9	60.5	89.8
Mm-SI–SII (6)	837.5	543.2[d]	1678.5[d]	2374.5	97.3	82.9	57.9	82.4

[a]Mm, Macaca mulatta; N, normal; SIp, partial SI lesion; SIt, total SI lesion; SII, SII lesion; SI-SII, combined SI-SII lesion.
[b]N, number of animals included in average score.
[c]Average only includes animals that reached criterion on all levels in acquisition.
[d]Some animals included in average never reached criterion in 20 or more sessions.
[e]Grains/linear inch.

SIZE ACQUISITION

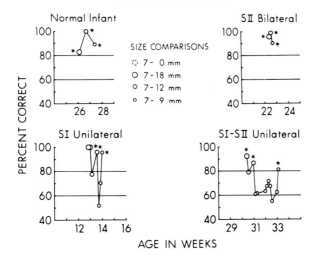

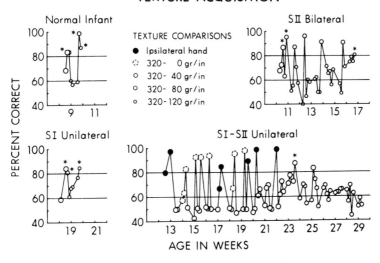

TEXTURE ACQUISITION

Figure 11. Acquisition curves for size and texture discrimination tasks for normal, SI-, SII-, and SI–SII-lesioned infant macaques. These behavioral data were obtained on the same apparatus described in Fig. 7. All handles were 3.8 cm long. Size handles varied from the correct handle of 7 mm diameter to 9, 12, and 18 mm in cross-sectional diameter. The texture handles were all 2 mm in diameter and covered by different grades of aluminum oxide abrasive, with the correct handle a smooth 320 grain/linear inch (gr/in) grade, and increasingly rough grades of 120, 80, and 40 gr/in. The first three comparisons on size and texture handles, with larger circles representing larger differences between handles, are illustrated in the legends. Training on the ipsilateral hand (signified by the filled circles) was used in initial training for the lesioned animals, and as a correction procedure when performance on the easiest-level task dropped below 60% correct over two consecutive sessions. Testing on the correct handle alone (7–0 mm and 320–0 gr/in), symbolized by the dashed circles, was used in early training and as a correction procedure. The asterisks near data points indicate when 80% criterion was first reached on each level. The normal, SI- and SII-lesioned infants reached criterion on all three levels of the size task but the SI–SII-lesioned infant was delayed and made more errors than others on the difficult-level size task. Similarly, the normal and SI-lesioned infants learned all levels of the texture tasks in a few sessions, whereas the SII-lesioned infant was significantly delayed on the difficult-level texture tasks. The SI–SII-lesioned infant reached criterion on the ipsilateral hand, and on the 320–0 and 320–40 gr/in comparisons, but not on the moderate and difficult level after 4 months of training. Table 2 gives the total number of errors made on each level for size and texture tasks, averaged across all animals for the normal and lesioned groups (Carlson, 1984a–c; Carlson and Burton, 1988).

recovery or sparing of function after total lesions, and appears to be a phenomenon similar to that seen after SI lesions in infant macaques. If the total SI lesion results in function being shifted to another area, is that area in the damaged or intact hemisphere and in a cortical or subcortical structure?

The first possibility to be examined was the role of the normal ipsilateral SI in recovery from a unilateral SI lesion in infants (Carlson and Burton, 1988). When removal of the opposite SI in an SI-lesioned infant did not reverse the observed recovery, the next area to be examined was SII in the damaged hemisphere. This required that we first explore the consequences of SII removal alone in an infant, as it was known that SII removal in an adult produced permanent impairment on size and texture tasks (Murray and Mishkin, 1984). Recent reports on thalamocortical (Friedman and Murray, 1986) and corticocortical connections (Friedman *et al.*, 1986) of SII suggest that VPI may provide the major thalamic input to SII, but that SI provides the critical source of low-threshold cutaneous input to SII (Pons *et al.*, 1986). These findings are consistent with Mishkin's (1979) serial model of tactile processing that SII projects to limbic cortex for higher cortical processing, and that SII lesions may interrupt the necessary connections between VPL, SI, and limbic cortex. However, when SII was removed in one or both hemispheres in infants, and tested first on texture, SII-lesioned infants made five times as many errors as normal infants, yet obtained normal thresholds after a few months of testing (Carlson and Burton, 1988). Both size acquisition and thresholds were at normal or above normal levels (see Fig. 11 and Table 2). The finding that SII lesions alone would not produce tactile deficits allowed for the next studies in which simultaneous or sequential SI–SII lesions were made in the same hemisphere in infants.

These combined lesions were the first to produce lasting tactile deficits in infants. The mild impairment seen after SI–SII lesions was similar to that following SI lesions for both size acquisition and size thresholds. However, on texture tasks, two infants failed to reach criterion on the moderate-level tasks and three other animals failed to reach criterion on the difficult-level task. The three animals tested on texture thresholds continued to show inferior performance on the moderate and difficult tasks. These results suggest that SI and SII are each capable of mediating texture in the infant, unlike in the adult, but that size discrimination may be mediated by other areas in addition to SI and SII in the infant. In the case of the infant, both SI and SII are not necessary but both are sufficient, unlike in the adult, where both are necessary but neither sufficient to mediate tactile discrimination (Carlson and Burton, 1988).

A mechanism that could explain both adult-level function in infants and the pattern of recovery or deficits following SI–SII lesions in infants requires sufficient thalamic input to SI or SII to mediate cutaneous-based texture tasks and non-cutaneous-based size tasks. Reports by Caminiti and Innocenti (1981) show that SI lesions in kittens cause some exuberant callosal connections between SII and SI in kittens (that normally retract late in development) to be maintained (see Innocenti, Volume 5 in this series). It has been shown that exuberant callosal connections exist between SI hand areas in fetal macaques, but retract before birth (Killackey and Chalupa, 1986). However, even if lesions in infant macaques were to maintain transient callosal connections, it would not explain the unilateral recovery mechanism that operates in our studies. A recent study of thalamic projections to SI in infant *Macaca* suggests that single thalamic neurons extend collateral projections to multiple areas in sensorimotor cortex in neonates, that are retracted in older infants and adults (Cheema *et al.*, 1986). These reports of exuberant collateral projections in the somatic sensory system of immature animals, and well known in other systems as well (O'Leary, 1989), suggested that such a developmental mechanism could be operating in the development of thalamic projections from VPL and VPI to SI and SII. A possible morphological basis for the normal and recovered function we found in infants could be a pattern of exuberant thalamic projections from VPL and VPI to both SI and SII, that mediates normal function in the neonate, and is stabilized following early SI or SII lesions, maintaining some input from thalamic neurons destined for both SI and SII in the single remaining area. Such a phenomenon could explain the equipotentiality of function, and the recovered or spared function, seen in the infant but not the adult macaque. The next set of experiments explores the pattern of thalamocortical projections in infant *Galago* as an initial effort to define recovery-of-function mechanisms.

5.3. Thalamocortical Projections in Infant and Adult *Galago*

In considering the possible basis (bases) for the recovery of function following removal of SI or SII, we reviewed the literature on developmental changes that occur in somatic sensory or other sensory or nonsensory regions of cortex in infant mammals. To explore the most promising possibility—exuberant, transient thalamocortical connections—we used a double-label strategy in infants and adult *Galago* (Carlson *et al.*, 1987) (Fig. 12). Following electrophysiological localization of SI and SII hand areas in the same hemisphere, two fluorescent dyes were injected and cells in the thalamus were examined for evidence of retrograde transport to the nuclei and cell bodies, indicating whether axons projected to one or both areas at different ages. Injections in infants produced double-labeled cells (in VPL and VPI primarily) in between 15 and 30% of the neurons, offering evidence for collateral projections to SI and SII at this age. In adults, similar injection produced no evidence of double-labeled cells, which suggests that such collaterals had retracted later in development. Our next step in this analysis is to demonstrate that some of the cells that project in both SI and SII in the infant are the same as those that maintain projections to the remaining somatic sensory area in the hemisphere sustaining an SI or SII removal in the infant. By use of temporal double-label techniques and the location of retrograde label in VPL or VPI, we intend to confirm that such a mechanism occurs in normal development and mediates recovered tactile function following early SI or SII lesions.

5.4. Early Tactile Deprivation and Tactile Discrimination Capacity in Infant *Macaca*

In previous studies we raised a single infant macaque with a gloved hand from birth to restrict tactile experience (Carlson, 1984a). With the glove deprivation procedure, the hand was held in a fisted position so that only small joint movements were possible and cutaneous stimulation was restricted to the digits touching the palm. As mentioned above, this procedure did not produce any impairment of discrimination capacity on size and texture tasks. Studies of visual deprivation in the first months of life have provided significant insight into normal developmental processes, most importantly concerning the role of interocular competition in the formation of ocular dominance columns (LeVay *et al.*, 1980). The classical studies of Harlow (Harlow and Harlow, 1973) demonstrated the critical role of tactile stimulation in the development of social behav-

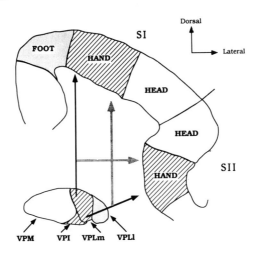

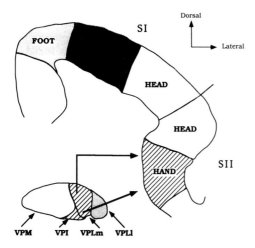

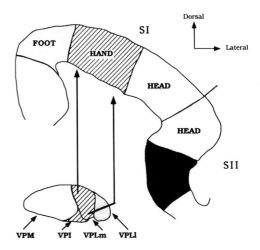

Figure 12. Illustration of a frontal view of the left hemisphere of an infant *Galago* showing the presumptive thalamocortical projection pattern from VPLm and VPI to the hand projection areas of SI and SII (Burton and Carlson, 1986; Carlson *et al.*, 1987). Based on the pattern of double-labeled cells after injections, it appears that single thalamic afferents project to both SI and SII in infants but not adults. If either SI or SII is removed in infants (signified by darkened cortical area), the collaterals to that lesioned area may retract, maintaining input from both ventral and dorsal portions of VPLm and VPI (which shows the same projection pattern as ventral VPLm) to the intact hand area, rather than to establish the normal adult pattern illustrated in Fig. 6. If early SI or SII lesions produce the thalamocortical projection pattern depicted in the lower half of this figure, the level of tactile function seen in normal and lesioned infants could be explained.

ior in infant macaques. Given these studies showing the neural and behavioral sequelae of early sensory deprivation, we have attempted to develop an analogous regime of "eye closure" for the somatic sensory system and use formal tests of tactile skills to evaluate sensory consequences.

In ongoing studies we are producing a reversible deafferentation by crush of the median and ulnar nerves innervating the glabrous hand and digits, to produce a temporary sensory deprivation in the hand in the first months of life. Studies of nerve crush in adult primates show that afferents will reinnervate the glabrous skin and obtain normal thresholds, receptive field properties, and submodality characteristics (Dykes and Terzis, 1979). Mapping studies of SI following nerve crush in adult primates also demonstrate normal recovery of topographic organization, as indicated by location, organization, and size of projection patterns from palm and digits (Wall *et al.*, 1983). The nerve crush strategy seems an appropriate method for obtaining reversible deprivation in the infant somatic sensory system in that both peripheral and central processes show restored function and organization in the adult. Observed differences in cortical organization or tactile capacity following nerve crush in infants would suggest a role for normal tactile activity in the ongoing developmental processes in the somatic sensory system. The elimination of sensory input to the glabrous hand areas in SI and SII in the first months of life should produce a temporary or lasting deficit if sensory input, or driven activity, is a critical variable in early postnatal maturation, as it has been shown to be in the visual system. Yet our preliminary studies suggest that this deprivation strategy, like the glove deprivation method, does not disrupt the normal development of tactile capacity in the infant.

For these studies, we developed a new discrimination apparatus that enables us to present a variety of textured surfaces using a tracking technique. This technique involves presentation of an easy comparison, followed by levels of increasing difficulty as the animal reaches 80% on each successive level. A series of ascending and descending levels of difficulty are presented during a single session until the threshold level is repeatedly determined. With this apparatus we have presented raised dot patterns (created by the Nyloprint letterpress technology), and found normal infants to have thresholds for these patterns equal to adult human subjects (Lamb, 1983). Using these dot patterns and sandpapers employed in earlier studies, we found normal texture thresholds in two infants following a median and ulnar nerve crush at 5 weeks of age (Carlson and Pearce, 1989). The areas of crush were 70 mm from the tips and appeared to produce a 10-week period of deprivation, with regeneration occurring at a rate of 1 mm a day. We trained both infants on size and texture tasks at 20 weeks and saw a slight delay in texture acquisition but thresholds measured by the older technique were normal (Carlson, 1984a). We are currently testing an infant with a crush 120 mm from the digit tips, which produced a 17-week deprivation of normal driven input.

Failure to produce lasting deficits after two deprivation procedures provokes questions as to whether the somatic sensory system requires tactile input for normal development as in the visual system. The eye closure deprivation technique appears to depend on the normal competition between thalamic input from the two eyes for the maintained pattern of thalamocortical synapses in cortex. It is not clear that competition exists between different types of somatic sensory inputs to cortex, in either the prenatal or early postnatal period. If there is competition, it could be between cutaneous and noncutaneous input, between hairy and glabrous input, between different digits or digits and palm fields or other variants of tactile afferent characteristics. Our own physiological studies in infant primates and published studies by Krubitzer and Kaas (1988) consistently show that receptive fields and SI organization do not differ from those in adults in any way to suggest mixed input from those categories of input found segregated in the adult. Our failure to find evidence for a critical period for the somatic sensory system in primates in the early postnatal weeks suggests that important activity-dependent events, if they do occur, may occur prenatally. Evaluation of the role of spontaneous or driven activity before birth may be necessary to understand the role of activity in the development of the somatic sensory system in primates.

6. Conclusions

Our developmental and comparative studies have been presented, along with earlier clinical and comparative studies on somatic sensory cortex and tactile capacity, to show the role that behavioral studies of normal and brain-lesioned primates have to play in modern studies of sensory cortex function. Our comparative studies show the patterns of SI and SII topography in prosimians and show that the simple SI pattern in *Galago* may limit the texture discrimination capacity of this species, just as an area 1 lesion in *Macaca* limits its tactile function. Our mapping study in *Saguinus* suggests that complex SI maps in Old and New World primates are not homologous, as evidence is lacking for such maps in species approximating early primate forms. Our behavioral studies with normal and area 1-lesioned New World primates suggest that the complex SI area in *Saimiri* and *Cebus* may not mediate the same level of texture capacity as in *Macaca*.

Developmental studies suggest that infant macaques have mature levels of tactile function in the first weeks of life, yet remarkable functional recovery follows selective SI or SII lesions at this age. The capacity of SI and SII to mediate function alone in infants leads us to consider the possible morphological basis for both the maturity and stability of tactile function in the young primate. The somatic sensory system in the infant primate also appears to be hardy enough to resist several forms of sensory deprivation during this same postnatal period. Results from developmental studies now suggest that examination and manipulation of the prenatal period may be critical to our understanding of the role of activity in the establishment of the advanced level of function seen in the newborn.

The most provocative questions that remain appear to have answers that must come from developmental studies. By what developmental mechanisms do the different patterns of SI organization come about, such that some species have a simple topography and others an expanded or complex topography? What, if any, role does neural activity play in the process of map formation which appears quite mature at birth? What are the mechanisms that stabilize the thalamocortical projection patterns of cutaneous and noncutaneous input to areas 3b, 1, and 2 and of separate SI and SII projections areas for the different digits? Understanding the relationship between developmental and phylogenetic sequences remains the most difficult, yet unquestionably the most interesting, issue in the study of brain and behavior relations in primates.

Several new theories of the developmental mechanisms that may mediate the expression of species differences in cortical organization have appeared recently. With the accumulating evidence as to the importance of regressive or selectional changes (cell death and collateral elimination) in development, Ebbesson (1984) proposed that more recent and complex thalamocortical patterns may be achieved primarily by the increased segregation of input. Such an evolutionary trend might be postulated to explain the apparent difference in the importance of VPL input to SII between *Macaca* and *Galago*. Increased differentiation and added complexity of input may occur by increased collateral elimination in development. Yet there is a multiplicity of other changes, such as increased size of subcortical and cortical cell numbers and novel interconnections, that relate to the tremendous diversity in central nervous systems of vertebrates that Ebbesson has studied and which he discusses in his review.

A second theory which takes a "selectionist" point of view toward the role of development in phylogeny is that of Edelman. In his book titled *Neural Darwinism* (1987), Edelman devised a theory of development, evolution, and perception that stresses the role of cell adhesion molecules in development and of "neuronal group selection" and "reentrant signaling" in neural function and perception. His theory rests on the distinction between "instructional" and "selectional" strategies that he championed in the immune system and which he now applies to the nervous system. He restricts his discussion of development to the cell adhesion molecules that he now studies, and his discussion of adult neural function, to the "dynamic" changes in SI maps of New World monkeys (Merzenich, 1985) and his approach to perception to a computer-based recognition network, called Darwin II. This theory seems to offer little in the way of real links between developmental processes and evolutionary biology but rather depends on analogies, metaphors, and computer simulations to create a theory in which "Lamarckian characteristics are superimposed upon a fundamental Darwinian base." Given that the driving force behind Edelman's (and Merzenich's, 1985) theories appears to be to minimize the contribution of genetics to both ontogenetic and phylogenetic processes, it is not surprising that Crick responds with the most thorough attempt to understand and evaluate this theory in his article titled "Neural Edelmanism" (1989). However, Crick responds, not as a molecular biologist, but rather as a neurobiologist concerned with lack of coherence in the concepts and representativeness in the evidence that Edelman presents. It would seem that any modern theory of development and evolution must account for the interaction of genetic and epigenetic factors as opposed to Edelman's theory which stresses epigenetic factors to the exclusion of genetic. Advances in molecular biology need not be ignored, or circumvented, by neurobiologists but rather exploited to gain insight into the exciting complexity of the development and evolution of brain and behavior in primates.

The greatest hope that the task of relating development and evolution is a solvable one comes from Gould's brilliant book, *Ontogeny and Phylogeny* (1977), in which he carefully presents the controversy over recapitulation and the modern alternatives to this archaic notion. He stresses the importance of molecular biology in the effort, particularly in the understanding of regulatory genes that effect the timing of developmental events. He stresses that large developmental, and species, differences can come from small variations in timing of developmental events. Contemporary workers have the advantages of a long history of ideas on this topic to consider as well as a variety of new techniques with which to test these theories. A genuine understanding of the developmental mechanisms leading to the evolution of brain and behavior in primates most certainly will require the integration of historical concepts and contemporary biological data as championed by Gould as opposed to the speculative and abstract approach attempted by Edelman.

Those of us interested in the development of the forelimb and central neural projections are in a favorable position to find answers to some enduring questions about development and evolution, as trophic factors have been discovered that may explain the variation in the size of cortical projection of tactile input (Purves, 1988), and other molecules that may determine the patterning of limbs (and possibly their neural correlates) have been identified (Brockes, 1989). This is not the time to ignore or deny the role of these molecular factors, but to study how they may interact with neural activity, and other epigenetic factors, to produce the variety of SI and SII maps established during fetal and neonatal stages of development in diverse primate species.

ACKNOWLEDGMENTS. This chapter is dedicated to the memory of Derek Denny-Brown in recognition of his major contributions to our understanding of sensory and motor systems in primates. His vital role in clinical training and research in neurology and his experimental studies of brain lesions in nonhuman primates were in the tradition of the "acutest intellects in medicine" quoted at the beginning of this chapter (Head and Holmes, 1911). His advice and encouragement in the early phases of my developmental studies provided both knowledge and inspiration.

The generous support of PHS funding from NIMH (MH24762, MH23652, MH40157) and NINDS (NS12090, NS14261, NS15070), and of NSF funding (BNS 79-14103, BNS 81-15044, BNS 86-17085) is acknowledged. Funds from the Milton Fund of Harvard University and the McDonnell Center for Study of Higher Brain Function of Washington University were used in partial support of the studies reviewed. Special thanks to Kim Fritz for her exquisite drawings and to Joe Gagliardi for his expert photography.

7. References

Adrian, E. D., 1941, Afferent discharges to the cerebral cortex from peripheral sense organs, *J. Physiol. (London)* **100:**159–191.

Barenne, J. G. D. de, 1916, Experimental researches on sensory localization in the cerebral cortex, *Q. J Exp. Physiol.* **9:**355–390.

Benjamin, R. M., and Welker, W. I., 1957, Somatic receiving areas of cerebral cortex of squirrel monkey (*Saimiri sciureus*), *J. Neurophysiol.* **20:**286–299.

Biegert, J., 1961, Volarhaut der Hände und Füsse, in: *Primatologia*, Volume II(3) (H. Hofer, A. H. Schultz, and D. Stark, eds.), Karger, Basel, pp. 1–326.

Brockes, J. P., 1989, Retinoids, homeobox genes, and limb morphogenesis, *Neuron* **2:**1285–1294.

Brodmann, K., 1909, Vergleichende Lokalisationslehre der Grosshirnrinde, in: *Ihren Prinzipien Dargestelt Auf Grund der Zellenbaus*, Barth, New York.

Broadmann, K., 1925, Bieträge zur histologischen Lokalisation der Grosshirnrinde. II. Mitteilung: Die Rindenfelder der niederen Affen, *J. Psychol. Neurol. Leipzig* **4:**177–226.

Burton, H., and Carlson, M., 1986, Second somatic sensory area (SII) in the prosimian primate, *Galago crassicaudatus*, *J. Comp. Neurol.* **247**:200–220.

Caminiti, R., and Innocenti, G. M., 1981, The postnatal development of somatosensory callosal connections after partial lesions of somatosensory cortex, *Exp. Brain Res.* **42**:53–62.

Campbell, A. W., 1905, *Histological Studies on the Localization of Cerebral Function*, Cambridge University Press, London.

Campbell, C. B. G., and Hodos, W., 1970, The concept of homology and the evolution of the nervous system, *Brain Behav. Evol.* **3**:353–367.

Carlson, M., 1981, Characteristics of sensory deficits following lesions of Broadmann's areas 1 and 2 in the postcentral gyrus of *Macaca mulatta*, *Brain Res.* **204**:424–430.

Carlson, M., 1984a, Development of tactile discrimination capacity in *Macaca mulatta*. I. Normal infants, *Dev. Brain Res.* **16**:69–82.

Carlson, M., 1984b, Development of tactile discrimination capacity in *Macaca mulatta*. II. Effects of partial removal of primary somatic sensory cortex (SmI) in infants and juveniles, *Dev. Brain Res.* **16**:83–101.

Carlson, M., 1984c, Development of tactile discrimination capacity in *Macaca mulatta*. III. Effects of total removal of primary somatic sensory cortex (SmI) in infants and juveniles, *Dev. Brain Res.* **16**:103–117.

Carlson, M., 1985, The significance of single or multiple cortical areas for tactile discrimination in primates, in: *Hand Function and the Neocortex* (A. W. Goodwin and I. Darian-Smith, eds.), Springer-Verlag, Berlin, pp. 1–16.

Carlson, M., Size and organization of primary somatic sensory cortex in relation to tactile discrimination capacity in primates: Old World prosimian, *Galago*, in preparation.

Carlson, M., and Burton, H., 1988, Recovery of tactile function after damage to primary or secondary somatic sensory cortex in infant *Macaca mulatta*, *J. Neurosci.* **8**:833–859.

Carlson, M., and FitzPatrick, K. A., 1982, Organization of the hand area in the primary somatic sensory cortex (SmI) of the prosimian primate, *Nycticebus coucang*, *J. Comp. Neurol.* **204**:280–295.

Carlson, M., Heurta, M. F., Cusick, C. G., and Kaas, J. H., 1986, Studies on the evolution of multiple somatosensory representations in primates: The organization of anterior parietal cortex in the New World callitrichid, *Saguinus*, *J. Comp. Neurol.* **246**:409–426.

Carlson, M., and Nystrom, P., 1986, Significance of topography in primary somatic sensory cortex (SI) for tactile discrimination capacity in Old and New World primates, *Soc. Neurosci. Abstr.* **12**:386.2.

Carlson, M., O'Leary, D. D. M., and Burton, H., 1987, Potential role of thalamocortical connections in recovery of tactile function following somatic sensory cortex lesions in infant primates, *Soc. Neurosci. Abstr.* **13**:25.2.

Carlson, M., and Pearce, M., 1989, Normal tactile function following early sensory deprivation in infant *Macaca*, *Soc. Neurosci. Abstr.* **15**:124.7.

Carlson, M., and Welt, C., 1980, Somatic sensory cortex (SmI) of the prosimian primate *Galago crassicaudatus*: Organization of mechanoreceptive input from the hand in relation to cytoarchitecture, *J. Comp. Neurol.* **189**:249–271.

Carlson, M., and Welt, C., 1981, Somatic sensory cortex (SmI) in prosimian primates, in: *Cortical Sensory Organization*, Volume 1 (C. N. Woolsey, ed.), Humana Press, Clifton, N.J., pp. 1–27.

Cheema, S. S., Darian-Smith, I., Darian-Smith, C., and Goodwin, A. W., 1986, Postnatal regressive changes in thalamic projections to somatic sensorimotor cortex of the macaque. A quadruple fluorescent dye tracer study, *Soc. Neurosci. Abstr.* **12**:1430.

Ciochon, R. L., and Chiarelli, A. B., 1980, Paleobiogeographic perspectives on the origin of the Platyrrhini, in: *Evolutionary Biology of New World Monkeys and Continental Drift* (R. L. Ciochon and A. B. Chiarelli, eds.), Plenum Press, New York, pp. 459–493.

Clark, W. E. L., and Boggon, R. N., 1935, The thalamic connections of the parietal and frontal lobes of the brain in monkey, *Philos. Trans.* **224B**:313–359.

Cole, J., and Glees, P., 1954, Effects of small lesions in sensory cortex in trained monkeys, *J. Neurophysiol.* **17**:1–13.

Corkin, S., Milner, B., and Rasmussen, T., 1970, Somatosensory thresholds: Contrasting effects of postcentral-gyrus and posterior parietal-lobe excisions, *Arch. Neurol.* **23**:41–58.

Crick, F., 1989, Neural Edelmanism, *Trends Neurosci.* **12**:240–247.

Critchley, M., 1953, *The Parietal Lobes*, Williams & Wilkins, Baltimore.

Dykes, R. W., and Terzis, J., 1979, Reinnervation of glabrous skin in baboons: Properties of cutaneous mechanoreceptors subsequent to nerve crush, *J. Neurophysiol.* **42**:1461–1478.

Ebbesson, S. O. E., 1984, Evolution and ontogeny of neural circuits, *Behav. Brain Sci.* **7**:321–366.

Edelman, G. M., 1987, *Neural Darwinism*, Basic Books, New York.

Felleman, D. J., Nelson, R. J., Sur, M., and Kaas, J., 1983, Organization of the somatosensory cortex in cebus monkey, *Brain Res.* **268:**15–26.

FitzPatrick, K. A., Carlson, M., and Charlton, J., 1982, Topography, cytoarchitecture and sulcal patterns in primary somatic sensory cortex (SmI) of the prosimian primate, *Perodicticus potto, J. Comp. Neurol.* **204:**296–310.

Friedman, D. P., and Murray, E. A., 1986, Thalamic connectivity of the second somatosensory area and the neighboring somatosensory cortical fields of the lateral sulcus of the monkey, *J. Comp. Neurol.* **252:**348–373.

Friedman, D. P., Murray, E. A., O'Neil, J. B., and Mishkin, M., 1986, Cortical connections of the somatosensory fields of the lateral sulcus of macaques. Evidence for a corticolimbic pathway for touch, *J. Comp. Neurol.* **252:**323–347.

Fritsch, G., and Hitzig, E., 1870, Über die Elektrische Erregbarkeit des Grosshirns, *Arch. Anat. Physiol. Wiss. Med.* **37:**300–332.

Gottlieb, G., 1972, Ontogenesis of sensory function in birds and mammals, in: *The Biopsychology of Development* (E. Tobach, L. A. Ronson, and E. Shaw, eds.), Academic Press, New York, pp. 67–128.

Gould, S. J., 1977, *Ontogeny and Phylogeny*, Harvard University Press, Cambridge, Mass.

Harlow, H. F., and Harlow, M. K., 1973, Social deprivation in monkeys, in: *Readings from the Scientific American: The Nature and Nurture of Behavior*, Freeman, San Francisco, pp. 108–116.

Head, H., 1920, *Studies in Neurology*, Oxford University Press, London.

Head, H., and Holmes, G., 1911, Sensory disturbances from cerebral lesions, *Brain* **34:**102–254.

Hirsch, J. F., and Coxe, W. S., 1958, Representation of cutaneous tactile sensibility in cerebral cortex of *Cebus, J. Neurophysiol.* **21:**481–498.

Jerison, H. J., 1967, *Evolution of the Brain and Intelligence*, Academic Press, New York.

Jones, E. G., 1985, *The Thalamus*, Plenum Press, New York.

Killackey, H. P., and Chalupa, L. M., 1986, Ontogenetic change in the distribution of callosal neurons in the postcentral gyrus of the fetal rhesus monkey, *J. Comp. Neurol.* **244:**331–348.

Krishnamurti, A., Sanides, F., and Welker, W. I., 1976, Microelectrode mapping of modality-specific somatic sensory cerebral neocortex in slow loris, *Brain Behav. Evol.* **13:**267–283.

Krubitzer, L. A., and Kaas, J. H., 1988, Responsiveness and somatotopic organization of anterior parietal field 3b and adjoining cortex in newborn and infant monkeys, *Somatosens. Mot. Res.* **6:**179–205.

Kruger, L., and Porter, P., 1958, A behavioral study of the functions of the Rolandic cortex in the monkey, *J. Comp. Neurol.* **109:**439–469.

Lamb, G. D., 1983, Tactile discrimination of textured surfaces: Psychophysical performance measurements in humans, *J. Physiol. (London)* **338:**551–565.

LeVay, S., Wiesel, T. N., and Hubel, D. H., 1980, The development of ocular dominance columns in normal and visually deprived monkeys, *J. Comp. Neurol.* **191:**1–51.

McKenna, T. M., Whitsel, B. L., and Dreyer, D. A., 1982, Anterior parietal cortical topographic organization in macaque monkey: A re-evaluation, *J. Neurophysiol.* **48:**289–314.

Merzenich, M. M., 1985, Sources of intraspecies and interspecies cortical map variability in mammals, in: *Comparative Neurobiology: Modes of Communication in the Nervous System* (M. S. Cohen and F. Strumwasser, eds.), Wiley, New York.

Merzenich, M. M., Kaas, J. H., Sur, M., and Lin, C.-H., 1978, Double representation of the body surface within cytoarchitectonic areas 3b and 1 in "SI" in the owl monkey *Aotus trivirgatus, J. Comp. Neurol.* **181:**41–74.

Merzenich, M. M., Nelson, R. J., Kaas, J. H., Stryker, M. P., Jenkins, W. M., Zook, J. M., Cynader, M. S., and Schoppman, A., 1987, Variability in hand surface representation in areas 3b and 1 in adult owl and squirrel monkeys, *J. Comp. Neurol.* **258:**281–296.

Minkowski, M., 1917, Etude sur la physiologie des circonvolutions rolandiques et pariétales, *Schweiz. Arch. Neurol. Psychiatr.* **1:**389–459.

Mishkin, M., 1979, Analogous neural models for tactual and visual learning, *Neuropsychologia* **17:**139–151.

Monakow, C. von, 1882, Über eininge durch Exstirpation in circumscripter Hirnrindenregionen bedingte Entwickelungshemmungen des Kaninchengehirns, *Arch. Psychiatr. Nervenkr.* **12:**141–156.

Murray, E. A., and Mishkin, M., 1984, Relative contributions of SmII and area 5 to tactile discrimination of monkeys, *Behav. Brain Res.* **11:**67–84.

Napier, J. R., and Walker, A. C., 1967, Vertical clinging and leaping—A newly recognized category of locomotor behaviour of primates, *Folia Primatol.* **6:**204–219.

Nelson, R. J., Sur, M., Felleman, D. J., and Kaas, J. H., 1980, Representations of the body surface in postcentral parietal cortex of *Macaca fascicularis, J. Comp. Neurol.* **192:**611–643.

O'Leary, D. D. M., 1989, Do cortical areas emerge from protocortex? *Trends Neurosci.* **12:**400–406.

Orbach, J., and Chow, K. L., 1959, Differential effects of resections of somatic sensory areas I and II in monkeys, *J. Neurophysiol.* **22:**195–203.

Paul, R. L., Merzenich, M., and Goodman, H., 1972, Representation of slowly and rapidly adapting cutaneous mechanoreceptors of the hand in Brodmann's areas 3 and 1 of *Macaca mulatta, Brain Res.* **36:**229–249.

Penfield, W., and Boldrey, E., 1937, Somatic motor and sensory representation in the cerebral cortex of man as studied by electrical stimulation, *Brain* **60:**389–443.

Pons, T. P., Friedman, D. P., Garraghty, J. B., O'Neill, J. B., and Mishkin, M., 1986, Somatic activation of neurons in the SII region of the macaque depends on postcentral somatosensory cortex, *Soc. Neurosci. Abstr.* **12:**798.

Powell, T. P. S., and Mountcastle, V. B., 1959a, The cytoarchitecture of the postcentral gyrus of the monkey, *Macaca mulatta, Bull. Johns Hopkins Hosp.* **105:**108–131.

Powell, T. P. S., and Mountcastle, V. B., 1959b, Some aspects of the functional organization of the cortex of the postcentral gyrus of the monkey: A correlation of findings obtained in a single unit analysis with cytoarchitecture, *Bull. Johns Hopkins Hosp.* **105:**133–162.

Purves, D., 1988, *Body and Brain: A Trophic Theory of Neural Connections,* Harvard University Press, Cambridge, Mass.

Radinsky, L., 1970, The fossil evidence of prosimian brain evolution, in: *The Primate Brain: Advances in Primatology,* Volume 1 (C. R. Noback and W. Montagna, eds.), Appleton–Century–Crofts, New York, pp. 209–224.

Randolph, M., and Semmes, J., 1974, Behavioral consequences of selective subtotal ablations in the postcentral gyrus of *Macaca mulatta, Brain Res.* **70:**55–70.

Rasmussen, T., and Milner, B., 1977, The role of early left-brain injury in determining lateralization of cerebral speech function, *Ann. N.Y. Acad. Sci.* **299:**355–369.

Ridley, R. M., and Ettlinger, G., 1976, Impaired tactile learning and retention after removals of the second somatic sensory projection cortex (SII) in the monkey, *Brain Res.* **109:**656–660.

Ridley, R. M., and Ettlinger, G., 1978, Further evidence of impaired tactile learning after removals of the second somatic sensory projection cortex (SII) in the monkey, *Exp. Brain Res.* **31:**475–488.

Robinson, C. J., and Burton, H., 1980, Somatotopographic organization in the second somatosensory area of *M. fascicularis, J. Comp. Neurol.* **192:**43–67.

Roland, P. E., 1976, Astereognosis, *Arch. Neurol.* **33:**543–550.

Roland, P. E., and Larsen, B., 1976, Focal increase of cerebral blood flow during stereognostic testing in man, *Arch. Neurol.* **33:**551–558.

Rose, J. E., and Mountcastle, V. B., 1959, Touch and kinesthesis, in: *Handbook of Physiology,* Section 1, Volume 1 (J. Field, H. W. Magoun, and V. E. Hall, eds.), American Physiological Society, Washington, D. C., pp. 387–429.

Ruch, T. C., and Fulton, J. F., 1935, Cortical localization of somatic sensibility. The effect of precentral, postcentral and posterior parietal lesions upon the performance of monkeys trained to discriminate weights, *Res. Publ. Assoc. Nerv. Ment. Dis.* **15:**289–330.

Ruch, T. C., Fulton, J. F., and German, W. J., 1938, Sensory discrimination in monkey, chimpanzee and man after lesions of the parietal lobe, *Arch. Neurol. Psychiatry* **39:**919–938.

Sanides, F., and Krishnamurti, A., 1967, Cytoarchitectonic subdivisions of sensorimotor and prefrontal regions and of bordering insular and limbic fields in slow loris (*Nycticebus coucang coucang*), *J. Hirnforsch.* **9:**225–252.

Semmes, J., and Mishkin, M., 1965, Somatosensory loss in monkeys after ipsilateral cortical ablation, *J. Neurophysiol.* **23:**473–486.

Semmes, J., and Porter, L., 1972, A comparison of precentral and postcentral cortical lesions on somatosensory discrimination in the monkey, *Cortex* **8:**249–264.

Semmes, J., Weinstein, S., Ghent, L., and Teuber, H.-L., 1960, *Somatosensory Changes after Penetrating Brain Wounds in Man,* Harvard University Press, Cambridge.

Smith, G. E., 1902, On the homologies of the cerebral sulci, *J. Anat.* **36:**309–319.

Smith, G. E., 1910, Some problems relating to the evolution of the brain, *Lancet* **1:**1–6; 147–153; 220–227.

Sur, M., Nelson, R. J., and Kaas, J. H., 1980, The representation of the body surface in somatic koniocortex in the prosimian (*Galago senegalensis*), *J. Comp. Neurol.* **180:**381–402.

Sur, M., Nelson, R. J., and Kaas, J. H., 1982, Representation of the body surface in cortical areas 3b and 1 of squirrel monkeys: Comparisons with other primates, *J. Comp. Neurol.* **211:**177–192.

Vogt, C., and Vogt, O., 1919, *Allgemeinere Ergebnisse unserer Hirnforschung*, Barth, Leipzig.

Walker, A. E., 1937, The thalamus in relation to the cerebral cortex, *J. Nerv. Ment. Dis.* **85:**249–261.

Wall, J. T., Felleman, D. J., and Kaas, J. H., 1983, Recovery of normal topography in the somatosensory cortex of monkeys after nerve crush and regeneration, *Science* **221:**771–773.

Welker, C., 1971, Microelectrode delineation of fine grain somatotopic organization of SmI cerebral neocortex in albino rats, *Brain Res.* **26:**259–275.

Whitsel, B. L., Petrucelli, L. M., and Werner, G., 1969, Symmetry and connectivity in the map of the body surface in somatosensory area II of primates, *J. Neurophysiol.* **32:**170–183.

Woolsey, C. N., 1943, "Second" somatic receiving areas in the cerebral cortex of cat, dog and monkey, *Fed. Proc.* **2:**55.

Woolsey, C. N., and Fairman, D., 1946, Contralateral, ipsilateral and bilateral representation of cutaneous receptors in somatic areas I and II of the cerebral cortex of pig, sheep and other mammals, *Surgery* **19:**684–702.

Woolsey, C. N., Marshall, W. H., and Bard, P., 1942, Representation of cutaneous tactile sensibility in the cerebral cortex of the monkey as indicated by evoked potentials, *Bull. Johns Hopkins Hosp.* **70:**399–441.

Index